Burns in Children: Pediatric Burn Management

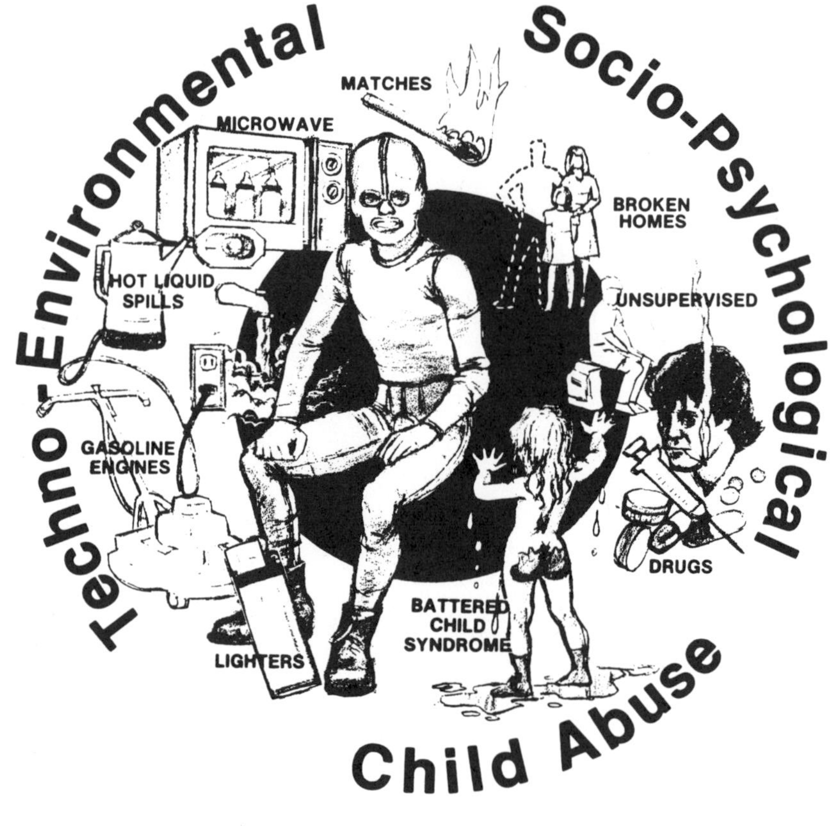

Techno-Environmental
Socio-Psychological
Child Abuse
MATCHES
MICROWAVE
BROKEN HOMES
HOT LIQUID SPILLS
UNSUPERVISED
GASOLINE ENGINES
DRUGS
BATTERED CHILD SYNDROME
LIGHTERS

Burns in Children: Pediatric Burn Management

HUGO F. CARVAJAL, M.D.
Professor of Pediatrics and Surgery
Director, Division of Pediatric Critical Care
University of Texas Medical School at Houston
Medical Director, Pediatric Critical Care Unit
Hermann Hospital
Houston, Texas
Formerly Chief of Pediatrics
Shriner's Burns Institute
Galveston, Texas

DONALD H. PARKS, M.D., F.R.C.S.(C.), F.A.C.S.
Associate Professor of Surgery
Director, Division of Plastic and Reconstructive Surgery
University of Texas Medical School at Houston
Director, Hermann Burn Center
Hermann Hospital
Houston, Texas
Formerly Chief of Surgery
Shriner's Burns Institute
Galveston, Texas

YEAR BOOK MEDICAL PUBLISHERS, INC.
Chicago • London • Boca Raton

1 2 3 4 5 6 7 8 9 0 K C 92 91 90 89 88

Library of Congress Cataloging-in-Publication Data

Carvajal, Hugo F.
Burns in children.

Includes bibliographies and index.
1. Burns and scalds in children. I. Parks, Donald H. II. Title. [DNLM: 1. Burns—in infancy & childhood. 2. Burns—therapy. WO 704 C331b]
RD96.4.C38 1988 617′.11′0088054 87–18891
ISBN 0–8151–1442–7

Sponsoring Editor: Nancy E. Chorpenning
Associate Managing Editor, Manuscript Services: Deborah Thorp
Copyeditor: Sally J. Jansen
Production Managers: Robert Allen Reedtz/Etta Worthington
Proofroom Supervisor: Shirley E. Taylor

To our parents
Hugo Sr., Delia, Stuart, and Mary, who guided our paths and filled our lives with love and confidence.

To our wives
Susan and Janice, for their unconditional support, love, and devotion, which made our task much easier and rewarding.

To our children
Brianna, Eric, Hugo III, Jessica, Karina, and Krisana, who willingly shared "their time" with our commitment to complete this book.

To all burned children
who have so bravely endured their injuries and have so greatly contributed to our education.

Contributors

Lory L. Alexander, R.N., M.S.
Clinical Nurse Specialist, University of Texas Medical Branch, Galveston, Texas

Ian J. Butler, M.D., F.R.A.C.P.
Professor of Neurology and Pediatrics, University of Texas Medical School at Houston, Houston, Texas

Hugo F. Carvajal, M.D.
Professor of Pediatrics and Surgery, Director, Division of Pediatric Critical Care, University of Texas Medical School at Houston; Medical Director, Pediatric Critical Care Unit, Hermann Hospital, Houston, Texas; Formerly Chief of Pediatrics, Shriner's Burns Institute, Galveston, Texas

Edwin A. Deitch, M.D.
Associate Professor of Surgery; Director, Division of Burns and Trauma, Louisiana State University School of Medicine, Shreveport, Louisiana

Mary K. East, M.D.
Instructor in Surgery, University of Michigan Medical School, Ann Arbor, Michigan

Patricia Fader, O.T.R.
Occupational Therapist, Department of Occupational Therapy, University of Texas Medical Branch, Galveston, Texas; Formerly Director of Occupational Therapy, Shriner's Burns Institute, Galveston, Texas

Irving Feller, M.D.
Professor of Surgery, Chief, Division of Burn Surgery, University of Michigan, Ann Arbor, Michigan

George J. Fuchs III, M.D.
Assistant Professor of Pediatrics, Division of Pediatric Gastroenterology, Louisiana State University School of Medicine in New Orleans, New Orleans, Louisiana

Wallace A. Gleason, Jr., M.D.
Associate Professor of Pediatrics, Director, The Children's Fund, Inc., Gastrointestinal Unit, University of Texas Medical School at Houston, Houston, Texas

John P. Heggers, Ph.D.
Professor of Surgery, Associate in Immunology and Microbiology, Director, Burn Center Laboratory, Wayne State University School of Medicine, Detroit, Michigan

Ian Alan Holder, Ph.D.
Professor of Research Surgery, Adjunct Professor of Microbiology and Molecular Genetics, University of Cincinnati College of Medicine; Director, Department of Microbiology, Shriner's Burns Institute, Cincinnati, Ohio

Joel H. Horovitz, M.D., F.R.C.S.(C.), F.A.C.S.
Director, Division of General Surgery, Maimonides Hospital, Brooklyn, New York

Claudella A. Jones, R.N.
Director of Professional Activities, Burn Center, University of Michigan Medical School, Ann Arbor, Michigan

Edward M. Kaye, M.D.
Assistant Professor of Pediatrics and Neurology, Boston Floating Hospital for Infants and Children, Boston, Massachusetts

Mary Knudson Cooper, Ph.D., L.P.C.
Clinical Assistant Professor of Pediatrics, University of Texas Medical School at Houston, Houston, Texas; Formerly Chief of Behavioral Sciences Division, Shriner's Burns Institute, Galveston, Texas; Assistant Professor of Psychiatry, University of Texas Medical Branch, Galveston, Texas

Steve Kohl, M.D.
Professor of Pediatrics, Program in Infectious Diseases and Clinical Microbiology and Department of Pediatrics, University of Texas Medical School at Houston, Houston, Texas

Stephen M. Larson, D.M.D.
Assistant Professor, Department of Anesthesiology, University of Texas Medical School at Houston, Houston, Texas

Hugo A. Linares, M.D.
Chief of the Division of Pathology Research, Shriner's Burns Institute; Clinical Assistant Professor of Pathology, University of Texas Medical Branch, Galveston, Texas

Harold R. Mancusi-Ungaro, Jr., M.D.
Director, University Hospital Burn Unit, Assistant Professor of Surgery, Division of Plastic and Reconstructive Surgery, University of Colorado Health Sciences Center, Denver, Colorado

Donald H. Parks, M.D., F.R.C.S.(C.), F.A.C.S.
Associate Professor of Surgery, Director, Division of Plastic and Reconstructive Surgery, University of Texas Medical School at Houston; Director, Hermann Burn Center, Hermann Hospital, Houston, Texas; Formerly Chief of Surgery, Shriner's Burns Institute, Galveston, Texas

Jai K. Prasad, M.D.
Instructor of Surgery, Department of Surgery, Division of Burn Surgery, University of Michigan, Ann Arbor, Michigan

Nancy B. Quay, R.N., M.S.
Clinical Education Specialist, Children's Medical Center at Dallas, Dallas, Texas

John Remensnyder, M.D.
Chief of Staff, Shriner's Burns Institute, Boston, Massachusetts; Associate Professor of Surgery, Harvard Medical School; Visiting Surgeon, Massachusetts General Hospital, Boston, Massachusetts

Martin C. Robson, M.D.
Professor of Surgery, Chairman, Division of Plastic Surgery, Director, Burn Center, Wayne State University School of Medicine, Detroit, Michigan

Margaret I. Saxon, M.S.
Programmer Analyst I, Burn Center, University of Michigan Medical School, Ann Arbor, Michigan

Beth A. Schindler, R.D., M.S.
Dietitian, Department of Dietetics, Hermann Hospital, Houston, Texas

Paul Silverstein, M.D., F.A.C.S.
Clinical Professor of Surgery, University of Oklahoma Health Sciences Center; Medical Director of the Burn Center, Baptist Medical Center of Oklahoma, Oklahoma City, Oklahoma

Wiley W. Souba, M.D., Sc.D.
Chief Resident, Department of Surgery, University of Texas Medical School at Houston, Houston, Texas

Cynthia M. Thomas, A.C.S.W., C.S.W.
Clinical Social Worker, Social Work Services, Hermann Hospital, Houston, Texas

Philip D. Thomson, Ph.D.
Director, The Burn Center Laboratory, Director, Clinical Laboratories, Department of Surgery, Division of Burn Surgery, University of Michigan Hospitals, Ann Arbor, Michigan

Ambrose M. Vallone, M.D.
Assistant Professor of Pediatrics, Division of Pediatric Critical Care, University of Texas Medical School at Houston, Houston, Texas

Thomas L. Wachtel, M.D.
Director, Burn Service GSMC, Director, Trauma Service GSMC, Clinical Associate Professor of Surgery, University of Arizona, Tucson, Arizona; Associate Clinical Professor of Surgery, University of California at San Diego, San Diego, California; Adjunct Professor of Engineering, Arizona State University, Tempe, Arizona

David J. Wainwright, M.D., F.R.C.S.(C.)
Assistant Professor of Surgery, University of Texas Medical School at Houston, Houston, Texas

Roberta Wilson, R.N.
Assistant Head Nurse, Burn Nurse Specialist, Oklahoma Children's Memorial Hospital, Division of Oklahoma Teaching Hospitals, Oklahoma City, Oklahoma

Robert A. Wolfe, Ph.D.
Associate Professor of Biostatistics, School of Public Health, University of Michigan, Ann Arbor, Michigan

R. M. Zuker, M.D., F.R.C.S.(C.), F.A.C.S.
Consultant in Plastic Surgery, Director, The Burn Unit, The Hospital for Sick Children, Toronto, Canada

Gerald T. Zwiren, M.D.
Clinical Assistant Professor of Surgery, Emory University School of Medicine; Department of Pediatric Surgery, Henrietta Egleston Hospital for Children, Atlanta, Georgia

Preface

The management of acute burn victims generally requires a multidisciplinary approach. In most cases, physicians from several disciplines must work in unison with other members of the health team in order to successfully retrieve the patient from the most catastrophic injury known. The complexity of the burn problem, the severity of its sequelae, and the endeavor for complete rehabilitation and reintegration of the patient into society also demands the participation of many basic and behavioral scientists. In the case of children, pediatricians and other personnel with special training in pediatrics constitute essential links and must join the team in their efforts. The team concept is therefore paramount to burn care and must be considered a sine qua non to optimal care and rehabilitation of all patients.

When the burned victim happens to be a child, the challenge to the burn team is even greater, and a competent and unified approach to patient care becomes mandatory. This is because the margins of safety are narrower in children, and therapeutic errors have greater consequences in infants and young children than in older children or adults.

Although physicians generally accept the concept that "children are different," there are times when specific pathologic conditions such as trauma or burns cross the boundaries of age and medical disciplines. Under these circumstances, the concept that "children are not merely little adults" is often overlooked and the focus is placed on pathology rather than on anatomic or physiologic differences between patients. This inadvertent omission can result in iatrogenic complications that are seldom recognized as preventable.

In the United States alone, 2 million burns occur annually, and of these, approximately 40% are children. Thirty to forty thousand burned children are hospitalized every year, and a considerable number succumb to their injuries. In burned children, the problems are unique, and different modalities of care must be developed and tailored to meet the needs of the patient. Extrapolation from adult norms is not always feasible or applicable, and lack of appropriate guidelines and standardization of therapy compound the problem.

Traditionally, burn injuries have fallen under the realm of surgery, and for the most part general surgeons and plastic surgeons have had to assume full responsibility for their care. It is time, however, for pediatrics as a discipline to take an active role in the care of the burned child and for pediatric subspecialists to share with the surgeons in this burden. This assumption of responsibility must be preceded by appropriate training of pediatricians in the field of Burn Medicine; thus, the care of the burned child must become part of the pediatric residency curriculum, and specific areas where input from pediatric subspecialists is needed must be acknowledged and further developed.

The recent worldwide development of pediatric critical care units offers a possible niche for pediatric burn victims who do not belong in adult burn care facilities. It also provides an ideal setting for the training of surgery and pediatric residents, medical and nursing students, and other members of the health care team. The need for continuous monitoring of the patient and care by specialized personnel further justifies the use of the pediatric intensive care setting for the management of the acutely burned child. In our hands such an approach has led to a significant reduction in burn morbidity and mortality and has successfully satisfied the needs of the patients and their families.

A textbook dedicated to outlining the principles of pediatric burn care is not only justifiable, but grossly overdue. Its main purpose would be to review and document the major physiologic differences between children and adults and propose effective treatment programs that take these differences into consideration. This book attempts to fulfill those objectives and as such it is intended for all members of the pediatric burn team, regardless of their training or expertise. As is usually the case with multiauthored textbooks, it was necessary to accommodate various writing styles as well as a certain amount of repetition. The latter was deemed valuable to strengthen some of the chapters and to allow the reader to benefit from the review of specific sections without having to read the book from "cover to cover."

The material is presented in seven major sections, the first of which is dedicated to burn prevention and epidemiology and is designed to provide information on the scope of the problems of pediatric burns, as well as actual data on who gets burned, how they get burned, and where. This type of epidemiologic review is essential to the development of prevention strategies and allocation of resources.

The sections on pathophysiology and acute care review our current knowledge on burn injuries in general and their impact upon pediatric populations. Specific management protocols are reviewed in detail. The section on surgery reviews the priorities of surgical management from the scene of the accident to complete autologous wound coverage at a tertiary care facility. The sections on immunology and infection and organ failure review common complications of burn injuries in pediatric patients and propose schemes for their management. Finally, the section on rehabilitation concerns itself with the psychosocial aspects of treatment, prevention, minimizing deformities, and reintegration of the child into his home, school, and society.

If this publication accomplishes nothing else but the recognition that pediatric burn patients have special needs and that treatment programs must be specifically designed to address those needs, our efforts will have been served. If in addition, it stimulates and recruits pediatricians and other health care professionals with expertise in children to join the burn team, our goal will have been fully satisfied.

HUGO F. CARVAJAL, M.D.
DONALD H. PARKS, M.D.,
F.R.C.S.(C.), F.A.C.S.

Acknowledgments

We wish to express our gratitude to Dr. George Krudy for his editorial assistance, and to Norma Jean Miller for her dedication and expert clerical assistance. To the many secretaries that spent multiple hours deciphering handwriting in formation and transforming dictation material into manuscript form, we extend our many thanks. The editors are indebted to all contributors who made this publication possible. They were selected with prior knowledge of their expertise in the field of pediatric burn care and their multiple contributions to the field of burn medicine in general.

We also wish to express our deepest appreciation to the many burned children who, having endured painful treatments and prolonged hospitalization, may have suffered further from our unintentional errors, while still contributing to our education.

HUGO F. CARVAJAL, M.D.
DONALD H. PARKS, M.D., F.R.C.S.(C.), F.A.C.S.

Contents

SECTION I

EPIDEMIOLOGY AND BURN PREVENTION

1 / Epidemiology of Burns in Children

MARY K. EAST, M.D.
CLAUDELLA A. JONES, R.N.
IRVING FELLER, M.D.
MARGARET I. SAXON, M.S.
ROBERT A. WOLFE, Ph.D.

Fires and burns are the leading cause of accidental death in the home for children ages 1 to 14 years. The National Burn Information Exchange (NBIE), a voluntary, physician-participation registry established in 1964, provides a means of collecting, storing, and analyzing data from specialized burn care facilities around the United States. As of October, 1985, 92,034 cases were on file from 133 burn care facilities; nearly 30,000 of these cases were children ages 1 to 18 years. Data are collected on a standard form, stored in a mainframe, and retrieved for annual reports to the members. These data serve as a baseline for relating survival and complications to severity factors and treatment modalities. Data can also be used for specific research projects and as a basis for prevention programs.

The NBIE data are used in this chapter to look at the epidemiology of burn accidents by who gets burned, how, and where, and how these factors relate to the outcomes of survival and length of stay. Strategies for prevention based on these data are also presented.

WHO GETS BURNED?

NBIE analysis of burns in newborns to children age 18 years show that infants and youngsters age birth through 4 years have a disproportionately high number of burn accidents (Table 1–1). This group accounts for nearly 52% of all pediatric burns.

The age distribution of the patients with burn injuries reported to the NBIE from 1964 to 1984 is shown in Figure 1–1. The high incidence of burn injuries in infants and toddlers is attributable to their total dependence on caretakers. The number of burn injuries tapers off for each year from age 3 to 16 years, but again rises as older adolescents enter the work force and sustain more injuries from car and motorcycle use and repair, as well as from improper use of flammable materials.[1]

The sex distribution of children with burn injuries is shown in Figure 1–2 with boys sustaining more injuries than girls in all age groups. The male to female ratio increases from 1.5 to 1.0 in the birth to 23-month age group to 3.5 to 1.0 in the 13- to 18-year age group.

Another method of looking at who gets burned is by victim type. Using NBIE data, Table 1–2 shows five victim types listed in order of frequency of occurrence. The majority of children burned are victims of their own actions, for example, a child playing with matches who accidently sets his or her clothing on fire. The second group comprises the innocent bystanders, for example, the child injured in a house fire caused by a gas leak and explosion. Analysis shows that the possibility of being this victim type grows less likely with age. The third group consists of intended victims—those deliberately injured by another child or adult. The least frequent victim type for children is the rescuer, for ex-

TABLE 1–1.
Epidemiology of Burns in Children—Who: Age Distribution, 1968–1984 (n = 29,448)*

AGE GROUP	NUMBER	%
0–23 mo	8,266	28
2–4 yr	7,080	24
5–12 yr	8,055	27
13–18 yr	6,054	21
Total	29,459	100

*From National Burn Information Exchange, Ann Arbor, Mich, June, 1985.

ample, the person burned during an attempt to save others trapped within a burning building. This group is not shown on the chart because of its infrequency.[2]

"Past medical history" includes those burn injuries caused or influenced by a preexisting illness or abnormality. While rare in the infant and toddler, it increases with age to 2.8% in the age group 13 to 18 years. The most common medical histories given were neurological abnormalities (68%), including mental retardation, decreased sensory or motor abilities such as cerebral palsy or paraplegia, and, most significantly, a history of seizure disorder. Other diagnoses include emotional abnormalities (about 21%), blindness (2%), drug addiction (5%) and alcohol abuse (2%). Suicide attempts account for less than 0.1% of all burn injuries, and suicide attempt as the cause of burn injuries among those patients with emotional problems has decreased by two-thirds since 1975. In general, the size of burn sustained in victims with a significant past medical history were of the same average size of burns in other victim types, but the length of stay for hospitalized patients was increased by approximately 50%. The mortality rate in patients with a significant medical history was 8% compared to the overall mortality rate of 5% for all victim types discussed. This difference was especially pronounced in

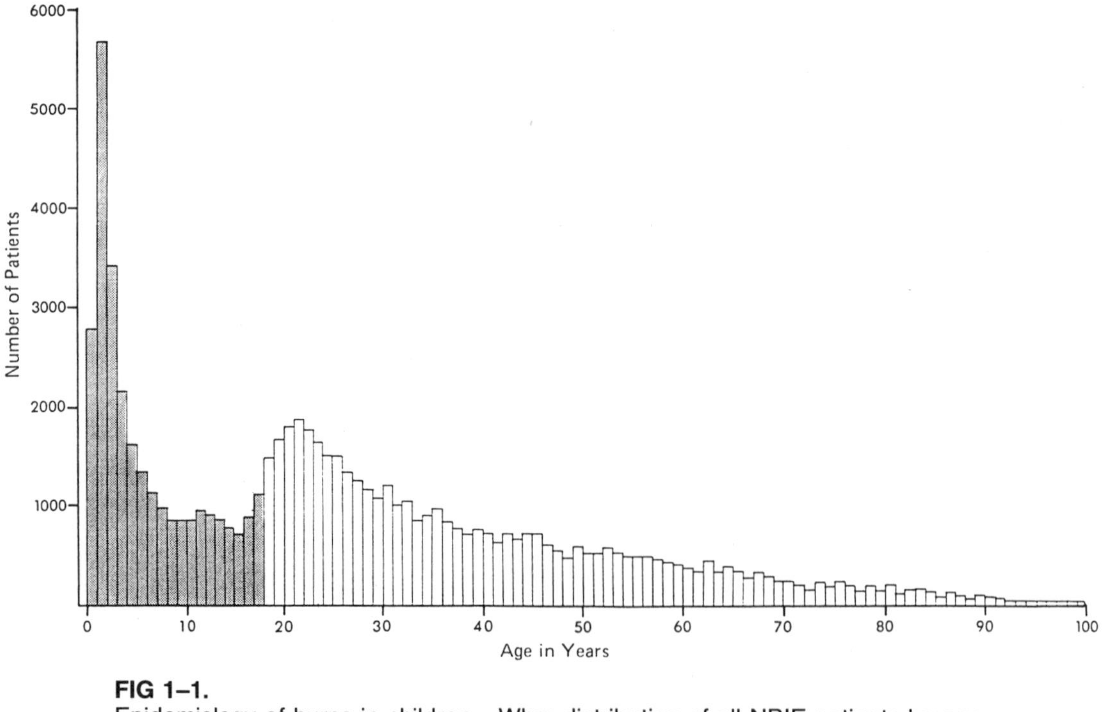

FIG 1–1.
Epidemiology of burns in children—Who: distribution of all NBIE patients by age, 1964–1984 (n = 75,540).

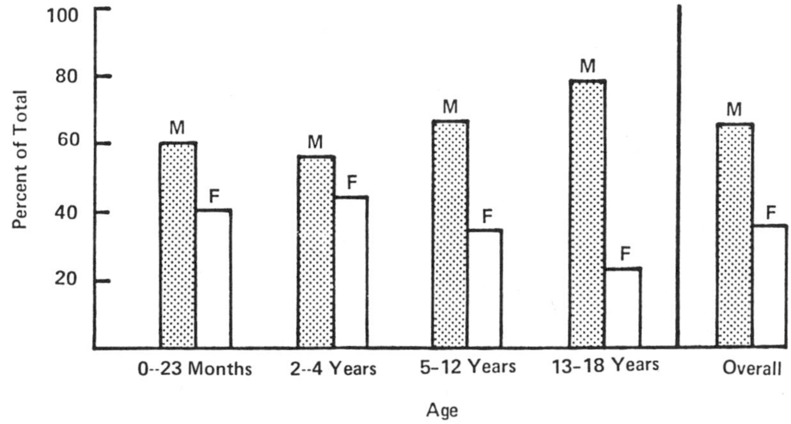

FIG 1–2.
Epidemiology of burns in children—Who: patient distribution by sex, 1964–1984 (n = 29,448).

the 1- to 23-month age group, with a mortality rate of 15% in patients with a significant medical history compared to 4% of all other victim types.

HOW ARE CHILDREN BURNED?

One way to look at how the burn injury occurred is by the type of agent causing the burn injury. Table 1–3 lists the burning agent by age group. Infants and toddlers are most frequently injured by scald burns (72%), while burns caused by flame and contact with hot solids equal about 25%. The majority of burns in this age group was sustained by pulling on objects or during play and play-learning behaviors.[3] Even though infants and younger children are more susceptible to sunburn, this type of injury accounted for less than 1% of all children admissions. By age two to four years, the frequency of scald injuries decreased to 54%, while that of burns caused by flames increased to 34%. Burn injuries in this group occurred mostly through play activities and include children beginning to experiment with matches and lighters. Burns caused by flame are the most common burn in the age groups 5 to 12 years and 13 to 18 years. For those children in the age group 5 to 12 years, the major activity listed when the burn accident occurred was playing or standing nearby when a fire occurred. The adolescent years include injuries caused during many and varied activities, such as igniting fires, riding in or driving vehicles, and during cleaning and repairing activities.

TABLE 1–2.
Epidemiology of Burns in Children—Who: Victim Types, 1964–1984 (n = 18,764)*

	VICTIM TYPE			
AGE	VICTIM OF OWN ACTION, %	INNOCENT BYSTANDER, %	INTENDED VICTIM, %	PAST MEDICAL HISTORY, %
0–23 mo	78	20	2	0.1
2–4 yr	76	20	3	0.3
5–12 yr	78	19	2	0.9
13–18 yr	83	12	2	2.8

*From National Burn Information Exchange, Ann Arbor, Mich, June, 1985

TABLE 1–3.
Epidemiology of Burns in Children—How: Distribution of Patients by Burning Agent, 1964–1984 (n = 27,094)*

AGE	TYPE OF BURNING AGENT				
	HOT LIQUID, %	FLAME, %	HOT SOLID, %	ELECTRICAL, %	CHEMICAL, %
0–23 mo	71.6	10.1	14.6	1.6	1.0
2–4 yr	53.6	33.6	7.8	2.7	1.0
5–12 yr	22.9	70.5	3.6	2.2	0.6
13–18 yr	20.2	69.3	4.3	3.8	2.0

*From National Burn Information Exchange, Ann Arbor, Mich, June, 1985

Ignition of fabric in a flame burn will significantly increase the size and depth of injury, length of hospital stay, cost of hospitalization, morbidity, and mortality resulting from the injury. NBIE research prompted federal legislation in the early 1970s to curtail sale of some flammable fabrics. In 1972 the United States Congress passed a Fabric Flammability Act requiring children's sleepwear sizes 0 to 6X to be flame resistant. Flame resistance was achieved through use of a chemical called TRIS. (In 1977 the United States Consumer Product Safety Commission banned TRIS in sleepwear because of possible carcinogenic properties, and other treatments were used for flame retardants.) However, the act served to significantly reduce the incidence of burns involving fabric ignition. The number of cases submitted to the NBIE with no fabric ignition involved in the accident has increased by 100% in the years 1975 to 1984. Also during that period the number of cases submitted with sleepwear ignition fell from 361 cases prior to 1975 to 38 cases from 1975 to 1984. The survival of those patients where there was fabric ignition has increased to 100% compared to an 82% survival rate before 1975.

WHERE DO ACCIDENTS OCCUR?

Table 1–4 addresses in detail the question of where these burn accidents occurred. In very young children nearly 94% of burn accidents occurred at home, indoors. This percentage decreases progressively with increasing age, with more injuries occurring outdoors, both at and away from home. During the adolescent years there is a significant increase in the burn injuries that occur while traveling in or on vehicles (11%) and at work (14%). The specific location of the accidents are shown in the diagrams in Figure 1–3. The kitchen is the most common site of injury for all age groups, followed by the bathroom for younger children, and the yard for older children. As the child grows older, and as the child becomes more independent, the location of the accident becomes more varied.

An analysis of the size and depth of burn as related to each age group was also compared for two time periods. The data show that both size of the total area burned and size of the full-thickness burn have decreased in recent years. It also shows that the percentage of full-thickness and total area burn increase as the child gets older.

SURVIVAL AND OUTCOME

Outcomes for the burn-injured child can be measured in several ways. Of immediate interest is, of course, survival and length of hospital stay (LOS) and after that the quality of the life of survivors. Survival curves, modeled by probit analysis, are shown in Figure 1–4 for all age groups in the NBIE data base by

TABLE 1–4.
Epidemiology of Burns in Children—Where: Distribution of Patients by Location, 1964–1984 (n = 23,781)*

	LOCATION OF ACCIDENT					
AGE	HOME—INDOORS, %	HOME—OUTDOORS, %	AWAY FROM HOME—INDOORS, %	AWAY FROM HOME—OUTDOORS, %	TRAVELING IN OR ON VEHICLE, %	AT WORK
0–23 mo	93.6	2.2	1.6	2.0	0.6	0
2–4 yr	84.4	8.7	2.0	3.6	1.4	0
5–12 yr	59.1	28.3	2.9	7.0	2.4	0.3
13–18 yr	37.9	21.2	4.4	12.0	11.0	13.5

*From National Burn Information Exchange, Ann Arbor, Mich, June, 1985

percent of total area burned. In Figure 1–5 survival is shown broken out by age group for children. (Both include children burned by all heat sources.) Figure 1–4, demonstrates that patients age 5 to 34 years have overall the best survival rate. People in this age group have greater stamina and endurance and generally better health and fewer incidences of past medical problems. The next best group for survival are the infants and children up to age 4 years and adults age 35 to 49 years. A closer look at survival in children (see Fig 1–5) reveals that older children (ages 13 to 18 years) have better survival rates, and survival is progressively worse the younger the patient.

Another outcome available for evaluation through NBIE data is the length of hospitalization; both for percent total body surface area burn (tba) and for percent full thickness

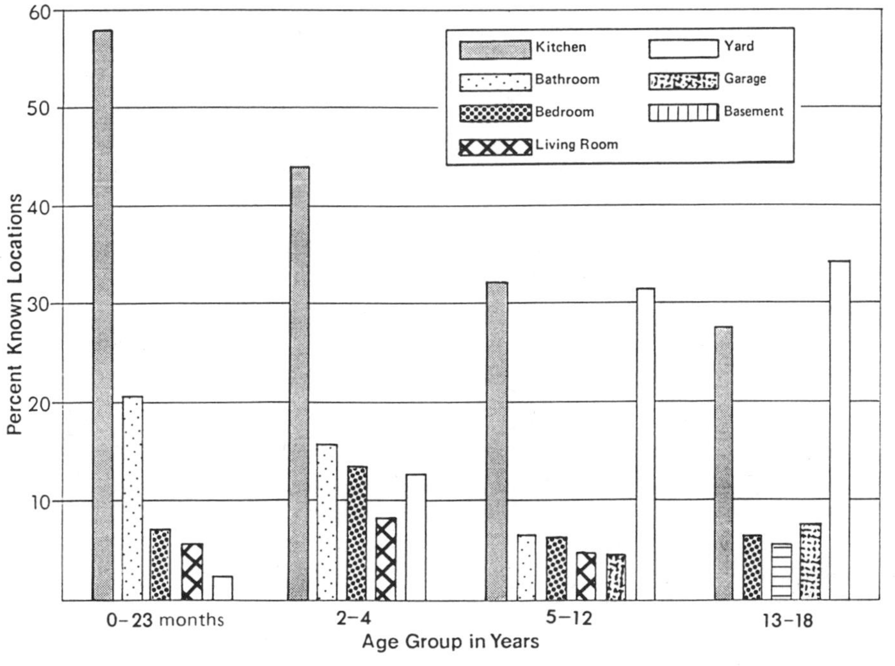

FIG 1–3.
Epidemiology of burns in children—specific location of burn accidents in the home.

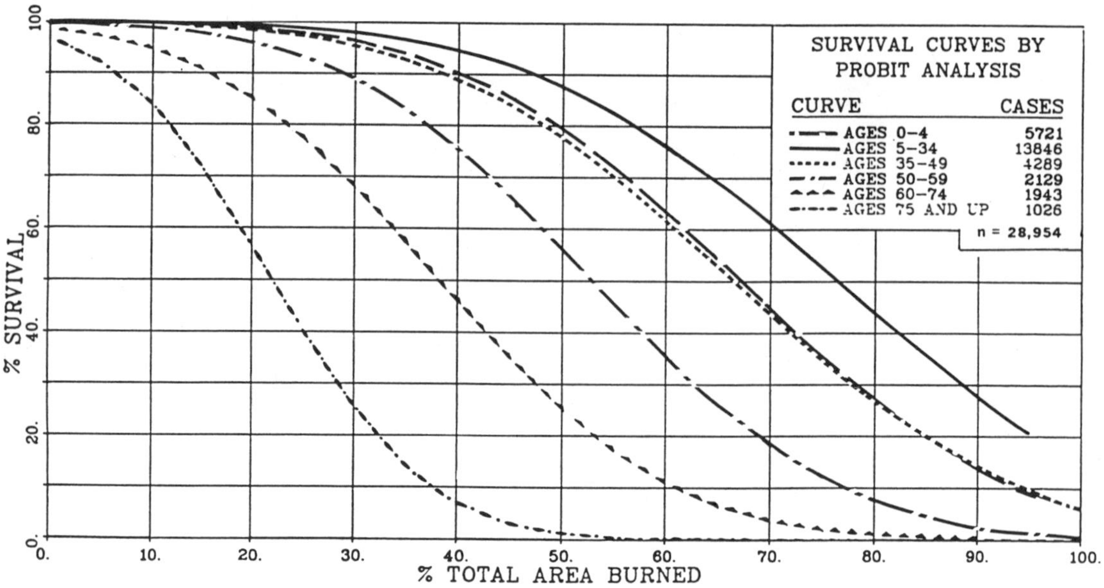

FIG 1–4.
Epidemiology of burns in children—burned patient survival age vs. total area burned, 1979–1984 (n = 28,954).

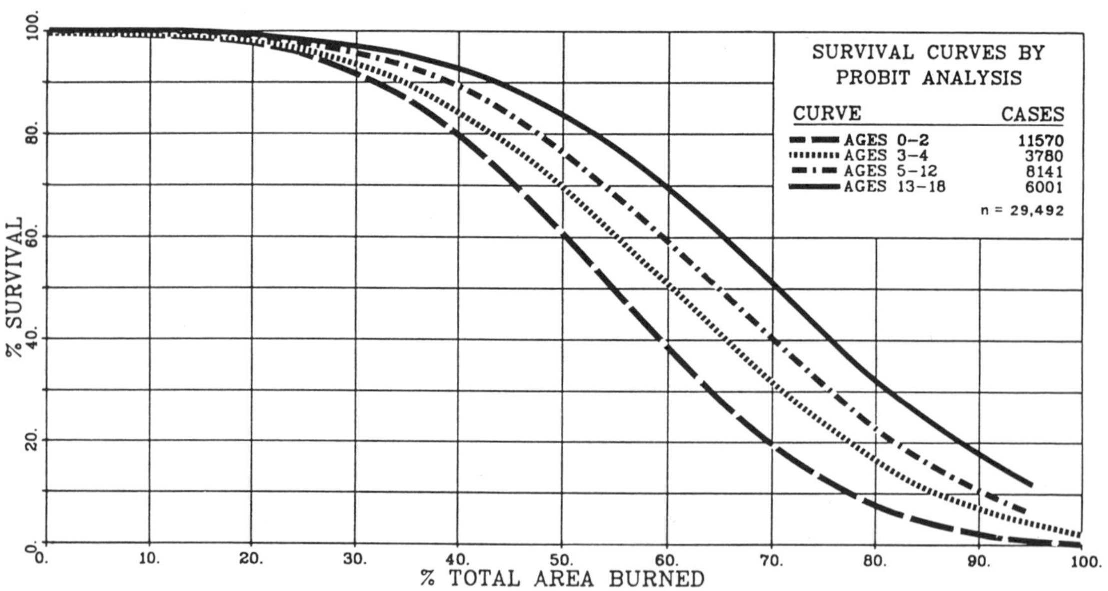

FIG 1–5.
Epidemiology of burns in children—burned children survival by age for all heat sources, 1964–1984 (n = 29,492).

burn. For the overall University of Michigan burn population in 1969, the average length of initial hospitalization (LOS) was 45 days. For the same period, for larger burns; those with a full thickness area greater than 20% tba, the average length of stay was 108 days. Obviously, as the size of the burn increases so does the length of stay, and the larger the full thickness injury the greater the morbidity and mortality. In 1969 the length of stay had decreased to 22 days and in 1985 it was an overall average of 19.6 days. The reduction in stay can be attributed to more organized care, better therapeutic agents, and smaller burn size with less full thickness area being admitted.

Not only is the overall size of burn decreasing somewhat as is LOS, but patients who do die are living longer before they die. The number of days between burn injury and death for fatalities was remarkably consistent among age groups, size of burn, and type of burning agent.[3] Most patients who died did so on the 16th to 18th day postburn, except for very small or very large burns. This number of days until death has increased from 15 days in the period 1964 to 1975 to 18 days in the period 1976 to 1984.

The quality of life enjoyed by burn survivors is a subject of considerable interest. We know that when appropriate care is given in specialized facilities the children tend to have self-esteem measurements similar to those of children in the general population. We also know that decreased LOS also correlates highly with better adjustment.[5, 6]

IF YOU DO THESE THINGS, YOU CAN PREVENT BURN ACCIDENTS

BATHROOM

- Set the temperature of your hot water heater at 124 degrees (F); a water temperature of 140 degrees can scald.
- Test the temperature of bath water before bathing babies and invalids. Run cold water first, then hot to desired warmness. Don't put baby in until all water is turned off.
- Never bathe a baby or youngster in hot water – their skin is too tender.
- Supervise toddlers and youngsters in the bathtub. If left unattended they could turn on the hot water and be scalded.

BEDROOM

- Keep the baby's or toddler's crib a safe distance from radiators, heaters and electrical outlets.
- Keep space heaters and vaporizers away from beds and curtains.
- Don't let cords dangle! Keep away from children's reach.
- Use fire-retardant sleepware for infants, toddlers and young children.
- Be careful when using heating pads – follow directions provided.
- NEVER SMOKE IN BED.
- Put People Protective Stickers on bedroom windows for each child, elderly or invalid sleeping there.

KITCHEN

COOKING

- Keep an eye on youngsters when you are cooking!
- COOK ON BACK BURNERS ONLY. This will prevent children from pulling boiling liquids off front burners.
- Keep handles of pots and pans turned in so children can't pull them off the edge of the stove or countertop.
- Supervise children when they are ready to learn to cook.
- Don't reach across a lit gas or electric burner.
- Don't store foods, especially cereal, over the stove – children could climb onto the stove to reach it.
- Don't set any hot liquids near the edge of a table or counter.

ELECTRICAL APPLIANCES

- Use only UL approved electrical appliances.
- NO DANGLING CORDS. Coil electrical appliance cords so children can't pull on dangling coffee pot or deep fryer cords.
- Unplug electrical appliances when not in use.
- Keep electrical appliances away from water.
- Never leave a hot iron unattended. Unplug it before you walk away.
- Cover electrical outlets to prevent children from sticking things into them.
- Don't overload extension cords.

BARBECUES

- Use only proper lighter fluid to light a barbecue, not gasoline or any other flammable fluid.
- Don't squirt barbecue lighter fluid on burning fires.
- Keep grill away from combustible walls or fences.
- Keep children away from barbecue fires.
- Don't throw hot embers on the ground – they could burn feet.

IN GENERAL

- Install heat and smoke detectors and keep them operating properly. Change batteries every Christmas, or as often as needed.
- HAVE A FIRE ESCAPE PLAN for all family members with a place to meet outside of the home. PRACTICE IT. Instruct babysitters of the plan.
- Keep fire and police numbers by the phone.
- If you smell gas or suspect a gas leak, open a window or door for fresh air and call the gas company or fire department for help. Do not light a match or turn on an electric light.
- Don't misuse or overload extension cords. If a toddler is in the home, don't use extension cords.
- Store corrosive chemicals ONLY in a safe place. Better yet, don't store them.
- Do not allow candles to burn unattended.
- Keep the fireplace screened.
- People with circulatory problems need to be especially careful using heating pads, space heaters, etc.

MATCHES

- Keep matches and lighters out of reach of toddlers and youngsters.
- Teach children at about age five that MATCHES ARE A TOOL. Teach proper use.

GASOLINE AND OTHER COMBUSTIBLE LIQUIDS.

- NEVER STORE gasoline and other combustibles. Buy a one-time-use quantity and replenish as needed.
- If you must store gasoline, store it in a locked utility shed away from the house.
- Never store it in the house or attached garage. Be sure there are NO nearby heat sources, eg. water heater, furnace, etc.
- Use combustible liquids ONLY with proper VENTILATION. Never repair gasoline engines inside the home, or in a closed garage.

Don't fill a hot engine in a lawn mower, snow blower or power boat; let it cool first.

FIG 1–6.
Measures that can prevent burn accidents.

PREVENTION ACTIVITIES

Anyone who has cared for or seen a child severely burned appreciates the need for vigorous prevention activities. Parents and caretakers of children need to be made aware of the simple, noncostly measures they can take to prevent needless accidents (Fig 1–6). Prevention of burns in infants and toddlers must be centered around prevention of scalds with the knowledge that these burns are incurred by the child playing or pulling on objects and occur most commonly in the kitchen as well as in the bathroom of the home.[6] These scald injuries occur primarily during meal preparation times and at bedtime when a mother is busy. A few steps to babyproof the house, taken before the baby becomes mobile, can prevent much grief and heartache.

Prevention for the preschooler also centers on the home environment but includes surveillance while in the immediate vicinity of the home. For this age group more burns are incurred from flame while playing with matches and lighters, although scalds still account for half of the burn injuries. Teaching this child that a match is a tool that requires proper usage is essential. The causes of burns in the older child and adolescent are multifactorial, and the incidence of burns occurring outdoors as well as away from home increases. The burns incurred are mostly from flame rather than scald or contact with hot solids and occur with increasing frequency in association with operation or repair of vehicles or use of flammable materials. These children benefit most from school-based prevention programs.

SUMMARY

In conclusion, analyses of nearly 30,000 pediatric burn patients entered into the NBIE between 1964 and 1984 provide a firm understanding of the epidemiology of childhood burns and serve as a basis for targeted prevention programs. A short summary of outcome as measured by mortality and length of hospital stay is also given and shows increased survival rates with increase in age of the child as well as the expected longer hospital stay with larger burns.

Accurate collection of data and analysis are required to define and establish methods of burn prevention, and the continued availability of reliable data is important for future studies designed to improve burn prevention methods.

REFERENCES

1. Feller I, Jones CA, James MH: Burn epidemiology: Focus on youngsters and the aged. *J Burn Care Rehabil* 1982; 3:285.
2. Green AR, Fairclough J, Sykes PJ: Epidemiology of burns in childhood. *Burns Incl Therm Inj* 1984; 10:368–371.
3. Feller I: Prevention of burns in 1 and 2 year olds. *NBIE Newsletter*, vol 1, no. 2, 1980.
4. Feller I: Improvements in burn care since 1965. *NBIE Newsletter*, vol 1, no. 1, 1980.
5. Bowden ML, Feller I, Tholen D, et al: Self-esteem of severely burned patients. *Arch Phys Med Rehabil* 1980; 61:449–452.
6. Knudson-Cooper MS: Adjustment of visible stigma: The case of the severely burned. *Soc Sci Med* 1981; 15B:31–44.
7. Jones CJ, Feller I: Burn prevention for children. *Offspring*, Fall 1980, pp 28–33.

2 / Prevention of Pediatric Burn Injuries

PAUL SILVERSTEIN, M.D.
ROBERTA WILSON, R.N.

ETIOLOGY OF PEDIATRIC BURNS

Children have historically been victims of a variety of environmental and sociopsychological hazards resulting in burns. They have often been exposed more to these hazards than adults because of their greater vulnerability to accidents due to their inability to recognize and evaluate hazardous situations. Because activities of daily living pose a greater danger to children than adults, researchers are devoting more time than previously to the study of technoenvironmental changes and sociopsychological situations, the two categories most commonly identifiable in the etiology of burn injuries to children.

Technoenvironmental

Technoenvironmental problems are the easiest to identify and control. Yesterday's children grew up in an environment less complicated than the technologically developed world experienced by today's youth. In the past, for example, children confronted hazards related to burns from the manufacture of lye soap and of preserves and from the cooking of foodstuffs over an open flame in the kitchen fireplace. Pouring boiling water into the washtub for the weekly bath or family laundry presented a common opportunity for careless injury. The use of kerosene lanterns and candles to light the home often led to rapidly spreading fires resulting from the ignition of straw mattresses and wooden household utensils and furniture. These historical hazards have changed with advances in technology and environmental modifications (Fig 2–1).

There are many pitfalls to which children are exposed as they grow both chronologically and developmentally. The microwave oven is a modern example. Microwave-heated baby formula warms unevenly from the center toward the periphery of the container. Undetected hot pockets can cause oral scald burns if the formula is not allowed to stand and equilibrate for several minutes before eating.[1]

Infants between the ages of 10 to 20 months learn to walk with the aid of anything they can grab to pull themselves into a standing position. Electrical appliance cords hanging over the edge of a table or countertop, or electrical cords from home tools become lethal objects when infants look for things to hold onto for stabilization while toddling. Frequent hazards are coffeepot cords hanging over the edge of a kitchen table, iron cords dropped over the end of an ironing board, and soldering iron cords in the home workshop.

Three- to 5-year-olds are fascinated by matches. A preschooler innocently becomes curious with a little stick that when struck gives off heat, light, flame, color, and odor. He senses nothing wrong or dangerous as he continues to explore and discover new areas in his environment.

A common danger for boys between the

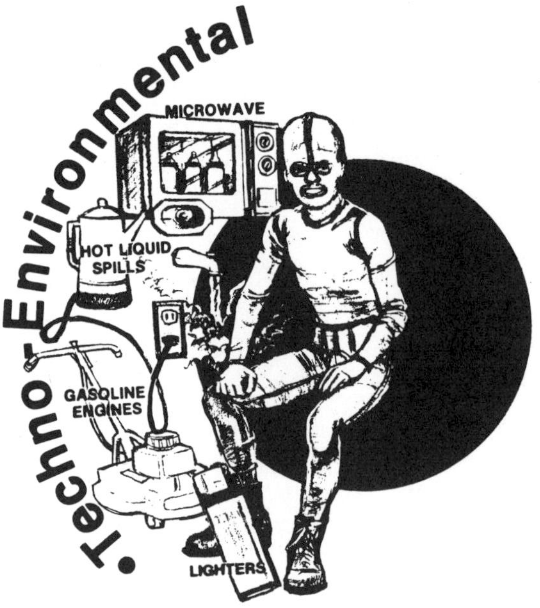

FIG 2–1.
Etiology of pediatric burns—technoenvironmental factors.

ages of 12 and 15 years is a small gasoline engine. As the preschooler is fascinated by the creation of fire and heat with the striking of a match, young teenage boys are equally entranced by starting an engine and making it run. Whether on a lawn mower, or a land, water, or recreational vehicle or model, a poorly adjusted engine can backfire through the carburetor and air filter and ignite fuel vapor or gasoline that might have been carelessly spilled over the sides of the engine. The great majority of burn accidents, therefore, are inflicted upon the child who is unaware of the technoenvironmental dangers to which he is exposed[2] (Table 2–1).

The child requires supervision and education by parents or other concerned, responsible members of the family unit. Practical demonstration of the safe use of technological innovations and their potential hazards will result in fewer accidents and more sensible risk-taking as a child matures. A more balanced assessment of reality thus becomes a way of life, rather than trial and error, which so often leads to death, disfigurement, or debilitating injury.

Children are especially traumatized by burn scar disfiguration, which makes them strangers to family members and friends at school. Disfigurement will bar most of them from developing normal relationships in adult life. Moreover, 54% of all children burned receive burns to the face, hands, or neck (Table 2–2). Since these areas are visible to other people, the disfigurement contributes to and results in a poor self-image[3] (see Table 2–2).

The vulnerability of children to burn trauma is exceeded only by deaths and injuries from automobile accidents and drowning.[4] In Great Britain, burns in children under the age of 15 years, and more significantly, under the age of 6, account for approximately one third of all childhood deaths (Table 2–3).[5] Burn trauma, the third major cause of childhood death, is related to the maturing of developmental skills from birth to adulthood. Children with less maturational development have more accidents than children with well-developed skills. Fewer accidents occur as a child increases in age to 21 years and into adulthood. Paradoxically both total body surface area burned and mortality rate increase as the child becomes a young adult between the ages of 20 and 24 years[6] (Table 2–4).

Over half of all fire injuries occur in the home,[7] most commonly in the kitchen and bathroom.[8] Most fire deaths of children expectedly stem from home fires. The Ohio National Fire Incident Reporting System noted that a preponderance of victims of all age groups are males[9] (Fig 2–2).

In a study undertaken at the University of California at Irvine, burns in children occurred most frequently from scalds, followed by flammable liquids, oil and grease, and matches[2] (Fig 2–3). Most of the scald burns occur in children 4 years old or younger, the age of the exploring child[2] (Fig 2–4). This group accounted for 75.5% of the total number of children scalded; moreover, 37.5% of these injuries occurred in children between

TABLE 2–1.
Burns to Children*

CAUSE	TOTAL BURNS	ADMISSIONS	TBSA† 30%	TOTAL DEATHS	DEATH TBSA 30%	TOTAL % MORTALITY	% MORTALITY INPATIENTS
Automobile, boat, plane, motorcycle	14	5	5	0	0	0	0
Chemical	10	2	5	0	0	0	0
Contact	27	2	0	0	0	0	0
Electrical	20	16	1	0	0	0	0
Firepit	15	10	0	0	0	0	0
Fireworks	11	1	0	0	0	0	0
Flammable liquids	50	22	4	1	1	2	4.5
Heaters	11	4	1	0	0	0	0
Housefire	17	8	4	2	2	11.8	25.0
Irons	11	3	0	0	0	0	0
Inhalation only	4	4	0	1	0	25.0	25.0
Oil and grease	38	17	1	0	0	0	0
Matches	28	21	3	0	0	0	0
Scalds	216	112	10	1	1	0.5	0.9
Sun, sunlamp, heating pad	32	1	0	0	0	0	0
Other	12	12	0	0	0	0	0
Totals	515	240	29	5	4	0.97	2.1

*From Jay KM, Bartlett RH, Dant R, et al: Burn epidemiology: A basis for burn prevention. *J Trauma* 1977; 17:946. Used by permission.
†TBSA = total burn surface area.

the ages of 1 and 2 years. Raine and Azmy[3] confirmed that in 650 children with thermal injuries, 472 patients (73%) were under 3 years of age (Fig 2–5), and 386 of these accidents (82%) were the result of scalding.

The source of the scalds varied[3] (Table 2–5). Jay and associates[2] disclosed that 75.5% of the children were burned in or near the kitchen, mostly by containers of hot liquids pulled onto themselves. And 12.5% of these scalds occurred in the bathroom when children were left unattended in the bath tub where the child or another sibling turned on the hot water (Table 2–6). In a New York study[10] of tap water burns, 50% of the victims were under the age of five years.

TABLE 2–2.
Percentage of Patients With Injuries to Each Part of Body*

PART OF BODY INJURED	% OF PATIENTS WITH INJURY TO BODY PART
Face	27
Neck	12
Chest	43
Trunk	15
Arms	34
Hands	15
Legs	28

*Modified from Raine P, Azmy A: A review of thermal injuries in young children. *J Pediatr Surg* 1983; 18:22. Used by permission.

The peak incidence for thermal injury to children is in the second year of life, a time of rapidly increasing mobility. It is also noted that infants and toddlers receive more scalds in the early morning hours with another peak of scalds in the late afternoon.[8]

The United States Consumer Product Safety Commission estimates that more than 2,600 people are treated for burns caused by scalding tap water every year. Exposure for 1 second to water at 158° F will cause a third-degree burn that requires skin grafting (Table 2–7).[11] Children who cannot distinguish between hot and cold water faucets suffer the greater number of tap water scalds (Table 2–8).[12]

Another identifiable threat causing scald

TABLE 2–3.
Demography, Vital Statistics, and the Pattern of Diseases in Childhood*

INTERNATIONAL DETAILED LIST NUMBERS	CAUSES OF DEATH	NUMBERS OF DEATHS BY AGE GROUP					RATES PER 100,000 POPULATION IN AGE GROUP				
		<1 YR	1–4 YR	5–9 YR	10–14 YR	0–14 YR	<1 YR	1–4 YR	5–9 YR	10–14 YR	0–14 YR
	(Population in thousands, Scotland, England, and Wales)	(630.7)	(2,651.0)	(4,106.4)	(4,472.9)	(11,861.0)	(630.7)	(2,651.0)	(4,106.4)	(4,472.9)	(11,861.0)
	All causes of death	8,711	1,506	1,145	1,179	12,541	1,381	56.8	27.9	26.4	106
	Accidents, poisoning, violence										
E890-99	Burns	8	64	23	19	114	1.3	2.4	0.6	0.4	1.0
E904	Hunger, thirst, exposure, neglect	20	—	—	—	20	3.2	—	—	—	0.2
E910	Drowning	9	47	52	23	131	1.4	1.8	0.3	0.5	1.1
E911-12	Inhalation of objects causing suffocation	133	29	5	6	173	21.2	1.1	0.1	0.1	1.5
E13	Mechanical suffocation	38	19	2	18	77	6.0	0.7	0.05	0.4	0.6
E950-59	Suicide	—	—	—	9	9	—	—	—	0.2	0.08
E960-69	Homicide and injuries purposely inflicted by other persons	30	41	14	15	100	4.8	1.5	0.3	0.3	0.8

*From Arneil GC, Forfar SO (eds): *Textbook of Paediatrics*. New York, Churchill Livingstone Inc, 1984, p 15. Used by permission.

TABLE 2–4.
Bull and Fisher's Grid of Approximate Probabilities for Various Combinations of Age and Area*

BODY AREA BURNED, %	PROPORTIONAL MORTALITY† BY AGE GROUP						
	0–4 YR	5–9 YR	10–14 YR	15–19 YR	20–24 YR	25–29 YR	30–34 YR
78 or more	1	1	1	1	1	1	1
73–77	.9	.9	.9	.9	.9	1	1
68–72	.9	.9	.9	.9	.9	.9	.9
63–67	.8	.8	.8	.8	.9	.9	.9
58–62	.7	.7	.7	.7	.8	.8	.8
53–57	.6	.6	.6	.6	.7	.7	.8
48–52	.5	.5	.5	.5	.6	.6	.7
43–47	.4	.4	.4	.4	.4	.5	.5
38–42	.3	.3	.3	.3	.3	.4	.4
33–37	.2	.2	.2	.2	.2	.3	.3
28–32	.1	.1	.1	.1	.2	.2	.2
23–27	.1	.1	.1	.1	.1	.1	.1
18–22	0	0	0	0	0	0	.1
13–17	0	0	0	0	0	0	0
8–12	0	0	0	0	0	0	0
3–7	0	0	0	0	0	0	0
0–2	0	0	0	0	0	0	0

*From Artz CP, Moncrief JA, Pruitt BA Jr: *Burns: A team approach.* Philadelphia, WB Saunders Co, 1979, p 20. Used by permission.
†The figures are proportional mortalities approximated to a single decimal point. Thus, 0.5 is equivalent to 50% mortality, and 1.0 means most probably a death.

burns to children is the microwave oven. The use of microwave ovens to heat infant formula for feedings has had serious consequences.[12a] A number of cases have been reported in which baby formula containers suddenly ruptured or broke when taken from the oven or while an adult was feeding the child! Both food and some dishes heated in microwaves have been found to be extremely hot. When the hot dish has been dropped or the food spilled when served, serious burn injuries have resulted. Parent education in the safe use of microwave ovens is necessary to reduce this type of accidental injury to children.

The second most identifiable etiology of burn injuries in children is single-ignition flame burns from flammable liquids, clothing, hot oil, or grease. Common sources of ignition are the kitchen stove, matches, space heaters, floor furnaces, outdoor fires, and household fires. A high percentage of accidents occur when children secretly do things forbidden by their parents, such as play with matches, gasoline, or cigarette lighters. Jealous children sometimes inflict injuries on their younger siblings.

When clothing ignition is involved in burn injuries, a greater percentage of the body surface is burned than in ignition burns when no clothing is involved. Clothing ignition will produce a burn two times the body surface area with six times the amount of third-degree loss resulting in a mortality four times the national average when compared with nonclothing ignition burns.[13] Burn injury due to clothing flammability has been greatly reduced due to federal requirements for the use of flame retardant material for children's sleepwear. The flammability standard of the Consumer Product Safety Commission (CS 191-53) was for years the only regulatory protection offered to the public. In 1967 Congress passed the first Flammable Fabrics Act

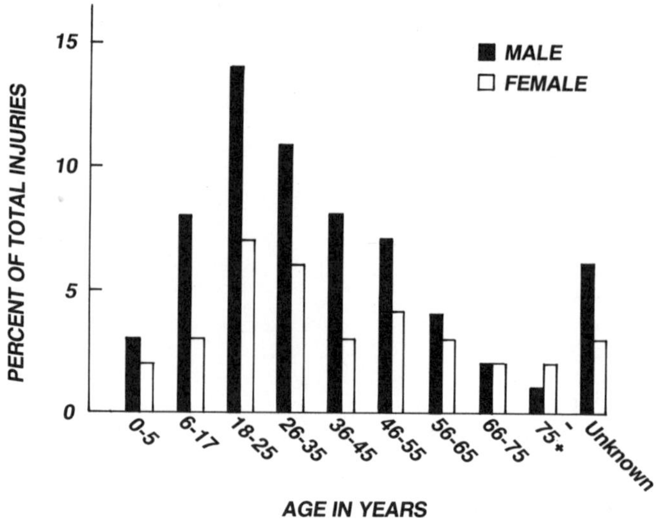

FIG 2–2.
Nonfatal fire injuries by age and sex. (From Carwile RH [ed]: *The 1984 Fire Almanac.* Quincy, Mass, National Fire Protection Association, 1983, p 152. Used by permission.)

Amendments. Since 1972 all children's sleepwear from size 0 to 6X have had to be flame resistant. In 1975 this regulation was expanded to include sizes 7 through 14. Most sleepwear for children was rendered nonflammable by chemical treatment. In 1977, however, the United States Consumer Product Safety Commission banned all production of TRIS-treated sleepwear following a complaint that TRIS-BP was carcinogenic in some species of animals.[14]

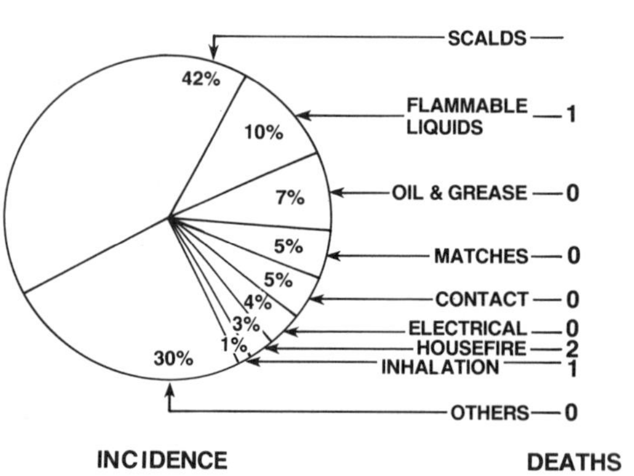

FIG 2–3.
Major causes of burn injury to children between 1972 and 1975. (From Jay KM, Bartlett RH, Dant R, et al: Burn epidemiology: A basis for burn prevention. *J Trauma* 1977; 17:946. Used by permission.)

Further reports[15] in 1979 by the Cooperative Industry Program on General Apparel Flammability added little to our knowledge of the influence of fabric content, weight, or garment style in determining clothing safety and flammability. However, the reports emphasized that loosely fitting, flowing garments are more susceptible to ignition, which results in serious flame injury, than close-fitting, short garments. Wool is the most flame resistant of the natural fibers. Most of the synthetic fibers will melt before they burn and can thus cause contact burns in addition to flame injury. Mixed blends of synthetic fibers and cotton will cause a combination of flame and melt injuries.

Flame burns resulting from residential fires account for over 2,000 pediatric deaths each year.[16] Most household fires occur between midnight and 6 A.M. when the occupants are sleeping and less able to respond quickly to emergency situations. Children are frequently the victims of someone else's carelessness, as demonstrated by fires caused by a dropped or nonextinguished cigarette smoked by adults, either in their own or an adjoining home. Most fire victims die as a result of inhalation of smoke, toxic gases, and products of combustion alone or combined with burns. Children under 9 years of age are

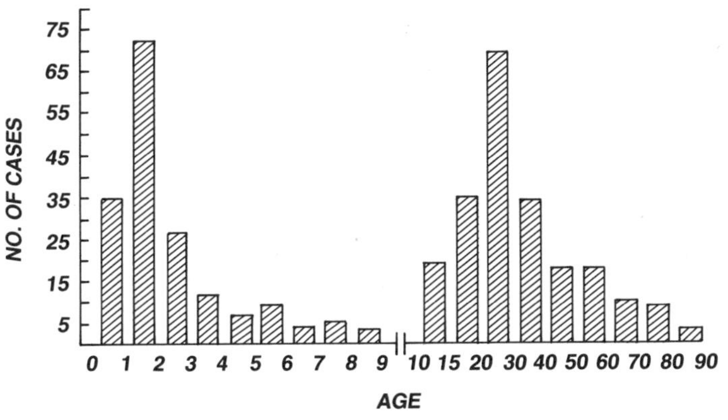

FIG 2–4.
Incidence of scald burns. (From Jay KM, Bartlett RH, Dant R, et al: Burn epidemiology: A basis for burn prevention. *J Trauma* 1977; 17:946. Used by permission.)

most vulnerable due to their inability to successfully escape.

Another common cause of thermal burns is the kerosene space heater. Although flammable fluid fires can cause severe injury, the kerosene itself is not the offender, since modern heaters are designed to shut off when bumped or knocked over. The real problem lies in the fact that the tops of these heaters may reach 200° to 300° F when the heater is lit. The potential for contact burn injury is great when the top of the unit is touched, or if a pan of water placed on top of the heater to increase humidity is subsequently knocked off.[17] Redesign of these units is imperative if this source of burn injury is to be extinguished. Recent popularity of wood-burning stoves has resulted in increased risks of injury by flame or contact burns and asphyxiation.

Sociopsychological

The second most identifiable major category influencing burn injuries in children is sociopsychological changes. This area is more difficult to investigate, define, and control. The child's greater vulnerability to accidents and the lack of coping skills have had serious

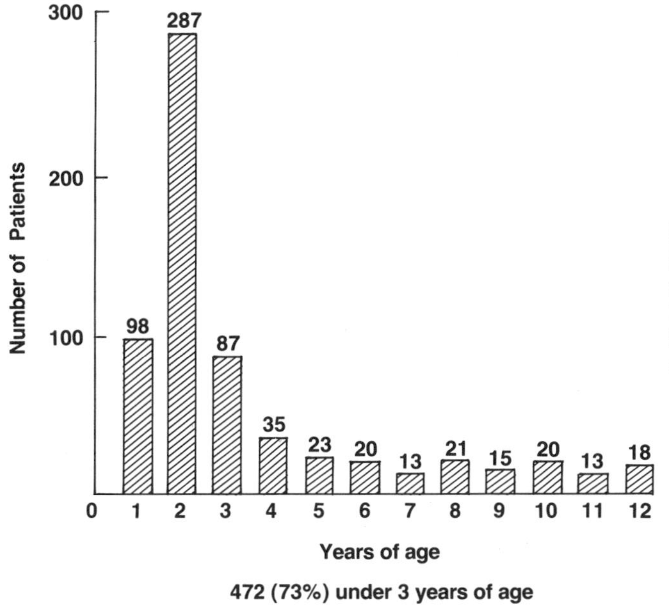

FIG 2–5.
Distribution according to age of 650 children with thermal injuries. (From Raine PA, Azmy A: A review of thermal injuries in young children. *J Pediatr Surg* 1983; 17:22. Used by permission.)

TABLE 2–5.
Percentage of 386 Scalds in Children due to Each Cause*

SOURCE OF SCALD	SCALDS, % (N = 386)
Water	48
Tea	33
Coffee	7
Soup	6
Fat	3
Milk	2
Other	1

*From Raine P, Azmy A: A review of thermal injuries in young children. *J Pediatr Surg* 1983; 17:22. Used by permission.

TABLE 2–7.
Immersion Time to Produce Full-Thickness Burns*

TIME	TEMPERATURE
1 sec	158° F
2 sec	150° F
10 sec	140° F
30 sec	130° F
1 min	127° F
10 min	120° F

*From Feldman KW, Schaller RT, Feldman JA, et al: Tap water scald burns in children. *Pediatr* 1978; 17:5–6. Used by permission.

life-long consequences. As the risks of other types of physical hazards have diminished, more attention has been focused on the effects of sociopsychological factors on burn injuries to children. This interest in child health and well-being concerns itself with understanding adaptive processes of the child to his total environment. Interpersonal relationships within the home and their connection to parenting skills are obviously involved with the health of children and can be considered part of preventive medicine and routine child care. Until recently, sociopsychological interactions have been often neglected or misunderstood. Full recognition of the importance and nature of these relationships is an integral part of any effective preventive health care program for children, parents, and society (Fig 2–6).

While technoenvironmental hazards are comparatively easy to study and comprehend, and to various degrees control, the human situation relating to burns in children is less well defined and more difficult to grasp. Nevertheless, the history of burn accidents clearly implicates the psychodynamic process in parent-child and in family group relationships. The results of human failings, such as haste, preoccupation, faulty judgment, and deliberate abuse create sociological strains and conflicts within the home or job environment. For instance, children and adults who have not progressed through normal stages of developmental behavior with respect to relationships and social responsibility are more likely to have accidents leading to death or permanent disability than children and adults who have developed well-defined coping skills, interrelational behavior, and social responsibility. Burned children frequently live

TABLE 2–6.
Childrens' Scalds: Where They Occur*

	NO.	% OF TOTAL
Kitchen related	145	75.5
Bath related	23	11.9
Unknown or other	24	12.5

*From Jay KM, Bartlett RH, Dant R, et al: Burn epidemiology: A basis for burn prevention. *J Trauma* 1977, 17:946. Used by permission.

TABLE 2–8.
Estimated Number of Scalds by Age*

AGE, YR	ESTIMATED NUMBER	% OF TOTAL	RELATIVE RISK[1]
<5	1,047	40.1	5.2
5–65	1,010	38.6	0.5
>65	558	21.3	2.1
Total	2,615	100.0	1.0

*From U.S. Consumer Product Safety Commission, Directorate for Hazard Identification and Analysis. Based on 1977 NEISS data and information supplied by the Bureau of the Census. Used by permission.

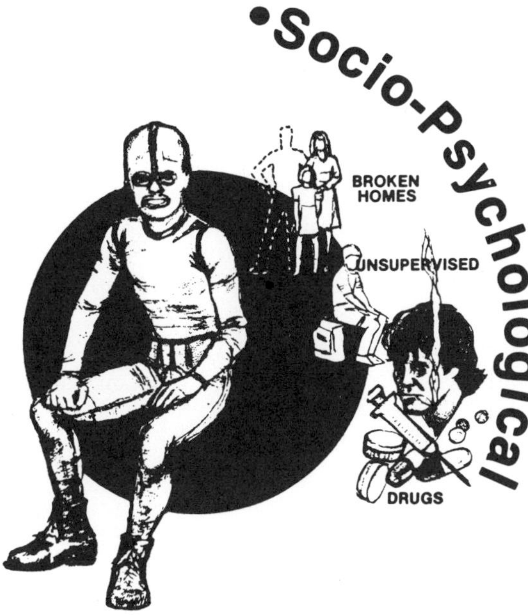

FIG 2–6.
Etiology of pediatric burns—sociopsychological factors.

in homes where separation, divorce, or job-related parental absence necessitates single parenting. Families in which both parents work outside the home are increasing in numbers. Parents in these families, of necessity, provide less supervision and practical education for their children, who are therefore more vulnerable to burn and other accidents.

This dereliction of supervision also parallels the demise of the extended family unit. It is increasingly uncommon for a kinsman to be available to care for the child of a working relative. Day care centers are not necessarily staffed with trained, loving attendants who have the time or interest to teach toddlers the hazards of hot liquids, matches, electricity, and cooking.

Another feature of a disintegrated family culture and stressed economic climate is the trend toward increased geographical separation and mobility of family members. Congested in-town transportation in large cities may extend the working day (and time away from children) by 1 to 3 hours. Prolonged parental absence from the home increases the vulnerability of children to accidents through inadequate supervision. In many cases, preadolescents returning from school are left to watch infants after the baby sitter leaves.

Disintegration of family relationships is exemplified by new evidence from unemployed mothers living in large cities. These mothers, especially if without a spouse, remain sociological strangers in their communities and tend to become isolated in their homes and apartments. In general, they have no one with whom to communicate or from whom they can seek advice. The situation is especially serious if the unemployed mother has moved from a rural area or a small town into a large city. Unemployed mothers, understandably, feel frustrated and insecure in the supervision of the development of their children. As a rule, a young or new mother separated from her husband can expect to receive little social or psychological support for herself or for her children from neighbors or community. Many of these mothers, under stress, find it difficult to cope with life. Children who grow in this environment tend to become emotionally disturbed and, in later life, demonstrate behavioral problems derived from sociopsychological factors that make them at high risk to burn injury.

Moreover, the risks to which a child is exposed depend on the cultural and economic climate into which the child is born and in which he or she matures. Children from poor or low middle-income families, for instance, are more likely to receive burns from a fuel oil heater sitting in the middle of a living room than a child in a higher-income family that enjoys a central heating system in its home.

Sociological or cultural situations in which drug use is common lead to psychological and metabolic changes resulting in careless supervision of children and burn accidents. This etiologic factor cannot be separated from the overall economic problems of the family.[8] The loss of extended parental supervision in families where both parents work or engage in adult social activities is also not easily resolved.

Child Abuse

Child abuse, more often referred to as the battered child syndrome, is gaining increasing exposure in the professional and lay press. Not only parents of lower socioeconomic classes or possessing psychotic traits or criminal-type personalities batter their children (Fig 2–7). *Nelson Textbook of Pediatrics*[18] reports that 90% of parents and adults responsible for battered children neither demonstrate psychotic disorders nor any criminal or antisocial behavioral patterns. The phenomenology of the battered child is seen by physicians and social workers as part of all socioeconomic classes including families from very prestigious social groups. Immature parents and adult care givers unable to blend kindness and affection with control and discipline exist throughout the social strata (Table 2–9).

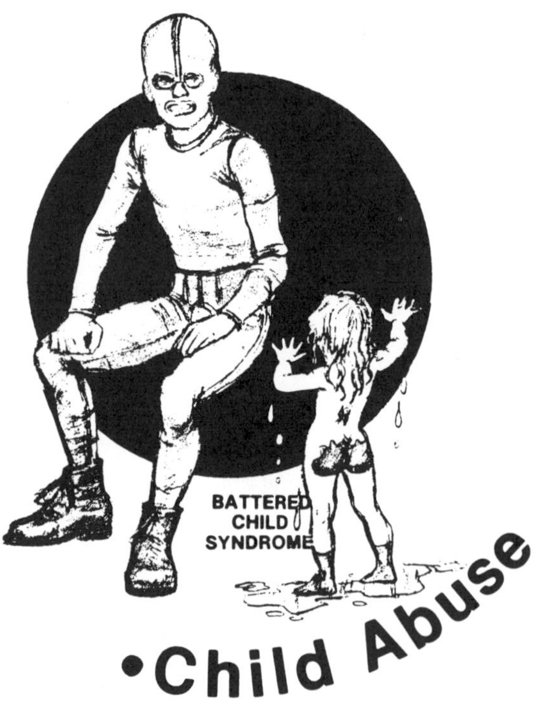

FIG 2–7.
Etiology of pediatric burns—child abuse.

When parents of an abused child are interrogated, they often justify physical abuse not only as a method of punishment, but also as a technique of teaching discipline. Ten percent of all cases of physical abuse involve burns.[24] Hight et al. write that 142 of 872 children (16%) had nonaccidental burns severe enough to "admit the burned child" to a hospital for treatment; moveover, of 1,518 cases of child abuse studied between 1972 and 1977, 136 children (9%) were confirmed as being intentionally burned.[19]

The most common burn to children is scalding, which accounts for 75% of all burns in patients ages 0 to 4 years, and 42% of all burns to children ages 4 years and older.[2] A common scalding technique is inflicted by the parent holding the child's legs against the abdomen and immersing the buttocks into boiling hot water. This torture has been "justified" as a means of discipline for enuresis or refusal to toilet train. The immersion burn reveals a noticeable, characteristic, sharply demarcated, circular burn around the buttock and/or abdomen with splattering of water on the hands, the feet, and other areas of the upper anatomy. This burn topography is not consistent with a child falling into a tub or sink filled with hot water or a child turning on hot water while sitting in a tub or sink. Other nonaccidental methods of burning include contact burns from hot metal objects and cigarettes.

TABLE 2–9.
Perpetrator of Child Abuse*

PERPETRATOR OF CHILD ABUSE	REPORTED CASES, %
Related care giver	90
Male friend of mother	5
Unrelated babysitter	4
Sibling	1

*Data from Behrman RE, Vaughan VC, Nelson WE (eds): *Nelson: Textbook of Pediatrics*. Philadelphia, WB Saunders Co, 1983, p 100. Used by permission.

Sociopsychological, medical, and criminal investigation of these cases revealed that family instability and an inability to deal with stress in crisis situations were important factors in the etiology of these injuries. The sociopsychological behavior patterns and education of the parents, adult care givers, and siblings were of primary concern for understanding the child abuse syndrome. Laws now exist in every state that require physicians to report all cases of suspected child abuse. The law further protects the physician from liability should the suspicions prove false.[20]

Juvenile Fire Setters

In many behavioral conduct disorders, the delinquent is injured while acting out impulsive behavior. The juvenile fire setter must be understood as a part of our society both as a burn victim and as an individual with a passive-aggressive personality disturbance.

Studies by Grustein,[21] and Machet and Mack[22] conclude that child fire setters demonstrate a complex syndrome of psychopathology relating to instinctive and defensive behavioral conduct disorders in which strong aggressive behavioral impulses and oral-sadistic drives[23] are aimed at destroying another person. Other studies conclude that many of these children suffer from mental illness ranging from a variety of behavioral conduct disorders to retardation and schizophrenia.[24] Dr. Gordon A. Heath writes that "childhood fire sett[ing], like other behaviors . . . is a true child psychiatric emergency."[24]

Another interpretation of juvenile pyromania views the disorder as an aggressive response to situational frustration and anxiety associated with factors found in the social disorganization of the family. It is common to discover that the parents of a child fire setter also exhibit behavioral maladjustments ranging from psychoneurosis to psychotic disorders. Interrogators of juvenile fire setters repeatedly describe exposure to angry parental disputes, which frequently erupt into violent physical struggles. Moreover, they may be witness to sadomasochistic sexual behavior between parents or a parent with another adult.

These sexual activities may be interpreted by the child as adult/parental aggressive behavior directed toward himself.[25] Children unable to assimilate, defuse, or understand the overwhelming panic aroused in these situations, as well as the fear of potential parental assault toward each other, act out their hostility toward peers and other children within the family. Pets, moreover, do not escape the displacement of a child's fear and aggression. Pets are often mistreated, battered, or killed by these children.[26] All of these behavior patterns are interpreted as an identification with a parental aggressor in an adverse family situation. The setting of fires by a child represents a plea to the community for help, attention, recognition, and social acceptance. Many child fire setters report an absence of parental affection, which leads to a lack of security within the home. In a survey conducted by Gruber et al.[27] 35% of fires set by children occurred after one or both of the parents withdrew from the child through divorce or separation.

INTERVENTION FOR BATTERED CHILDREN, CHILDHOOD FIRE SETTERS, AND THEIR FAMILIES

It is important to remember that children come into counseling with a variety of antisocial and behavioral conduct disorders associated with family and nonfamily sociopsychological problems. Coupled to this may be physiological brain disorders such as low IQ and certain physical handicaps. Each child and family then has specific problems requiring a treatment program unique to the individual situation.

First, the counselor must be comfortable and well adapted to society's norms. He cannot have poorly controlled antisocial impulses, and he must have a mature self-image (but not have too rigid a superego). These characteristics are very important because family members with antisocial and behavioral character disorders will not identify with an impulsive, rigid, opinionated counselor who does not himself enjoy life.

Second, group and individual counseling is necessary for all family members, including the battered child and the juvenile fire setter. The counseling program must emphasize the following:

1. The development of a sociopsychological value system for all family members.
2. The development of a good self-image.
3. A recreational-social life-style that creates newness, variety, enrichment, and a healthy enjoyment of life.
4. Assistance to all family members in feeling secure in relationships with each other and with nonfamily associations, and in being able to make decisions about these relationships.
5. That family members must minimize anxiety-provoking behavior with each other.

It is also important that the counselor not tolerate manipulative behavior directed between family members or toward himself. Manipulation of the counselor results in a lack of respect for his ability, values, and advice.

Third, new programs have been developed by various communities in cooperation with the Federal Emergency Management Agency to reduce the incidence of fire setting. Examples of two effective programs are those conducted by the San Francisco, Calif., Fire Department and the Upper Arlington, Ohio, Fire Department. The San Francisco program employs fire fighters who volunteer to work with and counsel delinquent youths to build the youths' self-esteem, strengthen relationships with the community, and teach the children less destructive ways to express anger. The Upper Arlington Fire Department's main thrust is to teach fire safety coupled with behavior modification and includes emphasis on fire prevention. For example, juvenile fire setters inspect buildings for fire safety and fire hazards and distribute fire hats to hospitalized children. Thus young patients become aware of their ability to help other children and give pleasure.[28] These programs employ multiple community resources to achieve a positive effect on solving the problems of abused children, the juvenile fire setter, and their families. Recognition and early intervention can alleviate and hopefully prevent long-term sociopsychological consequences.

PREVENTION

Educational programs aimed at specific identifiable and preventable etiological factors of burn injuries are essential. Use of mass media to develop positive behavior may be effective, but follow-up still is needed to determine its success. One media-based program, "Project Burn Prevention," was designed to measure the success of public education techniques in increasing awareness of burn dangers and reducing the incidence and the severity of burn injury. Funded by a United States Consumer Product Safety Commission grant, Elizabeth McLoughlin and associates[29] designated target areas of high-risk age groups and launched an educational barrage against flame burns because of their severity and against scalds because of their frequency. Through lectures, media presentations, printed materials, and controlled fire demonstrations, the defined population groups were saturated. Results and analysis of the impact of the program through follow-up testing and interviews indicate that "neither the school program nor the media campaign reduced burn incidence or severity . . . . Multiplicity of message, brevity of the campaign, and separation of the interventions are among possible reasons for the program's failure to significantly reduce burn injuries."[29]

Another program aimed at developing positive behavior modification is the National Fire Protection Association's "Learn Not to Burn Curriculum." Its goal is to reduce the incidence of burn injuries to children and to assist children in becoming safety-conscious adults. The project covers the school years kindergarten through eighth grade and concentrates on changing the behavior of the children most likely to become burn victims. Reduction of burn incidence and severity by prevention education is accomplished by instilling positive behavior patterns in the child and providing the entire family with additional instructions on proper procedure and reactions to a burn injury situation. "Operation EDITH (Exit Drills In The Home)," sponsored by the National Fire Protection Association and the Fire Marshal's Association of North America, is another program that can effectively teach positive behavior to accomplish burn and fire prevention. Support of legislation requiring approved smoke detectors in single and multifamily dwellings also can reduce the incidence and severity of burn injury.

The hazardous environment of the child can be changed through educational programs focused on the places where the accidents occur, specifically the kitchen and the bathroom. Parental awareness of the dangers should help reduce accidents. Strategies to eliminate the risk of burns in the kitchen include storing electrical appliance cords out of reach of small children, turning pot handles on the stove toward the wall, avoiding the use of tablecloths when hot items are served, placing hot food containers in the center of the table or well out of the reach of children, and avoiding holding young children in the lap while drinking hot beverages.

The hazardous areas of the bathroom and the kitchen need to be demonstrated to parents to render them burn-safe. For example, bathrooms and kitchens can be made scald-proof by the installation of scald-prevention faucets and of guards over heater vents, and by decreasing water temperature in hot water heaters to 120°F. Electrical outlets should be installed out of the reach of children, and unused wall receptacles should be protected by insertion of dummy plugs. Parents and baby-sitters need to be taught to never leave a bathing infant or child unattended. Placing locked gates in the doorway of the kitchen or the bathroom to keep infants and children out of unsupervised areas has also been helpful. Common sense must be reinforced through education.

There are no easy solutions that can be drawn from the sociological complexities of modern living. However, interesting observations can be made. First, technological progress can produce burn hazards of which parents and baby-sitters are not aware. Consumer protection agencies need to be adequately funded in order to continually test the safety of new home products, toys, and innovations. An age classification similar to that placed on toys can be developed for new technological devices. Second, it is important to understand the relationship between sociopsychological developmental problems of infancy and childhood and an accident-prone life pattern, which include being burned. Even if infant and child nurturing dilemmas experienced by parents are not always serious and sometimes only represent an expression of the parent's insufficient knowledge of their child's normal development, it seems wise and logical to regard these problems as warning signs. The perplexities of infant- and child-rearing should be identified as early as possible and be properly resolved through consultation and treatment in well-baby clinics and doctors' offices.

Based on clinical observations, Smith[8] strongly suspects that "the problems of cause and control of burn injury cannot be separated from the overall social and economic problems of the family." Federal, state, and private agencies established to promote the health and welfare of children must become more visibly concerned with educational needs through the publication and distribution of material directed toward the social and economic stumbling blocks encountered by today's families.

In addition to governmental commitment, the development of neighborhood and community involvement in burn prevention is necessary. Discussion groups can be facilitated and encouraged by burn center personnel, and literature organized by social, civic, and recreational clubs can be disseminated through partnerships with fire departments, the Red Cross, social welfare and medical offices, and other voluntary or local service organizations. Most established burn centers in the United States recognize their obligation to teach burn and fire prevention, as well as to provide care for the patient once he has been injured.

REFERENCES

1. Infant Nutrition Institute, Toronto, Ontario: Scalding baby food. *Can Nurse* 1985; 81(8):62.
2. Jay M, Bartlett RH, Danet R, et al: Burn epidemiology: A basis for burn prevention. *J Trauma* 1977; 17:943–947.
3. Raine PA, Azmy A: A review of thermal injuries in young children. *J Pediatr Surg* 1983; 18:21–26.
4. Halsey MN (ed): *Accident Prevention.* New York, McGraw-Hill Book Co (Blakiston Division), 1970, p 51.
5. Forfar JO, Arneil GC (eds): *Textbook of Paediatrics,* ed 3. New York, Churchill Livingstone, Inc, 1984, vol 1, p 15.
6. Artz CP, Moncrief JA, Pruitt BA Jr: *Burns: A Team Approach.* Philadelphia, WB Saunders Co, 1979, p 20.
7. Luther SL, Price JH: Burns and their psychological effects on children. *Sch Health* 1981; 419–422.
8. Smith EI: The epidemiology of burns. The cause and control of burns in children. *Pediatrics* 1969; 44(suppl):821–827.
9. Carwile RH (ed): *The 1984 Fire Almanac.* Quincy, Mass, National Fire Protection Association, 1983, p 152.
10. Baptiste MS, Feck G: Preventing tap water burns. *Am J Public Health* 1980; 70:727–729.
11. Feldman KW, Schaller RT, Feldman JA, et al: Tap water scald burns in children. *Pediatrics* 1978; 62:1–7.
12. Silverstein P, Lack BO: Art and science of burn care, in Boswick JA Jr (ed): *Epidemiology and Prevention.* Rockville, Md, Aspen Publications, 1987, p 16.

12a. Report of the Committee on Special Interests—Prevention. Annual Meeting of the American Burn Association, Chicago, April 9–12, 1986.

13. *Studies on Death, Injuries and Economic Losses Resulting From Accidental Burning of Products, Fabrics, or Related Materials,* Third Annual Report to the President of the United States and the Congress of the United States, prepared by the Department of Health, Education, and Welfare, Publication (FDA) 72-7013, 1971, p 36–37.
14. Bergman AG: Flame resistant sleepwear. *Pediatrics* 1977; 60:652–653.
15. May RS, DeClement FA: Evaluation of the final report (1979) of the Cooperative Industry Program on General Apparel Flammability. *J Burn Care and Rehabil* 3:279.
16. *Prepare for Disaster, Exit Drills in the Home,* Sherman Oaks, Calif, Alisa Ann Ruch Burn Foundation, 1980.
17. Rissmiller R: Kerosene heaters—A new burn threat to children. *Clin Pediatr* 1983; 22:203.
18. Schmitt BD, Kempe CH: Abuse and neglect of children, in Behrman RE, Vaughan VC III (eds): *Nelson Textbook of Pediatrics,* ed 12. Philadelphia, WB Saunders Co, 1983, p 100.
19. Hight RW, Bakalar HR, Lloyd JR: Inflicted burns in children. *JAMA* 1979; 242:517.
20. Randolph JG, Ravitch MM, Welch KJ, et al: *Injured Child—Surgical Management.* Chicago, Year Book Medical Publishers, 1979, p 407.
21. Grustein A: Stages in development of the control of fire. *Int J Psychoanal* 1952; 33:416.
22. Macht LB, Mack JE: The firesetter syndrome. *Psychiatry* 1968; 31:277–281.
23. Finichel O: *The Psychoanalytic Theory of Neurosis.* New York, WW Norton, 1945, pp 371–372.
24. Heath GA, Gayton WF, Hardesty VA: Childhood firesetting. *Can Psychiatr Assoc J* 1976; 21:229–237.
25. Nurcombe B: Children who set fires. *Med J Aust* 1964; 1(16):579–584.
26. Hellman DS, Blackman N: Enuresis, firesetting, and cruelty to animals. *Am J Psychiatr* 1966; 122:1431–1435.
27. Gruber AR, Heck ET, Mintzer E: Children who set fires: Some background and behavioral characteristics. *Am J Orthopsychiatry* 1981; 51:484–488.
28. Buchbinder L: The juvenile arsonist: What can fire departments do? *J Burn Care Rehabil* 1982; 3:299–300.
29. McLoughlin E, Vince CJ, Lee AM, et al: Project burn prevention: Outcome and implications. *Am J Public Health* 1982; 72:241–247.

SECTION II

PATHOPHYSIOLOGY

3 / Pathophysiology of the Burn Wound

MARTIN C. ROBSON, M.D.
JOHN P. HEGGERS, Ph.D.

Exposure of human skin to damaging levels of heat results in two types of injury: (1) an immediate direct cellular injury, and (2) a delayed injury due to progressive dermal ischemia. The skin can tolerate temperatures up to 40°C (104°F) for relatively long periods of time before apparent injury. Temperatures above this level, however, produce a logarithmic increase in tissue destruction.[1] The degree of tissue destruction correlates with both temperature and duration of exposure to the heat source. Thus, the depth of burning is determined by a combination of the burning agent, the temperature, and the duration of exposure (cell damage from protein denaturation occurs as result of high temperatures). Many of these changes are reversible. Only at temperatures exceeding 45°C (113°F) does denaturation exceed the capacity for cellular repair.[1] Nonetheless, the response of cells to heat is neither uniform nor static. The blood supply and local environment of the wound greatly determine the cellular response.

The classic description of Jackson[2] of three concentric zones of significant thermal injury in the burn wound provides a practical basis for discussion of local burn injury. The central area of the burn wound, that having most intimate contact with the heat source, is characterized by coagulation necrosis of the cells and is called the *zone of coagulation*. In this zone the temperature exceeds 45°C (113°F) and no cellular recovery is possible. The severity of the injury decreases from the surface of the skin to the deeper layers as well as concentrically from the central point of injury (Fig 3–1).

A labile area of injured cells, which may survive under ideal circumstances, extends concentrically from the central zone of coagulation. Although these cells show direct injury from the heat, the injury is not lethal to the cells. The progressive injury due to dermal ischemia occurs in this zone, designated by Jackson[2] as the *zone of stasis*. Before the mechanism of the progressive dermal ischemia was understood, and counteracting cells in the zone of stasis routinely necrosed within 24 to 48 hours following the burn.

Peripheral to the zone of stasis measures implemented, is the *zone of hyperemia*, which has sustained minimal injury. Cells in this zone will recover over a period of 7 to 10 days.

The initial cytologic evidence for thermal injury is a redistribution of the fluid and solid components of the cell nuclei. Imbibition of fluid results in nuclear swelling, membrane rupture, and pyknosis. Cell cytoplasm first becomes granular and then homogeneously coagulated. Progressive denaturation of cell protein occurs as temperatures rise. These changes in the thermally injured cell may be reversible since protein is constantly being denatured by the body and being replaced. However, as stated previously, at temperatures exceeding 45°C (113°F), this denaturation exceeds the reparative ability of the

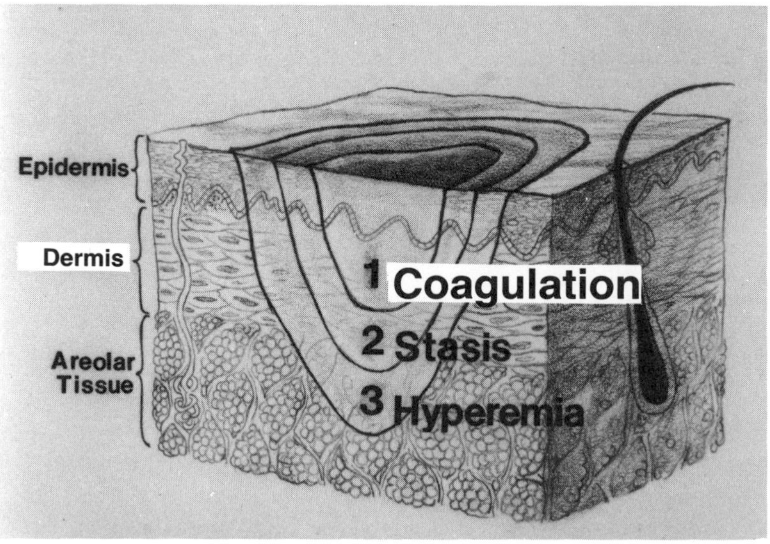

FIG 3–1.
Concentric zones of thermal injury. (Adapted from Jackson DM: The diagnosis of the depth of burning. *Br J Surg* 1953; 40:588.)

cell.[1] Therefore, reducing the temperature should reduce the denaturation of protein. Cells are also injured because of interference with vital metabolic processes. Thermolabile enzyme systems are blocked at approximately the same temperatures that effect protein denaturation.[3] The metabolic response of an individual cell varies, even within a homogeneous cell population. A decrease in enzyme activity below 50% of normal results in cell death, whereas lesser degrees of injury may be reflected in cell recovery.

Many investigators have shown that following the burn injury itself, changes continue to occur in the affected tissue. Whether these changes are manifestations of, or contribute to, ongoing damage, or whether they are evidence of reparative processes is not always clear. However, most investigators agree that significant tissue necrosis occurs for some time after the initial insult. Jackson[2] reported these changes in his description of the burn wound in which zone of stasis became devitalized in 24 to 28 hours like the central zone of coagulation. Order and Moncrief[4] demonstrated arteriographically that the wound was devascularized by 24 hours postinjury, although an earlier picture had shown patent vessels. Hinshaw[5] described progressive destruction of epithelial elements in follicles and sweat ducts over 24 to 48 hours. Some destruction was already evident in his first biopsies at 4 hours. Cotran and Remensnyder[6] described three types of small vessel reaction that depended on the intensity of the injury. The first, "immediate-transient" response, affecting mildly injured tissue, ended within 30 minutes postinjury. The "delayed-prolonged" response to more intense injury began 15 to 75 minutes postinjury, peaked at about 4 hours, and subsided by 8 hours after the burn. Progressive endothelial injury was observed by Ham and Hurley[7] over 24 hours, developing by 3 to 4 hours. Other changes, many of which are presumed to be associated with repair, were observed for 7 days. Branemark et al.[8] noted a decrease in flow through the small vessels within 5 to 7 minutes of the injury. Massiha and Monafo[9] demonstrated immediate compromise of the venous side of the microcirculation, which progressed for 24 hours. Whether all or some of these changes represent simple manifestations of damage that has already occurred or ongoing mechanisms of destruction postinjury is not clear. However, the burn wound does change progressively for at least 24 hours postinjury.

Cohnheim[10] was the first to describe the acute inflammation subsequent to thermal trauma. After immersing the ears of rabbits in water of different temperatures, he noted the initial quickening of local blood flow, then slowing, localized fluid exudation, leukocyte margination to vessel walls, and finally stasis of flow. Subsequent investigators have studied the role of the inflammatory reaction in tissue that is progressively destroyed subsequent to thermal injury. Sevitt[11] concluded that the inflammatory response contributed to the progressive tissue destruction by its effect on the microcirculation in burned areas. Leach et al.[12] noted that the full magnitude of tissue injury is not immediately apparent following thermal trauma, but becomes manifest at a later stage. Grant and Becker[13] used a laser beam to inflict microburns on selected areas in small vascular beds and showed that minimal endothelial injury induces white cell sticking, while severe injury evokes an additional platelet response.

The idea that the progressive changes in the burn wound may be related to inflammation led investigators to study the possible role of inflammatory mediators, specifically prostaglandins. These mediators, originally discovered[14, 15] in the 1930s in seminal fluid and lipid extract of sheep vesicular glands, were first called prostaglandins by von Euler.[11] For more than two decades, research was hampered by technology and lack of interest. Then in 1960, Bergstrom and his coworkers[17, 18] rekindled the interest by crystallizing two prostaglandins.

The observations by Ambache et al.[19] in 1965, while not related to burns, were the first indication that prostaglandins played some role in the inflammatory process. Early reports clearly indicated the presence of a substance with biological activity in human blister fluid. However, its identity remained obscure. For a long time investigators had postulated that burned skin forms some kind of "burn toxin." In 1973, the toxic factors in the burned skin were isolated and characterized.[20]

Anggard and his colleagues[21, 22] first demonstrated the role of prostaglandins in thermal injury in 1970. In an experimental model they showed that the lymph fluid draining from the scalded paw of a dog contained prostaglandins, mainly prostaglandin E_2 (PGE_2). Subsequent studies in the guinea pig scald model revealed a prostaglandin-like material in concentrations 24 to 40 times that of the control skin.

Investigators concentrated their efforts on explaining the role of PGE_2 and PGF_{2a} in a thermal injury. Using acidic lipid extracts of burn wound secretions collected over a 3-week period, Arturson[23] showed biologic activity equivalent to 5.0 to 30 ng/ml of PGE_2. The highest levels was observed during the first 24 hours postinjury. These amounts were considered far above those necessary for biologic activity.

Anggard, Arturson, and Jonsson showed[22] that lymph flow in the scalded dog paw could be reduced 30% to 40% in the animal treated with indomethacin. An efflux of prostaglandins initially persisted for 150 minutes in the lymph from untreated animals. A second efflux occurred 3 to 5 hours posttrauma. Treated animals showed no efflux of prostaglandins (PGE_2).

Therapeutic manipulation of the zone of stasis of the burn wound using prostanoid inhibitors was attempted to delineate the pathophysiology of the thermal injury. Heparin, an anticoagulant once thought to have some therapeutic value for the burn wound, was examined in the thermal injury. Using arteriography, Noble et al.[24] showed that heparin was of no value in preventing dermal necrosis. Later Carr[25] showed that heparin had no effect on prostanoid derivatives with the exception of PGE_1, for which it was antagonistic.

In 1979 and 1980 two independent groups

of investigators[26–28] isolated thromboxane from burn blister fluids. The thromboxane concentration varied from 1.45 to 6.04 ng/ml with a mean concentration of 1.7 ng/ml. Prostaglandin E_2 levels did not exceed 0.53 mg/ml. These findings, while somewhat perplexing, rekindled the efforts to further delineate the true pathophysiology of the thermal injury. Since thromboxane is a potent platelet aggregator and vasoconstrictor counteracting the action of PGI_2, the finding suggests that PGE_2 and PGF_{2a} were present in exudates and tissue fluids of burns in a steady-state relationship because of their bidirectional activity, and that this homeostasis was essential to the preservation and integrity of the cell.

Investigators have used specific thromboxane synthetase inhibitors in an attempt to reverse dermal necrosis. Dermal microcirculation, xenon 133 washout, and immunohistochemical assays have been performed.[30, 31] Data from these studies clearly indicate that thromboxane synthetase inhibition with imidazole, dipyridamole, and methimazole preserved dermal microcirculation, as determined by india ink perfusion to the subpapillary plexus and by xenon 133 washout (half-life was 12.7 minutes for controls and 4.6 minutes for the test group). An immunohistochemical assay showed that although PGE_2 and PGF_{2a} remained present in the tissue, thromboxane accumulation was prevented within 24 hours in the treated groups of burned animals, whereas in the control animals, thromboxane levels were greatly elevated.[28, 31] The treated animals healed with little or no evidence of injury, whereas the control group remained denuded.

When thromboxane synthetase is inhibited, platelet adherence is reduced, leukocytes and red blood cells are prevented from sticking to vessel walls, and vessels dilate.[29] In the small-sized burn used in the experiments discussed, the pathologic changes in the microvasculature only occurred in the burned area, since xenon 133 clearance times were normal in the unburned areas. The blockage of formation of only one metabolite of arachidonic acid, thromboxane, prevented the vascular changes in the burn wound, allowed dermal perfusion, and yet allowed other prostaglandins to be formed. This circumvents any possible detrimental effects that would occur using steroidal or nonsteroidal anti-inflammatory agents. If a similar pathophysiology of the progressive injury is confirmed in humans, a specific antithromboxane or other inflammatory-mediator blocking agent may possibly prove beneficial in preventing progressive dermal ischemia and in increasing the ultimate amount of skin salvaged.

In addition to understanding the direct cellular and progressive ischemic responses to heat, it is important to describe macroscopic or clinical observations concerning the extent of injury to determine treatment of the burn wound. The number of cells in the skin that are destroyed or injured is reflected in the functional capacity of the skin. Thus, the vertical depth of burning is important. The superficial or first-degree burn is characterized solely by pain and redness. Within a few days, the outer layer of injured cells peels away from totally healed subjacent skin with no residual scarring.

The second-degree burn is best subclassified as either a superficial partial-thickness or deep partial-thickness burn. The superficial partial-thickness injury is characterized by blister formation. Breaking or removal of the blisters results in weeping of fluid from the burn surface. However, since the basal layers of the dermal portion of the skin are uninjured, regeneration of the superficial injured layers is prompt. If no secondary infection or subsequent insult occurs, these burns usually heal in 14 to 17 days. The more serious deep partial-thickness burn, however, is often indistinguishable from a full-thickness or third-degree burn. Such a wound comprises many areas of only marginally viable tissue. Injury to the dermis is subtotal. Nonetheless, survival of the remaining dermis and the associated epidermal appendages is in jeopardy unless optimal conditions for preservation of these elements can be maintained. Such wounds may heal spontaneously, though healing may require 3 to 4 weeks. On the other hand, these wounds may become deeper with the progressive dermal ischemia and convert to full-thickness necrosis. Even if healing occurs, the resultant epithelium is often of poor quality and injured by minor trauma. Hypertrophic scar formation is not an infrequent sequela of such an injury. These wounds present the most treatment options.

In the third-degree or full-thickness burn, the skin is totally destroyed through the full thickness of the dermis. Such a wound cannot heal spontaneously. Restoration of the integrity of the skin over such a wound can be accomplished only by ingrowth of epithelium from the margins of the wound or by grafting skin from nonburned areas of the body.

Finally, fourth-degree burns consist of injuries involving not only total destruction of the skin but injury or destruction of subjacent tissues such as subcutaneous fat, fascia, muscle, or bone. Closure of such wounds often necessitates not only skin grafts but often local or regional flaps to definitively cover the wound.

The most important requirement for successful treatment of the burned patient remains the effective treatment and ultimate healing of the burn wound. The multisystemic responses of the burn patient, and ultimately his death or survival, are closely related to the successful management of the burn wound. Thus, an understanding of the pathophysiology of the local burn injury itself is paramount to the successful treatment of the burn victim.

REFERENCES

1. Moritz AR, Henrique FC, Jr: Studies of thermal injury: The relative importance of time and surface temperature in the causation of cutaneous burns. *Am J Pathol* 1947; 23:695.
2. Jackson DM: The diagnosis of the depth of burning. *Br J Surg* 1953; 40:588.
3. Cruickshank GND, Hershey FB: The effect of heat on the metabolism of guinea pigs' ear skin. *Ann Surg* 1960; 151:419.
4. Order SE, Moncrief JA: *The Burn Wound.* Charles C Thomas, Publisher, Springfield, Ill, 1965.
5. Hinshaw JR: Early changes in the depth of burns. *Ann NY Acad Sci* 1968; 150:548.
6. Cotran RS, Remensnyder JP: The structural basis of increased vascular permeability after graded thermal injury—light and electron microscopic studies. *Ann NY Acad Sci* 1968, 150:495.
7. Ham KN, Hurley JV: An electron microscope study of the vascular response to mild thermal injury in the rat. *J Pathol Bacteriol* 1968; 95:175.
8. Branemark PI, Breine U, Joshi M, et al.: Part I. Pathophysiology of the thermal burns. Microvascular pathophysiology of burned tissue. *Ann NY Acad Sci* 1968; 150:474.
9. Massiha H, Monafo WW: Dermal ischemia in thermal injury: The importance of venous occlusion. *J Trauma* 1974; 14:705.
10. Cohnheim J: Local disturbance of the circulation, in Cohnheim J: *Lectures on General Pathology.* London, New Sydenham Society, 1889, pp 109–171.
11. Sevitt S: Inflammatory changes in burned skin: Reversible and irreversible effects and their pathogenesis, in Sevitt S: *Burns, Pathology, and Therapeutic Implications.* London, Butterworth & Co, 1957.
12. Leach EH, Peters RA, Rossiter RJ: Experimental thermal burns especially the moderate temperature burn. *Q J Exp Physiol* 1943; 32:67–86.
13. Grant L, Becker FF: Mechanisms of inflammation I: Laser induced thrombosis—a morphlogic analysis. *Proc Soc Exp Biol Med* 1965; 119:1123.
14. Goldblatt MW: Properties of human seminal plasma. *J Physiol (Lond)* 1935; 84:208–218.
15. Kurzrok R, Lieb C: Biochemical studies of human semen: II. The action of semen on the human uterus. *Proc Soc Exp Biol Med* 1930; 28:268–272.
16. von Euler VS: On the specific vasodilating and plain muscle stimulating substances from accessory genital glands in man and certain animals (prostaglandin and vesiglandin). *J Physiol (Lond)* 1936; 88:213–243.
17. Bergstrom S, Eliasson R, von Euler VS, et al: Some biological effects of two crystalline prostaglandin factors. *Acta Physiol Scand* 1959; 45:133–144.
18. Bergstrom S, Sjovall J: The isolation of prostaglandin E from sheep prostate glands. *Acta Chem Scand* 1960; 14:1701–1705.
19. Ambache N, Kavanagh L, Whiting J: Effect of mechanical stimulation on rabbits' eyes: Re-

lease of active substance in anterior chamber perfusates. *J Physiol (Lond)* 1965; 176:378–408.

20. Allgower M, Cueni LB, Stadtler K, et al: Burn toxin in mouse skin. *J Trauma* 1973; 13:95.
21. Anggard E:. *Proceedings of the Fourth International Congress on Pharmacology*, vol 4. Basel, Schwabe and Co Publishers, 1970.
22. Anggard E, Arturson G, Jonsson CE: Effect of prostaglandins in lymph from scalded tissues. *Acta Physiol Scand* 1979; 80:46–51.
23. Arturson G: Arachidonic acid metabolism and prostaglandin activity following burn injury, in Ninneman J (ed): *Traumatic Injury: Infection and Other Immunologic Sequelae*. Baltimore, University Park Press, 1983, pp 55–78.
24. Nobel GHS, Robson MC, Krizek TJ: Dermal ischemia in the burn wound. *J Surg Res* 1977; 23:117–125.
25. Carr J: The anti-inflammatory action of heparin: Heparin as an antagonist to histamine, bradykinin and prostaglandin E_1. *Thromb Res* 1979; 16:507–516.
26. Jonsson CE, Granström E, Hamberg M: Prostaglandins and thromboxanes in burn injury in man. *Scand J Plast Reconstr Surg* 1979; 13:45–47.
27. Heggers JP, Ko J, Robson MC, et al: Evaluation of burn blister fluid. *Plast Reconstr Surg* 1980; 65:798–804.
28. Heggers JP, Loy GL, Robson MC, et al: Histological demonstration of prostaglandins and thromboxanes in burned tissue. *J Surg Res* 1980; 28:110–117.
29. Heggers JP, Robson MC: Prostaglandins and thromboxanes, in Ninnemann J (ed): *Traumatic Injury: Infection and Other Immunologic Sequelae*. Baltimore, University Park Press, 1983, pp 79–102.
30. DelBeccaro EJ, Robson MC, Heggers JP, et al: The use of specific thromboxane inhibitors to preserve the dermal microcirculatiön after burning. *Surgery* 1980; 87:137–141.
31. Robson MC, DelBeccaro EJ, Heggers JP, et al: Increasing dermal perfusion after burning by increasing thromboxane production. *J Trauma* 1980; 20:722–725.

4 / Chemical Burns in Children

HAROLD R. MANCUSI-UNGARO, JR., M.D.

Chemical burns and chemical injuries create a particular threat to children. Chemical burns not only constitute a special threat to limb but pose an added danger to life because of the potential for systemic toxicity. Such toxicity is amplified by the relatively low body weight and ease with which a large expanse of body area can be exposed to toxic chemicals in a child. The danger is further augmented by the ubiquity of toxic substances in the modern household. Pediatricians and other medical professionals who deal with children and parents on a regular basis need to be aware of the potential hazards as much to prevent such injuries as to treat them once such tragedies occur.

Burns are classified into four major categories according to mechanism of injury. The first and foremost category includes the thermal burns, i.e., flame burns, contact burns, and scald burns, including scalds from contact with molten metals and minerals, and hot liquid chemicals. Electrical injuries provide a different mechanism of injury but essentially constitute a thermal burn as the electrical injury is transformed into heat. Similarly, radiation burns are produced by absorption and transformation from a different part of the electromagnetic spectrum. In short, thermal, electrical, and radiation burns denature the skin and underlying tissues through the absorption of energy.

Chemical burns are different. While the skin becomes denatured, the process occurs through chemical disruption and alteration of physical properties. Additional considerations regarding the mechanism of injury add to the uniqueness. In particular, the potential for local and systemic toxicity must be addressed when chemical burns are treated.

Because the injury process is different, chemical injuries carry with them an increased morbidity and mortality. In the United States, 2 million people are burned each year, and 8,000 people die. Meanwhile, 60,000 chemical injuries occur that lead to 3,000 deaths. Although the latter mortality figures reflect not only cutaneous but also ingestion injuries, the two forms of injury often accompany each other. In any case, while chemical burns account for only 3% of the burns, chemical injuries produce a comparably greater mortality.

The potential for exposure to dangerous chemicals is ubiquitous (Table 4–1). Noxious agents exist throughout the home as well as in the workplace. Strong alkalies and acids are used in the home for cleansing. The hydroxides and carbonates or caustic sodas of sodium, potassium, ammonium, lithium, barium, and calcium can be found in anything from oven cleaners to drain cleaners and paint removers. Both sodium hydroxide and sodium carbonate are included in the reagents of a common urine testing kit (Clinitest) for diabetics. Another corrosive, lime, is a common soil additive spread on lawns and collected in many garden sheds. Even cement acts as a caustic when left in contact with the skin.

Acids contribute to the action of many household products. Hydrochloric acid is the most active ingredient in many bathroom cleansers, while oxalic acid is a common rust

TABLE 4–1.
Sources of Exposure to Harsh Chemicals in the Home (With Selected Common Examples by Brand Name)

MECHANISM OF INJURY				
CORROSION	DEHYDRATION	OXIDATION	DENATURATION	VESICATION
Lye/Caustic soda	Sulfuric acid	Hypochlorite	Hydrofluoric acid	Gasoline
Drain cleaner (Drāno,	Drain cleaner	Swimming pool	Rust remover	Fuel
Liquid Plumr)	(Instant Power)	chlorinator	(Quaker House)	Solvent
Oven cleaner	Hydrochloric acid	(Burn Out)	Carburetor/metal cleaner	Dimethysulfoxide
(Easy-Off)	(muriatic acid)	Mildew remover (X-14)	(Continental Con-Coil)	(DMSO)
Paint remover	Swimming pool pH			Veterinary
(Red Devil)	Masonry cleaner			Anti–inflammatory
Diabetic urine test kit	Toilet bowl cleaner			Methyl bromide
(Clinitest)	(Lysol)			Soil sterilizer
Lime	Oxalic acid			Fumigant
Phenol	Rust remover (Zud)			insecticide
Disinfectant				
(1-Stroke)				

remover. Concentrated hydrochloric acid (muriatic acid) is the main compound used to decrease pH in home swimming pools; and concentrated sulfuric acid is the "industrial-strength" drain cleaner found in hardware stores. Hydrofluoric acid, a stronger acid yet, constitutes the main ingredient in a household rust remover and a common carburetor cleaner. In the workplace, the use of hydrofluoric acid requires the use of special protective garments, ranging from total neoprene suits to specially tested, flawless rubber gloves. Yet, in the home it may be used without simple rubber gloves or eye protectors.

Burns can be produced by chemicals other than acids and alkalies. While household bleach contains dilute hypochlorite, this oxidizing agent is another chemical found in concentrated form for use in the home swimming pool. Similarly, phenols appear in varying concentrations in a variety of disinfectants. Finally, hydrocarbons in the form of gasoline pose a danger, and not simply from flammability; prolonged contact with gasoline produces a chemical burn.

FIRST AID

Primary Therapy: Stop the Process

The primary therapy for all burns is "stop the process." In fires, the adage is "stop, drop, and roll." In chemical burns, stopping the process can be both complex and time-consuming because of the mechanism of injury.

The severity of a chemical injury depends on five factors: (1) chemical strength of the agent, (2) quantity of the agent, (3) manner and duration of skin contact, i.e., progression, (4) penetration, and (5) mechanism of action.

Although the distinction is not always obvious, chemical agents can be divided into five categories based on mechanism of action and/or effect: (1) corrosion, (2) dehydration, (3) oxidation, (4) denaturation, and (5) vesication. Household burns generally involve corrosives or dehydrating chemicals. Corrosives produce protein denaturation with erosion and ulceration. Such agents included lye, phenol, white phosphorous, and dichromates. Dehydration comes about when strong acids, such as sulfuric acid and hydrochloric acid, rob the tissues of water. Oxidizing agents include chromic acid, hypochlorite, and potassium permanganate; the process of oxidation of the skin involves chemicals rather than fire. In denaturation, new chemical bonds are set up, thus fixing or stabilizing the tissues; the action of tannic acid in tanning offers a prime example. Finally, vesicants produce blisters by liberating tissue amines. Exposure to such agents is not common, although gasoline and dimethyl sulfoxide (DMSO) fall into this category. The less common vesicants include the halogenated hydrocarbons, cantharides, and military gases.

Whatever the chemical agent, first aid consists of removing saturated clothing from the victim and irrigating the wound with massive amounts of water. The water can be running, or it can be in a large tank. The volume of water dissipates the heat generated by dilution of the agent. Water irrigation constitutes immediate first aid and should continue at the scene for 20 to 30 minutes and thereafter for 2 to 12 hours. Up to 48 hours of continuous irrigation may be necessary for burns involving the eye (Figs 4–1 through 4–3). In short, no agent has been found superior to water. Irrigation should be continued for up to 6 hours for acids and for the longer periods for alkalies. The extended period of irrigation for alkalies is necessitated by the bonding of alkalies to tissue proteins. A general rule of thumb includes irrigation until the patient himself notices a decrease in pain, burning, or stinging. Measurement of skin surface pH is also often helpful. While prolonged irrigation is therapeutic, it is less helpful when copious irrigation is not instituted within the first hour following the injury.

Although each case must be individualized and the potential for toxicity of each agent expeditiously investigated, chemical neutralization is not recommended since it produces

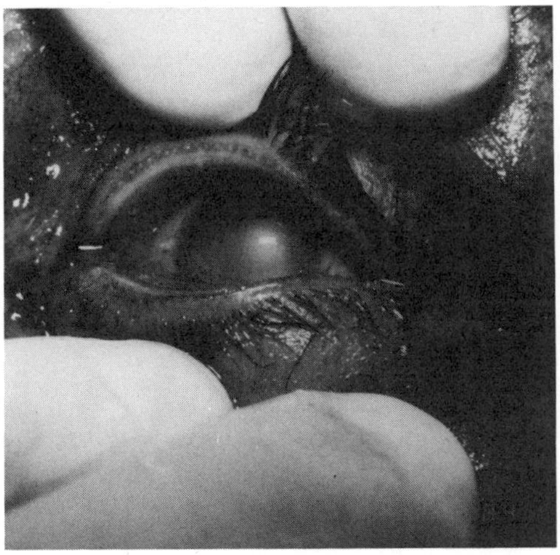

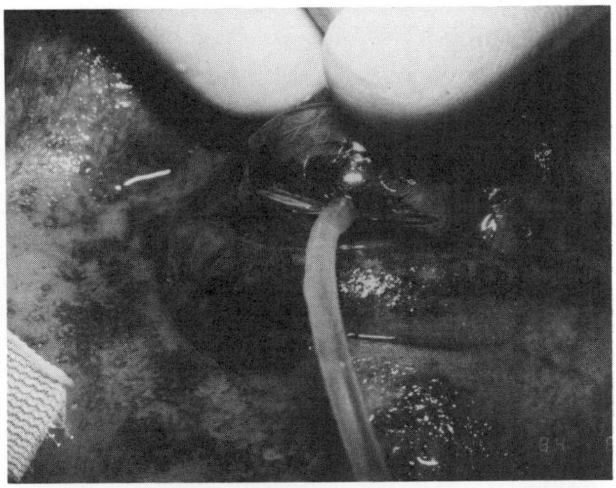

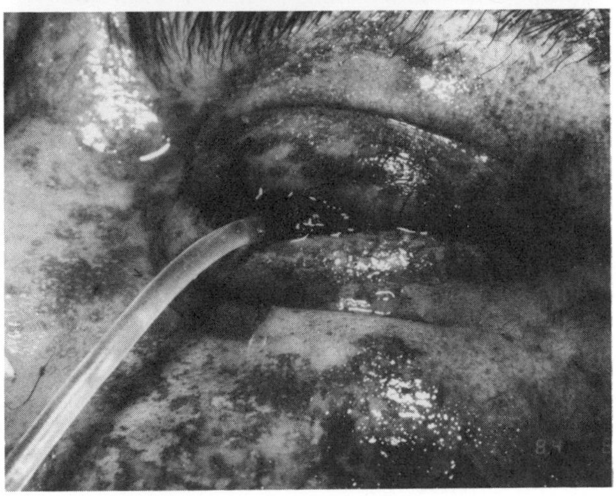

FIG 4–1 (above).
Alkali burn to the eye.
FIG 4–2 (above right).
Alkali burn to the eye. Placement of a Morgan lens under the eyelids and over the globe.
FIG 4–3 (right).
Alkali burn to the eye. Continuous irrigation is facilitated by placing a Morgan lens under the eyelids and over the globe.

heat and furthers tissue necrosis. The one exception to this rule is hydrofluoric acid.

Hydrofluoric acid is the strongest of the inorganic acids. It produces injury from the highly ionized acid moiety. Further injury comes about from penetration and binding of the fluoride ion (Figs 4–4 through 4–6). Within the soft tissues, the fluoride becomes insoluble only as calcium or magnesium fluoride. In short, it penetrates until it combines with the bone and/or systemic calcium and magnesium. Treatment, therefore, is aimed at precipitating the insoluble salts of calcium and magnesium, and occasionally ammonium. Immediate treatment, as with all burns, includes massive and copious irrigation with water for 20 to 30 minutes at the scene. Following this immediate period of irrigation, flushing the surface with aqueous benzalkonium (Zephiran), a quaternary ammonium compound, helps precipitate any residual fluoride and seems to reduce the stinging pain of the burn. Then, if available, a topical salve incorporating magnesium hydroxide and magnesium sulfate in a water-soluble base is applied during the time the victim is transferred to professional care. Professional care consists of assessing the size of and treating the injury. For burns involving less than 20% of the total body surface area, a solution of 10% calcium gluconate solution is injected directly into the burn and its immediate periphery at a dose of approximately 0.5 ml/sq cm. In addition, some authorities[9] have experimented with the 24-hour application of compresses moistened with a 50:50 dilution of calcium gluconate and DMSO. Such compresses do not, however, supplant the need for injection therapy with calcium gluconate.

One final note with regard to first aid: the rescuer should avoid injury to himself. When removing saturated clothing and hosing down the victim, remember that contact with the victim's clothing, the victim himself, or materials at the scene can make the rescuer a secondary victim. Furthermore, emergency room personnel should be reminded to wear gloves and/or protective clothing during their efforts to irrigate and resuscitate the victim.

Be Aware of Early Respiratory Complications

The early treatment of chemical burns, as with all injuries, begins with the ABCs, i.e., checking (A) airways, (B) breathing, and (C) circulation. Secure the airway as necessary, either with simple positioning, a mechanical airway, or endotracheal tube. If ventilation is required, be wary of mouth-to-mouth resuscitation; the rescuer should avoid injury to himself. Proceed with cardiopulmonary resuscitation (CPR) as necessary; but, again, the rescuer should avoid injury to himself caused by contact with the patient, his clothing, or the scene of the injury.

In addition to the usual reasons to be aware of the ABCs, chemical injuries can be particularly noxious to the cardiopulmonary system. A history of the injury at the scene should include the question of enclosed space, the mechanism of injury, and the nature of exposure. History should determine the risk of exposure to vapors of strong acids, ammonia, hypochlorite, or even cyanide gas. In addition, certain organic agents may produce an allergic response. Whatever the potentially offending agent, compromise of the upper airway may not be immediate. Rather, upper airway edema may ensue within 12 to 24 hours.

EXTENT AND DEGREE

The extent of injury of a chemical burn follows the total body surface area nomograms as with thermal injuries. However, the extent needs to be reassessed at frequent intervals during the initial period of treatment. The involved area may appear to increase if exposed areas are overlooked and omitted from irrigation. On the other hand, the estimate of the area involved may actually diminish in response to prolonged hydrotherapy. Indeed, hydrotherapy may influence the progression of the injury. It may determine whether an

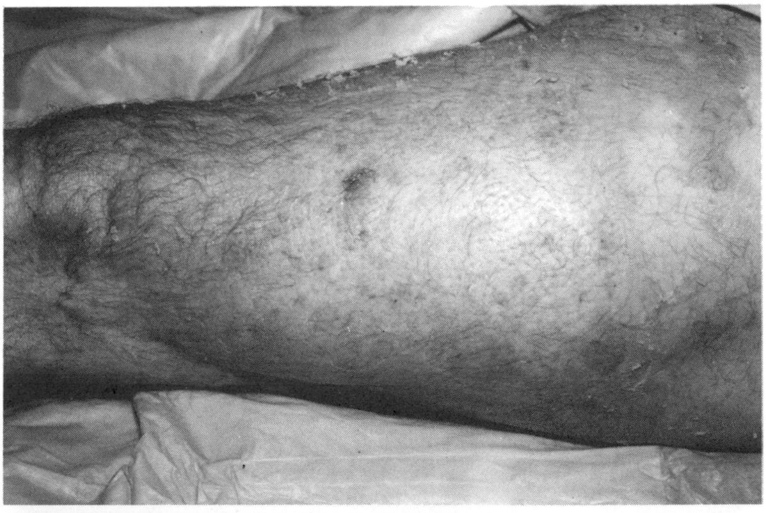

FIG 4–4
Hydrofluoric acid burn. Initial presentation.

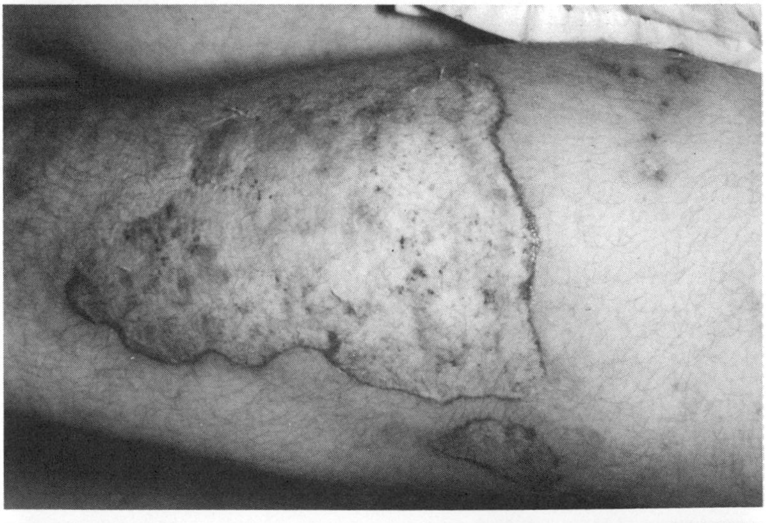

FIG 4–5
Hydrofluoric acid burn. Progression of injury at 48 hours (same patient as in Fig 4–4).

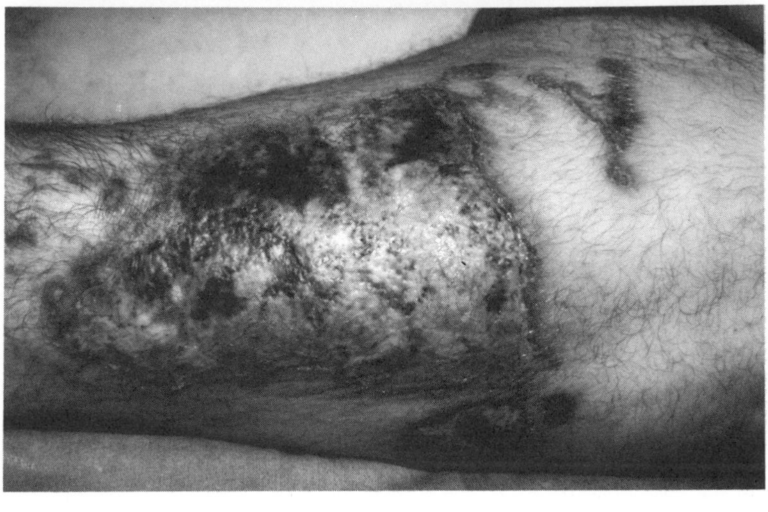

FIG 4–6
Hydrofluoric acid burn 1 week postinjury. The lesion has progressed despite appropriate treatment, including injection with calcium gluconate (same patient as in Figs 4–4 and 4–5).

affected area remains a first-degree burn or goes on to produce blistering and more severe denaturation.

As with thermal burns, severity of a chemical injury can be discussed in terms of degrees or depth of injury. However, initial appearances are often deceiving. A first-degree chemical burn appears reddened like sunburn. Similarly, second-degree or partial-thickness burns may appear blistered, pink, and moist (Fig 4–7). Likewise, a third-degree burn may seem dry and anesthetic. However, the mechanism of the injury may vary from self-limited penetration, as the chemical bonds and hardens the superficial skin, to one of progressive penetration and destruction. For instance, phenol tends to remain superficial, while nitric acid proceeds to obliterate the surface anatomy (Figs 4–8 and 4–9).

With thermal burns, one considers extent and degree as part of the criteria for admission to hospital. In the case of chemical injuries, a chemical burn is a special burn, the extent of which cannot be appreciated at the time of initial presentation. Therefore, chemical injuries, especially those to children, warrant admission to a hospital.

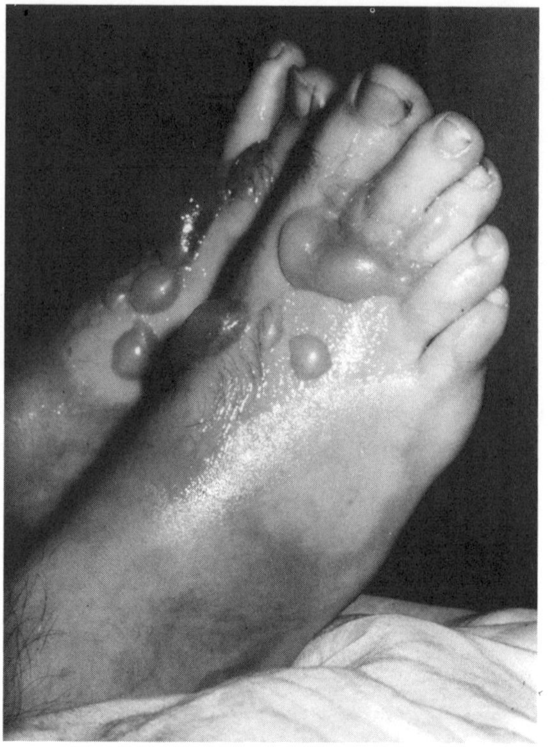

FIG 4–7.
Second-degree burn from methyl bromide appears blistered, pink, and moist. (From Jarowenko DG, Mancusi-Ungaro HR Jr: The care of burns from methyl bromide (case report). *J Burn Care Rehab* 1985; 6:119–123. Used by permission.)

EMERGENCY ROOM CARE

As with thermal injuries, chemical burns require reassessment in the emergency room. Such reassessment includes a detailed estimate of extent of involved body surface area and degree of severity. It also provides an opportunity to weigh the patient and reassess the requirements for fluid resuscitation. A detailed history must be taken and a physical examination performed. However, throughout this reassessment and resuscitation, the emergency room staff must not lose sight of the progressive nature of the injury and continue with copious irrigation. As stated before, throughout the emergency room procedures, the staff must avoid injury to themselves from any residual chemicals.

Time in the emergency room must also be spent looking for other injuries. Besides the obvious possibility of injuries secondary to related trauma, chemical burns have their own peculiar risks. For one, ingestion must be ruled out. Lye burns to the face require a physical examination, including the mouth. Any evidence of ingestion must also suggest the possibility of inhalation.

TOXICITY

Certain chemical burns carry a high probability of systemic toxicity or derangement of normal parameters. For example, hypocalcemia can result from significant absorption of oxalic and hydrofluoric acid. In the case of hy-

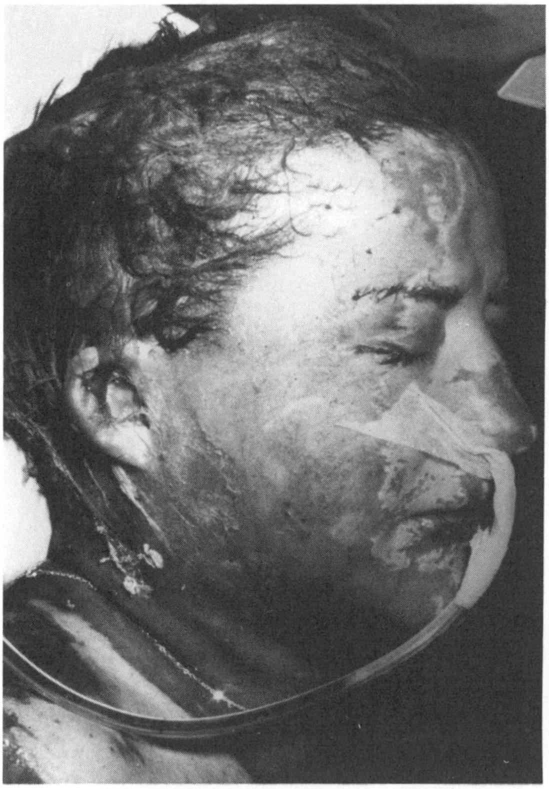

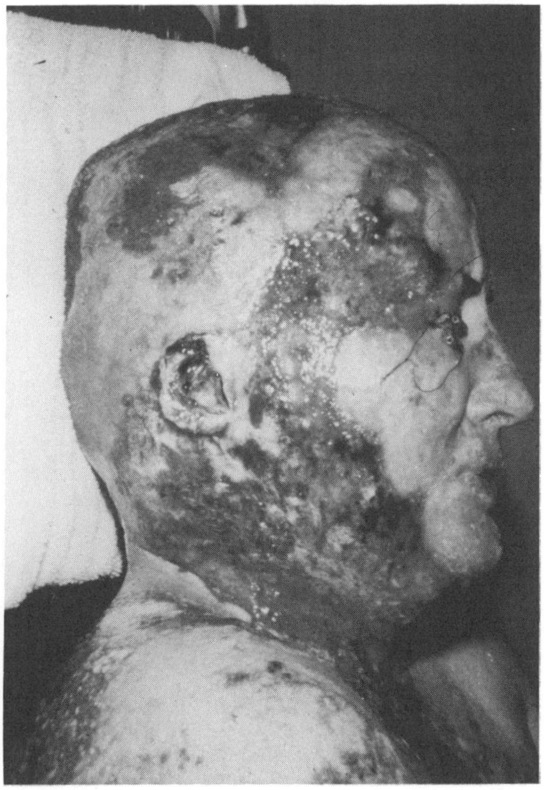

FIG 4–8 (left).
Third-degree nitric acid burn. Discolored skin at initial presentation.
FIG 4–9 (right).
Third-degree nitric acid burn. Discolored skin becomes a full-thickness loss with time.

drofluoric acid burns, the fluoride ion tends to bind serum calcium, but treatment with injectable calcium gluconate may shift the balance in the opposite direction. Methemoglobinemia and hemolysis occur from significant absorption of cresol.

The physician must bear in mind that absorption comes about not only through the skin but also through the inhalation of vapors. As ingestion should suggest the possibility of an inhalation injury, the inhalation of vapors is in fact a form of ingestion. More serious toxicity, such as hepatic necrosis and nephrotoxicity, results from the absorption of tannic acid, and to a lesser degree from chromic, formic, and picric acids, as well as metallic phosphorous.

GASOLINE

Gasoline burns require special attention and deserve special mention. Contact burns from gasoline tend to produce trivial-appearing, second-degree exfoliation (Fig 4–10). However, the absorption of gasoline through the skin can lead to multiple organ-system failure and death. The odor of gasoline on the breath following cutaneous absorption of the hydrocarbon is an ominous physical finding. Systemic toxicity progresses with upper airway obstruction within 6 hours. By 24 hours hepatic enzymes are elevated and urine output has dropped. Nephrotoxicity becomes progressive. The absorption of the hydrocarbon destroys not only the surfactants of the

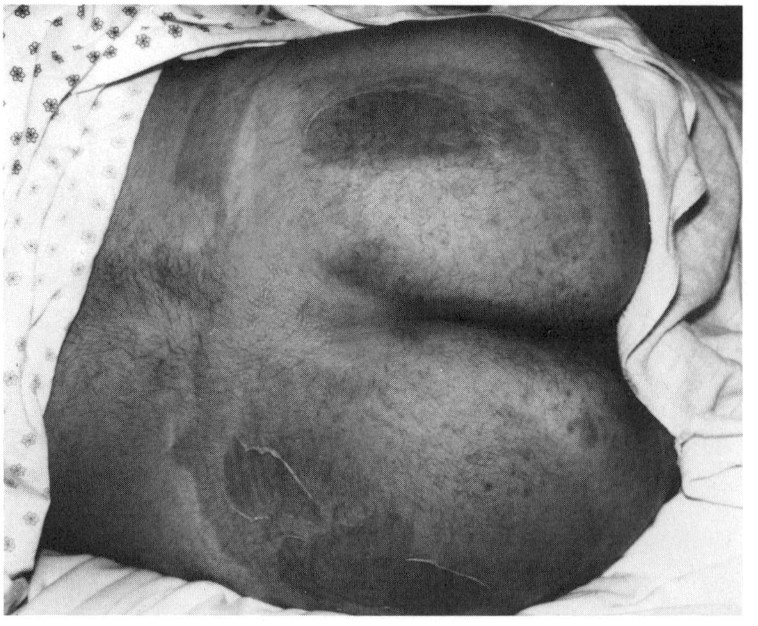

FIG 4–10.
Contact burn from gasoline produces a superficial, partial-thickness burn injury.

respiratory tract but continues to poison all membranes. Gastrointestinal (GI) disturbances, neurologic changes, and cardiomyopathy follow pulmonary, hepatic, and renal failure. Death usually ensues within a week.

In addition to the basic toxicity of the hydrocarbon itself, leaded gasoline carries the added toxicity of tetraethyl lead. Because the lead is organically bound, the serum levels are unreliable. Urine must be examined for toxic levels of lead. Levels of greater than 150 micrograms of lead in a 24-hour urine suggest severe lead toxicity. Treatment should include administration of either British antilewisite (BAL) or ethylenediaminetetraacetate (EDTA) for 5 days followed by a 10 to 14-day course of penicillamine.

Finally, gasoline burns carry the added danger of potential injury to the medical team. Avoid ignition accidents!

TAR AND MOLTEN MINERALS

In the category of special burns, tar burns present a direct contrast to gasoline burns. Molten tar or asphalt constitutes a simple scald burn. The material itself has no toxicity from absorption. Emergency care givers should cool the molten material with cold water taking care to avoid chilling the victim. Efforts to remove the hardened tar with vigorous cleansing only serve to avulse the interface between heat-damaged and heat-injured cells, thus deepening the burn. The material itself is not toxic and is relatively sterile. Hence, no vigor need be exerted to remove the substance. Rather, the wound should be gently cleansed with soap and water and then dressed with a petrolatum-based ointment. Triple antibiotic ointment (bacitracin-polymixin B-neomycin) is readily available in the hospital setting; it provides the necessary solvent combined with anti-infective agents. Dressings can then be changed at frequent intervals with gradual separation of the tar and often spontaneous healing of the burn. Once all of the tar is removed, the physician can reassess the need for any surgical treatment.

Most molten minerals including metals can be managed in a manner similar to tar burns. While the petrolatum will not dissolve the offending agent, it will with time provide an interface between the mineral and the skin, thus allowing spontaneous and atraumatic separation.

WOUND CARE

The depth of injury may not be apparent immediately after the accident. Once defined, second-degree or partial-thickness injuries can be allowed to heal by conservative methods. Large blisters should be debrided to remove any absorbed and dissolved chemical in the blister fluid. Removing blisters and dressing with a biologic membrane (such as Biobrane) often diminishes pain. Third-degree injuries should be allowed to demarcate and then be debrided and closed surgically. Appropriate topical antibacterials should be used as with a thermal injury.

RECOVERY AND REHABILITATION

The initial hospital course may require support of vital functions. During the period of healing and/or demarcation, vital functions should be maintained by appropriate physical therapy, splinting, and surgical intervention.

SUMMARY: OBSERVE THE DISTINCTION

As stated, chemical burns constitute a special burn. They are not self-limited but rather represent the possibility for progressive injury. Emergency care includes stopping the process by removing saturated clothing and irrigating with massive amounts of water. With the exception of burns from hydrogen fluoride or hydrofluoric acid, chemical burns need not be neutralized. In handling all victims of chemical injuries, avoid injury to the rescuer. Beyond emergency care and the progressive nature of the injury, chemical injuries carry the added danger of systemic toxicity. Accordingly, as with all trauma, begin with the ABCs. In due course, determine the degree of absorption through the skin, inhalation of toxic vapors, or ingestion of toxic substances. Chemical injuries in children require observation in the hospital by skilled personnel.

BIBLIOGRAPHY

1. Beesinger DE, Mancusi-Ungaro HR Jr: Dealing with hydrofluoric acid injuries. *Industrial Chemical News* 1983; 4:34.
2. Demling RH, Buerstatte WR, Perea A: Management of hot tar burns. *J Trauma* 1980; 20:242.
3. Gruber RP, Laub DR, Vistnes LM: The effect of hydrotherapy on the clinical course and pH of experimental cutaneous chemical burns. *Plast Reconstr Surg* 1974; 55:200–204.
4. Hunter GA: Chemical burns of the skin after contact with petrol. *Br J Plast Surg* 1968; 21:337–341.
5. Jarowenko DG, Mancusi-Ungaro HR Jr: The care of burns from methyl bromide (case report). *J Burn Care Rehabil* 1985; 6:119–123.
6. Jelenko C III: Chemicals that "burn." *J Trauma* 1974; 14:65–72.
7. Mancusi-Ungaro HR Jr, Blackwell SJ: The care of burns from molten sulfur: Presentation of a burn to the right hand. *J Burn Care Rehabil* 1983; 4:280–281.
8. Proctor NH, Hughes JP: *Chemical Hazards of the Workplace*. Philadelphia, JB Lippincott, Co, 1978.
9. Reus W, Zachary LS, Gottlieb J, Heggers JP, et al: Treatment of experimental hydrofluoric acid burns. Proceedings of the 16th Annual Meeting of the American Burn Association, San Francisco, 1984, pp 149–150.
10. Shewmake SW, Anderson BG: Hydrofluoric acid burns: A report of a case and review of the literature. *Arch Dermatol* 1979; 115:593–596.
11. Simpson LA, Cruse CW: Gasoline immersion injury. *Plast Reconstr Surg* 1981; 67:54–57.
12. Tepperman PB: Fatality due to acute systemic fluoride poisoning following a hydrofluoric acid skin burn. *J Occup Med* 1980; 22:691–692.

5 / Chemical Burns of the Esophagus and Stomach in Children

GERALD T. ZWIREN, M.D.

Chemical burns of the esophagus and stomach in children are usually the result of accidental ingestion of a strong alkali such as lye or the ingestion of an acid, mainly hydrochloric acid or sulfuric acid. Children under 5 years are the most frequent victims; an estimated 5,000 children ingest lye products every year.[1] Approximately 10% to 20% will have severe burns resulting in stricture.[2] The incidence of acid ingestion is lower, probably because strong acids are used less around the house. Lye causes damage by liquefaction necrosis, which may progress transmurally. Contact of a strong alkali with the esophagus for 10 seconds may produce severe damage to the esophageal wall.[2] Strong acids such as hydrochloric acid or sulfuric acid cause a coagulation necrosis, which forms an eschar, which may limit further damage. Lye usually burns the esophagus, and acid burns the stomach, but this is not an invariable rule.[4, 5]

CAUSTIC BURNS

The critical factor in strong alkali ingestion is the amount of the alkali, i.e., whether it is liquid or solid, the volume, the concentration, and the pH. Liquid lye is particularly dangerous, and a single agent, Liquid PlumR, introduced around 1967, reportedly accounted for 17% of the lye injuries in children.[1] The concentrations of sodium hydroxide in these products vary from 30.5% (Liquid PlumR) to 98% (granular Drāno).[1] Clinitest tablets are another concentrated source of lye that produces severe burns when swallowed.[2, 6] The critical pH is 12.5. The various pH values are listed in Table 5–1. Government laws, such as the Federal Hazardous Substance Act of 1970, reduced the percentage of sodium hydroxide allowed in lye products to less than 10%, but this concentration is still severely destructive, particularly in liquid form. Even 0.5% sodium hydroxide can produce a stricture.[7] Many of the lye products are available at the neighborhood grocery store. Unfortunately, laws requiring labeling and packaging standards do not prevent the transfer of lye products to a soft drink bottle, and the label warnings are of no value to preschool children.

Pathophysiology

Lye or strong alkalies produce damage to the oropharynx, larynx, esophagus, and mediastinum by liquefaction necrosis. A tracheoesophageal fistula and gastric perforation with peritonitis may occur. Haller[2] described the stages of a burn. The first stage, lasting 1 to 4 days, consisted of acute necrosis and cellular death with an inflammatory response. The second stage, the 5th through 14th day, consisted of ulceration and granulation along with neovascularization and fibroblast proliferation with collagen deposition. In the last stage, the 15th through the 90th day, stricture formation and cicatrization followed when collagen contraction occurred, adhesions developed and scarring took place, and the epithelium was replaced. The scar contracts for months (Ta-

TABLE 5–1.
pH and Viscosity of Commercial Compounds Compared to Laboratory Solutions*

COMPOUND	pH (METER)	pH (PAPER)	VISCOSITY
Water	7.0	7.0	1.24
Basic H	3.5	4.0	1.54
Ammonia	12.5	12.0	1.28
Liquid PlumR	14.0	12.0	1.54
Bleach	11.4	11.0	1.43
Zep Drain Aid	14.0	12.0	5.09
Drain Kleen	14.0	12.0	4.36
Liquid Drāno	14.0	12.0	2.17
Drain Mate	8.2	6.0	1.15
Zepomatic	11.6	12.0	1.47
Zep laundry compound	12.6	12.0	2.07
30% NaOH	14.0	12.0	6.24
10% Ammonia	12.5	12.0	1.28
28% Ammonia	13.0	12.0	1.036

*From Vancura EM, Clinton JE, Ruiz E, et al: Toxicity of alkaline solutions. *Ann Emerg Med* 1980; 9:118–122. Used by permission.

ble 5–2). Much of the information on lye burns of the esophagus is from animal experiments. Butler et al.[8] instilled 20% sodium hydroxide in a segment of dog esophagus for 60 seconds. He noted varying degrees of injury, but stricture occurred in the deep third-degree burns only. Bosher et al.[9] noted that in dogs the bacterial invasion was not a decisive factor in the pathogenesis of stricture. According to Haller, et al.[4], the cat esophagus most closely compares with the human esophagus, particularly that of a child.

Clinical Presentation

The clinical presentation varies with the severity and site of the lye burn. Oral and pharyngeal burns are associated with drooling, blister formation, and pain. Laryngeal burns may be accompanied by dyspnea, which may be severe enough for a tracheostomy. Esophageal burns may cause dysphagia. Gastric damage from perforation may result in a shock-like picture. Damage to the thoracic esophagus with perforation and tracheoesophageal fistula may produce respiratory symptoms and shock. The presence or absence of oral burns is no indication that esophageal burns are present. Between 25% and 50% of patients with oral burns will have esophageal injuries,[10] but 10% to 15% of patients with no oral burns will have esophageal burns.[2]

TABLE 5–2.
Progressive Pathogenesis of Esophageal Lye Burn Injuries

STAGE	WEEK	PATHOGENESIS
1	1	Liquefaction necrosis and inflammation
2	2	Granulation and fibroblast proliferation
3	3	Fibrous replacement and replacement of squamous cell lining; stricture

Diagnosis

The history of ingestion of a strong alkali with or without clinical presentation should be sufficient to warrant early esophagoscopy. This should be done within 24 hours of the burn injury to establish the presence and severity of lye injury. A rigid or flexible esophagoscope can be used. The main advantage of a flexible scope is that the entire esophagus is more easily and possibly more safely evaluated.[11] Some have advocated esophagoscopy only to the point of visible burns, thereby lessening the chance of perforation. Barium studies of the acute burn do not provide additional important information except as a baseline. The acute burns of the esophagus fall into three categories: First-degree, characterized by hyperemia, edema, and superficial erosion; second-degree, characterized by erythema, blister formation, and superficial ulceration with fibrinous exudate; and third-degree, characterized by deep ulceration, loss of epithelium, and evidence of granulation tissue.[10]

Treatment

The use of emetics is to be avoided since violent emesis may cause esophageal damage. Dilution therapy is probably of no value since the damage is produced within 10 to 15 seconds. Similarly, dilute acids are of no known value. The airway should be assessed initially as damage to the airway may be the most life-threatening event. Severe compromise of the airway from epiglottic or laryngeal edema may require a tracheotomy. A gastrostomy is indicated if oral intake is not possible and for later use in dilatation as will be discussed. Intravenous fluids should be started to provide volume support in the event of hypotension and for administering antibiotics and steroids. A shock-like state may indicate perforation of a viscus. If a burn is established at esophagoscopy, then the steroids and antibiotics should be started. If there is a delay in the esophagoscopy, then the steroids and antibiotics should be administered prior to the procedure, since steroids have little antifibroblastic effect 48 hours after ingestion.[12] This is not a universally accepted therapy, and some feel that first-degree burns do not need therapy; the therapy is inconclusive in second-degree burns, and third-degree burns will not be changed at all.[13] The evidence in favor of the use of steroids for their antifibroblastic effect and antibiotics for the prevention of bacterial invasion is based on experimental and clinical evidence, which is not overwhelmingly conclusive. Rosenberg et al.,[14] Haller et al.,[4, 15] Weisskopf[16] and others[17] have not shown clear clinical or experimental evidence of their value. In a review[6] of 270 patients with lye burns, 53% (66 of 124) of the untreated patients and 24% (34 of 140) of those patients treated with steroids and antibiotics developed strictures. Until studies on comparable data are available, the early use of steroids and antibiotics is indicated. The Salzer method[2, 18] of early repeated daily dilatations have few advocates.[13] Bosher,[9] in dog experiments, concluded that early dilatations were harmful to the healing process. The steroids and antibiotics should be continued for at least 4 weeks, and a barium (Ba) swallow should follow to evaluate the presence of strictures. Symptomatic strictures are an indication for dilatation. Many methods of dilatation exist either antegrade, using bougies or by balloon catheter under fluoroscopic guidance,[19] or retrograde via the gastrostomy, using Tucker dilators or other instruments. Retrograde dilatation, however, requires the placement of a string down the esophagus. We prefer to insert the string at esophagoscopy, placing a filiform and follower through the scope and advancing the filiform into the stomach. The filiform tip is retrieved through the gastrostomy opening, a string is tied to it, and the string is withdrawn through the mouth. The string can then be internalized by the method of Tepas and Golladay.[20] Retrograde dilatations can later be done using the Tucker dilators, which are much safer than the antegrade dilators. The antegrade dilators are more likely to perforate the esophagus because of the maze-like strictures caused by the lye burns. In children, we perform the dilatation under general anesthesia to lessen the fright and avoid the pain of these procedures. Figure 5–1 is a flow chart of the treatment of a lye burn.

In certain severe lye burns with full-thickness injury and extension of the lye burn to

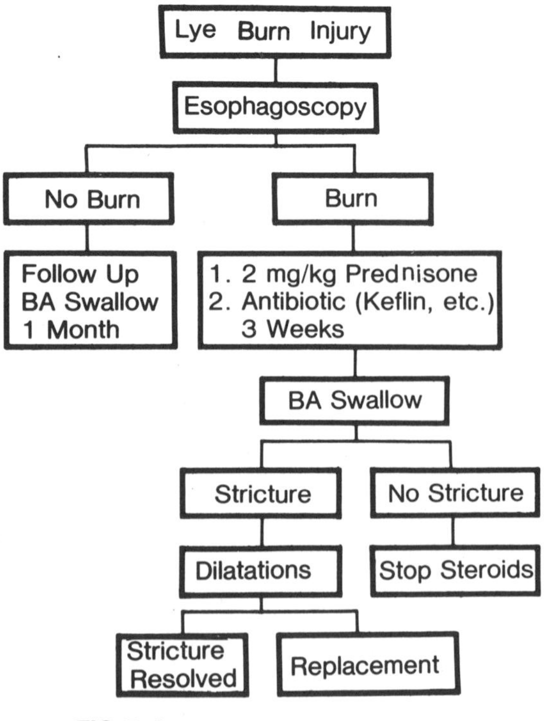

FIG 5–1.
Schema of treatment for a lye burn.

the mediastium, a thoracotomy may be indicated for drainage and diversion procedures. If a tracheoesophageal fistula is present then an upper esophagostomy, isolation of the fistula within a tube of esophagus, oversewing of the distal esophagus, and a gastrostomy should be done according to the method of Burrington and Raffensperger.[21] They reported the fistula closed spontaneously in most instances but that esophageal replacement was needed at a later date.

Dilatation for a diagnosed stricture of the esophagus should be based on the symptoms in the child. Dysphagia, emesis, and excessive salivation are all indications for esophagoscopy and dilatation. Foreign material and food impacted at the stricture may cause sudden worsening of symptoms and require esophagoscopic removal and subsequent dilatation. The success of dilatation in resolving strictures of the esophagus is variable and unpredictable; some resolve after repeated dilatations, and others remain refractory. In our experience, deep third-degree burns usually result in strictures that eventually require replacement therapy. Discontinuance of the dilatation is based on repeated recurrence of symptoms after frequent dilatations, with little or no progress in the caliber of the esophagus. A serious perforation is another indication for replacement. If the child's frequent hospitalizations and dilatations interfere with his or her life-style, school, or work, then replacement should be considered.

Alternative methods of treating the stricture of the esophagus include direct steroid injections,[22] intraluminal stents,[23] and the use of a lathyrogen called β-aminopropionitrile (BAPN), which has been shown experimentally to decrease the tensile strength of collagen fibrils in established strictures. The use of BAPN described by Madden et al.,[24] is experimental, and clinical trials are not yet available.

Esophageal Replacement

The colon is the main organ used for replacement of the esophagus. The right colon with a terminal segment of ileum is ideally suited for replacement, but the left colon is equally as good and preferred by some surgeons. The colon, however, is considered a conduit and does not have intrinsic peristalsis when used for replacement. In three cases of lye burn strictures in children, we have used the right colon to replace the entire esophagus up to the hypopharynx with eventual good results. The complications of colon interposition include anastomotic leakage, 25% redundancy with occasional aspirations, bleeding peptic ulcer of the colon, anastomotic stricture, and intestinal obstruction.[25] Occasionally necrosis of the colon from vascular occlusion occurs. The reported mortality in colon replacement for benign diseases is approximately 5%.[25] Other organs used are the jejunum, a gastric tube, a vascularized patch of colon, and a free graft of jejunum with microvascular anastomosis, particularly in cervical strictures.[6] Primary resection of a narrow stricture is used, but frequently the damage involves too long a segment for adequate normal margins to be anastomosed.

Removal of the damaged esophagus following replacement is advised by some authors, mainly because of the increased incidence of carcinoma in a diseased esophagus. Tucker and Yarington[26] cited the increase as 1,000-fold or between 2% to 5% over a 20-year period. They cited a 15-year-old boy who later developed cancer following a lye burn injury of the esophagus of 12 years' duration.

ACID BURNS OF THE ESOPHAGUS AND STOMACH

The accidental ingestion of strong acids is relatively rare in children. Thirty-four adult patients with gastric injuries from acid ingestion were reported from 1960 to 1969 by Maull et al.[27] The ingestion of a toilet cleanser containing hydrochloric acid and scattered reports of mineral acid ingestion, such as nitric and sulfuric acids, have been noted.[28] Acids are supposed to lick the esophagus and burn the stomach. While this is generally true, severe damage from acid burns has affected the esophagus. Clinically significant esophageal injury occurs in 6% to 20% of cases of acid ingestion.[27] The rapid passage of the acid and the supposed resistance of the esophageal mucosal epithelium have been cited as factors in the sparing of the esophagus. The stomach is the main organ injured by acid ingestion.

Pathophysiology

Acids produce coagulation necrosis. This necrosis forms an eschar, which limits further damage. In contrast, the liquefaction necrosis produced by a strong alkali progresses transmurally. As with alkali burns, the form of the acid, i.e., liquid or solid; ph; the concentration; the amount; and duration of contact are important factors in the extent of the injury. A full stomach at the time of the injury and the spasm of the pylorus from the burn tend to produce damage to the pyloric area, while acid in an empty stomach produces damage to the body of the stomach. Dilution of concentrated sulfuric acid with an equivalent amount of water results in temperature elevations to 80°C.[27] Neutralization results in even greater heat production.[27] This heat could be a significant factor in causing damage if these treatment modalities were used.

Acid burns are classified in the same way as alkaline burns, namely superficial, deep, and transmural. Superficial burns or first-degree burns are characterized by superficial mucosal hyperemia, edema, and superficial sloughing. Deep or second-degree burns involve transmural damage, and third degree-burns extend beyond the wall and involve paraesophageal tissues such as the mediastinum and pleural and peritoneal cavities.[5] Because of the sloughing, a perforation is more likely to occur, and septic shock and death may follow these events. If the burn does not result in perforation, scarring from the necrosis may result in antral or pyloric cicatrization, and a linitis plastica picture or a pyloric stricture may result. Necrosis of the entire stomach and portions of the esophagus have been reported.[29, 30]

Clinical Presentation

Oral or pharyngeal tissue injuries may be present. Respiratory symptoms from laryngeal or tracheal injury and edema may occur. Hematemesis, midepigastric abdominal pain, and a rigid abdomen from peritonitis may occur. In severe cases, septic shock, renal failure, and death may result. A late complication is the stricture formation, which then produces gastric outlet obstructive symptoms such as early satiety, bloating, and vomiting.

Radiographic Findings

Muhletaler et al.[31] described the esophageal radiographic findings in strong acid ingestion. He studied a group of Peruvian patients who ingested 27% muriatic acid in suicide attempts. He described three phases. In the first phase, mucosal and submucosal edema, atony, and dilatation occurred. Three of this group of patients underwent emergency laparotomy due to the presence of free air or emphysematous gastritis. In the second phase, 10 to 16 days postinjury, an esophagram showed narrowing and mucosal ulcerations with submucosal edema and atony. In the chronic phase, 20 to 30 days after ingestion of the acid, esophageal stenosis was seen in almost all of these patients. Significant dilatation of the esophagus in the acute phase is considered similar to the toxic dilation of the colon. They conclude that severe esophageal injury can occur with acid ingestion. A simple x-ray may show air in the mediastinum or evidence of aspiration. An abdominal x-ray must be obtained to see if free air, which would signify a perforated viscus, is present.

Treatment

No standardized method of treatment of acid ingestion exists, partly due to the lack of experimental information and the low incidence of clinical cases of this condition. Penner,[28] in an excellent review, stated that the acids do not produce their entire injury instantaneously as alkalies do, and therefore therapy should be directed toward preventing additional injury. Emetics may produce increased contact time by the regurgitation of acid and are therefore contraindicated. He also states that injury may occur as long as 90 minutes after ingestion. Dilution and neutralization therapy may cause significant and potentially injurious heat production and is contraindicated. Nasogastric suction and removal of the acid is a rational approach. Antacids are recommended, but their effect is not documented, nor is the therapeutic effect of steroids and antibiotics well documented. Steroids may decrease the protective effect of inflammation, increasing the danger of perforation, and therefore may be contraindicated. Surgical intervention with resection of the damaged viscus may be wise in selected instances in which the damage is overwhelming or the dissolution of tissue appears imminent. Respiratory compromise is treated by intubation or tracheostomy, depending on the severity of the damage to the larynx or trachea. Long-term parenteral nutrition is a valuable adjunctive measure.

Localized strictures involving the antrum or pylorus are treated by partial gastrectomy with a Billroth I procedure. With gastroenterostomy the damaged portion is retained, which may result in bleeding from the inflamed mucosa. Also, the gastroenterostomy may result in stomal bleeding, a common complication. Massive resection of the stomach has been done with jejunum or colon replacement.[30, 32]

REFERENCES

1. Leape LL, Ashcraft KW, Scarpelli DG, et al: Hazard to health—liquid lye. *N Engl J Med* 1971; 284:578–581.
2. Haller JA Jr: Corrosive strictures of the esophagus, in Ravitch M, Welch KJ, Benson CD, et al (eds): *Pediatric Surgery,* ed 3. Chicago, Year Book Medical Publishers, 1979, pp 473–475.
3. Borja AR, Ransdell HT Jr, Thomas TV, et al: Lye injuries of the esophagus: Analysis of ninety cases of lye ingestion. *J Thorac Cardiovasc Surg* 1969; 57:533–538.
4. Haller JA Jr, Andrews HG, White JJ, et al: Pathophysiology and management of acute corrosive burns of the esophagus: Results of treatment in 285 children. *J Pediatr Surg* 1972; 6:578–583.
5. Goldman LP, Weigert MD: Corrosive substance ingestion: A review. *Am J Gastroenterol* 1984; 79:85–90.
6. Zwiren GT, Andrews HG, Hester TR Jr: Progress in treating lye burn injuries of the esophagus in children, in Brooks BF (ed): *The Injured Child.* Austin, University of Texas Press, 1985, pp 113–125.
7. Vancura EM, Clinton JE, Ruiz E, et al: Toxicity of alkaline solutions. *Ann Emerg Med* 1980; 9:118–122.
8. Butler C II, et al: Morphologic aspects of experimental esophageal lye strictures: I. Pathogenesis and pathophysiologic correlations. *J Surg Res* 1984; 17:232–244.
9. Bosher LH Jr, Burford TH, Ackerman L: The pathology of experimentally produced lye burns and strictures of the esophagus. *J Thorac Surg* 1951; 21:483–489.
10. Rosenow EC III, Bernatz PE: Chemical burns of the esophagus, in Payne WS, Olsen AM (eds): *The Esophagus.* Philadelphia, Lea and Febiger, 1974, pp 139–146.
11. Sugawa C, Mullins RJ, Lucas CE, et al: The value of early endoscopy following caustic ingestion. *Surg Gynecol Obstet* 1981; 153:553–556.
12. Tewfik TL, Schloss MD: Ingestion of lye and other corrosive agents—a study of 86 infant and child cases. *J Otolaryngol* 1980; 9:72–77.
13. Webb WR, Koutras P, Ecker RR, et al: An evaluation of steroids and antibiotics in caustic burns of the esophagus. *Ann Thorac Surg* 1970; 9:95–102.
14. Rosenberg N, Kunderman PJ, Vroman L, et al: Prevention of experimental esophageal stricture by cortisone; control of suppurative complications by penicillin. *Arch Surg* 1953; 66:593–598.
15. Haller JA Jr, Bachman K: The comparative effect of current therapy on experimental caustic burns of the esophagus. *Pediatrics* 1964; 34:236–245.
16. Weisskopf A: Effects of cortisone on experimental lye burn of the esophagus. *Ann Otol Rhinol Laryngol* 1952; 61:681–689.
17. Reyes HM, Lin CY, Schlunk FF, et al: Experimental treatment of corrosive esophageal burns. *J Pediatr Surg* 1974; 9:317–327.
18. Oakes DM, Sherck JP, Mark JBD: Lye ingestion: Clinical patterns and therapeutic implications. *J Thorac Cardiovasc Surg* 1982; 83:194–204.
19. Ball WS, Strife JL, Rosenkrantz J, et al: Esophageal strictures in children: Treatment

by ballon dilatation. *Radiology* 1984; 150:263–264.

20. Tepas JJ III, Golladay ES: An improved method for retaining retrieval line in children undergoing repeated esophageal dilatation. *J Pediatr Surg* 1978; 13:371.
21. Burrington JD, Raffensperger JG: Surgical management of tracheoesophageal fistula complicating caustic ingestion. *Surgery* 1978; 84:329–334.
22. Holder TM, Ashcraft KW, Leape LL: The treatment of patients with esophageal strictures by local steroid injections. *J Pediatr Surg* 1969; 4:646–653.
23. Mills LJ, Estrera AS, Platt MR: Avoidance of esophageal stricture following severe caustic burns by the use of an intraluminal stent. *Ann Thorac Surg* 1979; 28:60–65.
24. Madden JW, Davis WM, Butler C: Experimental esophageal lye burns. II. Correcting established strictures with beta-amino propionitrile and bougienage. *Ann Surg* 1973; 178:277–284.
25. Postelthwait RW: Colonic interposition for esophageal substitution. *Surg Gynecol Obstet* 1983; 156:377–383.
26. Tucker JA, Yarington CT: The treatment of caustic ingestion. *Otolaryngol Clin North Am* 1979; 12:343–349.
27. Maull KI, Scher LA, Greenfield LJ: Surgical implications of acid ingestion. *Surg Gynecol Obstet* 1979; 148:895–898.
28. Penner GE: Acid ingestion: Toxicology and treatment. *Ann Emerg Med* 1980; 9:374–379.
29. Berry WB, Hall RA, Jordan GL: Necrosis of the entire stomach secondary to ingestion of a corrosive acid: Report of a patient successfully treated by total gastrectomy. *Am J Surg* 1965; 109:652–655.
30. Canti T: Personal communication, 1985.
31. Muhletaler CA, Gerlock AJ Jr, de Soto L, et al: Acid corrosive esophagitis: Radiographic findings. *AJR* 1980; 134:1137–1140.
32. Chong GC, Beahrs OH, Payne WS: Management of corrosive gastritis due to ingested acid. *Mayo Clin Proc* 1974; 49:861–865.

SECTION III

ACUTE CARE

6 / Controversies in Fluid Resuscitation and Their Impact on Pediatric Populations

HUGO F. CARVAJAL, M.D.

Fluid therapy remains a major controversial issue in the field of burn medicine. Lack of agreement exists not only in regard to the quantity and composition of the fluids to administer, but also in regard to the choice and significance of the guidelines used to monitor the patient's state of hydration. All three areas of controversy are intimately linked to one another; thus, even though the issue regarding the quantity of fluids is critical to burn resuscitation, the amount of fluid infused is dependent on the composition of the hydrating solution and ultimately on the guidelines that are used to assess the effectiveness and end point of therapy.

QUANTITY OF FLUIDS: THE BURN FORMULA

Several formulas designed to aid the physician in estimating the quantity of fluid required by burn victims have been proposed (Table 6–1). These have been reviewed in detail by Davis.[35] The estimates of some of the early formulas were based on the weight of the patient, the total serum protein level, or the hematocrit.[15, 42, 43, 60, 73] In the early writings, the extent of the burn was felt to be important, but it was not consistently taken into consideration until 1947, when Cope and Moore[33] popularized the surface area formula and proposed that fluids be given in relation to the size of the burn. These investigators also proposed the current rate of fluid administration that advocates one half of the total estimates to be given during the first 8 hours and the other half during the subsequent 16 hours. Their method allowed 75 ml of plasma and 75 ml of crystalloid for every 1% of body surface burned, plus maintenance fluids, which for an average-sized adult amounted to approximately 2,000 ml/24 hours. According to Davis,[35] some of the first few patients treated with this program were fluid-overloaded; thus a limit equivalent to 10% to 12% of the body weight in liters (one half of the extracellular fluid space) was subsequently introduced as the maximum 24-hour-fluid allowance.

The Evans formula, derived from some of the human studies of Cope and Moore[33] as well as from experimental animal studies, was developed in 1952. Evans et al.[44] recommended equal amounts of colloid (plasma) and crystalloid for a total fluid intake for the first 24 hours postinjury of 2 ml/kg/% of body surface area (BSA) burned plus 2,000 ml to replace normal fluid losses (average adult). The authors further recommended that a ceiling for burn size (50% of body surface) be used.

The Brooke formula developed by Reiss et al.[98] agreed with the estimates of the Evans formula in regard to the volume of fluid but decreased the amount of colloid allowed by one half. Maintenance fluid allowance (water or 5% dextrose in water), and ceilings for

TABLE 6–1.
Formulas to Estimate Fluid Requirements in Burned Patients

AUTHOR	FORMULA TO ESTIMATE FLUID NEEDS	HYDRATING SOLUTION	RATE OF FLUID ADMINISTRATION AND SPECIAL INSTRUCTIONS
Cope and Moore (1947)	150 ml/% BSA* *burned*/24 hr + "maintenance fluids"	1/2 plasma and 1/2 crystalloid, 5% dextrose in water	Half during first 8 hr and half during subsequent 16 hr; ceiling: 10%–12% of body weight in liters
Evans et al. (1952)	2 ml/kg/% BSA *burned*/24 hr + 2,000 ml/24 hr (maintenance fluids)	1/2 plasma and 1/2 crystalloid, 5% dextrose in water	Half during first 8 hr and half during subsequent 16 hr; ceiling: 50% burn
Gelin (1952)	<30% burn = 2 ml/kg/% BSA *burned*/48 hr† 30%–60% burn = 2.5 ml/kg/% BSA *burned*/48 hr† >60% burn = 3 ml/kg/% BSA *burned*/48 hr†	Dextran (low molecular weight)	
Reiss et al. (1953)	2 ml/kg/% BSA *burned*/24 hr + 2,000 ml/24 hr (maintenance fluids)	1/4 plasma and 3/4 crystalloid, 5% dextrose in water	Half during first 8 hr and half during subsequent 16 hr; ceiling: 50% burn
Eagle (1956)	30 ml/% BSA *burned*/48 hr + 10% of body weight in kg/48 hr + 4,000 ml/sq m BSA/48 hr	Dextrose 5% 0.66 N saline containing 20 gm of human serum albumin per liter	Ceiling: 50% burn; burns <15% do not administer the fluid equivalent to 10% of the body weight
Batchelor et al. (1961)	Mean (children) 3 ml/kg/% BSA *burned*/24 hr† Range (children) 1–5 ml/kg/% BSA *burned*/24 hr†	Plasma and blood only	Too wide a variation to rely on a single figure formula
Welch (1962)	A. 1.5 ml/kg/% BSA *burned*/24 hr + B. 1 ml/kg/% BSA *burned*/24 hr + C. 1,500 ml/sq m BSA	a. Plasma b. Normal saline c. Dextrose 5% in water	Rate: 1/3 first 8 hr, 1/3 second 16 hr, 1/3 second day
Baxter and Shires (1968)	4 ml/kg/% BSA *burned*/24 hr†	Crystalloids only (isotonic salt solutions)	Half during first 8 hr and half during subsequent 16 hr; no ceiling
Carvajal (1975)	5,000 ml/sq m BSA *burned*/24 hr + 2,000 ml/sq m *total* body surface/24 hr	Dextrose 5% lactated Ringer's solution containing 12.5 gm of human serum albumin per liter	Half during first 8 hr and half during subsequent 16 hr; no ceiling
Pruitt (1979)	3 ml/kg/% BSA *burned*/24 hr†	Crystalloids only (Isotonic salt solutions)	Half during first 8 hr and half during subsequent 16 hr; no ceiling
Bowser and Caldwell (1983)	2 ml/kg/% BSA *burned*/24 hr	Hypertonic lactated saline	Ceiling: 50% burn

*BSA indicates body surface area
†Total fluid intake—no separate allowance for maintenance fluids.

burn size remained identical to those proposed by Evans et al.[44]

The formulas of Cope and Moore,[33] Evans et al.,[44] and Reiss et al.[98] are the original prototypes of what we have termed "two-figure formulas." This term refers to the estimation of burn-related losses separately from maintenance fluid requirements (two independent formulas). This manipulation offered a safeguard for the very small or very extensive burns, a safeguard not afforded by "single-figure formulas" such as the one proposed by Gelin[51] in 1952. According to Gelin, who used dextran exclusively as the hydrating solution, patients with burns of less than 30% of the BSA required 2 ml/kg/% of BSA burned; those with moderate-sized burns (30% to 60% of BSA) required 2.5 ml/kg/% of BSA burned; and those with severe burns (>60%) needed 3 ml/kg/% of body surface burned during the entire period of early fluid resuscitation (first 48 hours).

Up to this point, fluid resuscitation programs had been designed for the adult burn victim with "proportionately smaller quantities" recommended for children. In 1956, Eagle[39] for the first time proposed a complicated formula for hydration of burned children. This initial effort used a combination of BSA in square meters, weight, and percent of BSA burned to arrive at fluid estimates for burn-related losses (edema and evaporative losses) and maintenance fluid requirements.[39, 40] In 1961, Batchelor et al.[10] emphasized the need to consider the size of the patient and the extent of the burn for rehydration of burned children. Though these investigators used only plasma and blood for resuscitation, they noted that when expressed in relation to weight and percent of BSA burned, the amount of plasma required by pediatric burn patients varied widely (1 to 5 ml/kg/% of BSA burned). They pointed out that while fluid intake for their patients averaged 3 ml/kg/% of BSA burned, adherence to such a figure was not recommended for burned children due to the wide variation encountered.[10]

In 1961, Metcoff et al.[80] reported data on four burned children subjected to detailed fluid and electrolyte balance studies. Using a modification of the Evans formula, these investigators observed that oliguria persisted for 12 hours (9 to 10 ml/sq m of body surface per hour) despite "adequate resuscitation" and suggested "an excess of antidiuretic hormone" as a possible explanation for their findings. They stressed the need to consider BSA in estimating fluid requirements and attributed some of the edema to excessive sodium administration.

The large surface area to weight ratio of children in comparison to adults was emphasized by Haynes[62] in 1965. Recognizing that the Evans formula was not optimal for hydration of burned children, and to minimize errors in fluid therapy, Haynes advocated continuous bedside monitoring of the patient and frequent hematocrit determinations.[62, 66] For the lack of a better estimate, this investigator also recommended adherence to the 50% burn ceiling.

Single figure formulas such as the Parkland formula[13] or the modified Brooke formula[96] have received increased attention in recent years and have enjoyed worldwide popularity. However, in pediatric patients these formulas are often inaccurate, and major modifications of the initial resuscitation plan are often necessary.[66, 94] The modified Brooke and Parkland programs recommend the administration of lactated Ringer's solution in quantities of 3 and 4 ml/kg/% BSA burned for the first 24 hours postinjury, respectively. One half of the estimate is given during the first 8 hours and the other half during the subsequent 16 hours. According to these programs, protein replacement is not begun until the fourth 8 hour period (second day).

One of the problems with formulas that make no separate allowances for maintenance fluid requirements and burn-related losses (edema and evaporation) stems from the fact that in children maintenance fluid requirements are not directly proportional to the weight of the patient. Hence, different formulas would need to be developed for patients of different ages and sizes. Estimation of burn-related losses (edema and evaporation) on the basis of body weight may also be inaccurate because the losses are primarily related to the extent of tissue injury and not to the patient's weight.[23, 33, 39, 80] Let us assume, for example, that we are dealing with a 1-year old, 10-kg child who has suffered a 15% scald burn (see Table 6–1). Average maintenance fluid requirements for a child this size should be approximately 800 ml/24 hours,[47, 111] but the burn would obviously increase his 24-hour fluid needs beyond that level. However, for this hypothetical case the Parkland formula would only recommend 4 ml/kg/% of BSA burned per 24 hours, or 4 × 10 × 15 = 600 ml/24 hours. A 600 ml/24 hour–allowance is obviously inadequate, as it does not even meet daily maintenance fluid requirements. The same child with burns of 30%, 45%, 60%, 75%, and 90% of his body surface would receive, according to the Parkland formula, progressively greater but not necessarily more accurate quantities of fluid (Table 6–2). If the normal average fluid requirements for children are subtracted from the first 24-hour fluid estimates, as calculated by the Parkland formula, the volume of fluid allotted to replace burn-related losses would vary between −200 to 2,800 ml, depending on the size of the burn (see Table 6–2). Thus, according to the estimates depicted in Table 6–2, doubling the burn size from 30% to 60% of BSA would increase the fluid allowances for replacement of burn-related losses by fourfold (400 to 1,600 ml), while doubling the burn size from 45% to 90% of BSA would only increase the fluid allowance by less than threefold (1,000 to 2,800 ml). The same estimates in a 4-year-old or a 12-year-old child would also result in significantly different proportions. When the amount of fluid allowed for burn-related losses is expressed in relation to the surface area burned, the inaccuracies of single-figure formulas become evident; the fluid estimates in relation to the burned area (in square meters) become increasingly higher as the weight of the patient or the size of the burn increases (Fig 6–1). Thus, unless single figure formulas are corrected for age and burn size, they tend to underhydrate the small child or the child with small burns and overhydrate the older child with extensive injuries. Since the proponents of these formulas advocate that no ceiling for burn size be used, and since a leaky vascular bed can lead to accumulation of large quantities of fluid in the interstitium, significant hydration errors can go unrecognized. While this criticism also applies to other fluid formulas that base their estimates on weight, the errors are minimized by estimating burn-related losses and maintenance fluid requirements separately.[66,94] Further refinements can be achieved by relating fluid needs to the surface area burned in square meters (% burn × body surface area) and estimating maintenance fluid requirements in relation to total body surface area.[23] According to this program, which uses a composite burn solution, total fluid requirements for the first 24 hours postburn can be calculated on the basis of 5,000 ml/sq m of body surface burned per 24 hours (burn-related losses), plus 2,000 ml/sq m of total body surface per 24 hours (maintenance fluid requirements). This approach has been recommended because most of the edema fluid accumulates in the injured skin,[19] and evaporative fluid losses are proportional to the surface area burned.[74] The use of two separate figures to calculate burn-related fluid losses and maintenance fluid requirements makes the surface area formula suitable for burns of all sizes and assures that all burn patients regardless of age receive fluids in proportion to the size of their injury. Figure 6–1 shows that while the ratio of total fluid estimate to maintenance fluid requirements increases in proportion to the size of the injury, with the surface area formula the increments are equivalent for all age groups but vary widely with the Parkland formula. With the surface area formula a child with a 60% surface area burn will be estimated to require a volume of fluids for the first 24 hours postinjury equiva-

TABLE 6–2.
Comparison Between First Twenty-Four Hour Fluid Estimates (Parkland Formula) and Average Maintenance Requirements in Burned Children and Adults

AGE, WEIGHT, AND TOTAL BODY SURFACE	BSA* BURNED, %	PARKLAND FORMULA FLUID ESTIMATE (4 ml/kg/% burn/24 hr)	AVERAGE MAINTENANCE FLUID REQUIREMENTS, ML†	ALLOWANCE FOR BURN-RELATED LOSSES		
				QUANTITY	% OF MAINTENANCE	ML/SQ M BSA BURNED
1 yr, 10 kg, 0.46 sq m	15	600	800	−200	−25	−2,780
	30	1,200		400	50	2,780
	45	1,800		1,000	125	4,630
	60	2,400		1,600	200	5,550
	75	3,000		2,200	275	6,110
	90	3,600		2,800	350	6,480
4 yr, 16.5 kg, 0.68 sq m	15	990	1,200	−210	−18	−2,060
	30	1,980		780	65	3,820
	45	2,970		1,770	148	5,780
	60	3,900		2,760	223	6,760
	75	4,950		3,750	312	7,350
	90	5,940		4,940	412	8,070
12 yr, 40 kg, 1.3 sq m	15	2,400	2,250	150	6	770
	30	4,800		2,550	113	6,540
	45	7,200		4,950	215	8,460
	60	9,600		7,350	326	9,420
	75	12,000		9,750	433	10,000
	90	14,400		11,750	522	10,040
20 yr, 70 kg, 1.86 sq m	15	4,200	3,250	950	29	3,405
	30	8,400		5,150	158	9,229
	45	12,600		9,350	288	11,170
	60	16,800		13,550	417	12,142
	75	21,000		17,750	546	12,714
	90	25,200		21,950	675	13,112

*BSA indicates body surface area.
†Calculated on the basis of 1,750 ml/sq m of body surface per day.

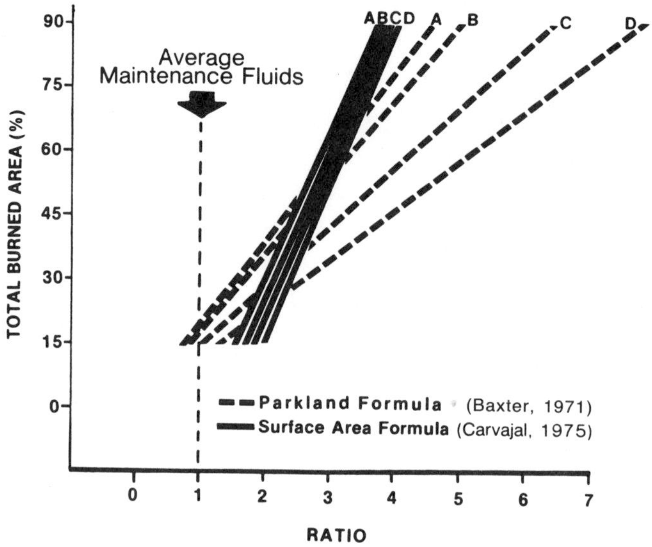

FIG 6–1.
Relationship between total fluid estimate (first 24 hours postburn) and recommended maintenance fluid allowance in burned children. Notice that while the ratio of total fluid estimates to maintenance fluid requirements increases as the size of the burn increases, the relationship between these two variables remains constant for all ages with the surface area formula, but varies widely with the Parkland formula (A = 1-year-old burn patient, B = 4-year-old, C = 12-year-old, D = 20-year-old).

lent to three times his average maintenance fluid requirements (300% of maintenance) regardless of age. Baxter and Shires,[13] on the other hand, would estimate progressively larger proportions as the child gets older (200% for a 1-year-old child, up to 417% for a 20-year-old adult).

COMPOSITION OF THE HYDRATING SOLUTION

The basic issues regarding the composition of the hydrating fluids are whether hypertonic or isotonic salt solutions should be used for burn resuscitation and whether or not colloids need to be added to the various mixtures. The studies in humans by Monafo,[82] Caldwell and Bowser,[20] and Jelenko et al.,[67, 68] as well as the experimental animal work of Fox et al.[48, 50] and Markley et al.,[77] suggest that when hypertonic salt mixtures are used, the total quantity of fluid can be curtailed and edema can be minimized. Although on the surface such an approach seems plausible, concern exists regarding the occurrence of undesirable side effects such as hypernatremia and hyperosmolality, which (particularly in children) can lead to intracellular dehydration,[71] cerebral hemorrhage,[46] hyperosmolar coma, and inhibition of lipolysis.[41]

The addition of plasma or albumin to resuscitation fluids has been recommended by many investigators,[26, 39, 44, 64, 65, 68, 75, 98, 108] but it has also been criticized on the assumption that the burn-induced increase in vascular permeability and the consequent extravasation of proteins persist for up to 36 hours postinjury.[12, 76, 77, 86, 87] The main concern is that protein administration during the first 24 hours may increase protein accumulation in the interstitium and thus trap water. In 1948 Cope and co-workers[32] found that following a burn injury, the capillary membrane allowed the passage of albumin (molecular weight, 69,000) into the interstitium. This and other studies[99] confirmed the original work of Underhill et al.,[115] Field et al.,[45] Blalock,[16a] and provided the basis for much of the controversy regarding colloid vs. crystalloid fluid resuscitation.

During the last decade the validity of these original investigations has been questioned[19, 29, 30] since evidence contradicts the earlier findings. Using radioactive isotopes (iodine 131[^{131}I]) and autoradiographic techniques to demonstrate albumin extravasation in burned animals, Brouhard et al.[19] were able to duplicate the findings of Cope et al.[32] (Fig 6–2), but also demonstrated that when the radioactive tracer was administered intravenously at different times after the burn (0, 2.5, 5.5, 11.5, 17.5, 23.5, 35.5, and 47.5 hours after the injury) and the animals were killed by decapitation exactly 30 minutes later, a completely different pattern for albumin extravasation was noted (Fig 6–3). These data suggested that effective transcapillary sieving of albumin molecules into burned skin (second-degree burns) essentially stops (in the rat) at approximately 8 hours postinjury, but that a significant portion of the albumin that leaks prior to this time remains extravascular for at least 48 hours. An alternative though less likely explanation for the findings would be that a balance between albumin extravasation and extraction of albumin from the interstitium via lymphatics occurs at 8 hours postinjury. In a subsequent investigation, Carvajal et al.[30] further documented their previous observations, but this time with more extensive burns in a scald burn model that required fluid resuscitation (Fig 6–4). This study also demonstrated that edema of injured tissues was maximal at 3 hours postburn and persisted beyond 24 hours postinjury (Figs 6–5, 6–6). In contrast to the burned tissues neither albumin extravasation nor water accumulation was observed in unburned tissues.[30] Other studies designed to determine the effect of burn depth on vascu-

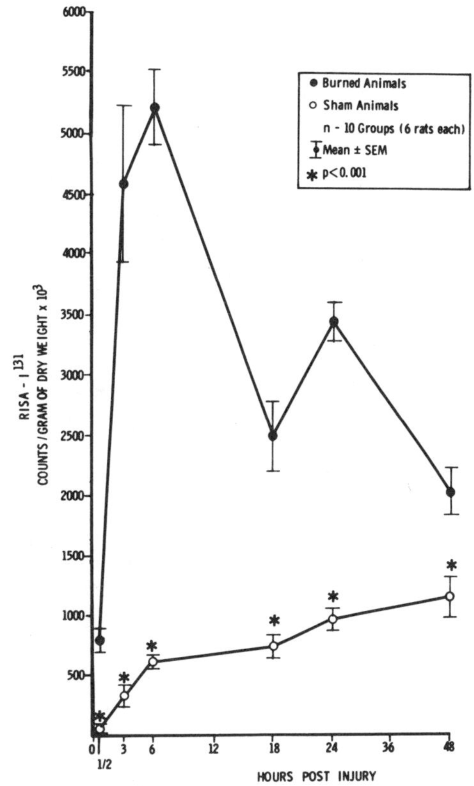

FIG 6–2.
Cumulative levels of radio-iodinated serum albumin (RISA-^{131}I) (counts per minute per gram of dry tissue) in skin from burned and control animals. In each instance RISA-^{131}I was administered immediately after the burn. (From Brouhard BH, Carvajal HF, Linares HA: Burn edema and protein leakage in the rat: I. Relationship to time of injury. *Microvasc Res* 1978; 15:221–228. Used by permission.)

lar permeability[29] revealed almost identical findings and only a minimal effect of burn depth upon microvascular sieving of albumin molecules (Fig 6–7). These studies also demonstrated that burn edema occurred rapidly and was of similar severity for superficial as well as deep burns (Fig 6–8). While extrapolation from rats to humans may not be possible, data from 30 pediatric burn patients with burns of 20% to 92% of their body surface[30] indicate that when albumin is added to resuscitation fluids (12.5 gm/L) from the onset of resuscitation, the serum albumin levels are

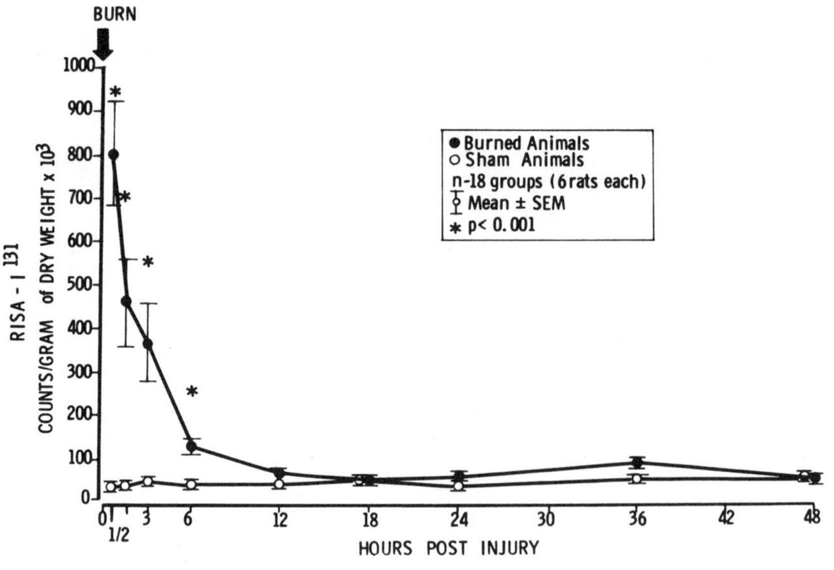

FIG 6–3.
RISA-^{131}I (in counts per minute per gram of dry tissue) in skin from burned and control animals, 30 minutes after injection (30 minutes to 48 hours after a burn). (From Brouhard BH, Carvajal HF, Linares HA: Burn edema and protein leakage in the rat: I. Relationship to time of injury. *Microvasc Res* 1978; 15:221–228. Used by permission.)

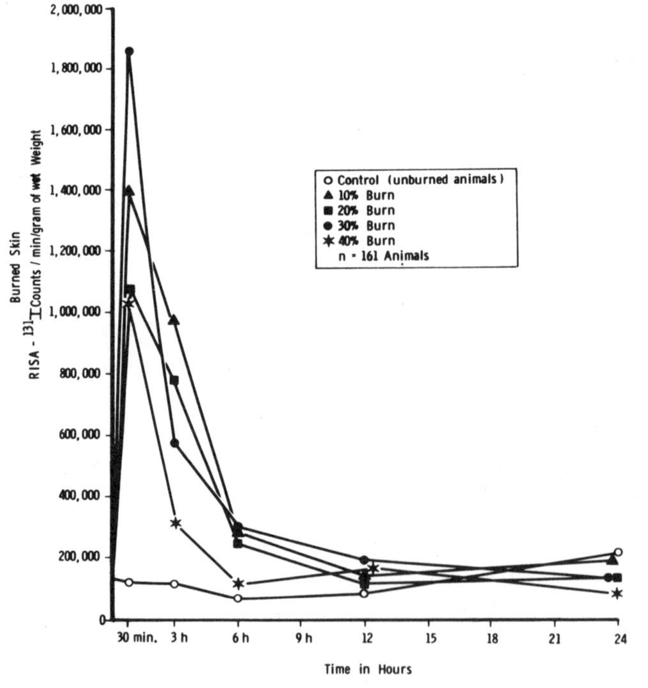

FIG 6–4.
Composite graph comparing RISA-^{131}I counts (albumin leakage) in skin from unburned rats and burned skin from rats subjected to 10%, 20%, 30%, and 40% partial-thickness scald burns. By 12 hours postinjury, no differences between the rats in the experimental and control groups can be demonstrated, $P > .01$. (From Carvajal HF, Linares HA, Brouhard BH: Relationship of burn size to vascular permeability changes in rats. *Surg Gynecol Obstet* 1979; 149:193–202. Used by permission.)

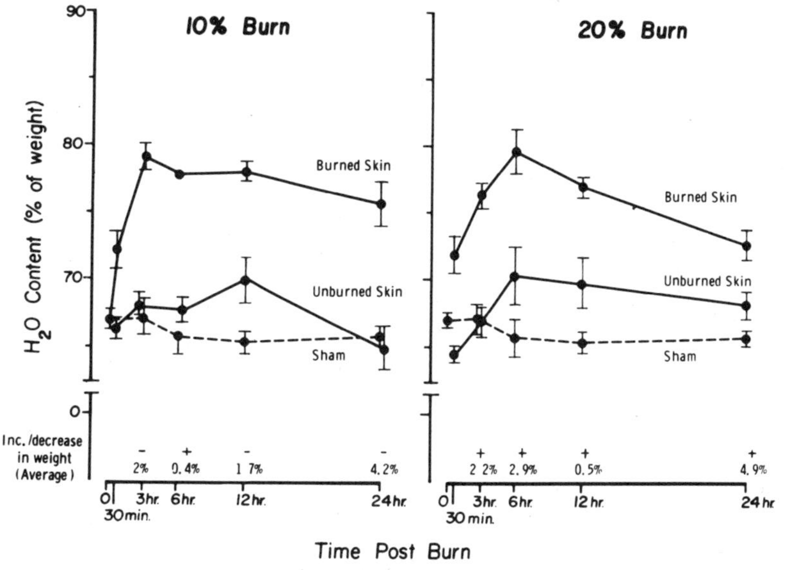

FIG 6–5.
Water (H_2O) content expressed as percent of weight of burned and unburned skin from burned (10% and 20% of BSA burned) and control (sham) animals. The weight of the animals expressed as percent change from control is also shown on the graphs. (From Carvajal HF, Linares HA, Brouhard BH: Relationship of burn size to vascular permeability changes in rats. *Surg Gynecol Obstet* 1979; 149:193–202. Used by permission.)

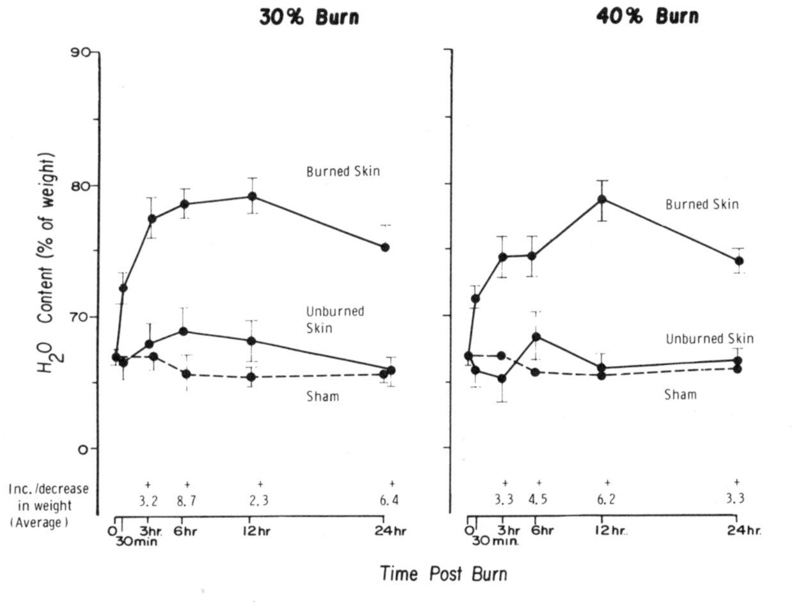

FIG 6–6.
Water (H_2O) content expressed as percent of weight of burned and unburned skin from burned (30% and 40% of BSA burned) and control (sham) animals. The weight of the animals expressed as percent change from control is also shown on the graphs. (From Carvajal HF, Linares HA, Brouhard BH: Relationship of burn size to vascular permeability changes in rats. *Surg Gynecol Obstet* 1979; 149:193–202. Used by permission.)

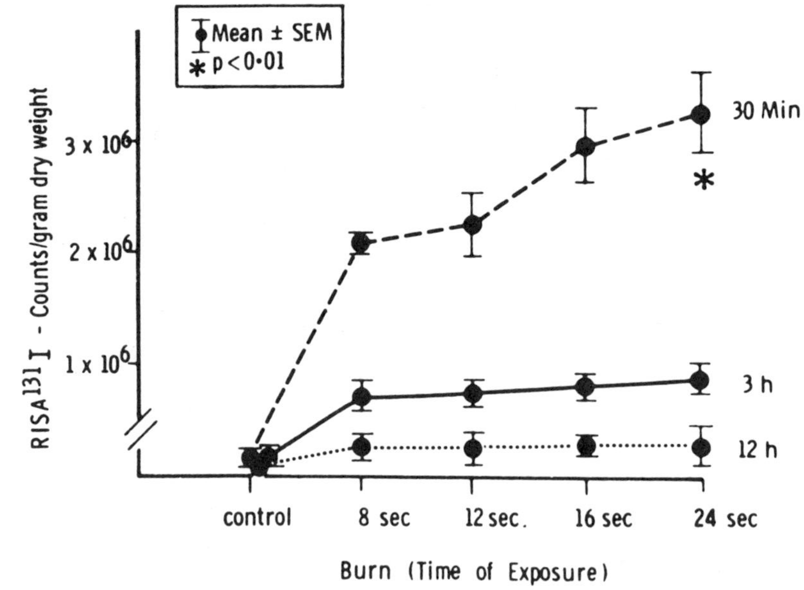

FIG 6–7.

RISA-131I extravasation of control (unburned) skin and burned skin of different depths, at 30 minutes, 3 hours, and 12 hours postinjury. Notice that at 30 minutes after injury, the 24 second-burn resulted in significantly higher RISA-131I counts than the burns of lesser severity. RISA-131I leakage was no longer demonstrable by 12 hours postinjury. (From Carvajal HF, Linares HA: Effect of burn depth upon edema formation and albumin extravasation in rats. *Burns* 1980; 7(2):79–83. Used by permission.)

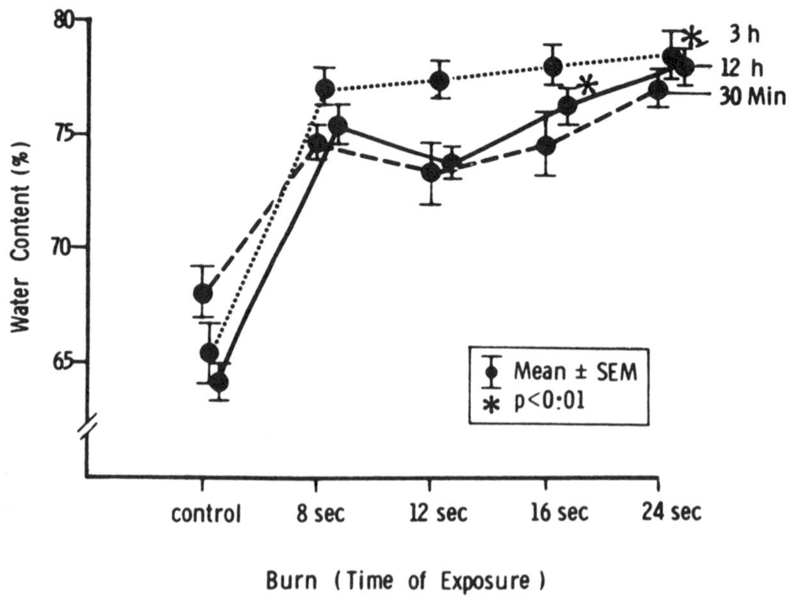

FIG 6–8.

Water content (percent) of control (unburned) skin and burned skin of different depths at 30 minutes, 3 hours, and 12 hours postinjury. Notice that at 12 hours after injury the 16- and 24-seconds burns resulted in a higher skin water content than the 12- and 8-seconds burns. (From Carvajal HF, Linares HA: Effect of burn depth upon edema formation and albumin extravasation in rats. *Burns* 1980; 7(2):79–83. Used by permission.)

maintained within the normal range (Fig 6–9), edema is curtailed, and the clinical condition of the patient is much improved. Although these studies did not quantitate albumin in the extravascular space, they suggested that at least some of the exogenous albumin remained intravascular (otherwise, albumin levels would have been markedly decreased). These studies also showed that the portion of albumin that leaked and presumably remained trapped in the tissues did not markedly affect edema formation (Fig 6–10). Thus, if the phenomenon of increased vascular permeability is indeed transient and of therapeutic significance for only the first 6 hours after the burn, withholding albumin or plasma beyond this point would not only lack experimental support, but could be detrimental to the patient. Holleman et al.[65] have shown that when plasma proteins are not replaced, the colloid osmotic pressure of plasma decreases, fluid escapes the intravascular space, and hypovolemia as well as peripheral edema develop.

A decrease in microvascular integrity may not be the only mechanism responsible for volume shifts.[38, 56] Capillary endothelial cell gaps and other electron microscopy findings can be demonstrated within minutes of the injury, but their role in the formation of edema is unclear. Hypoproteinemia leads to a reduction in colloidosmotic pressure, and indirectly (through depletion of interstitial protein stores) it may also result in an increased fluid conductivity.[38] These and any other changes mediated by histamine, serotonin, leukotrienes, prostaglandins, or oxygen radicals could lead to efflux of fluid from the intravascular compartment and the development of edema, but the latter may or may not be related to extravasation of proteins. In other words, it is conceivable that while coexisting, during the first few hours after the injury, protein extravasation and interstitial edema may be independent of one another. If, as reported by Baxter in 1974,[10a] the disturbance in the cell membrane manifested by decreased transmembrane potentials and decreased adenosinetriphosphatase is secondary to hypovolemia and tissue ischemia, then cellular sodium influx[10a] and intracellular edema could well be another unrelated or loosely associated phenomenon.

The use of hypertonic salt solutions in burn resuscitation was first suggested by Moyer et al.[89] in 1944. Using a severely scalded dog burn model, these investigators observed that a longer period of survival could be achieved

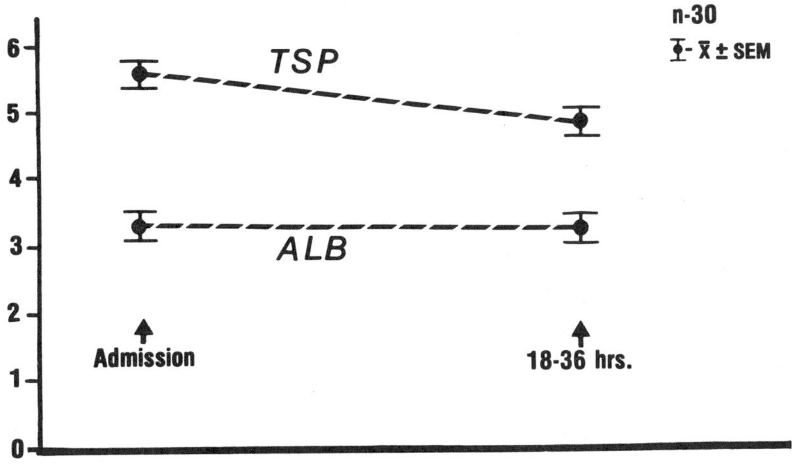

FIG 6–9.
Total serum protein *(TSP)* and serum albumin *(ALB)* levels (gm/dl) on admission and at 18–36 hours postinjury in thirty acutely burned children resuscitated according to the surface area formula and program.[23]

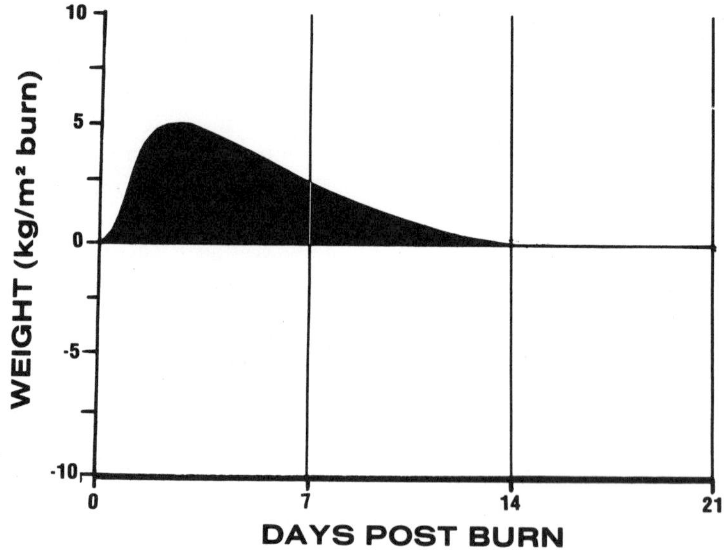

FIG 6–10.
Weight profile in 30 acutely burned children resuscitated according to the fluid program outlined by Carvajal.[23]

with the intravenous administration of solutions containing 129 mEq of sodium chloride and 25 mEq of sodium bicarbonate/L than with hypotonic salt solutions or plasma.[89] Subsequent animal studies by Fox and Baer[48] and Moyer et al.[90] suggested that heat-injured cells avidly trapped sodium. These observations provided the basis for the first clinical trials of hypertonic lactated saline (HLS) in burn resuscitation.[82a] Using solutions containing 300 or 250 mEq of sodium per liter and 200 and 100 mEq of racemic lactate, respectively, Monafo reported that "successful resuscitation" could be achieved in either adults or children with extensive burn injuries (Table 6–3). In these original studies, the aim of resuscitation was to maintain urine production at a rate of 30 ml/hour in adults and proportionately less hourly volumes, in children (actual figures in children were not reported).

Based on their published data regarding sodium and water intake (Table 6–4), we have estimated (assuming a normal weight-for-height ratio) that the children in Monafo's studies[82a] received fluids with an average concentration of sodium of 187 mEq/L for the first and second 24 hours postinjury. Although higher than in the hypotonic or isotonic resuscitation programs, this concentration of sodium is significantly below what has been generally associated with the HLS resuscitation regimen. A lower concentration of sodium results from the simultaneous administration of hypotonic salt solutions, which although part of the HLS program, is not commonly recognized.

Another aspect of the HLS program, the

TABLE 6–3.
Survival Rates in Patients With Burns Resuscitated by Hypertonic Lactated Saline*

PATIENTS	SURVIVED, %	BURNED BSA OF SURVIVORS, %	DIED, %	BURNED BSA OF DECEASED, %	DEATHS DURING SHOCK PHASE (0–72 HR), %
Adults (n=81)	36 (n=29)	40	64 (n=52)	64	?
Children (n=25)	88 (n=22)	33	12 (n= 3)	64	?
Total (n=106)	48 (n=51)	37	52 (n=55)	64	20 (n=21)

*Adapted from Monafo WW, Chuntrasakul C, Ayvasian V: *Am J Surg* 1973; 126:778–783.

TABLE 6–4.
Sodium and Water Intake in Burned Patients Resuscitated With Hypertonic Lactated Saline*

	Sodium Intake (mEq/kg/% of BSA burned)			Water Intake (ml/kg/% of BSA burned)		
Survivors Only	1st 24 hr	2nd 24 hr	Total	1st 24 hr	2nd 24 hr	Total
Adults (n = 29)	0.49	0.19	0.68	1.96	1.5	3.46
Children (n = 22)	0.74	0.41	1.15	3.94	3.04	6.98

*Adapted from Monafa WW, Chuntrasakul C, Ayvasian V: *Am J Surg* 1973; 126:778–783.

significance of which has not been fully appreciated, is that its proponents accept low hourly urine volumes (c 30 ml/hour) as indicative of adequate hydration.[20, 82] Since the end point of successful resuscitation according to the original HLS program is the attainment of a urine flow rate of 30 ml/hour in the adult (correspondingly less for children), the amount of fluid "required" to reach the expected goal is obviously less than in patient whose therapy is expected to result in higher urine volumes (Figs 6–11 and 6–12). Animal studies that have compared HLS to other regimens for burn resuscitation (Fig 6–12) and that have adhered to stricter guidelines for fluid and sodium administration have failed to demonstrate significant differences in hourly urine production.[25, 83, 85] However, since in humans fluid intake has been reported to be curtailed by HLS resuscitation, a *relative* diuresis has been assumed to occur.[20, 82, 82a]

Thus, even though animal studies have not documented an increase in urine production, it makes perfect physiologic sense that such an increase should occur, unless other factors such as excessive secretion of antidiuretic hormone (ADH) are able to counteract the expected response. The administration of HLS and the resultant increase in serum osmolality can be equated to certain pathologic conditions such as diabetic ketoacidosis; hyperosmolar, nonketotic coma; or osmotherapy.[5] In other words, the presence of an osmotically active substance in plasma, whether sodium, glucose, mannitol, or urea, should increase extracellular fluid osmolality and favor fluid movement out of the intracellular compartment (Fig 6–13). Thus, the intravascular volume is expanded, glomerular filtration increases, and the reabsorptive capacity of the renal tubule is exceeded; the net effect is diuresis, natriuresis, and loss of other plasma constituents as well.[52, 95] Excessive kaliuresis

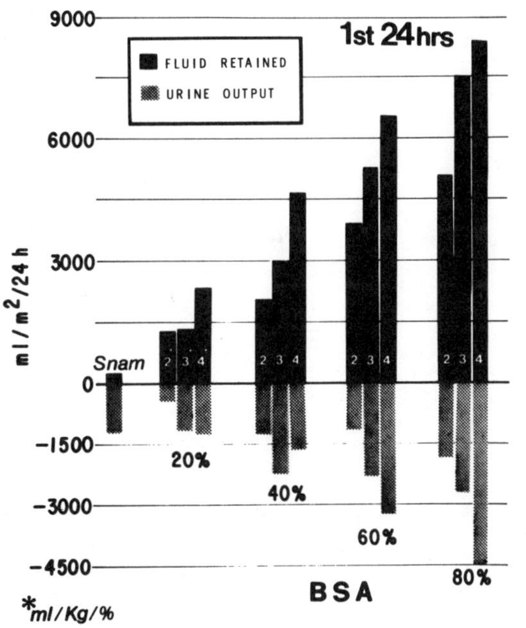

FIG 6–11.
Effect of total fluid intake on urine production in burned sheep (20%; 40%; 60%; or 80% of BSA burned) resuscitated with 2, 3, or 4 ml/kg/% of BSA burned/24 hours of an isotonic colloid-containing solution (Carvajal HF, unpublished data, 1983).

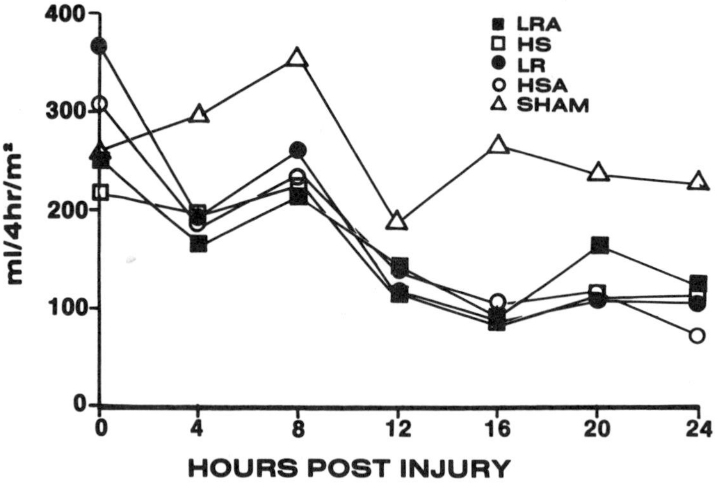

FIG 6–12.
Urine output in burned sheep (40% of BSA burned) successfully resuscitated with equal quantities (2.3–2.5 ml/kg/% of BSA burned/24 hours) of 5% dextrose in lactated Ringer's solution containing 12.5 gm of HS albumin per liter (LRA), hypertonic lactated saline (HS), dextrose 5% in lactated Ringer's solution (LR) and hypertonic lactated saline containing 12.5 gm of HS albumin per liter (HSA). Sham (nonburned animals) received maintenance fluids only (crystalloids). (Adapted from Carvajal HF: What is the ideal burn resuscitation solution? Proceedings of the 12th Annual Meeting of the American Burn Association, San Antonio, Texas, 1980, p 39.)

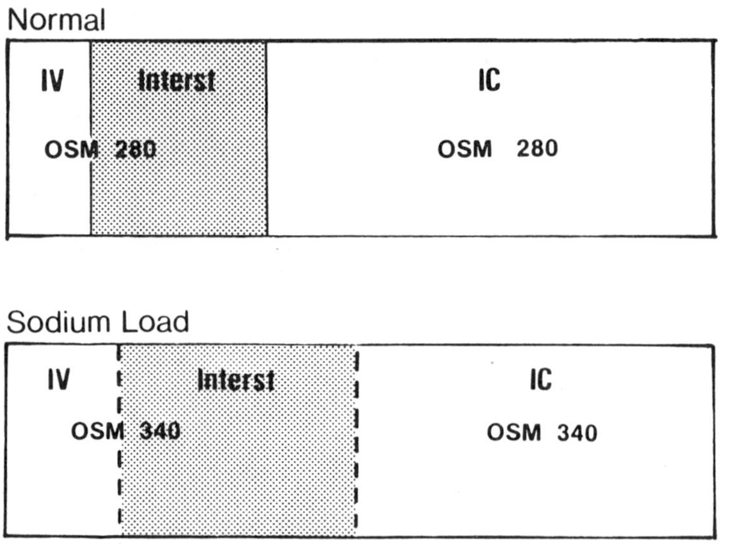

FIG 6–13.
Diagram depicting the effect of a sodium load on the volume of body fluid compartments. By virtue of being an extracellular ion, the quantity of sodium, rather than the resulting change in osmolality, determines the relative volumes of intracellular *(IC)* and extracellular fluid compartments. The effect of sodium upon intravascular *(IV)* and interstitial *(Interst)* fluid compartments is proportional to the original volume of each compartment prior to administration of sodium.

with consequent hypokalemia, for example, has been reported with the use of HLS in burn resuscitation.[27, 84, 85]

Although patients treated with the HLS program are described as hemodynamically stable, animal studies have revealed that the cardiac output is usually restored at a slower rate with HLS[25, 85] than with other solutions. When comparable amounts of fluid are administered, isotonic solutions containing albumin have resulted in a better hemodynamic response. Figure 6–14 depicts the changes in cardiac index observed in burned sheep (40% burn model) resuscitated with *equal* amounts of lactated Ringer's solution (LR), lactated Ringer's solution plus albumin (LRA), hypertonic lactated saline (HLS), and hypertonic lactated saline plus albumin (HLSA) as well as sham controls. In this study[25] fluid intake was maintained constant. Thus the hydrating solution rather than the guidelines of resuscitation was the independent variable.

The HLS program has undergone significant modifications since its inception. First, it was observed that the solution containing 300 mEq of sodium, 200 mEq of racemic lactate, and 100 mEq of chloride often resulted in hypernatremia and metabolic alkalosis;[82] thus, the intermittent and simultaneous administration of free water or lactated Ringer's solution was recommended.[82] Subsequently, a reduction in the concentrations of sodium and racemic lactate in the resuscitation fluids (250 and 100 mEq/L, respectively) and a corresponding increase in the chloride concentration to 150 mEq/L was proposed. Despite these changes, the intermittent administration of *hypotonic* solutions was still necessary whenever the serum sodium exceeded 150–160 mEq/L.[82a]

While the original program had no mecha-

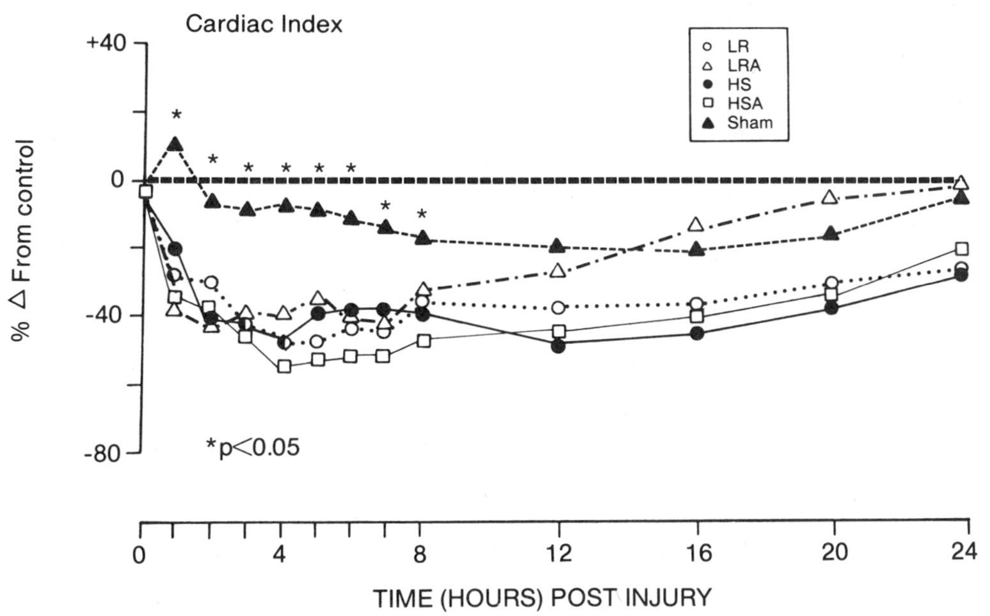

FIG 6–14.
Cardiac index changes in burned sheep (40% of BSA burned) resuscitated with equal quantities (2.3–2.5 ml/kg/% of BSA burned/24 hours) of 5% dextrose in lactated Ringer's solution containing 12.5 gm of HS albumin per liter (LRA), hypertonic lactated saline (HS), dextrose 5% in lactated Ringer's solution (LR), and hypertonic lactated saline containing 12.5 gm of HS albumin per liter (HSA). Sham (nonburned animals) received maintenance fluids only (dextrose 5% 0.33% sodium chloride injection).[27]

nism to estimate fluid needs, in subsequent writings a single figure formula (2 ml HLS/kg/% BSA burned) was proposed to estimate fluid requirements for the first 24 hours postinjury.[20] For the second 24 hours, 0.6 ml HLS/kg/% BSA burned *plus* replacement of insensible water losses (Haldane solution) was recommended.[20] According to recent publications, the overall sodium concentration of hydrating fluids has been decreased even further.[83] Thus, while the modified HLS program is better tolerated by most patients at present, it still lacks obvious advantages over conventional therapy. Fluid intake and overall weight gain are reportedly minimized, but burn edema does not change,[106] and edema in nonburned areas may actually increase (Fig 6–15). Furthermore, since the HLS program results in an increase in osmolality for all fluid compartments and since sodium is an extracellular ion, expansion of the extracellular space at the expense of intracellular fluids is the net result. Whatever protection to the intravascular volume is derived from the excess sodium, it is only transient and to a large extent dependent on the ability of the kidneys to excrete the sodium load. Thus, it is possible that some of the benefits that have been attributed to resuscitation with HLS may be related to the acceptance by their proponents of a state of relative dehydration and uneven distribution of water among body fluid compartments, rather than to any specific properties of the sodium ion.

A mild diuresis as well as a tendency to kaliuresis and presumably loss of other minerals has no therapeutic merit.[27] In a recent study in severely burned children, HLS was com-

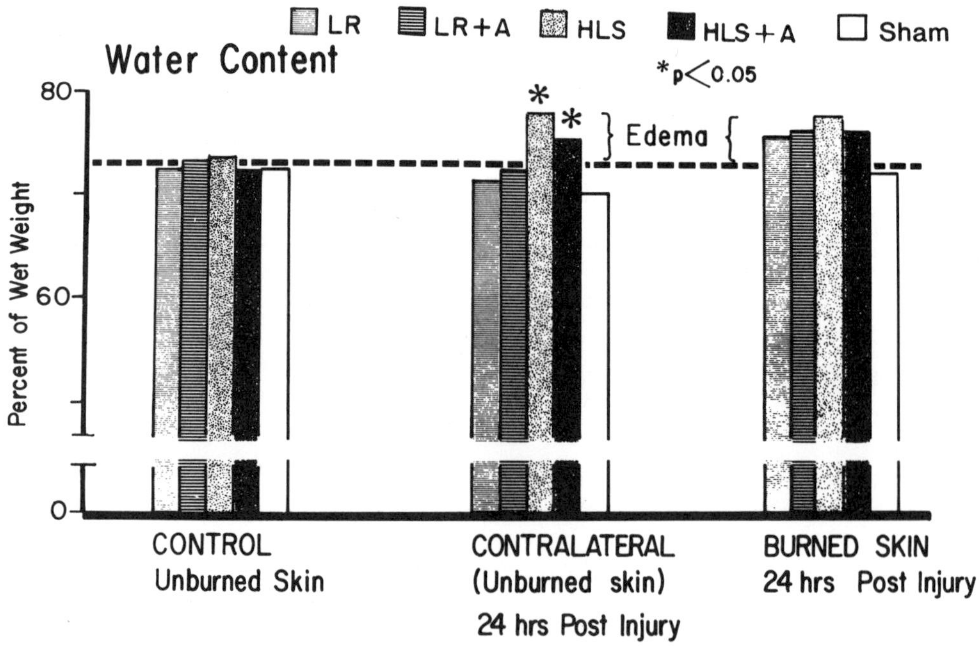

FIG 6–15.
Percent water content ([wet weight − dry weight] × 100/wet weight) of control (prior to burn), burned and contralateral skin from burned sheep (40% of BSA burned) resuscitated with equal quantities (2.3–2.5 ml/kg/% of BSA burned/24 hr) of 5% dextrose in lactated Ringer's solution containing 12.5 grams of HS albumin per liter (LRA), hypertonic lactated saline (HS), dextrose 5% in lactated Ringer's solution (LR), and hypertonic lactated saline containing 12.5 grams of HS albumin per liter (HSA). Sham animals received maintenance fluids only (dextrose 5% 0.33% sodium chloride injection.)[27]

pared to hypotonic as well as colloid-containing fluids.[17] However, the study groups were not comparable in regard to age (median age was 3 years for the colloid, 5 years for the hypotonic, and 12 years for the HLS groups), and the guidelines used to estimate fluid requirements and evaluate the objectives of treatment were different for each group. Furthermore, most of the data (weight gain, fluid intake, urine production, and sodium intake and output) were reported as group means, and only in relation to body weight and percent of BSA burned. Because the HLS group was older (and therefore had a decreased surface area-to-weight ratio), it could have been predicted a priori to have required less fluid. In another study,[84] crystalloid solutions containing sodium in concentrations of less than 150 mEq/L, 150 to 199 mEq/L and greater than 199 mEq/L were compared to one another in their ability to maintain body homeostasis and urine values in the range of 0.5 to 1.0 ml/kg/hour. Although mortality was high (42%) for all groups (thirty-one of seventy-four patients died) and seven patients died within 48 hours of injury, a positive correlation between water and sodium intake and mortality was reported. Since the urine output ranged between 0.5 to 1.0 ml/kg/hour for all patients and no differences between groups were demonstrated in this regard, the data presented can be interpreted two different ways: (1) either the urine output did not reflect the level of hydration, and death resulted from overhydration, or (2) excess water and sodium administration is deleterious to the burn patient and leads to increased mortality.

Though both of these possibilities could be invoked and could be linked to one another, the data reported do not allow for further conclusions to be drawn. However, the assumptions that excessive water and sodium administration in the form of hypotonic solutions were responsible for the increased mortality may not be appropriate without first demonstrating that the same resuscitation solution at lower volumes is also associated with a high mortality. In other words, it is quite possible that the increased morbidity and mortality in this study were secondary to iatrogenic factors, rather than to the composition of the resuscitation fluids.

According to Bowser and Caldwell,[17] "The major therapeutic effect of HLS, other than its volume replacing value, is secondary to the sustained hypernatremia and the consequent increase in serum osmolality." The authors theorize that the increased osmolality of the extracellular fluid results in a fluid shift from the intracellular to the extracellular compartment. This shift inhibits edema formation and improves kidney function by an "osmotic diuresis" effect, which counteracts the antidiuresis so characteristic of burn trauma. The studies of Sokawa et al.[106] and Carvajal[25, 27] suggest that at least some of these assumptions are incorrect. The latter studies have shown that edema in neither injured nor uninjured tissue is minimized by increasing the sodium content of resuscitation fluids. By virtue of being an extracellular ion, the *quantity* of *sodium*, rather than the resulting change in osmolality is what determines the volume of the respective fluid compartments (see Fig 6–13). Thus as the sodium content of intravascular and interstitial fluid compartments increase, so does their volume. In other words, from a physiologic standpoint, edema in the interstitium should be directly proportional to its sodium content, and HLS resuscitation should enhance rather than diminish edema of the tissues (see Fig 6–15), whether injured or not.[95] Since the water content of the intracellular compartment is decreased by the consequent increase in extracellular fluid osmolality and outward fluid shift, "cellular edema" is decreased, but only in cells that have a normally functioning sodium/potassium pump.

Caldwell and Bowser[20] postulate that the osmotic diuretic effect of a sodium load counteracts the antidiuretic effect of ADH may not be appropriate either, without first documenting that such indeed occurs. Our studies[25] in burned sheep resuscitated with

HLS as well as with other hydrating solutions suggest that such an assumption could be incorrect. In these studies, HLS resuscitation did not increase urine volume (see Fig 6–12), nor did it significantly lower urine osmolality (Fig 6–16); the latter effect is the hallmark of osmotic diuresis.[52]

Thus, from a theoretical standpoint, it is difficult to conceive that HLS resuscitation, which results in hypernatremia, hyperosmolality, increased interstitial edema, delayed restoration of cardiac output, natriuresis (rejection of a significant portion of the sodium given), kaliuresis, and no obvious improvement in urine output, offers any therapeutic advantages to the burn victim. Furthermore, the persistent increase in serum osmolality should be viewed with concern as it is poorly tolerated by children; cerebral hemorrhage, idiogenic osmol formation and rebound cerebral edema, circulatory congestion, and inhibition of lipolysis are potential complications that deserve investigation in pediatric populations.

The addition of 12.5 gm of albumin to each liter of HLS containing 240 mEq sodium and 120 mEq each of chloride and lactate (HLSA) for burn resuscitation was first proposed by Jelenko et al.[68] These investigators compared the effects of three different solutions (LR, HLS, and HLSA) on burn resuscitation in adult burn victims. Fluids were administered according to a demand program, and the objectives of resuscitation were to maintain mean arterial pressure between 60 and 100 mm Hg and a urine flow rate of 30 to 50 ml/hour. Although several hemodynamic and physiologic parameters were measured, the objectives of resuscitation were varied depending on the composition of the hydrating fluids. According to Jelenko et al.,[67, 68] patients in the HLSA group "required" less fluids, were resuscitated over a shorter period of time, were able to tolerate oral fluids earlier, and required shorter periods of ventilatory support than those in the other two groups. However, since the resuscitation guides used by Jelenko et al. have not re-

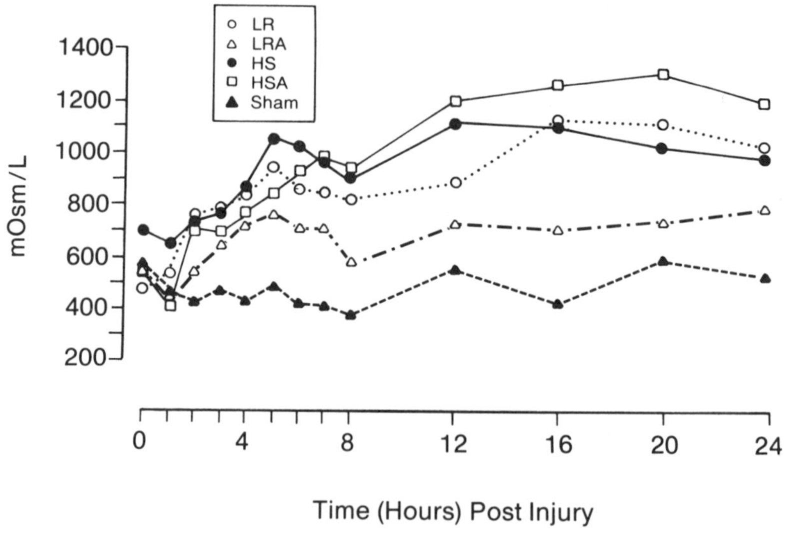

FIG 6–16.
Urine osmolality in burned sheep (40% of BSA burned) resuscitated with equal quantities (2.4–2.5 ml/kg/% of BSA burned) of 5% dextrose in lactated Ringer's solution containing 12.5 gm of HS albumin per liter (LRA), hypertonic lactated saline (HS), dextrose 5% in lactated Ringer's solution (LR), and hypertonic lactated saline containing 12.5 gm of HS albumin per liter (HSA). Sham (unburned animals) received maintenance fluids only (dextrose 5% 0.33% sodium chloride injection). A persistently high urine osmolality for all groups studied (except the sham group) is indicative of persistent ADH secretion and speaks against an osmotic diuretic effect.[27]

ceived widespread acceptance, and since treatment objectives varied between groups, interpretation of these results must await further studies. For example, urine production was one of the variables used to guide resuscitation, but it was significantly different among groups; it should have been equal. Though the actual values were not reported, central venous pressure differences among groups occurred. Again, this was one of the variables used to judge the adequacy of resuscitation. Also, the mean arterial pressure range of 60 to 110 mm Hg chosen to guide fluid administration is too wide to presume equal hemodynamic balance for all patients studied. Furthermore, studies in burned animals (sheep) have questioned the validity of mean arterial pressure and hourly urine volume measurements to guide fluid resuscitation (Fig 6–17) and have failed to demonstrate significant advantages from the use of HLSA over other conventional treatments.[25]

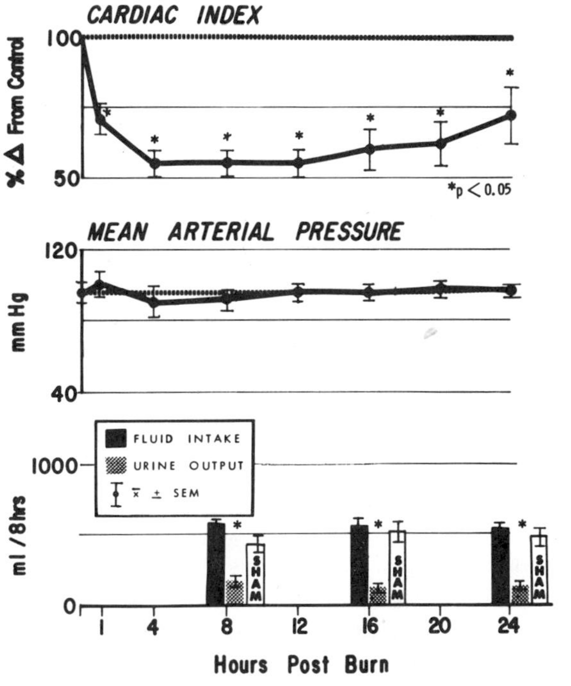

FIG 6–17.
Relationship between cardiac index, mean arterial pressure, fluid intake, and urine output in six sheep subjected to full-thickness burn injuries (40% of BSA burned) who received only maintenance fluids (1,500 ml/sq m/24 hours) consisting of dextrose 5% in 0.33% sodium chloride injection. Notice that despite significant change in cardiac index and oliguria (as compared to sham controls), the mean arterial pressure remains unchanged. (From Carvajal HF: The optimal composition of burn resuscitation fluids. Submitted for publication, 1984.)

RESUSCITATION GUIDELINES

Lack of agreement also exists in regard to the choice of resuscitation guides. For example, some investigators use hourly urine volume exclusively as the guide of hydration. Others such as Haynes[63] recommend frequent measurements of hematocrit to detect hemoconcentration or volume expansion; monitoring of central venous pressure has been recommended by Moncrief[87] and Hall,[59] and Jelenko et al.[67, 68] has proposed the use of mean arterial pressure. Invasive monitoring, including measurement of the cardiac index and ventricular stroke work index, has also been used at some institutions.[2, 3, 4, 78, 79]

The basic problem is that the resuscitation objectives of the various programs have not been adequately defined. Hence, the guidelines used to evaluate success or failure have become the subject of criticism. For example, if the goal of therapy is to prevent the development of renal insufficiency, this should not be equated with urine production equal to or greater than 50 ml/hour. The same may be accomplished with lesser quantities of fluids and a less pronounced diuresis. Likewise, if the objective of resuscitation is to restore cardiac output to normal, the time factor during which this should be accomplished must be defined. Rapid fluid infusion and other therapeutic interventions could accomplish this goal within 4 hours, but unacceptable complications such as pulmonary edema or excessive peripheral edema may not justify it, particularly if a slower return of the cardiac output to normal is associated with a lower morbidity.

Some of the difficulties associated with interpretation of much of the published studies have been recently illustrated by Carvajal.[27] In this study, burned sheep (20%, 40%, 60%, and 80% BSA burned) were resuscitated with a total 24 hour fluid intake equivalent to either 2, 3, or 4 ml/kg/% area of burn. The rate of fluid administration was fixed (one half during the first 8 hours and the other half during the subsequent 16 hours) and only one solution (lactated Ringer's plus 12.5 gm of human serum albumin per liter) was used. Several clinical and hemodynamic variables were measured at frequent intervals, and the animals were killed at 24 hours postinjury. A sham group of animals (nonburned) was subjected to the same experimental manipulations and received maintenance fluids during the same time interval. Figure 6–11 depicts the total fluid intake and average urine volume excreted during the 24-hour study. When compared to the sham animals, all groups, with the exception of the 20% burned surface area–2 ml/kg/% group, had adequate urine production and presumably were adequately resuscitated. While an increase in fluid intake was associated with an increase in urine output, progressively greater quantities of fluid were retained in the body, thus increasing body weight (Fig 6–18).

Since the animals with burns of 60% and 80% increased their urine output by twofold to threefold as compared to the sham controls, one would have assumed that the diuresis represented an attempt of the body to eliminate the excess fluid. However, measurements of water clearance revealed that an antidiuretic effect was still present (negative water clearances) and that water was reabsorbed even at high rates of urine production (Fig 6–19). These data support the contention that inappropriate secretion of ADH is at least partly responsible for the state of antidiuresis that characterizes the burn injury. It also suggests that high urine volumes in burned victims may be associated with retention of inappropriate quantities of fluids and do not necessarily reflect optimal hemodynamics. Thus, recognition of the state of antidiuresis may be more important than selection of any

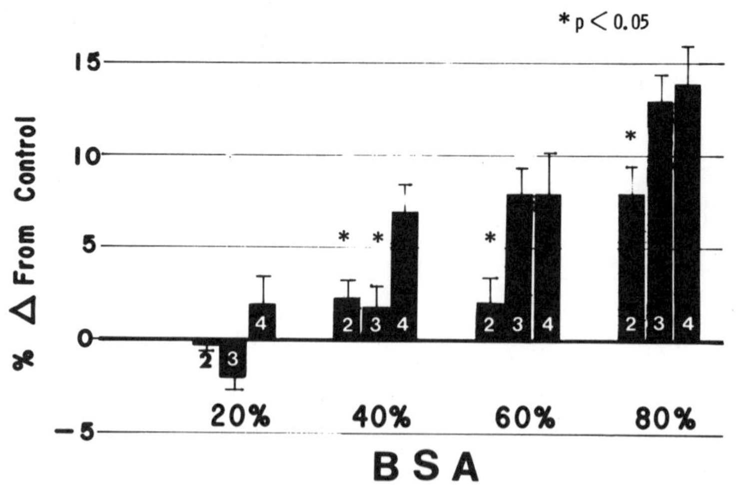

FIG 6–18.
Weight change (percent change from control value) in burned sheep (20%, 40%, 60%, and 80% of BSA burned) resuscitated with either 2, 3, or 4 ml/kg/% of BSA burned/24 hours of an isotonic colloid-containing solution. Notice that as the intake of fluid increases, so does the weight of the animal at the completion of experiment (24 hours postinjury). (From Carvajal HF: The optimal quantity of fluids in burn resuscitation. Submitted for publication.)

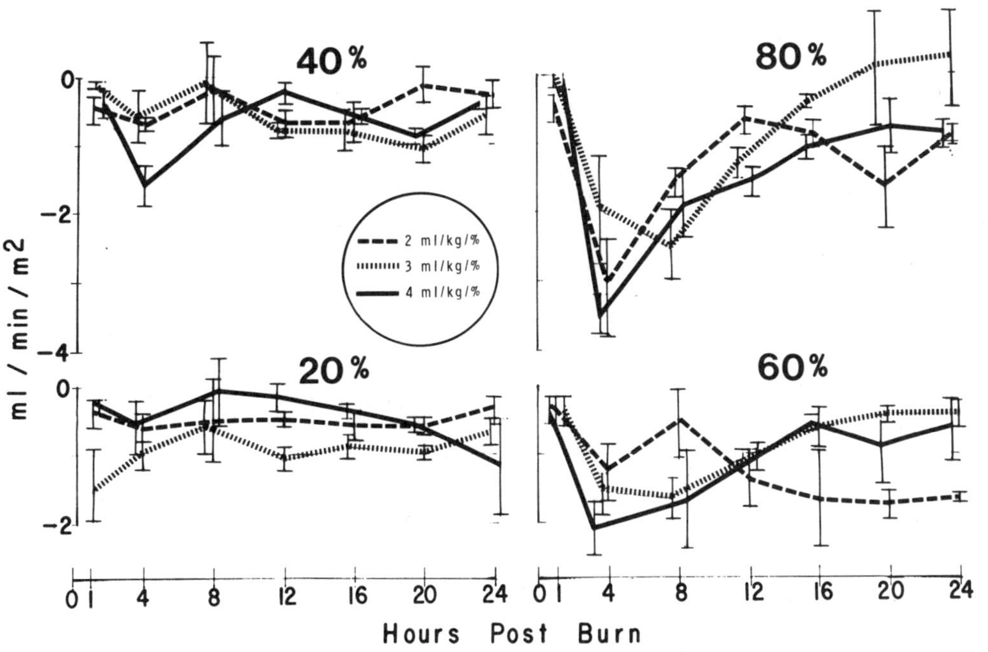

FIG 6–19.
Water clearance (CH_2O) in burned sheep (BSA burned 20%, 40%, 60%, 80%) resuscitated with 2, 3, 4 ml/kg/% of BSA burned of an isotonic salt solution (lactated Ringer's) containing 12.5 gm of albumin/liter. Notice that CH_2O remains in the negative range, despite significant diuresis (see Fig 6–11 also) indicating persisting secretion of antidiuretic hormone. (From Carvajal HF: The optimal quantity of fluids in burn resuscitation. Submitted for publication, 1984.

given fluid formula or fluid composition in the process of preventing edema formation (Fig 6–20).

SUMMARY OF CONTROVERSIES IN BURN RESUSCITATION

Quantity of Fluids

Although no agreements in regard to the quantity of fluids needed for resuscitation have been reached, investigators have become aware of the dangers of overhydration, and a tendency toward a reduction in fluid intake and curtailment of edema formation represents a common goal.

In general, fluid resuscitation formulas based on weight are inadequate to estimate fluid requirements in burned children. Estimates based on BSA and BSA burned appear better suited for this purpose, as they introduce greater accuracy and consistency for children of all ages and burns of different sizes.

The objectives of resuscitation must be carefully defined in order to prevent excessive fluid administration. Hourly urine output correlates poorly with the state of hydration and should be used only in conjunction with other hydration guidelines. Invasive monitoring is seldom if ever needed to hydrate burned children as it may introduce additional morbidity.

Composition of the Hydrating Solution

Significant differences exist among the compositions of the various solutions that are currently advocated for fluid resuscitation of the burned patient. These differences are of

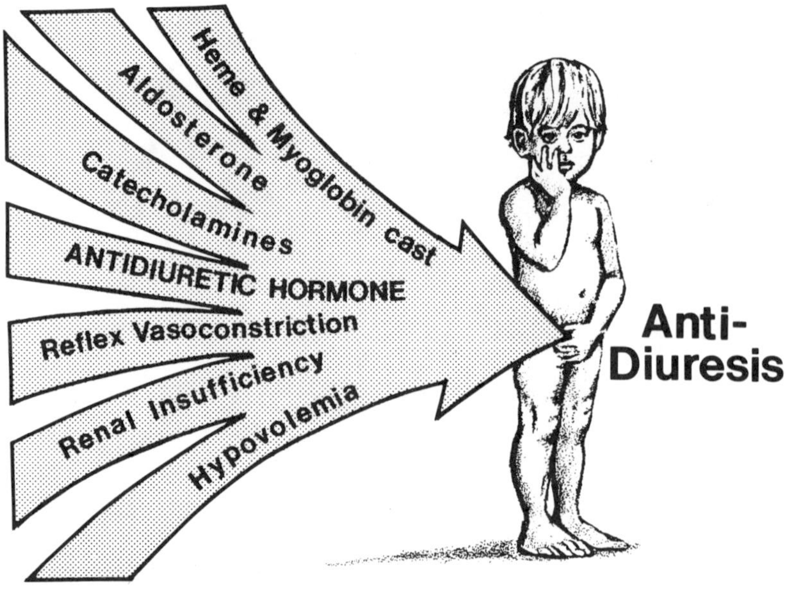

FIG 6–20.
Antidiuresis.

such magnitude that the effect of the various solutions on body homeostasis is likely to be dramatically different. Multiple human and animal studies have been performed to document the effectiveness of one therapy over another, but several confounding factors have impeded proper interpretation of results.

In general, colloid-containing fluids, though more expensive, exert a more rapid and complete resuscitation than do crystalloids, even during the first 24 hours postinjury. Colloid-containing fluids restore hemodynamics with lesser infusate volumes, minimize edema formation, and maintain cardiac, pulmonary, renal, and gastrointestinal function.

Hypertonic salt solutions offer no theoretical or practical advantages to the pediatric burned patient and may even be deleterious. Thus, the following generalizations regarding resuscitation fluids for burned children seem valid:

1. The concentration of sodium should be isotonic or slightly hypotonic.*
2. Bicarbonate or lactate should be added to combat acidosis and facilitate the preparation of a more physiologic fluid mixture (sodium/chloride 3:2 ratio).
3. The concentration of albumin in resuscitation fluids should be 1 to 1.5 gm/100 ml.
4. The addition of carbohydrate seems desirable to provide a protein-sparing effect.

The advantages of using a composite solution are as follows:

1. Only one type of solution is required for resuscitation.
2. Fluid, electrolytes, and proteins are given simultaneously in quantities that approximate the losses.
3. The total quantity of fluids required for 24 hours may be prepared in advance, and therefore only the rate of infusion may need adjustment.

Guides to Resuscitation Therapy

The major controversy regarding the guides to resuscitation is whether or not hourly urine volume accurately reflects the state of hydration and whether or not a given level of urine

*Children less than 1 year of age require less quantities of sodium (70 to 80 mEq/L).

production must be or can be maintained by altering the rate of fluid administration.

A well-hydrated, unburned child on maintenance fluids should produce an average of 650 ml of urine per square meter of body surface per day. This is equivalent to an average of 30 ml/hr/sq m of body surface. Thus, no burned child should be expected to exceed this figure (except during the diuretic phase). The burned patient is in a state of antidiuresis (see Fig 6–20). This is primarily related to the secretion of antidiuretic and other hormones in response to trauma, pain, fear, apprehension, and abnormal postures and positions, as well as to the effects of various drugs. During the acute phase, exaggerated sympathetic responses also contribute to a reduction in urine production. Thus, in the burn patient it is impossible to determine how much urine should be produced or should be considered normal. The expected amount is obviously below 30 ml/hr/sq m, but the the exact figure is unknown. What is known, however, is that attempts to force diuresis by excessive fluid administration often leads to a positive water balance, excessive edema, and cardiopulmonary congestion.

In the burn patient, urine output varies widely from one hour to another and is better evaluated when expressed over a period of 4 hours and in relation to body surface area. Various clinical and laboratory guidelines must be correlated before a decision to increase or decrease the rate of fluid administration is made. In general, the lower the amount of urine production that is expected, the lower the quantity of fluid that is required for resuscitation.

REFERENCES

1. Agarwal N, Petro J, Salisbury RE: Physiologic profile monitoring in burned patients. *J Trauma* 1983; 23:577–583.
2. Aikawa N, Martyn JAJ, Burke JF: Pulmonary artery catheterization and thermodilution cardiac output determination in the management of critically ill burned patients. *Am J Surg* 1978; 135:811–817.
3. Aikawa N, Ishibiki K, Nalto C, et al: Individualized fluid resuscitation based on haemodynamic monitoring in the management of extensive burns. *Burns Incl Therm Inj* 1982; 8:249–255.
4. Agarwal N, Petro J, Solisbury R: Physiologic profile monitoring in burned patients. *J Trauma* 1983; 23:577–583.
5. Arieff AI, Guisado, R, Lazarowitz VC: The pathophysiology of hyperosmolar states, in Andreoli TE, Grantham JJ, Rector FC Jr (eds): *Disturbances in Body Fluid Osmolality.* Baltimore, Williams & Wilkins Co, 1977, pp 277–250.
6. Arturson G: Prostaglandins in human burn wound secretions. *Burns* 1977, 3:112.
7. Arturson G, Jonsson CE: Transcapillary transport after thermal injury. *Scand J Plast Reconstr Surg* 1979; 13:29–38.
8. Arturson G, Hedlund A: Primary treatment of 50 patients with high tension electrical injuries. *Scand J Plast Reconstr Surg* 1984; 18:111–118.
9. Artz CP: The Brooke formula, in Polk HC Jr, Stone HH (eds): *Contemporary Burn Management.* Boston, Little, Brown & Co, 1971, pp 43–51.
10. Batchelor ADR, Kirk J, Sutherland AB: Treatment of shock in the burned child. *Lancet* 1961; 1:123–127.

10a. Baxter CR: Fluid volume and electrolyte changes of the early post-burn period. *Clin Plast Surg* 1974; 1:693.

11. Baxter CR: Controversies in the resuscitation of burn shock. *Curr Concepts Therm Care* 1982; 5:5–14.
12. Baxter CR: Crystalloid resuscitation of burn shock, in Polk HC Jr, Stone HH (eds): *Contemporary Burn Management.* Boston, Little, Brown & Co, 1971, pp 7–32.
13. Baxter, CR, Shires GT: Physiological response to crystalloid resuscitation of severe burns. *Ann NY Acad Sci* 1968; 150:874–893.
14. Barter FC, Schwartz WB: The syndrome of inappropriate secretion of antidiuretic hormone. *Am J Med* 1967; 42:790.
15. Black DA: Treatment of burn shock with plasma and serum. *Brit Med J* 1940; 2:693–697.
16. Blaha J: Experience of children's burns treatment. *Acta Chir Plast* 1982; 24(4):226–34.

16a. Blalock A.: Experimental shock: VIII. The importance of the local loss of fluid in the production of the low blood pressure after burns. *Arch Surg* 1931; 22:610.

17. Bowser BH, Caldwell FT Jr: The effect of resuscitation with hypertonic vs. hypotonic vs. colloid on the wound and urine fluid and electrolyte losses in severely burned children. *J Trauma* 1983; 23:916–923.

18. Brouhard BH, Carvajal HF: Effect of inhibiting prostaglandin synthesis of edema formation and albumin leakage during thermal trauma in the rat. *Prostaglandins* 1979; 17:939–946.
19. Brouhard BH, Carvajal HF, Linares HA: Burn edema and protein leakage in the rat. I. Relationship to time of injury. *Microvasc Res* 1978; 15:221–228.
20. Caldwell FT, Jr, Bowser BH: Critical evaluation of hypertonic and hypotonic solutions to resuscitate severely burned children: A prospective study. *Ann Surg* 1979; 189:546–552.
21. Carvajal HF: Acute management of burns in children. *South Med J* 1975; 68:129–131.
22. Carvajal HF: Fluid therapy for the acutely burned child. *Compr Ther* 1977; 3:17–24.
23. Carvajal HF: A physiologic approach to fluid therapy in severely burned children. *Surg Gynecol Obstet* 1980; 150:379–384.
24. Carvajal HF: Acute management of severely burned patients. *ER Rep* 1980; 1:45–48.
25. Carvajal HF: What is the ideal burn resuscitation solution? Proceedings of the 12th Annual Meeting of the American Burn Association, San Antonio, Texas, 1980, p 39.
26. Carvajal HF: Management of severely burned patients: Sorting out the controversies. *Emerg Med Rep* 1985; 6:89–96.
27. Carvajal HF: The optimal composition of burn resuscitation fluids. Submitted for publication.
27a. Carvajal HF: The optimal quantity of fluids in burn resuscitation. Submitted for publication.
28. Carvajal HF, Brouhard BH, Linares HA: Effects of antihistamine antiserotonin and ganglionic blocking agents upon increased capillary permeability following burn trauma. *J Trauma* 1975; 15:969–975.
29. Carvajal HF, Linares HA: Effect of burn depth upon edema formation and albumin extravasation in rats. *Burns*1980; 7:79–83.
30. Carvajal HF, Linares HA, Brouhard BH: Relationship of burn size to vascular permeability changes in rats. *Surg Gynecol Obstet* 1979; 149:193–202.
31. Carvajal HF, Reinhard JA, Traber DL: Renal and cardiovascular functional response to thermal injury in dogs subjected to sympathetic blockade. *Circ Shock* 1976, 3:287–298.
32. Cope O, Graham JB, Moore FD, Ball MR: The nature of the shift of plasma protein to the extravascular space following thermal trauma. *Ann Surg* 1948; 128:1041–1055.
33. Cope O, Moore FD: The redistribution of body water and the fluid therapy of the burned patient. *Ann Surg* 1947; 126:1010.
34. Cuono CB: Early management of severe thermal injury. *Surg Clin North Am* 1980; 60:1021–1033.
35. Davis JWL: *Physiological Responses to Burning Injury*. London, Academic Press, 1982.
36. Demling RH: Burn edema, Part I. Pathogenesis: *J Burn Care Rehabil* 1982; 3: 138–148.
37. Demling RH: Fluid resuscitation after major burns. *JAMA* 1983; 250:1438–1440.
38. Demling RH: Improved survival after massive burns. *J Trauma* 1983; 23:179–84.
39. Eagle JF: Parenteral fluid therapy of burns during the first 48 hours. *NY J Med* 1956; 56:1613–1618.
40. Eagle JF, Schenk WG, Shim W: Parenteral fluid therapy of burns (use of a single solution during the first 48 hours). *JAMA* 1960; 174:1589–1592.
41. Eklund J, Hallberg D: Hyperosmolality and lypolysis: An experimental study with reference to hypernatremia in burned patients. *Acta Chir Scand* 1970; 136:91–93.
42. Elkinton JR, Wolffe WA, Lee WE: Plasma transfusions in the treatment of the fluid shift in severe burns. *Ann Surg* 1940; 112:150–157.
43. Elman R: The therapeutic significance of plasma protein replacement in severe burns. *JAMA* 1941; 116:213–216.
44. Evans EI, Purnell OJ, Robinett PW, et al: Fluid and electrolyte requirements in severe burns. *Ann Surg* 1952; 135:804–816.
45. Field ME, Drinker CK, White JC: Lymph pressures in sterile inflammation. *J Exp Med* 1932; 56:363–370.
46. Fimberg L: Pathogenesis of lesions in the nervous system in hypernatremic states. *Pediatrics* 1959; 23:40–45.
47. Fimberg L, Kravath RE, Fleischman AR: *Water and Electrolytes in Pediatrics*. Philadelphia, WB Saunders Co, 1982.
48. Fox CL Jr, Baer H: Redistribution of potassium, sodium, and water in burns and trauma and its relation to the phenomena of shock. *Am J Physiol* 1947; 151:155–167.
49. Fox CL Jr, Lasker SE, Winnfield JM: Rationale of early fluid and sodium therapy of extensive burns, in Ellison ER, Fieren SR, Mulholland JH (eds): *Current Surgical Management*. Philadelphia, WB Saunders Co, 1957, vol 2, pp 402–418.
50. Fox, CL Jr, Stanford JW: Comparative efficacy of hypo-, iso-, and hypertonic sodium solutions in experimental burn shock. *Surgery* 1974; 75:71–79.
51. Gelin LE: Macrodex and oxygen in the pri-

mary treatment of extensive burns. *Acta Chir Scand* 1952; 103:351–352.

52. Gennari FJ, Kassirer JP: Osmotic diuresis. *N Engl J Med* 1974; 291:714–720.
53. Gennari, FJ: Serum osmolality uses and limitations. *N Engl J Med* 1984; 310:102–105.
54. Goodwin CW, Long JW, Mason AD, Pruitt BA Jr: Paradoxical effect of hyperoncotic albumin in acutely burned children. *J Trauma* 1982; 21:63.
55. Goodwin CW, Dorethy J, Lam V, et al: Randomized trial of efficacy of crystalloid and colloid resuscitation on hemodynamic response and lung water following thermal injury. *Ann Surg* 1983; 197:520–531.
56. Granger ND, Gabel JC, Drake RE: Physiologic basis for the clinical use of albumin solutions. *Surg Gynecol Obstet* 1978; 146:97–104.
57. Griffiths RW, Laing JE: A burn formula in clinical practice. *Ann R Coll Surg Engl* 1981; 63:50–53.
58. Griffith RW: A low volume burn resuscitation regimen: Assessment of performance of probit analysis. *Br J Surg* 1981; 68:225–228.
59. Hall KVN, Sorensen B: The treatment of burn shock—results of a five-year randomized controlled clinical trial of dextran 70 vs. Ringer's lactate solution. *Burns* 1978; 5:107–112.
60. Harkins HN, Cope O, Evans EW, et al: Fluid and nutritional therapy of burns. *JAMA* 1945; 128:475–479.
61. Harms BA, Bodai BI, Kramer GC, et al: Microvascular fluid and protein flux in pulmonary and systemic circulations after thermal injury. *Microvasc Res* 1982; 23:77.
62. Haynes BW: The management of burns in children. *J Trauma* 1965; 5:267–277.
63. Haynes BW Jr: Early fluid treatment of severe burns: Hemodynamic alterations and the use of dextran and blood. *Ann NY Acad Sci* 1968; 150:907–911.
64. Hilton JG: Effects of fluid resuscitation on total fluid loss following thermal injury. *Surg Gynecol Obstet* 1981; 152:441.
65. Holleman JH, Gabel JC, Hardy JD: Pulmonary effects intravenous fluid therapy in burn resuscitation. *Surg Gynecol Obstet* 1978; 147:161–166.
66. Hutcher N, Haynes BW Jr: The Evans formula revisited. *J Trauma* 1972; 12:453–458.
67. Jelenko C III, Solenberger RI, Wheeler ML, Callaway BD: Shock and resuscitation. III. Accurate refractometric COP determinations in hypovolemia treated with HALFD. *JACEP* 1979; 8:7–11.
68. Jelenko C III, Williams JB, Wheeler ML, et al: Studies in shock and resuscitation, I. Use of hypertonic albumin-containing fluid demand regimen (HALFD) in resuscitation. A physiologically approrpiate method. *Crit Care Med* 1979; 7:157–167.
69. Jenkinson LR: Fluid replacement in burns. *Ann R Coll Surg Engl* 1982; 64:336–338.
70. Kramer GC, Gunther RA, Nerlich ML, et al: Effect of Dextran-70 on increased microvascular fluid and protein flux after thermal injury. *Circ Shock* 1982; 9:529–541.
71. Kravath RE, Aharon AS, Abal G, et al: Clinically significant physiologic danger from rapidly administered hypertonic solutions: Acute osmol poisoning. *Pediatrics* 1970; 46:267–275.
72. Kreusser W, Rice E: The phosphate-depletion syndrome. *Contre Nephrol* 1978; 14:162–174.
73. Lam CR: Plasma therapy of burns. *Ann Surg* 1941; 113:1089.
74. Lamke LO, Nilsson GE, Reithner HL: The evaporation water loss from burns and the water vapor permeability of grafts and artificial membranes used in the treatment of burns. *Burns* 1977; 3:159–165.
75. Larson DL, Abston S, Goldman AS: The burned child. *Texas Med* 1971; 67:58–67.
76. Markley K, Bocanegra M, Bazan A, et al: Clinical evaluation of saline solution therapy in burn shock. *JAMA* 1956; 161:1465–1473.
77. Markley K, Smallman E, Milliken C: The efficacy and toxicity of iso-, hypo-, and hypertonic sodium solutions in the treatment of burn shock in mice. *Surgery* 1964; 57:698–703.
78. Martyn JA, Snider MT, Farago LF, et al: Thermodilution right ventricular volume: A novel and better predictor of volume replacement in acute thermal injury. *J Trauma* 1981; 21:619–626.
79. Martyn JA, Snider M, Szyfelbein S, et al: Right ventricular dysfunction in acute thermal injury. *Ann Surg* 1980; 191:330–335.
80. Metcoff J, Buchman H, Jacobson M, et al: Losses and physiologic requirements for water and electrolytes after extensive burns in children. *N Engl J Med* 1961; 265:101–111.
81. Micheels J, Alsbjörn B, Sørensen B: Laser doppler flowmetry: A new noninvasive measurement of microcirculation in intensive care? *Resuscitation* 1984; 12:31–39.
82. Monafo WW: The treatment of burn shock by the intravenous and oral administration of hypertonic lactated saline solution. *J Trauma* 1970; 10:575–586.

82a. Monafo WW, Chuntrasakul C, Ayvasian V: Hypertonic sodium solution in the treatment of burn shock. *Am J Surg* 1973; 126:778–783.
83. Monafo WW, Halverson JD, Schechtman K: The role of concentrated sodium solutions in the resuscitation of patients with severe burns. *Surgery* 1984; 95:129–134.
84. Moyland JA, Rechler JM, Mason AD: Hypertonic lactate saline resuscitation in thermal injury. *Surg Forum* 1971; 22:49.
85. Moyland JA, Rechler JM, Mason AS: Resuscitation with hypertonic lactate saline in thermal injury. *Am J Surg* 1973; 125:580.
86. Moncrief JA: Effects of various fluid regimens and pharmacologic agents on the circulatory hemodynamics of the immediate postburn period. *Ann Surg* 1966; 164:723–752.
87. Moncrief JA: Burns. *N Engl J Med* 1973; 288:444–454.
88. Moss GS: Plasma albumin and postoperative ileus. *Surg Forum* 1967; 333–336.
89. Moyer CA, Coller FA, Iob V, et al: A study of the interrelationship of salt solutions, serum, and defibrinated blood in the treatment of severely scalded anesthetized dogs. *Ann Surg* 1944; 120:367–376.
90. Moyer CA, Margraft HW, Monafo WW: Burn shock and extravascular sodium deficiency—treatment with Ringer's solution with lactate. *Arch Surg* 1965; 90:799–811.
91. Moyland JA, Mason AD, Rogers PW, et al: Post burn shock: A critical evaluation of resuscitation. *J Trauma* 1973; 13:354–358.
92. Moyland JA, Rechler JM, Mason AD: Hypertonic lactate saline resuscitation in thermal injury. *Surg Forum* 1971; 22:49.
93. Moyland JA, Rechler JM, Mason AD: Resuscitation with hypertonic lactate saline in thermal injury. *Am J Surg* 1973; 125:580.
94. O'Neill JA: Fluid resuscitation in the burned child—a reappraisal. *J Pediatr Surg* 1982; 17:604–607.
95. Pitts RF: *Physiology of the Kidney and Body Fluids.* Chicago, Year Book Medical Publisher, 1968.
96. Pruitt BA Jr: Fluid and electrolyte replacement in the burned patient. *Surg Clin North Am* 1978; 58:1291–1312.
97. Pruitt BA Jr: Fluid resuscitation for extensively burned patients. *J Trauma* 1981; 21:690–692.
98. Reiss E, Stirman JA, Artz CP, et al: Fluid and electrolyte balance in burns. *JAMA* 1953; 152:1309–1313.
99. Roberts JC, Courtice FC: Measurements of protein leakage in the acute and recovery stages of thermal injury. *Aust J Exp Biol Med Sci* 1969; 47:421–433.
100. Schwartz S: Consensus summary on fluid resuscitation. *J Trauma* 1979; 19:876–877.
101. Settle JA: Urine output following severe burns. *Burns* 1974; 1:23–42.
102. Second conference on supportive therapy in burn care. Fluid resuscitation. *J Trauma* 1981; 21 (suppl):686–699.
103. Shimazaki S, Hoshioka T, Tanaka N, et al: Body fluid changes during hypertonic lactated solution for burn shock. *J Trauma* 1977; 17:38.
104. Shires GT: NIH Consensus development conference. Supportive therapy in burn care. Concluding remarks by the chairman. *J Trauma* 1979; 19(suppl):935–936.
105. Shoemaker WC, Czer LC: Evaluation of the biologic importance of various hemodynamic and oxygen transport variables. *Crit Care Med* 1979; 7:424–431.
106. Sokawa M, Monafo E, Dietz F: The relationship between experimental fluid therapy and wound edema in scald wounds. *Ann Surg* 1981; 193:237–244.
107. Sotos JF, Dodge PR, Meara P, et al: Studies in experimental hypertonicity: I. Pathogenesis of the clinical syndrome, biochemical abnormalities, and cause of death. *Pediatrics* 1960; 26:925–938.
108. Stone HH: The composite burn solution, in Polk HC Jr, Stone HH (eds): *Contemporary Burn Management.* Boston, Little, Brown & Co, 1971, pp 93–104.
109. Stark H, Weinberger AH, Ben-Basset M: Persistent hyponatremia and inappropriate antidiuretic hormone secretion in children with extensive burns. *J Pediatr Surg* 1979; 14:149.
110. Stratta R, Saffle JR, Kravitz M, Ninnenmann JL, et al: Exchange transfusion therapy in pediatric burn shock. *Circ Shock* 1984; 12:203–212.
111. Talbot NB, Crawford JD, Butler AM: Medical progress: Homeostatic limits to safe parental fluid therapy. *N Engl J Med* 1953; 248:1100–1108.
112. Tranbaugh RF, Lewis FR, Christensen JM, et al: Lung water changes after thermal injury—the effects of crystalloid resuscitation and sepsis. *Ann Surg* 1980; 192:479–490.
113. Traber DL, Bohs CT, Carvajal HF, et al. Nicotinic acid-mannitol supplement in postburn resuscitation: A double blind study in sheep. *Burns* 1979; 5:299–307.
114. Turner R, Carvajal HF, Traber DL: Effects of ganglionic blockade upon renal and cardiovascular dysfunction induced by thermal injury. *Circ Shock* 1977; 4:103–113.
115. Underhill FP, Kapsinow R, Fisk ME: Studies

on the mechanism of water exchange in the animal organism: II. Changes in capillary permeability produced by a superficial burn. *Am J Physiol* 1930; 95:315–324.
116. Welch KJ: Thermal burns, in Benson CD, Mustard WT, Ravitch MM, (eds): *Pediatric Surgery*. Chicago, Year Book Medical Publishers, 1962, vol 1, pp 53–70.
117. Worden GD, Stratta RJ, Saffle JR, et al: Plasma exchange therapy in patients foiling to resuscitate from burn shock. *J Trauma* 1983; 23:945–951.
118. Yoshioka T, Maemura K, Ohhashi Y, et al: Effect of intravenously administered fluid on hemodynamic change and respiratory function in extensive thermal injury. *Surg Gynecol Obstet* 1980; 151(4):503–507.
119. Zarins CK, Rice CL, Peters RM, et al: Lymph and pulmonary resp. to isobaric reduction in plasma oncotic pressure in baboons. *Circ Res* 1978; 43:925–930.

7 / Resuscitation of the Burned Child

HUGO F. CARVAJAL, M.D.

EMERGENCY MEASURES

It is imperative that care be administered in an orderly fashion (Table 7–1). The number one priority of care is establishment of an adequate airway. This is particularly important in case of flame burns when the injury is incurred indoors (enclosed space), and the possibility of smoke inhalation exists. All unconscious patients must be intubated immediately, and those with physical evidence of smoke inhalation should undergo careful evaluation of the respiratory system to determine whether or not an artificial airway is needed.[49] Severe bronchospasm and progressive edema of the upper airway are common complications of smoke inhalation or inhalation of heated air or steam and must be anticipated.[43] All patients requiring cardiopulmonary resuscitation (CPR) at the site of the accident, regardless of the severity or time factor, must remain intubated and mechanically ventilated for 3 to 5 days postinjury.

Simultaneously with evaluation of the respiratory status, cardiac hemodynamics must be assessed, and the patient must be inspected for previously unrecognized injuries. An intravenous (IV) line is then inserted, and administration of isotonic fluids or plasma is begun. It is important to record the type and amount of fluid remaining in IV bags that are exchanged. A safe rate of fluid administration (unlikely to result in complications) is 600 ml/sq m of body surface per hour, or 20 ml/kg/hour. This rate can be maintained for up to 2 hours until more precise calculations for fluid therapy can be made. Simultaneously, the stomach should be emptied via a nasogastric tube to prevent dilatation, vomiting, and/or aspiration of gastric contents, and a small quantity of an antacid left in the stomach (i.e., Maalox, 30 ml/sq m of body surface) to retard the development of stress ulcers.[7, 36, 46, 57]

An indwelling urinary catheter is then inserted (closed system), the bladder emptied, and the time noted. A complete urinalysis is usually obtained at this time, but it is preferable to await the production of a fresh urine sample. Since the quantities of fluids and medications to be administered are better estimated according to the size of the patient and the extent of the injury, the weight and height must be measured carefully and the body surface area (BSA) in square meters calculated (Fig 7–1). Whenever possible, weight should be obtained before dressings, bedclothing, or restraints are applied and afterward, as well. Thereafter, the wounds are cleansed and debrided, their depth assessed, and the extent of second- and third-degree burns is estimated using body surface charts corrected for age (Fig 7–2).

Since an accurate assessment of the extent of the injury is essential to successful fluid resuscitation, whenever possible the wounds should be mapped by two independent observers (Fig 7–3). The "rule of nines" designed for adults is not applicable to children. A modified version, originally proposed by Parks et al.,[41] may be used under field conditions to estimate the extent of the burn, but it is not optimal. The most accurate method, which takes into consideration appropriate body proportions for age, was described by Lund and Browder.[35] The body proportions corresponding to the age groups depicted in

TABLE 7–1.
Priorities of Medical Procedures in the Emergency Phase of Pediatric Burn Injuries*

PROCEDURE	INDICATION	COMMENT
Establish an adequate airway	Burns of the face Laryngeal edema Smoke inhalation	Intubate early; beware of bronchospasm; avoid emergency tracheostomy
Examine for trauma to head, skeleton, or nervous system	Loss of consciousness Explosions	Remove clothing; radiologic examination helpful
Begin intravenous infusion	To prevent or correct intravascular dehydration	Use isotonic fluids
Empty stomach through a nasogastric tube	To prevent gastric dilation, vomiting, or aspiration	Follow with antacids at 1–2 hr intervals
Insert an indwelling Foley catheter	To monitor hourly urine output	Use a closed drainage system; beware of a state of antidiuresis
Examine the burn wound	To estimate depth and extent	Use burn charts corrected for age
Clean, debride, and dress the burn area	To minimize microbial colonization	Use topical antimicrobial therapy
Administer medications	To treat infections; to prevent tetanus; for sedation and analgesia	Use intravenous route for sedation
Begin fluid, electrolyte, and protein administration	To replace antecedent deficits and concurrent losses	Use isotonic fluids containing colloid and appropriate formulas to estimate fluid requirements

*Adapted from Carvajal HF, Goldman AS: Burns, in Vaughan VC III, McKay RJ (eds): *Nelson Textbook of Pediatrics*, ed 10. Philadelphia, WB Saunders, 1975, pp 279–284. Used by permission.

Figure 7–2 are thus used to evaluate the extent of the injury (second- and third-degree burns only). Severe burns exceeding 60% of the body surface are more conveniently mapped by estimating the nonburned areas.

Circumferential deep second- or third-degree burns must be evaluated and their tourniquet effect recognized to avoid limb ischemia or respiratory embarrassment resulting from chest wall involvement. Whenever appropriate, escharotomies must be performed early, as edema is bound to decrease blood supply and further compromise circulation to viable tissues.[41] The wounds are then cleansed, debrided, and covered with dressings saturated with an antimicrobial agent (see Chapter 9, "Topical Antimicrobials"). If there are no injuries to the central nervous system, sedatives may be given, preferably by the IV route. For analgesia, morphine (0.05 to 0.1 mg/kg of body weight) may be given, but in most cases valium (5 mg/sq m of body surface, per dose, q 6–8 hours) is sufficient to control pain and anxiety.

Although the risk of tetanus following burns is small, we continue to recommend tetanus prophylaxis in the form of tetanus toxoid (diphtheria-pertussis-tetanus vaccine [DPT]) for children less than 6 years of age and tetanus-diphtheria vaccine (TD) for older children and adults if 5 years have elapsed since the last booster injection. Passive protection with tetanus immunoglobulin (TIG) is indicated only when the patient has had less than two previous injections of tetanus toxoid. The recommended dose for TIG is 250 to 500 units

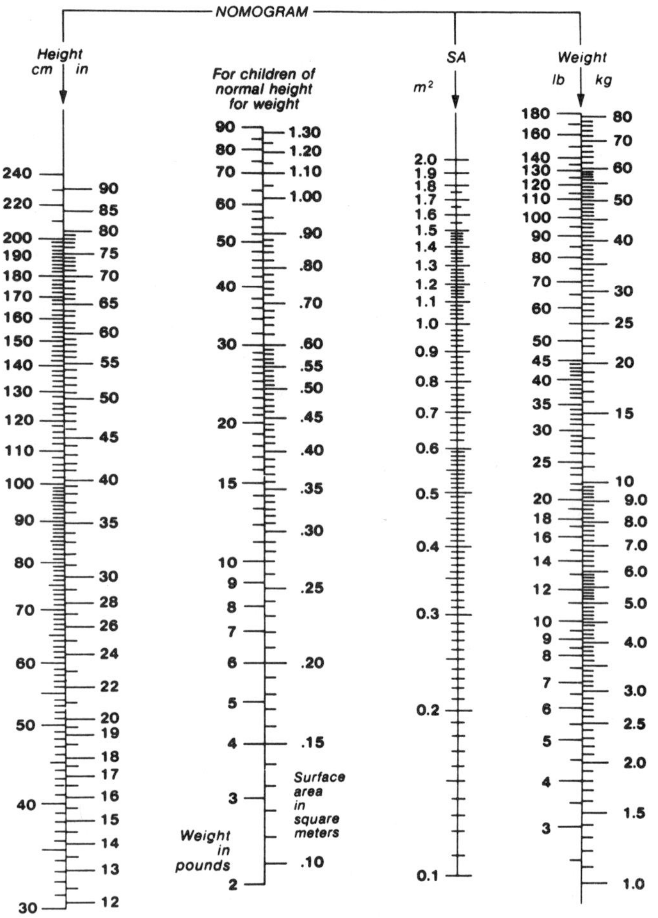

FIG 7–1.
Surface area nomogram.

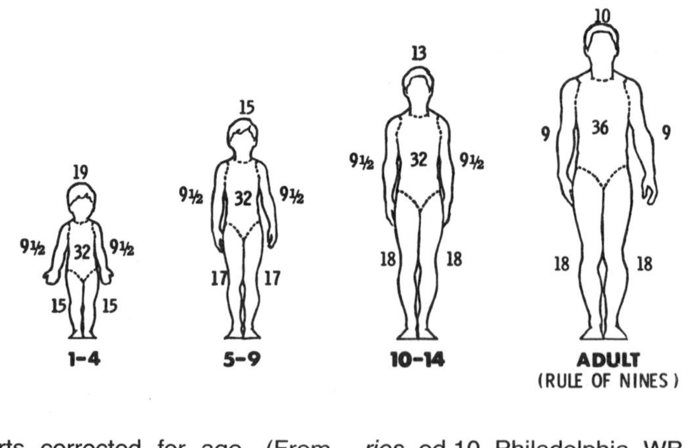

FIG 7–2.
Body surface charts corrected for age. (From Carvajal HF, Goldman AS: Burns, in Vaughan VC III, McKay RJ (eds): *Nelson Textbook of Pediatrics,* ed 10. Philadelphia, WB Saunders Co, 1975, pp 279–284. Used by permission.)

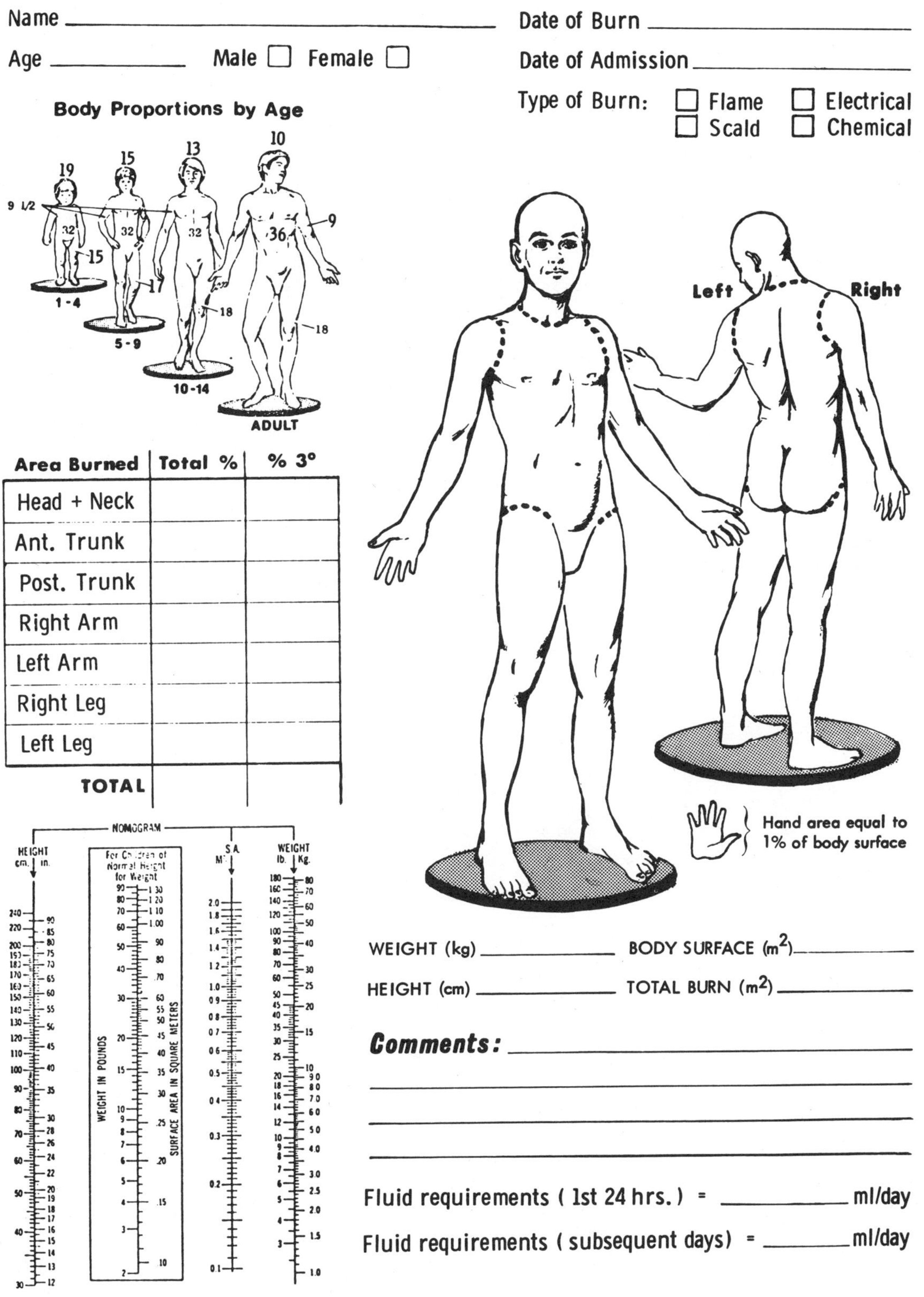

Name ______________________ Date of Burn ______________________

Age __________ Male ☐ Female ☐ Date of Admission ______________________

Type of Burn: ☐ Flame ☐ Electrical ☐ Scald ☐ Chemical

Area Burned	Total %	% 3°
Head + Neck		
Ant. Trunk		
Post. Trunk		
Right Arm		
Left Arm		
Right Leg		
Left Leg		
TOTAL		

WEIGHT (kg) __________ BODY SURFACE (m^2) __________

HEIGHT (cm) __________ TOTAL BURN (m^2) __________

Comments: ______________________

Fluid requirements (1st 24 hrs.) = __________ ml/day

Fluid requirements (subsequent days) = __________ ml/day

FIG 7–3.
Burn assessment chart. (From Carvajal HF: Fluid therapy for the acutely burned child. *Compr Ther* 1977; 3:17–24. Used by permission.)

Physical Findings in Acute Dehydration

Severity of Dehydration	Mucose Membrane	Skin Turgor	Fontanelle	Heart Rate	Urine Output	Sensorium	Respirations	Body Temp.
Mild (3-5% Acute Weight Loss)	*Dry	*Decreased	N	N	N	N	N	N
Moderate (6-10% Acute Weight Loss)	Dry	Decreased	*Sunken	*Tachycardia	*Oliguria	*Lethargy	*Tachypnea	*Fever
Severe (11-15% Acute Weight Loss)	Parched	Poor	Sunken	Tachycardia	*Periods of Anuria (6-12 hrs.)	*Stupor and Irritability	*Deep and Pauseless (Kussmaul)	*Fever
Extreme (> 16% Acute Weight Loss)	Parched	Poor	Sunken	Rapid and Thready Pulse	Anuria for > 12 hours	*Coma Moribund	*Slow and Shallow	Fever or *Hypothemia

*Indicates physical findings required to acertain the diagnosis.

Severity of Dehydration	Tears	Eyes	Blood Pressure	Peripheral Circulation
Mild (3-5% Acute Weight Loss)	N	N	N	N
Moderate (6-10% Acute Weight Loss)	N	N	N	N
Severe (11-15% Acute Weight Loss)	*Absent	*Sunken	*Hypotension	*Decreased Perfusion
Extreme (> 16% Acute Weight Loss)	Absent	Sunken	Shock	*Mottling and Cyanosis

FIG 7–4.
Dehydration assessment chart.

given intramuscularly. A single dose of benzathine penicillin (1.2 million units intramuscularly) is also recommended to eradicate β-hemolytic streptococci and prevent colonization of the wounds with this organism.

OBJECTIVES OF FLUID RESUSCITATION

The ultimate goal of fluid resuscitation is restoration of body homeostasis. This is achieved by replacing antecedent deficits and concurrent losses of fluid, electrolytes, and protein resulting from the burn. In addition, normal water and electrolyte losses must be simultaneously replaced. Exaggerated losses resulting from the injury itself, the abnormal physiologic state, or certain treatment modalities must be anticipated and replaced before significant deficits develop.

Depending on the extent and severity of the injury and the time elapsed before therapy is instituted, the burned child is at risk of developing variable degrees of intravascular volume deficits. The physical findings that are associated with mild to extreme dehydration are depicted in Figure 7–4.

In an effort to minimize and protect the body from the effects of dehydration and volume contraction, compensatory mechanisms are brought into play.[18] These mechanisms remain operational until fluid and electrolyte balance is restored. Thus the objectives of therapy must be coordinated with and complement the body's attempt to compensate for the physiologic derangement. For example, if as a result of the injury, severely damaged capillaries are "physiologically amputated" from the rest of the body by preferential perfusion of nondamaged vessels,[30] fluid therapy should not interfere or counteract this response. This is particularly important when considering the time interval during which replacement of losses must be accomplished. Animal studies have demonstrated that restoration of cardiac output to normal can be attained within a few hours of the burn,[39, 55] but the physiologic cost of such an accomplishment has not been fully evaluated. Even in the presence of significant fluid deficits, rapid fluid infusion may worsen, instead of improve, the physiologic derangement.[44]

Specifically, fluid resuscitation should attain and maintain a normal or near normal state of hydration in all body fluid compartments, correct acid-base imbalances, and restore cardiovascular, pulmonary, and renal hemodynamics. However, these objectives should be accomplished at the least possible physiologic cost and without adding further pathology *(primum non nocere)*. Restoration of perfusion pressures should lead to maximal oxygenation of injured and noninjured tissues; it should facilitate spontaneous healing, prevent wound conversion, minimize bacterial colonization of the wound, and prepare the injured areas for early grafting (Table 7–2).

Rehydration should be accomplished without overloading the circulation and preferably over a period of 24 hours. Attempts to replace deficits over shorter periods of time are usually fraught with multiple complications, including excessive edema formation, and should be discouraged.

It must be emphasized that restoration of fluid and electrolyte balance and organ function does not necessarily imply a return to normal of all physiologic variables. Oliguria, for example, may persist for 48 to 72 hours or even longer after the burn as a result of excessive secretion of antidiuretic hormone (ADH).[7] Cardiac output may increase beyond preburn levels within 24 hours of the injury and a state of hypercatabolism may persist for several days after the burn. Thus, the physician's expectations should take into consideration not only the physiologic makeup of the child, which differs significantly from that of the adult, but also the specific responses of the various organs to the burn injury.

TABLE 7–2.
Objectives of Fluid Resuscitation

General
To replace antecedent and concurrent deficits of fluid, electrolytes, and proteins, and restore body homeostasis
To anticipate and replace maintenance fluid and electrolyte requirements before significant deficits develop
To prevent or minimize organ dysfunction and edema formation
Specific
To attain and maintain a normal or near normal state of hydration in all body fluid compartments
To correct acid-base imbalance
To restore and preserve cardiovascular, pulmonary, and kidney function
To restore perfusion pressures for maximal oxygenation of injured and noninjured tissues, in order to attain spontaneous healing of as much burned area as possible; to prevent wound conversion; to minimize wound colonization; and to prepare the injured areas for early grafting

During this time, errors in fluid therapy may have grave consequences. Underhydration can prolong the state of shock, worsen the metabolic acidosis, and induce organ dysfunction, while overhydration fosters edema formation and pulmonary congestion.

Accurate prediction of fluid requirements is particularly difficult in burned children because most fluid resuscitation formulas have been designed for adult individuals (e.g., Brooke and Parkland formulas), and their estimates of fluid needs are based solely on body weight and percentage of body surface burned. Furthermore, current versions of these formulas make no separate allowances for maintenance fluids and the fluid needed to replace burn-related losses; thus they tend to underhydrate small children and to overestimate fluid requirements for the large or obese child. (See Chapter 6, "Controversies in Fluid Resuscitation and Their Impact on Pediatric Populations.") Similar errors are also likely to be committed at the extremes of burn size. For these and other reasons we do not recommend the use of "single-figure" formulas such as the Parkland or the modified Brooke formula for hydration of burned children.

Compared to adults, children (and particularly infants) have high rates of heat exchange relative to size and weight and high rates of water exchange in relation to total body water.[13] Muscle water and electrolyte composition is also different in children compared to adults.[14, 15] Children also require relatively larger volumes of urine for excretion of waste products, and insensible water losses when expressed in terms of body weight are significantly greater in children than in adults.[18] For these reasons, estimates of fluid and electrolyte requirements based on energy expenditures of body surface rather than body weight offer greater accuracy, consistency, and simplicity.

FLUID REPLACEMENT PROGRAM FOR CHILDREN

A program for fluid replacement specifically designed for children, which takes into consideration the physiologic responses associated with the burn injury, was developed by Carvajal[5] in 1975. We have used this program to hydrate burned children for over 10 consecutive years and continue to obtain excellent results.[7, 8] The key features of this program follow.

Estimate of Total Fluid Requirements

Fluid requirements are estimated according to a simplified formula[6] based on total BSA and BSA *burned* in square meters. The BSA is estimated taking into account the patient's height and weight and a standard surface area nomogram (See Fig 7–1). The extent of the burn is estimated using body proportions corrected for age (see Fig 7–2); and the BSA burned is calculated by multiplying the percent burn times the BSA.

Total fluid requirements for the first day are estimated as follows:

5,000 ml/sq m of body surface *burned* per 24 hours (burn-related losses)
+
2,000 ml/sq m of total *body surface* per 24 hours (maintenance fluids)

Half of the 24-hour fluid allowance is administered during the first 8 hours, and the other half during the subsequent 16 hours (Fig 7–5). No ceiling for burn size is used. All fluids (composite burn solution) are administered intravenously and with the exception of an antacid (Maalox, 30 ml/sq m of BSA per hour for the first 24 hours), the patient receives nothing by mouth. Fluid received prior to arrival at a center for definitive care must be reviewed and whenever appropriate, adjustments are made. (See section on pitfalls of fluid therapy during the first 24 hours.)

EXAMPLE.—A one-year-old child (10 kg) with a BSA of 0.47 sq m sustained full-thickness flame burns to approximately 35% of his body surface. Despite having received 100 ml of lactated Ringer's solution during the first hour postinjury, he appeared dehydrated on admission. The following calculations are used to determine total fluid requirements:

1. Fluids received during the initial evaluation period (lactated Ringer's solution, saline, or plasma) need not be included in the calculation of requirements for the first 24 hours. These fluids may be given at rate of approximately 20 ml/kg/hour or 600 ml/sq m/hour for 1 to 2 hours.
2. Estimation of first 24 hours' requirements:
   Burn-related losses (5,000 ml/sq m of body surface *burned* per 24 hours)

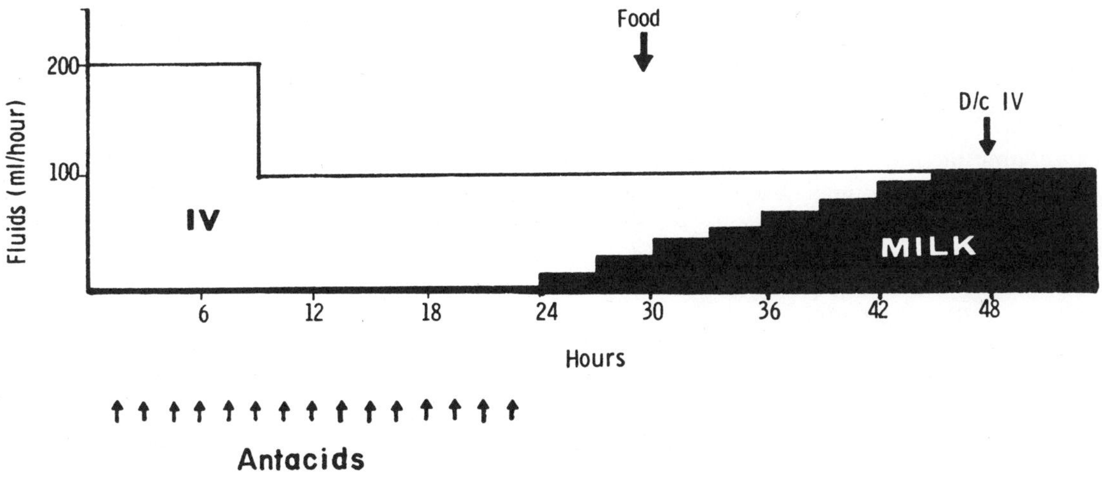

FIG 7–5.
Rate of fluid administration. Half of the first day fluid estimate is administered intravenously (IV) during the first 8 hours postinjury. The other half is given during the subsequent 16 hours. Homogenized milk by mouth and food are begun during the second day. Only antacids are given per orum during the first day. D/c = discontinue. (From Carvajal HF: A physiologic approach to fluid therapy in severely burned children. *Surg Gynecol Obstet* 1980; 150:379–384. Used by permission.)

Hypothetical example: 5,000 × 0.47 × 0.35 = 820 ml/24 hours

Maintenance fluids (2,000 ml/sq m of *total* body surface per 24 hours)

Hypothetical example: 2,000 × 0.47 = 940 ml/24 hours

Thus in this hypothetical case total estimates for the first 24 hours, (burn-related losses plus maintenance fluids) are 820 ml + 940 ml = 1,760 ml.

3. Half of the estimated amount (880 ml) is given during the first 8 hours, and the other half during the subsequent 16 hours.

   Hypothetical example:

   First 8 hours = 110 ml/hour
   Second 8 hours = 55 ml/hour
   Third 8 hours = 55 ml/hour

Although this method for estimating fluids offers definite advantages in children, it still provides only reasonable estimates of the quantities of fluid needed for the first 24 hours postinjury. Successful resuscitation of the child requires not only the use of an appropriate formula, but also a clear understanding of the fluid therapy program as a whole and particularly the methods used to assess the hydration status of the patient.

Composition of Hydrating Solution

The program we follow uses only one hydrating solution (composite solution) for the first 24 hours. This is an isotonic glucose-containing solution to which a *moderate* amount of colloid (human serum albumin) is added. The solution is prepared by mixing 50 ml of 25% human serum albumin (12.5 gm) with 950 ml of 5% dextrose in lactated Ringer's injection. The electrolyte, glucose, and protein content of this mixture are as follows:

Na^+	132.0 mEq/L
Cl^-	109.0 mEq/L
Lactate	26.6 mEq/L
K^+	3.8 mEq/L
Glucose	47.5 gm/L
Albumin	12.5 gm/L

In infants less than 1 year of age, the concentration of sodium in the hydrating solution must be lowered; otherwise, hypernatremia is likely to develop in the second or third day postinjury. In this age group (less than 12 months of age), we recommend a solution prepared by mixing 930 ml of 5% dextrose and 0.33% sodium chloride injection, 20 ml of sodium bicarbonate injection (1 mEq/ml) and 50 ml of 25% human serum albumin. The final composition of this mixture is shown in the following tabulation.

Na^+	81 mEq/L
Cl^-	61 mEq/L
HCO_3^-	20 mEq/L
K^+	0
Glucose	46.5 gm/L
Albumin	12.5 gm/L

Since large amounts of potassium are released from injured cells into extracellular fluids, *no additional potassium should be added to the hydrating solutions during the first 12 to 24 hours* postburn and certainly not before normal kidney function has been ascertained. After the first 12 to 24 hours 20 to 30 mEq of potassium *phosphate* may be added to each liter of IV fluids. The use of phosphate instead of chloride is recommended to prevent the development of significant hypophosphatemia and its consequential effects on cell function (Table 7–3). Plasma and urine glucose levels should be monitored and in the rare cases of intolerance,[1, 50] glucose must be omitted from the hydrating fluids. However, in children, this is not usually a problem.

TABLE 7–3.
Effects of Phosphate Depletion on Cell Metabolism*

Somatic Cell
Decreased function
Adenosine triphosphate (ATP) depletion
Erythrocytes
Inhibition of glycolysis
ATP depletion
Decreased 2, 3-diphosphoglyceric acid (DPG)
Tissue hypoxia
Changes in intracellular cation concentration
Spherical shape
Decreased survival
Leukocytes
Decreased chemotaxis
Decreased phagocytic activity
Platelets
Decreased function

*Adapted from Kreusser W, Ritz E: The phosphate-depletion syndrome. *Contrib Nephrol* 1978, 14:162–174.

A major advantage of using a composite solution is that fluids, electrolytes, and albumin can be simultaneously replaced in quantities that approximate the patient's losses. The rate of infusion, then, is the only adjustment necessary, and the total volume needed can be prepared in advance. This method also avoids so-called "piggy-backs" and allows more accurate control of fluid intake.

Guidelines to Fluid Resuscitation

Monitoring the results of fluid therapy in the burned patient represents a significant challenge to the burn team. This is because no single criterion can be used to predict the state of hydration consistently or accurately, and it becomes necessary that as many indicators as possible be correlated before making a decision to increase or decrease the quantities of fluid to be administered (Table 7–4).

TABLE 7–4.
Noninvasive Guides to Fluid Resuscitation Therapy in Burned Children

Vital signs
Pulse
Respiration
Temperature
Blood pressure
Physical examination
General appearance
State of sensorium
Peripheral circulation (venous capillary filling)
Body weight
Laboratory data
Hematocrit
Bun,* UUN*
Blood pH and gases
Serum and urine osmolality
Serum and urine electrolytes
Urine specific gravity
Fluid losses
Gastric losses
Urine volume at 2-4 hr intervals
Stool losses (diarrhea)

*BUN indicates blood urea nitrogen; UUN, urine urea nitrogen.

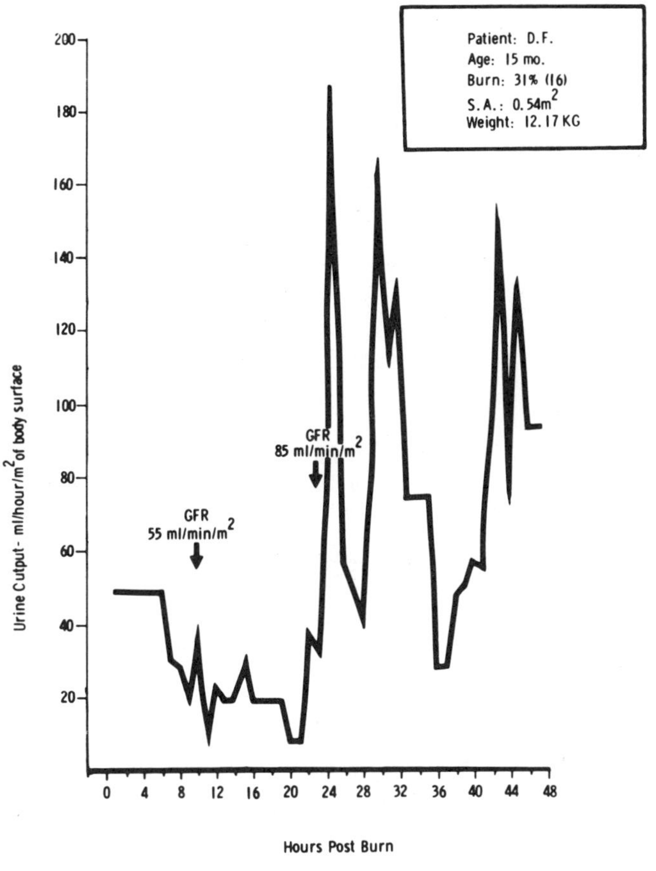

FIG 7–6.
Hourly urine output in a 15-month old infant who sustained a 31% burn scald and was successfully resuscitated using the surface area formula and program for fluid replacement. Notice that hourly urine volume varied widely, despite constant fluid administration and normal glomerular filtration rate.

The hourly urine volume is not a good predictor because the kidneys are under the influence of exaggerated hormonal responses, which for the most part correlate poorly with the state of hydration (Figs 7–6 and 7–7).

Under most circumstances, normally functioning kidneys are able to excrete water and sodium loads over a relatively short period of time (3 to 6 hours). However, if excessive quantities of ADH are secreted, oliguria may persist despite intravascular volume expansion. While in most other conditions this would soon lead to cardiopulmonary congestion and even heart failure,[19, 24] in burned patients the increase in vascular permeability effectively removes the excess fluid from the circulation. Burn edema develops, and the fluid administered follows the path of least resistance, which in the presence of the syndrome of inappropriate antidiuretic hormone (SIADH) would be the interstitial or even the intracellular fluid compartments (Fig 7–8). Although urine production cannot be completely disregarded, it must be recognized that at least during the immediate postburn period an obligatory oliguria (antidiuresis) is part of the overall clinical response (Fig 7–9).

Human[7] and animal studies[11] have further shown that the hourly urine volume varies greatly from one hour to another despite constant fluid administration (see Figs 7–6 and 7–7). This may be due to intermittent secretion of ADH, rapid degradation of the hormone, and/or reflex-mediated changes in renal hemodynamics.[11, 55]

Despite marked fluctuations in hourly urine volume, relatively constant 8-hour volumes (Fig 7–10) are often attained.[6] This ob-

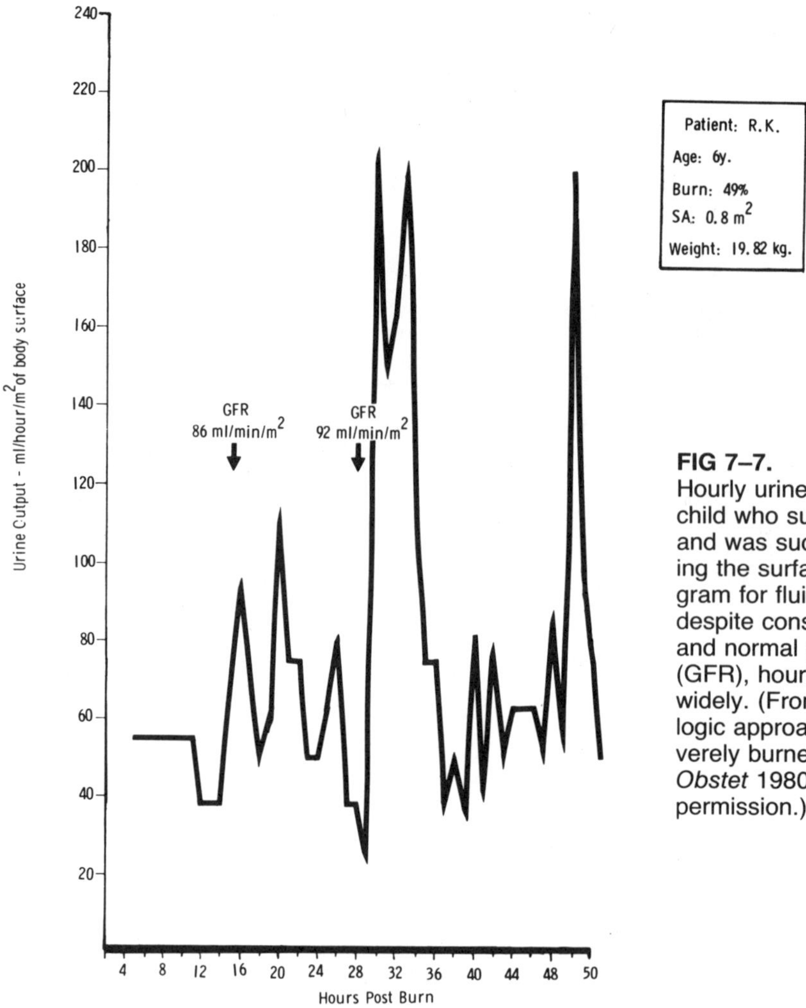

FIG 7–7.
Hourly urine output in a 6-year-old child who sustained a 49% flame burn and was successfully resuscitated using the surface area formula and program for fluid replacement. Notice that despite constant fluid administration and normal glomerular filtration rate (GFR), hourly urine volumes varied widely. (From Carvajal HF: A physiologic approach to fluid therapy in severely burned children. *Surg Gynecol Obstet* 1980, 150:379–384. Used by permission.)

servation supports the contention that under conditions of stress, the kidneys cannot be depended upon to correct errors in hydration.[38] Thus the physician's expectations regarding urine production should be in line with the functional capacity of the kidney under hormonal and sympathetic influences. Fluid pushes should be avoided, as they can result in rapid expansion of the intravascular compartment, which may in turn lead to increased losses of fluid into the interstitium (see Fig 7–8).

Although none of the many variables used to guide hydration are consistently accurate by themselves, when several variables are correlated as a group, and trends instead of individual measurements are used, the state of hydration can be more precisely assessed (see Table 7–4). The general appearance of the patient and the state of sensorium provide valuable information regarding fluid balance. For example, a conscious and alert child who is responsive to commands is usually well hydrated; the lethargic, thirsty, and anxious patient with decreased capillary filling and/or evidence of peripheral vascular insufficiency (cold, dry, discolored, and mottled skin) is obviously dehydrated (see Fig 7–4). A rapid, thready pulse and a high respiratory rate would also be indicative of volume contrac-

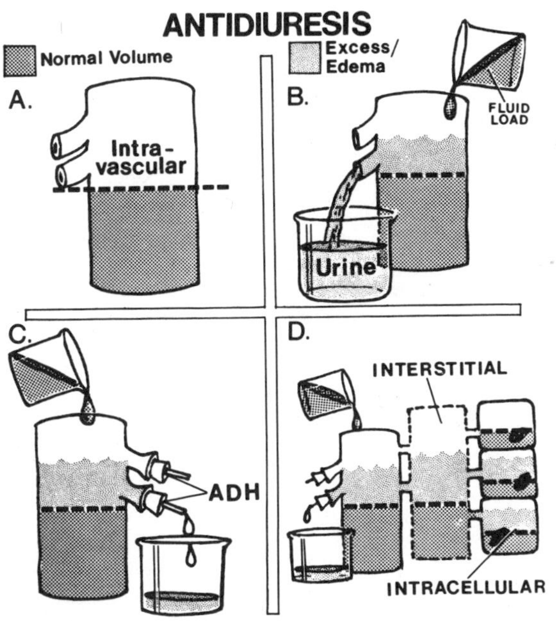

FIG 7–8.
Schematic representation of normal fluid volume *(A)* and the effect of an intravenous fluid load in a normal individual *(B)*, in the presence of exaggerated secretion of ADH *(C)*, and exaggerated ADH secretion plus increased vascular permeability and disruption of the cell membrane as seen in burn injuries *(D)*. In the latter condition, the path of least resistance for a fluid load is the interstitial (burn edema) and intracellular compartments (cell edema), rather than excretion via the kidney.

tion. The mean arterial pressure does not change significantly until the degree of volume deficit exceeds 11% to 12% of normal, but in most cases a reduced pulse pressure can be an early clue of intravascular volume deficit. In the absence of renal failure, a moderate increase in blood urea nitrogen (BUN) would be indicative of a reduction in renal blood flow and glomerular filtration rate characteristic of dehydration. A hypercatabolic state and/or renal insufficiency can be ruled out by measuring urine urea nitrogen (UUN), urine and plasma osmolality, and urinary electrolytes. In the presence of oliguria, a high urine sodium greater than 30 mEq/L, coupled with isosthenuria (urine osmolality ~300 mOsm/L), and a UUN/BUN ratio of less than 10 would be indicative of acute renal failure, while dehydration is characterized by a low urinary sodium, high urine osmolality, and a UUN/BUN ratio in excess of 20.

A high hematocrit due to fluid, electrolytes, and protein escaping the intravascular compartment is usually seen during the immediate postburn period.[7, 23] As the intravascular volume is restored the hematocrit progressively declines (Fig 7–11). Failure to demonstrate this change would be indicative of persistent volume deficit. Certain variables can be misleading. For example, a rising spe-

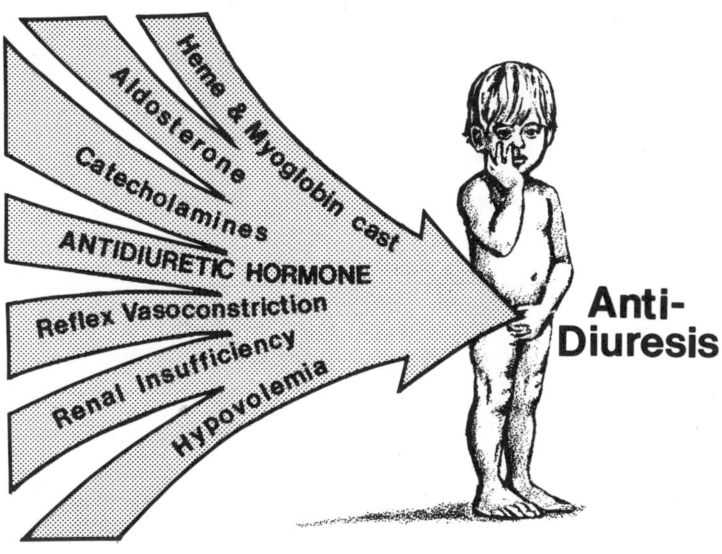

FIG 7–9.
Factors responsible for reduced urine production in burned patients.

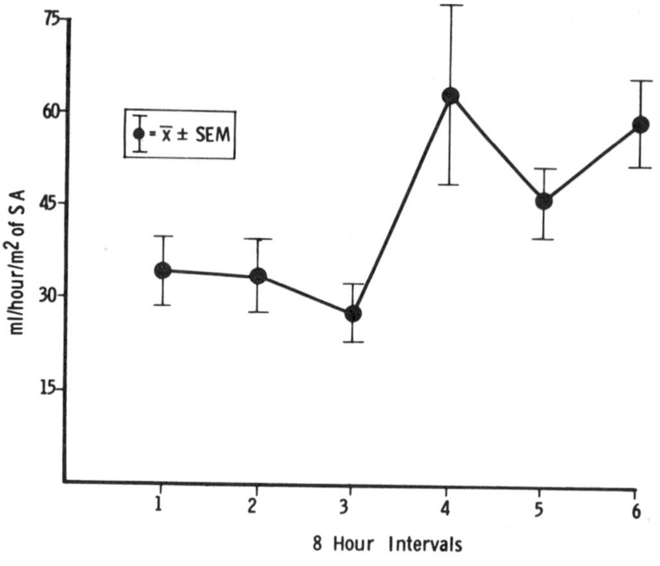

FIG 7–10.
Relatively constant 8-hour urine volumes. Urine volumes at 8-hour intervals in ten children with extensive burns (31%–90% BSA burned) who were successfully resuscitated according to the surface area formula. (From Carvajal HF: Fluid therapy for acutely burned child. *Compr Ther* 1977; 3:17–24. Used by permission.)

cific gravity or urine osmolality usually indicates secretion of ADH, but not necessarily volume contraction.[24] If present, the latter can be confirmed by demonstrating a reduced urinary sodium (<20 mEq/L). Measurements of blood pH and gases also provide valuable information. In the absence of hypoxemia, the presence of a metabolic acidosis indicates poor peripheral perfusion, reduced kidney function, and lactic acid production.[42] A blood pH that is normal or progressing toward normal levels would be indicative of adequate perfusion and tissue oxygenation. Although the weight of the patient does not provide much information regarding the state of hydration, a baseline weight should be obtained. This measurement becomes increasingly more important after the second to third day postinjury.

PITFALLS OF FLUID THERAPY DURING THE FIRST 24 HOURS

Although fluid formulas should be considered only guides to resuscitation, agreement between the predicted (surface area formula)

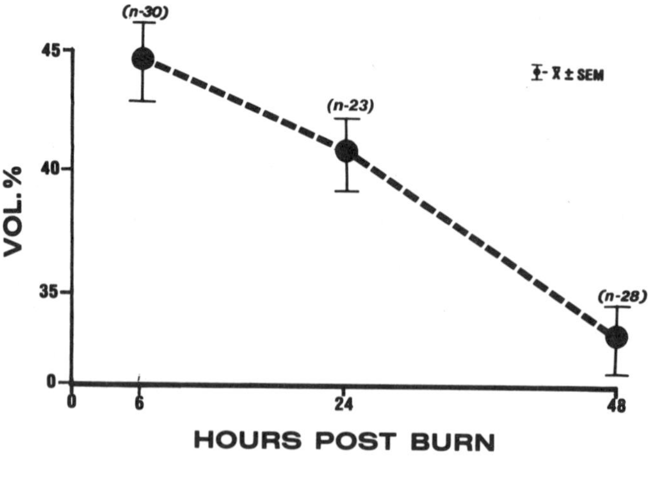

FIG 7–11.
Progressive drop in hematocrit as seen in 30 acutely burned children hydrated according to the surface area program (Adapted from Carvajal HF: A physiologic approach to fluid therapy in severely burned children. Surg Gynecol Obstet 1980; 150:379–384.)

and actual amounts of fluid needed for "successful" resuscitation has been excellent in children with burns up to 92% of their body surface, and seldom has it been necessary to alter the original fluid therapy plan because of underhydration or overhydration (Table 7–5). Nonetheless, errors can be committed. A discussion of the most frequent errors follows.

Errors in Measuring Body Surface Area

Surface area is better estimated with the use of standard nomograms (see Fig 7–1), which take into account the weight and height of the child. Most nomograms provide scales for weight in pounds and kilograms and for height in inches and centimeters. Thus, these variables must be carefully plotted to avoid errors. Some nomograms also allow for estimation of surface area based on weight alone (see Fig 7–1), and mathematical formulas (Lowe's formula) are also available to perform this calculation:

$$\text{Body surface area (sq m)} = 0.1 \times (\text{Wt}^2[\text{kg}])^{1/3}$$

The user must recognize that estimates based on weight alone may incur significant error unless the individual height and weight are in the 50th percentile for age.

Occasionally, particularly in critically ill children, weight measurements may not be possible or appropriate, and the weight has to be estimated. A simple rule of thumb to estimate the 50th percentile weight based on age (up to 10 years of age) is as follows:

$$\text{Female weight (kg)} = [\text{age (years)} \times 2] + 8$$
$$\text{Male weight (kg)} = [\text{age (years)} \times 2] + 9$$

Errors in Estimating the Extent of the Burn

Only second- and third-degree burns should be taken into account when estimating the total area burned. First-degree burns characterized by erythema (flash burns) should not be included. The use of appropriate body proportion charts corrected for age (see Fig 7–2) and careful mapping of the wounds (see Fig 7–3) by two independent observers should minimize errors in this regard.

Failure to Make Appropriate Corrections When Fluid Therapy Is Delayed or Fluid Administration Has Been Excessive

When fluid therapy is delayed or the patients have received insufficient quantities of fluids, they are often dehydrated and require extra fluids to rapidly expand their contracted intravascular volume, restore cardiovascular and renal hemodynamics, and combat acidosis. In most cases 20 ml/kg of body weight of an isotonic solution with or without colloid, administered over an hour will accomplish this goal.

Restoration of renal hemodynamics may not occur right away in the patient who has incurred a severe dehydration. Correction of acid/base imbalance and return of blood pressure to levels near normal should be considered a reasonable objective, which once attained should satisfy the initial resuscitation efforts. Thereafter, hydration should proceed as if the patient had just been burned and no delays had taken place (Fig 7–12).

On the other hand, patients who have received excessive quantities of fluids have already developed significant edema. For practical purposes, this fluid is not readily accessible to the circulation, and care must be exercised in making adjustments to the rate of fluid administration. Attempts to compensate for the extra fluid administered are not well tolerated, and in most cases it is better to disregard the excess fluids and proceed with the hydration plan (see Fig 7–10).

Failure to Make Appropriate Corrections in Cases of Vasomotor Nephropathy (Acute Renal Failure)

Though a rare occurrence, acute renal insufficiency manifested by anuria, marked oliguria, isosthenuria, and natriuresis should be

TABLE 7–5.
Relationship Between Age, Weight, Body Surface Area (BSA), Fluid Intake, Maximum Weight Gain (Edema), and Extent of the Burn in 30 Burned Children*

						FLUID INTAKE—FIRST 24 HR		FLUID INTAKE—SECOND 24 HR		
	BSA BURNED, %	THIRD-DEGREE BURN, %	AGE, YR	WEIGHT, KG	BSA, SQ M	PREDICTED†, ML	ACTUAL, ML	PREDICTED†, ML	ACTUAL, ML	MAX WEIGHT GAIN KG/SQ M BURNED
$\bar{x}$	46.0	23.0	7.0	28.5	0.98	4,130	3,968††	3,146	3,126	4.1
SEM	3.6	4.2	0.9	3.1	0.07	314	296	243	231	0.3
SD	19.8	23.2	4.8	17.0	0.40	1,720	1,620	1,332	1,266	1.7
Range	20–92	0–83	0–15	8–70	0.4–1.65	1,350–9,100	1,250–7,870	1,035–7,100	960–6,300	1.3–8.0

*From Carvajal HF: A physiologic approach to fluid therapy in severely burned children. *Surg Gynecol Obstet* 1980, 150:379–384. Used by permission.
†Predicted on the basis of the surface area formula.
††Equivalent to 3 ml/kg/% BSA burned/24 hr.

recognized early and before excessive fluid administration is undertaken.[27] If renal insufficiency develops, appropriate *reductions* in fluid intake to compensate for the lack of urine production (expected urine output should be 30 ml/sq m of body surface per hour) should be implemented to avoid overhydration.[34]

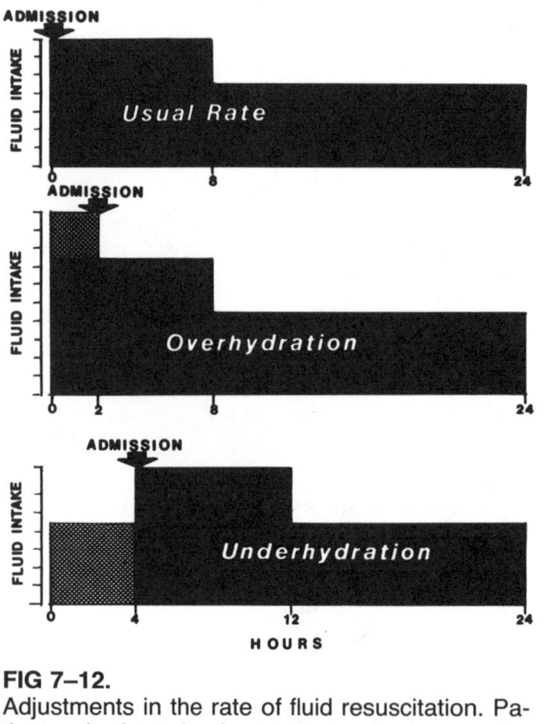

FIG 7–12.
Adjustments in the rate of fluid resuscitation. Patients who have inadvertently received excessive fluids must be adjusted to the usual rate without attempting to compensate for the excess fluid already received (overhydration). Delayed resuscitation or underhydration is usually managed by rapidly correcting the intravascular deficit over an hour and initiating resuscitation as if the patient had just been burned (underhydration).

Failure to Recognize That a State of Antidiuresis Is Invariably Present During the First 24 Hours Postinjury

Urine production equivalent to 120 ml/sq m of body surface per 4 *hours* (average 30 ± 15 ml/sq m of body surface per hour) must be considered adequate. Higher urine volumes are unlikely to be achieved without significant overhydration. As many variables as possible should be correlated before a decision is made to increase or decrease the rate of fluid administration. Fluid pushes are seldom, if ever, indicated.[7]

Failure to Recognize That Infants Under 1 Year of Age Require Lower Concentrations of Sodium in Hydrating Fluids

Infants have a large surface area-to-mass ratio (twofold to threefold as compared to the adult) and thus a high rate of heat exchange (water exchange). For example, the surface area-to-weight ratio for a 3-kg child is 0.2:3 or 0.07 and that for a 70-kg adult is 1.9:70 or 0.027. Thus, the infant's weight is only 4% that of the adult, but his surface area is 11% of the adult's. These differences become narrower as the child gets older, but remain significant for the first 5 years of life. In infants obligatory fluid losses are magnified by higher metabolic rates, higher osmolar loads presented to the kidney, and relatively immature kidney function. All of these factors decrease the infant's and young child's margin of safety and favor the occurrence of dehydration and electrolyte imbalance if intake of fluid is curtailed or relatively hypertonic solutions are administered. Thus we recommend that the concentration of sodium and chloride in resuscitation fluids for children under 1 year of age be reduced, but some children between 12 and 24 months of age have relatively immature kidney function and may require similar adjustments, as well.[53]

Failure to Recognize That Smoke Inhalation Requires Adjustments in Fluid Therapy

Although several authors recommend a reduction in the volume of fluids to be administered to patients with evidence of smoke inhalation, this may or may not be indicated. Pulmonary edema is a common early complication of smoke inhalation, which in most cases is not preventable.[33] If present, pulmonary edema may, depending on its severity, increase fluid requirements. However, edema fluid is not static, and in most cases pulmonary lymph flow increases to compensate for the increased fluid flux through damaged pulmonary capillaries.[58] What is often overlooked is that the administration of fully humidified air-oxygen mixtures to mechanically ventilated patients significantly reduces their pulmonary insensible losses, and they may effectively end up with a positive fluid balance. Also, positive-pressure ventilation and high positive end-expiratory pressure (PEEP) levels decrease venous return to the heart and produce discomfort and anxiety, all of which increase the secretion of ADH and result in a further reduction in the production of urine. Thus in general, mild smoke inhalation may increase fluid requirements by increasing the respiratory rate, the work of breathing, and, consequently, energy expenditure. On the contrary, patients with severe smoke inhalation often need mechanical ventilatory support, analgesics, and muscle relaxants, which may actually decrease their insensible water losses. These patients may require a reduction in the volume of resuscitation fluids.[25, 51] In the latter case, we usually recommend a reduction in fluid intake of approximately 500 ml/sq m of body surface area per 24 hours; while in cases of mild smoke inhalation, we monitor the patient closely and are more willing to increase fluid intake from the total amount estimated by the surface area formula.

Failure to Recognize That Electrical Injuries Result in Considerably More Tissue Damage Than Is Apparent and Thus Require More Fluids for Resuscitation

The severity of an electrical injury is dependent on the extent and depth of the skin damage caused by the electrical arc and the type and amount of cell and organ damage.[3] While the degree and extent of surface damage is obvious, damage to deep structures is practically impossible to assess accurately and may be compared to crush injuries.[2] Complete destruction and obliteration of capillaries and surrounding structures complicate matters further as the degree of fluid and protein extravasation (edema formation) is related not only to the extent of tissue damage, but also to the patency of the blood vessels at the site of the injury. The development of hemoglobinemia and myoglobinemia and formation of casts, which may completely obstruct the renal tubules and often lead to severe oliguria and renal failure, add further confusion to the diagnostic dilemma.

Fortunately and despite the difficulties discussed above, most electrical injuries are limited to small areas of the body. Extensive electrical burns are usually fatal, with most patient's dying at the scene of the accident. Thus, from the fluid resuscitation standpoint, there is leeway, and prevention of renal insufficiency becomes the most important priority.[2, 17] Our approach to the management of these patients is to overestimate the injury by 25% to 50% and to ensure a forced diuresis, aimed at flushing the renal tubules of myoglobin and hemoglobin by-products. This can be attained by the administration of either mannitol in doses of 0.5 to 1.0 gm/kg of body weight or furosemide, 1 mg/kg of body weight, or both, at repeated intervals for as long as hemoglobinuria or myoglobinuria are evident. In most cases, a high fluid intake plus the administration of these two diuretics is sufficient to clear the abnormal proteins from the urine and obviate renal insufficiency.

We do not use sodium bicarbonate, hypertonic saline, or acetazolamide therapy, nor do we attempt to maintain the urine output at any given level. In the rare case in which severe oliguria or anuria unresponsive to diuretic therapy develops and the condition of the patient does not allow for a clinical assessment of the degree of volume deficit, hemodynamic monitoring with the Swan-Ganz catheter is used to guide subsequent fluid replacement and ensure hemodynamic stability.

FLUID, ELECTROLYTE, AND PROTEIN REPLACEMENT DURING THE SECOND AND SUBSEQUENT DAYS

Fluid and Electrolyte Replacement

In children, fluid requirements during the second day postinjury and subsequent days amount to approximately three quarters of the first day estimates. This volume is slightly higher than what has been recommended for adult individuals.[54] The differences are due to the large surface area-to-mass ratio of children as compared to adults, their higher rates of heat exchange, and their increased obligatory fluid losses. Despite the increased fluid requirements, maximum weight gain (edema) usually occurs within 2 to 3 days postinjury. Thereafter a daily reduction in weight should follow (diuretic phase) until the 13 to 14 day postburn, at which point the patient's preburn weight (dry weight) is usually attained (see weight profile, Fig 6–10, Chapter 6 "Controversies in Fluid Resuscitation").

After the first 24 hours, and once capillary permeability has been restored, fluid losses resulting from the injury occur primarily in the form of burn exudate and evaporation of fluids through denuded skin. Thus, for the second and subsequent days, we recommend that fluid needs be estimated as follows:

3,750 ml/sq m of *body surface burned* per day (burn-related losses)
+
1,500 ml/sq m of total body *surface area* per day (maintenance fluids).

Since water loss by evaporation is electrolyte-free, sodium requirements after the first 48 hours are markedly curtailed and can be satisfied by administering *oral* or *IV* solutions with a sodium concentration of 50 mEq/L. This concentration of sodium has been found to be optimal for children over 1 year of age, but infants have difficulties handling sodium loads and solutions containing 35 to 40 mEq/L are better tolerated. Potassium requirements after the first day are usually satisfied by administering solutions with concentrations of 30 to 40 mEq/L. Potassium phosphate instead of potassium chloride is preferred in order to replace phosphate deficits, which burned children frequently incur. The addition of phosphate instead of chloride also allows the preparation of more physiologic fluid mixtures (sodium-to-chloride ratios of 3:2). Increased requirements for potassium are particularly prominent during the diuretic phase where excessive sodium delivery to the distal nephron leads to significant kaliuresis. These losses should be anticipated and replaced to prevent intestinal hypomotility and intolerance to enteral feedings.

Milk Program

According to our fluid resuscitation program[26] the transition from IV (composite burn solution) to oral fluids is accomplished in most cases during the second postburn day. Beginning at 24 hours postburn, homogenized milk, or in the case of infants, a comparable substitute (infant formula), is offered hourly. Depending on the patient's tolerance, which in most cases is acceptable, the amount of milk (starting with one sixth of total hourly fluid intake) is increased at 4-hour intervals and simultaneously the intravenous (IV) fluids are proportionally decreased (see Fig 7–5). The objective is to maintain total fluid intake (oral + IV) constant. If for some reason the voluntary consumption of milk is limited, nasogastric tube feedings are used instead. The milk program not only reduces the incidence of stress ulcers, but also helps to meet the caloric demands of the burned patient. Ideally, by the end of 48 hours, oral fluid administration replaces IV therapy completely. It is important to recognize that a methodic and progressive increase in milk administration with a corresponding decrease in IV fluids is going to result in approximately equal quantities of IV and oral fluids for the second postburn day (Fig 7–13). Since the concentration of sodium in IV fluid is 132 mEq/L for children over 1 year of age, and milk contains 25 mEq of sodium per liter, the average concentration of sodium for all fluids received during the *second day* is 78 mEq/L [(132 + 25)/2] for children over 1 year of age and correspondingly less for infants [(81 + 25)/2].

Experience with over 200 acutely burned children has demonstrated that when carefully followed, this program results in an optimal fluid and electrolyte balance. If, on the other hand, the quantity of IV fluids during the second day exceeds oral fluids, or vice versa, variable degrees of hypernatremia or hyponatremia, respectively, are likely to develop. Thus, assuming strict adherence to the resuscitation program, the average concentrations of sodium for resuscitation fluids for days 1, 2, and 3 postinjury should be 132, 78, and 50 mEq/L; *most patients with burns over 20% of their body require sodium supplementation beginning on day 3* (25 mEq for every liter of milk consumed). Sodium in the form of sodium chloride tablets or 3% sodium chloride elixir may be used for this purpose (four to six divided doses per day). The risk of hyperosmolality is low, but patients on high-calorie, high-protein feedings who sustain extensive evaporative water losses must be monitored frequently for this possibility.

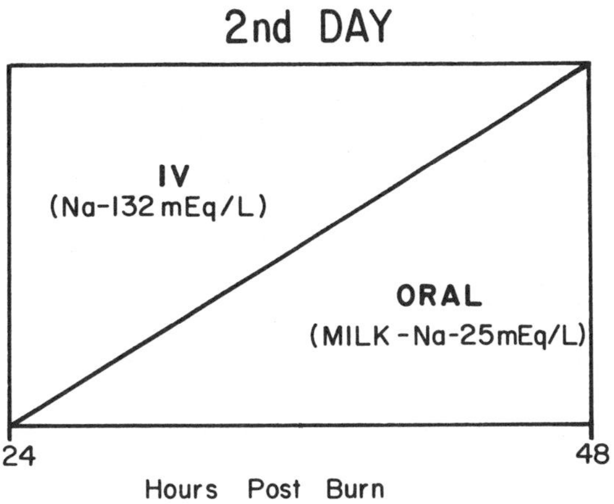

FIG 7–13.
Schematic representation of fluid intake during the second day (24 to 48 hours postinjury), surface area formula and program for fluid resuscitation. Strict adherence to the program should result in equal amounts of intravenous and enteral fluids and a total concentration of sodium of approximately 78 mEq/L.

Albumin and Blood Replacement

The loss of albumin, and to a lesser degree other serum proteins in the form of burn exudate, continues beyond the first 24 hours and remains significant until the third to fourth week after burning. Grafting and healing of autologous skin rapidly reduces the losses of nitrogen in exudate. In burns over 20% of the body surface, these losses exceed the synthetic ability of the liver and hypoalbuminemia develops. The consequences of hypoalbuminemia are manyfold[21, 32, 37, 47, 52, 58] and beyond the scope of this chapter. Suffice it to say that significant hypoalbuminemia, even when associated with compensatory increases in α_2-macroglobulins, leads to a reduction in colloid osmotic pressure, intravascular volume contraction, and edema formation.[21] Hypoalbuminemia is also associated with intestinal wall edema, "appropriate" ADH secretion, impaired absorption of water and nutrients from the gastrointestinal (GI) tract, and paralytic ileus.[40] In general, when the colloid osmotic pressure (COP) is below 14 mm Hg, enteral diets are poorly tolerated. Also, secondary hyperaldosteronism usually becomes manifest at this level of COP. To avoid this, we replace albumin losses to maintain a colloid osmotic pressure above 15 mm Hg. In the absence of septicemia or heavy colonization of the burn wound with bacteria, which increases exudate formation and albumin losses, the amount of human serum albumin necessary to maintain COP greater than 15 mm Hg is approximately 100 gm/sq m of body surface *burned per week* (three divided doses). In most cases we administer albumin as a 5% solution in 5% dextrose and 0.33% sodium chloride injection over 3 to 6 hours and at 2- to 3-day intervals. On the days when the patients receive albumin or plasma, the oral fluids are correspondingly decreased. This program for protein replacement is seldom necessary beyond 3 to 4 weeks postinjury and rarely needed, except in infants, when the total burn is less than 20% to 25% of the body surface.

Blood loss as a direct result of the injury or complications thereof *needs to be replaced during the second to fifth day after the burn;* timing depends on the severity of the anemia. Unless the patient is actively bleeding or has severe concomitant hypoproteinemia, packed-cell transfusions are better tolerated than whole blood. The usual dose is 10 ml/kg of body weight administered over 3- to 4-hour period. Unless active bleeding is present, the maximum amount of blood that we recommend over a single 24-hour period is 15 ml/kg of body weight. Packed cells in larger quantities frequently result in cardiopulmonary congestion or dangerous hypertension.

Mild anemia (hemoglobin 8.5 to 10 gm/dl) is usually well tolerated and unless a surgical procedure under general anesthesia is anticipated, blood transfusions are not necessary.[48] Oxygen-carrying capacity, oxygen delivery, and oxygen extraction by the tissues are adequate at these levels of hemoglobin, and transfusions of blood offer no advantages. If anything, blood transfusions eliminate the stimulus to erythropoiesis and may indirectly increase the dependency on exogenous blood administration.

REFERENCES

1. Allison P, Hinton P, Chamberlain MJ: Intravenous glucose tolerance, insulin, and free fatty acid levels in burned patients. *Lancet* 1968; 2:1113–1116.
2. Arturson G, Hedlund A: Primary treatment of 50 patients with high tension electrical injuries: I. Fluid administration. *Scand J Plast Reconstr Surg* 1984; 18:111–118.
3. Baxter CR: Present concepts in the management of major electrical injury. *Surg Clin North Am* 1970; 50:1401.
4. Baxter CR, Shires GT: Physiologic response to crystalloid resuscitation of severe burns. *Ann NY Acad Sci* 1968; 150:874.
5. Carvajal HF: Acute management of burns in children. *South Med J* 1975; 68:129–131.
6. Carvajal HF: Fluid therapy for the acutely burned child *Compr Ther* 1977; 3(3):17–24.
7. Carvajal HF: A physiologic approach to fluid therapy in severely burned children. *Surg Gynecol Obstet* 1980; 150:379–384.
8. Carvajal HF: Management of severely burned patients: Sorting out the controversies. *Emerg Med Rep* 1985; 6:89.
9. Carvajal HF, Goldman AS: Burns, in Vaughan VC III, McKay RJ (eds): *Nelson Textbook of Pediatrics*, ed 10. Philadelphia, WB Saunders Co, 1975.
10. Carvajal HF, Parks D: Survival statistics in burned children *J Burn Care Rehabil* 1982; 3:81–84.
11. Carvajal HF, Reinhart JA, Traber DL: Renal and cardiovascular functional response to thermal injury in dogs subjected to sympathetic blockade. *Circ Shock* 1976; 3:287.
12. Clark AM: Burns in childhood. *World J Surg* 1978; 2:175.
13. Darrow DC: The significance of body size. *Am J Dis Child* 1959; 98:416.
14. Dubois J: Variations in water and electrolyte composition of muscle and skin in infants suffering acute dehydration. *Pediatr Res* 1972; 6:219–230.
15. Dubois J: Water and electrolyte content of human skeletal muscle—variations with age. *Rev Europ Etud Clin Biol* 1972; 17:505.

16. Durtschi MB, Kohler TR, Finley A, et al: Burn injury in infants and young children. *Surg Gynecol Obstet* 1980; 150:651.
17. Eklund J: Renal regulation of body osmolal balance in burns: A clinical and experimental study with special reference to hyperosmolality. *Acta Chir Scand* 1970; 410(suppl).
18. Fimberg L: Interrelationships between electrolyte physiology, growth, and development, in Fimberg L, Kravath RE, Fleischman AR (eds): *Water and Electrolytes in Pediatrics.* Philadelphia, WB Saunders Co, 1982; p 3.
19. Friedman AL, Segar WE: Antidiuretic hormone excess. *J Pediatr* 1979; 94:521.
20. Gilmore JP: Cardiovascular changes of the burned dog following the infusion of intravenous solutions. *Am J Physiol* 1957; 190:513.
21. Granger ND, Gabel JC, Drake RE, et al: Physiologic basis for the clinical use of albumin solutions. *Surg Gynecol Obstet* 1978; 146:97.
22. Gump FE, Kinney JM: Energy balance and weight loss in burned patients. *Arch Surg* 1971; 103:442.
23. Haynes BW Jr: The management of burns in children. *J Trauma* 1965; 5:267–277.
24. Hays RM: Antidiuretic hormone. *N Engl J Med* 1976; 295:659.
25. Heimbach DM: Smoke inhalation: Current concepts. *Top Emerg Med* 1981; 3(suppl 3):75–83.
26. Hildreth M, Carvajal HF: Caloric requirements in burned children: A simple formula to estimate daily caloric requirements. *J Burn Care Rehabil* 1982; 3:78–80.
27. Hodson EM, Kjellstrand CM, Maver ME: Acute renal failure in infants and children: Outcome of 53 patients requiring hemodialysis treatment. *J Pediatr* 1979; 93:756–761.
28. Holleman JH, Gable JC, Hardy JD: Pulmonary effects of intravenous fluid therapy in burn resuscitation. *Surg Gynecol Obstet* 1978; 147:161–166.
29. Hutcher N, Haynes BW Jr: The Evans formula revisited. *J Trauma* 1972; 12:453–458.
30. Jelenko C III, Williams JB, Wheeler ML, et al: Studies in shock and resuscitation: I. Use of hypertonic albumin-containing fluid demand regimen in resuscitation: A physiologically appropriate method. *Crit Care Med* 1979; 7(suppl 4):157–167.
31. Kreusser W, Ritz E: The phosphate-depletion syndrome. *Contrib Nephrol* 1978; 14:162–174.
32. Lewis RT: Albumin: Role and discriminative use in surgery. *Can J Surg* 1980; 23:322–328.
33. Li N, Yang ZC, Jiang KY, et al: Effect of intravenous infusion on development of pulmonary oedema after inhalation injury. *Burns Incl Therm Inj* 1983; 9:394–400.
34. Liebermann E: Management of acute renal failure in infants and children. *Nephron* 1973; 2:193–208.
35. Lund CL, Browder NC: The estimation of areas of burns. *Surg Gynecol Obstet* 1944; 79:352.
36. McAlhany JC Jr, Czaja AF, Pruitt BA Jr: Antacid control of complications from acute gastroduodenal disease after burns. *J Trauma* 1976; 16:645.
37. Marty AT: Hyperoncotic albumin therapy. *Surg Gynecol Obstet* 1974; 139:105–108.
38. Metcoff J, Buchman H, Jacobson M et al: Losses and physiologic requirements for water and electrolytes after extensive burns in children. *N Engl J Med* 1961; 265:101–111.
39. Moncrief JA: Effect of various fluid regimens and pharmacologic agents on the circulatory hemodynamics of the immediate postburn period. *Ann Surg* 1966; 164:723–752.
40. Moss GS: Plasma albumin and postoperative ileus. *Surg Forum* 1967; 18:333–336.
41. Parks DH, Carvajal HF, Larson DL: Management of burns. *Surg Clin North Am* 1977; 57:875–894.
42. Perkin RM, Levin DL: Shock in the pediatric patient: II. Therapy. *J Pediatr* 1982; 101:319–332.
43. Phillips AW, Cope O: The revelation of respiratory tract damage as a principal killer of the burned patient. *Ann Surg* 1962; 155:1.
44. Pruitt BA Jr: Fluid resuscitation of burn patients: Does clinical 'success' necessitate 'excess'? *South Med J* 1976; 69:1399.
45. Pruitt BA Jr: Advances in fluid therapy and the early care of the burn patient. *World J Surg* 1978; 2:139.
46. Pruitt BA Jr, Goodwin CW Jr: Stress ulcer disease in the burned patient. *World J Surg* 1981; 5:209–222.
47. Rackow EC, Fein AI, Leppo J: Colloid osmotic pressure as a prognostic indicator of pulmonary edema and mortality in the critically ill. *Chest* 1977; 72:709–713.
48. Rice CL, Moss GS: Blood and blood substitutes: Current practice. *Adv Surg* 1979; 13:93.
49. Robinson NB, Hudson LD, Robertson HT, et al: Ventilation and perfusion alterations after smoke inhalation. *Surgery* 1981; 90:352–363.
50. Rosenberg SA, Brief DK, Kinney JM, et al: The syndrome of dehydration, coma, and severe hyperglycemia without ketosis in patients convalescing from burns. *N Engl J Med* 1965; 272:931–938.
51. Scheulen JJ, Munster AM: The Parkland formula in patients with burns and inhalation injury. *J Trauma* 1982; 22:869–871.
52. Skillman JJ: The role of albumin and oncoti-

cally active fluids in shock. *Crit Care Med* 1976; 4:55–61.

53. Spitzer A: Renal physiology and functional development, in Edelmann CM Jr (ed): *Pediatric Kidney Disease*. Boston, Little, Brown & Co, 1978; pp 3–25.
54. Stone HH: The composite burn solution, in Polk HC Jr, Stone HH (eds): *Contemporary Burn Management*. Boston, Little, Brown & Co, 1971, pp 93–104.
55. Turner R, Carvajal HF, Traber DL: Effects of ganglionic blockade upon the renal and cardiovascular dysfunction induced by thermal injury. *Circ Shock* 1977; 4:103–113.
56. Vaughan VC: Developmental pediatrics, in Behrman RE, Vaughan VC III (eds): *Nelson Textbook of Pediatrics*. Philadelphia;, WB Saunders Co, 1983; pp 10–38.
57. Watson LC, Abston S: Prevention of upper gastrointestinal hemorrhage in 582 burned children. *Am J Surg* 1976; 132:790.
58. Zarins CK, Rice CL, Peters RM, et al: Lymph and pulmonary response to isobaric reduction in plasma oncotic pressure in baboons. *Circ Res* 1978; 43:925–930.

8 / Initial Management of the Burn Wound

R. M. ZUKER, M.D., F.R.C.S.(C.)

An open burn wound as opposed to intact skin facilitates bacterial access and, as such, acts as the common denominator for burn sepsis and the majority of deaths of burn victims being treated in hospitals. In the initial stages, however, the burn wound itself does not constitute a major threat to survival. In this chapter, the initial management of the burn wound at the scene of injury, in the emergency room, and in the hydrotherapy treatment room will be discussed. Special problems relating to blister formation, eschar constriction, compartment syndrome, and the burn dressing will be dealt with in detail.

AT THE SCENE

At the scene of injury attention should be directed toward cessation of the burning process. After all materials in contact with the burn area (clothes, bracelets, rings, etc.) have been removed, the temperature of the affected parts should be reduced to room temperature by soaking in cold water.[4, 5, 8, 15, 18] This not only prevents progressive protein coagulation but also helps in reducing pain. The wound is then covered with a clean towel or sheet until it is reevaluated in the local emergency room.

IN THE EMERGENCY ROOM

Children with burns in excess of 10% of the body surface area or a lesser injury with significant involvement of the face, hands, perineum, or feet should generally be managed in the hospital. A child with associated soft tissue or skeletal injuries as well as suspected inhalation burns also requires hospitalization. Sadly, social circumstances in which ongoing child abuse or inadequate supervision may further threaten the life of the child may also necessitate hospitalization. In these situations, the wound is simply covered and the patient taken to the hydrotherapy treatment room.

Children with minor injuries not requiring hospitalization may be treated as an outpatient. Scald burns are particularly suitable for outpatient management if the social situation permits. Loose debris should be removed, blisters appropriately dealt with, as will be described later in this chapter, and the wound carefully dressed.

Skin damaged by scald burns, particularly those on flat, nonmobile surfaces, may be suitable for temporary biological or biosynthetic skin substitutes (see Chapters 14 and 15, "Burn Wound Coverings and Biologic Dressings," and "Immunologic Considerations in the Burned Child"). Early and watertight application, however, is imperative as is careful, frequent follow-up. Murky fluid accumulation often signals infection and requires removal of the dressings as well as frequent dressing changes and application of topical antimicrobials.

The outpatient management of minor superficial burns may also be carried out using an antimicrobial ointment such as Polysporin (Burroughs Wellcome) followed by petrolatum-impregnated mesh gauze, moist gauze, dry gauze, and bandage. The patient should be seen again in 3 to 4 days and the wound inspected for signs of infection. If the wound is clean, the same dressing routine can be repeated at 3-day intervals until the superficial wound epithelializes (10 to 14 days). Involved joints are best managed by immobilization with bulky dressings. Rigid splints are virtually never indicated in the initial management in children, although their later use is often helpful.

IN THE HYDROTHERAPY TREATMENT ROOM

The patient who requires hospitalization is transferred to the hydrotherapy treatment room where certain steps in burn-wound management are carried out (Table 8–1). It is preferable for the burn unit to be notified of the expected admission in advance.

EVALUATION AND DOCUMENTATION

The burn tub (with appropriate liners) is prepared with salinized water. The patient is gently placed in the tub and the burn wound carefully evaluated for its extent and depth. This is then accurately documented (see burn assessment charts in Chapter 7, Figs 7–1 to 7–3.

DEBRIDEMENT; CARE OF BLISTERS

Loose debris, necrotic tissue, and broken blisters are then debrided and wound cultures taken. It is preferable to allow blisters that are intact to remain so.[18] The moist, sterile, plasmatic environment of the blister is far better for wound healing and reepithelialization than anything we can provide (Fig 8–1). If, however, the blister breaks, it is best to debride it (Fig 8–2). Proliferating bacteria could become "locked in" between the dermis and the blister ceiling and cause further tissue necrosis to potentially viable elements. In young children blisters over mobile flexion creases have little or no chance of remaining intact for over a few hours. These are best dealt with by early initial debridement.

At this point the extent and depth of the burn wounds are reassessed and the previous documentation adjusted, if necessary. It is clear that for this to be done accurately, application of topical agents must be delayed.

DISTAL PERFUSION AND ESCHAR CONSTRICTION.—With the ongoing and expected intracellular and interstitial edema that follow the burn injury, a thick, dense, circumferential eschar can lead to significant problems in distal perfusion.[7, 11, 12, 14] This internal swelling coupled with an unyielding cover will first

TABLE 8–1.
Initial Management of the Burn Wound

Evaluation and documentation
Debridement
Care of blisters
Distal perfusion and eschar constriction
Dressing of the wound

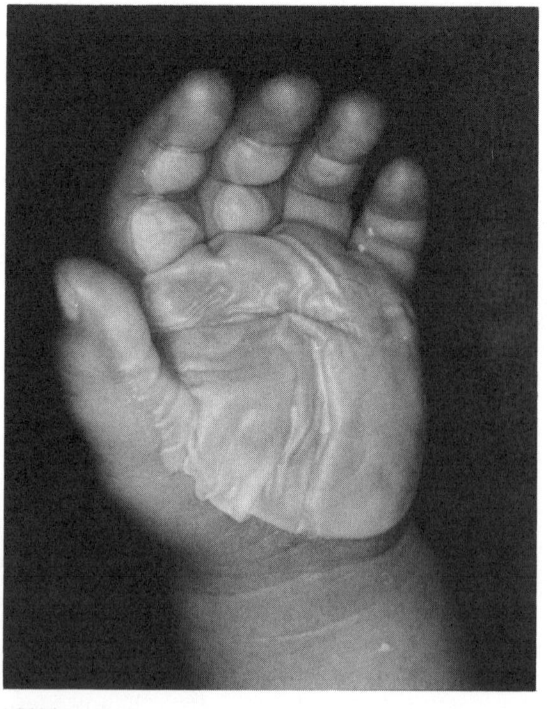

FIG 8–1.
Burn to palm—blister can be left intact.

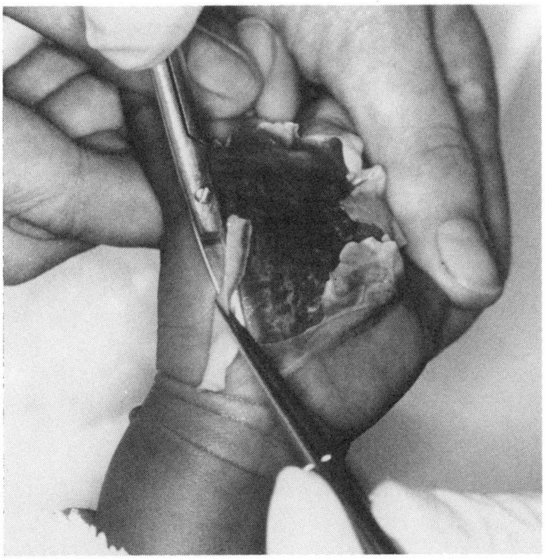

FIG 8–2.
Burn to palm—broken blister should be debrided.

lead to venous insufficiency (Fig 8–3). When this diagnosis is made or very strongly suspected, release of the constricting eschar is indicated. The eschar is simply incised longitudinally down to subcutaneous fat from the proximal area of the eschar to the distal. Midmedial and midlateral incisions are made. Often further intervening incisions are needed as well (Fig 8–4). As the nerve endings in the eschar are nonfunctional, escharotomy can be easily carried out in the treatment room or at the bedside with no anesthetic. In children, light sedation helps alleviate anxiety. Bleeding is usually not a problem and can be controlled with gentle pressure.

Only rarely is there a need to incise deeper than the subcutaneous fat when carrying out an escharotomy. The constricting culprit is the eschar, not the fascia. However, if escharotomy is delayed, a compartment syndrome could become established.[7, 11, 12, 14] The pathophysiology is the same as that of a tight cast. In this situation, escharotomy alone may not be sufficient to solve the problem (as cast re-

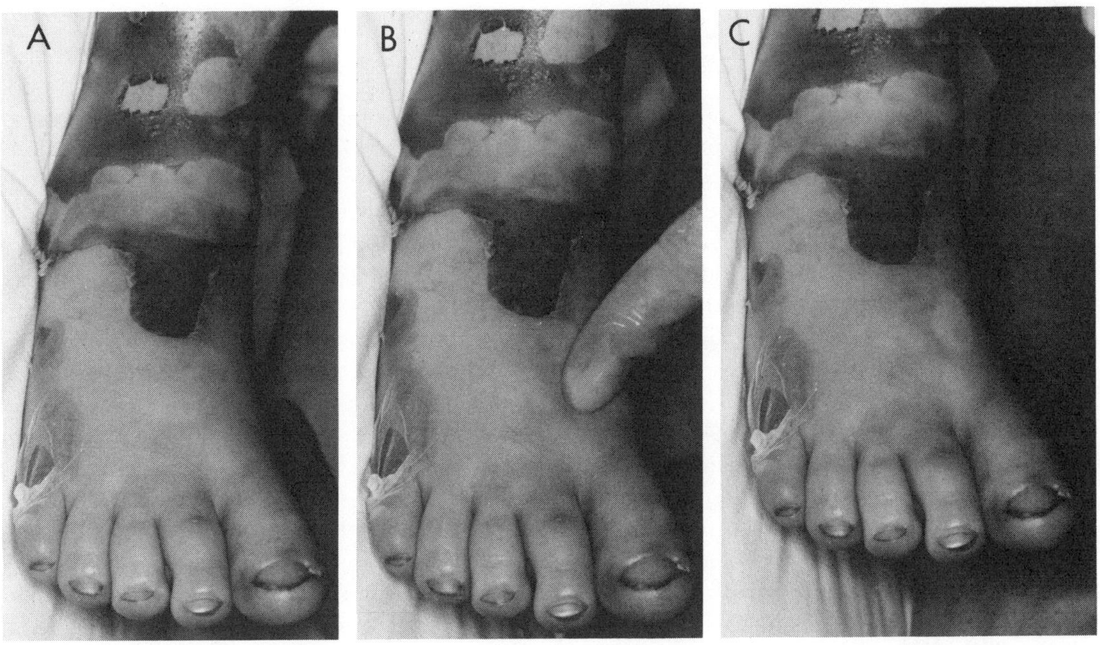

FIG 8–3.
Compromised circulation to foot, **(A).** Finger pressure on the foot, **(B).** Slowed capillary refill, indicating vascular compromise, **(C).**

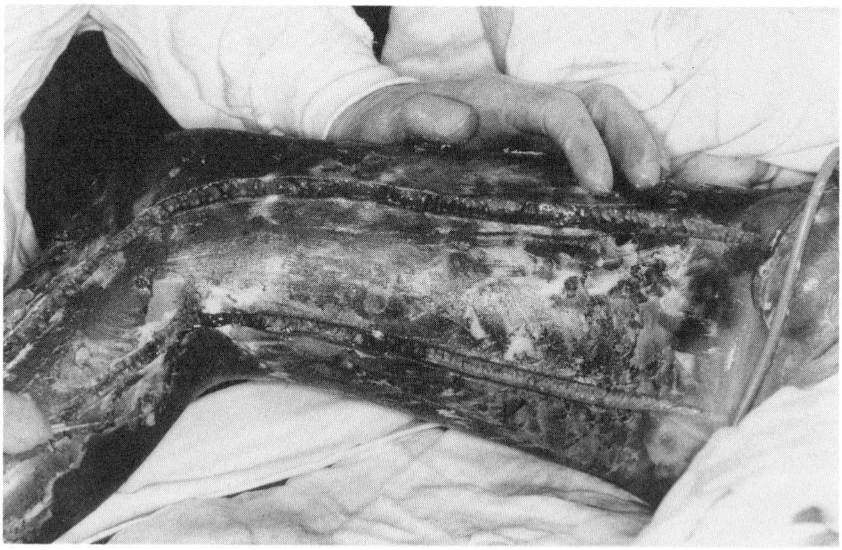

FIG 8–4.
Escharotomy of compromised limb.

moval will not alleviate compartment syndrome), and fasciotomy will be needed. Following the trend of the wick catheter is most helpful. Fasciotomy is more likely required when associated skeletal trauma or major soft-tissue injury is superimposed on the burned extremity. It is almost always required in high-voltage electrical injury, not only at the primary site of involvement, but also along the injury in the extremities. Fasciotomy should be carried out in the operating room under general anesthesia. All involved compartments must be decompressed along with the epimysium of the muscle groups.

Eschar constriction may not be limited to the limbs. Circumferential burns of the chest and upper abdomen with a tight, constricting eschar may limit lung expansion. Although in infants and children lung expansion occurs mainly through diaphragmatic movement, one should be on the alert for signs of hypoxia (irritability, confusion, tachypnea). Blood gases will confirm the diagnosis and truncal escharotomies should be done at once. Longitudinal incisions along the anterior axillary lines are most effective and should be combined with a transverse incision at the costal level (Fig 8–5). Further incisions paralleling these should be made until respiratory function is uncompromised.

THE WOUND AND ITS DRESSING.—Major strides have been made in reducing the incidence of burn-wound sepsis by the use of topical antimicrobials. The application of these agents combined with twice-daily hydrotherapy and careful debridement constitutes basic, initial-wound management.

The burn wound as described by Jackson[10] consists of three concentric zones of injury (see Chapter 3). The outermost and most superficial is known as the zone of hyperemia. Barring intervening infection, this will heal spontaneously in about 1 week. The innermost and deepest is known as the zone of coagulation. Injury in this zone is lethal to its cellular components and, depending on its depth, may heal spontaneously (through surviving underlying skin appendage elements), epithelialize from adjacent epidermal elements, or require surgical resurfacing. The intervening zone, the zone of stasis, may survive despite damage to its microvasculature. It is imperative that management of the burn

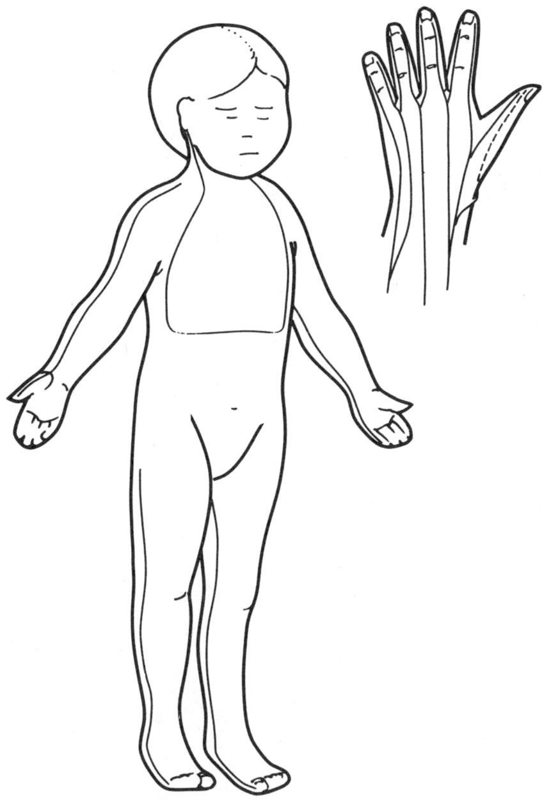

FIG 8–5.
Preferred escharotomy sites—additional incisions may be needed.

wound not further compromise this zone[17] but rather provide as optimal an environment as possible for tissue survival. Clinically this translates into maintenance of optimal peripheral perfusion with adequate oxygenation. Thus, ischemia from underhydration and also as a result of excessive edema from overhydration should be avoided. Hypoxia from respiratory compromise clearly will diminish marginal tissue survival. Overventilation in patients on respirators will cause hypocarbia resulting in peripheral vasoconstriction, which also may reduce tissue viability. Similarly, hypothermia is a potent peripheral vasoconstrictor and should be avoided.

Locally, the zone of stasis can be adversely influenced by infection and dessication.[19] Antimicrobials "buttered" on the burn wound to 3 to 5 mm thick with the gloved hand (Fig 8–6,A) have a significant effect in decreasing bacterial flora and thus in reducing the risk of infection. Our current agent of choice is silver sulfadiazine cream[13] with gentamicin cream being reserved for those children with sulfa allergy. The wound is then covered with moist saline gauze (Fig 8–6,B), then dry gauze, and held in place with Kling bandage and loose netting (Fig 8–6,C). This outer netting must be secure enough to hold the gauze in place, particularly in toddlers, but must not be constricting. Custom adaptation from varying widths can accommodate any dressing need. Avoidance of constriction is critical, however, and in difficult areas such as the neck and perineum, other means of fixation (e.g., taping) or the open method may be best. Facial burns constitute a special situation in young children as a cream easily rolls off or is easily rubbed off or even eaten by the child. An ointment such as Polysporin (Burroughs Wellcome) is preferred with the wound left open. This ointment is reapplied whenever it is rubbed off and also with major dressing changes.

The major dressing changes are carried out in conjunction with hydrotherapy in the burn tub twice daily. Loose, necrotic debris is gently removed and the wound cleansed. At this point astute observers will recognize signs of infection or conversion (see Chapter 13). Great care is taken to avoid desiccation of the wound as otherwise viable elements can in this way be destroyed. The wound is redressed as indicated previously.

THE FUTURE

Our current efforts in wound care are directed toward avoiding ischemia or hypoxia from systemic events, and locally in providing as optimal an environment as possible for wound healing.[2] We now know, however, that the burn progresses, and the injury worsens with time.[3] Drugs to combat this progression are currently being evaluated (aspirin, dipyridamole, and other thromboxane inhibi-

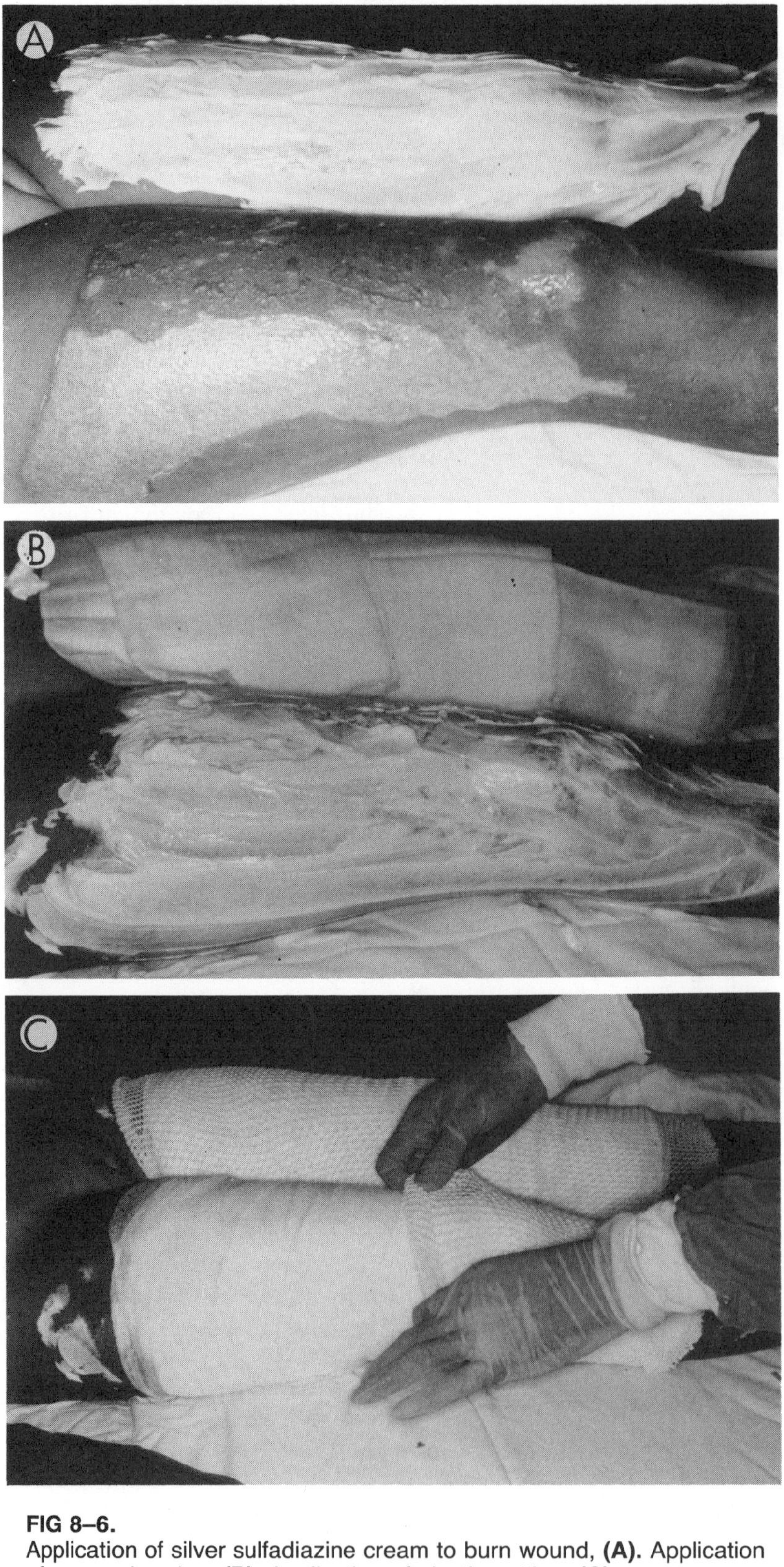

FIG 8–6.
Application of silver sulfadiazine cream to burn wound, **(A).** Application of gauze dressing, **(B).** Application of elastic netting, **(C).**

tors).[6, 9, 16] Although the precise reason for this progression remains unknown, the search for endogenous mediators of local and systemic effects continues. The mediators may be products of tissue destruction[8] or perhaps a result of the host defense response.[1] Once the factors responsible for the progression of the burn injury are better understood, our efforts can be directed toward their neutralization, rather than simply providing an optimal environment for nature's wound healing process.

REFERENCES

1. Arturson MG: The pathophysiology of severe thermal injury. *J Burn Care Rehabil* 1985; 6:129–146.
2. Boykin JV, Eriksson E, et al: Microcirculation of a scald burn: An in vivo experimental study of the hairless mouse ear. *Burns* 1980; 7:335–338.
3. deCamara DL, Raine TJ, London MD, et al: Progression of thermal injury: A morphological study. *Plast Reconstr Surg* 1982; 69:491–499.
4. deCamara DL, Raine TJ, Robson MC: Ultrastructural aspects of cooled thermal injury. *J Trauma* 1981; 21:911–919.
5. deCamara DL, Robson MC: New microscopic evidence of cooling of the burn wound. *Surg Forum* 1980; 31:553–555.
6. Del Beccaro EJ, Robson MC, Heggers JP, et al: The use of specific thromboxane inhibitors to preserve the dermal microcirculation after burning. *Surgery* 1980; 87:137–141.
7. Gaspard DJ, Kohl RD: Compartmental syndromes in which the skin is the limiting boundary. *Clin Orthop* 1975; 113:65–68.
8. Heggers JP, Robson MC, London MD, et al: Cooling and the prostaglandin effect in thermal injury. *J Burn Care Rehabil* 1982; 3:350–354.
9. Heggers JP, Robson MC: Prostaglandins and thromboxane, in Wachtel TL (ed): *Critical Care Clinics Symposium on Burns.* 1985; 1:59–77.
10. Jackson DM: The diagnosis of depth of burning. *Br J Surg* 1953; 40:588–596.
11. Matsen FA: Compartmental syndrome: An unified concept. *Clin Orthop* 1975; 113:8–14.
12. Mubarak SJ, Hargens AR: Acute compartment syndromes. *Surg Clin North Am* 1983; 63:539–565.
13. Ollstein RN, McDonald C: Topical and systemic antimicrobial agents in burns. *Ann Plast Surg* 1980; 5:386–392.
14. Patman RD: Compartmental syndromes in peripheral vascular surgery. *Clin Orthop* 1975; 113:103–110.
15. Raine TJ, Heggers JP, Robson MC: Cooling the burn wound to maintain microcirculation. *J Trauma* 1981; 21:394–397.
16. Robson MC, Del Beccaro EJ, Heggers JP, et al: The effect of prostaglandins on the dermal microcirculation after burning and the inhibition of the effect by specific pharmacological agents. *Plast Reconstr Surg* 1979; 63:781–787.
17. Robson MC, Kucan JO, Paik KI, et al: Prevention of dermal ischemia after thermal injury. *Arch Surg* 1978; 113:623–625.
18. Saranto JR, Rubayi S, Zawacki B: Blisters, cooling, antithromboxanes, and healing in experimental zone-of-stasis burns. *J Trauma* 1983; 23:927–933.
19. Zawacki BE: Reversal of capillary stasis and prevention of necrosis in burns. *Ann Surg* 1974; 180:98–102.

9 / Topical Antimicrobials

THOMAS L. WACHTEL, M.D.

Topical agents are used for the initial control of burn-wound infection[60] and to prevent burn-wound sepsis.[36] Most of the morbidity and mortality from a major burn is the result of infection of the wounds by bacteria or fungi. Morbidity from both large and small burn wounds is related directly to infection. Large burn wounds are at a proportionately greater risk. Bacterial infection may deepen a dermal burn and thus delay spontaneous healing or even cause conversion to a full-thickness injury.

The rationale for using topical chemotherapy stems from the type of pathologic lesion created by thermal injury.[30] Portions of the skin undergo complete coagulation necrosis in varying depths and as a result become avascular. Surrounding and often intermixed with these areas are zones of stasis where the blood supply is equivocal, and the wounds may either reepithelialize or progress to complete necrosis. Therefore, a large portion of the burn remains ischemic initially if not avascular permanently. Adjacent to these areas are areas of hyperemia in which the vascularity is increased. In full-thickness burns confluent thrombosis of arterioles, capillaries, venules, and even larger vessels is characteristic. Thrombosis is incomplete in partial-thickness burns with gradual reestablishment of the dermal circulation in the deeper, viable segments of the dermis.

Immediately after the victim suffers a burn injury, the wound is essentially sterile. Contamination by soil or water may occur after the accident as a result of first aid measures or during transport.[30] Surface colonization predominated by staphylococci begins in a few hours in all burns. Shortly thereafter, the number of organisms, primarily from the hair follicles, increases and the organisms invade through the membrane at the base of the hair follicle into the perifollicular tissue and beyond.

After 3 to 5 days, gram-negative organisms predominate, and the more virulent strains begin active invasion of the unburned tissues. Gram-negative organisms spread mainly via the lymphatics. Hematogenous spread is uncommon in the early phases, occurring more commonly at a later time as the organisms invade the lumen of the blood vessels.[42] The vascular, destructive nature of the burn predisposes the burn site to bacterial invasion by precluding effective delivery of the body's host-defense mechanisms to the local scene and preventing systemic antibiotics from penetrating the flat eschar. This is particularly true of the wound surface closest to the heat source, which is predictably the most severely injured and the original site of most burn-wound infections. For this reason antimicrobial agents are best used topically. A number of effective topical antimicrobials have been used to control the surface colonization.[1, 2, 6, 10, 12, 13, 15, 20, 25, 30, 47]

Before the use of effective topical antibacterial agents, the reported mortality resulting from burn injuries was 38% to 45% of patients admitted to burn centers. The use of appropriate topical therapy reduced the mortality in a typical burned patient population to 14% to 24%[36] and significantly altered the incidence of burn-wound sepsis.[1, 11, 28, 34, 37, 38, 39, 41, 44, 49] The most striking reduction in mortality from the decreased incidence of burn wound sepsis has been in children below the age of 15 years. In this age group studies have demonstrated a 33% reduction in burn-wound sepsis (35% to 2%).[33] In fact, there has been a reduction in overall mortality in all series reported in which children under the age of 15 years were a significant portion of the patient population.[31, 33]

The characteristics of an ideal topical chemotherapeutic agent for the treatment of the burn wound are listed in Table 9–1. No topical agent now available fulfills all of these criteria.[51] All possess relative advantages and disadvantages. None will sterilize the burn wound or totally prevent bacterial proliferation.[33, 34, 37] As with several other components of burn care, the therapeutic regimen used for topical antimicrobial bacterial control is controversial.[34, 40, 52, 63] In practice, many of the topical agents have proved to be clinically effective when applied appropriately during the periods that they have been utilized in a plethora of burn facilities.

TABLE 9–1.
Characteristics of an Ideal Topical Chemotherapeutic Agent

Painless on application
Prevents desiccation
Nonallergenic
Penetrates burn wound to sufficient depth
Achieves bacteriologic control/bactericidal
Does not inhibit reepithelialization
Does not injure viable cells

Initially, these antimicrobials were primarily 0.5% silver nitrate solution[38, 39] and mafenide.[22, 23, 32, 47, 53, 54] Now, many other topical agents are available.[7, 12, 26–28, 30, 57] Currently, the most popular topical agent in use is silver sulfadiazine.[11] It is applied in an open fashion or on fine mesh gauze and held in place with elastic net dressings in a semiclosed fashion (Fig 9–1).[60, 61]

No single optimal method of burn wound

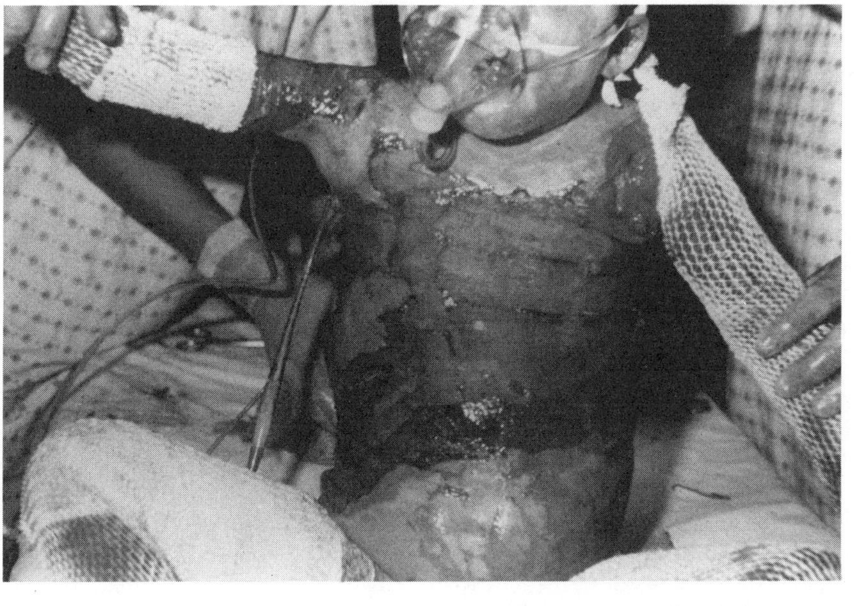

FIG 9–1.
Semiclosed method of burn dressing to a 4-year-old child. Topical agent, applied to fine mesh gauze prior to the dressing change, is placed over the burn wound and held in place with elastic net as shown on the arms and legs.

treatment has been devised to date, and therefore no universally applicable and acceptable technique has been described.[32] This chapter describes the use of the topical antimicrobial agents available. These recommendations are made with full realization that the use of topical antimicrobial agents is limited to supportive treatment that allows the burn wound to heal spontaneously or to assisting the burn surgeon in the grafting techniques that are necessary to close full-thickness burn wounds by controlling bacterial proliferation prior to and during these operative procedures.

SELECTION AND APPLICATION OF THE TOPICAL ANTIMICROBIAL

The selection of the topical agent applied to the burn wound is determined by the nature of the burn wound to be treated and the characteristics of the agent. The prime factors for consideration are the site of the burn, the size and depth of the burn, and the type of bacterial flora to be treated. The agent should be applied to large burns as soon as possible after the burn injury so only enough time has elapsed for a burn care expert to assess the size and depth of the wound.[30] It is important that the topical agent used be strictly and adequately applied and reapplied so proliferation of bacteria can be controlled or a stepwise reduction in the bacterial count obtained. The agent should keep or decrease the count of the intraeschar bacterial population to below 100,000 organisms per gram of tissue[19] and prevent invasion of subjacent unburned tissue.[58] The agent selected should possess a clinical record of efficacy, which includes its effect on the microflora of burn wounds of varying magnitude as well as the mortality attendant to the use of the agent.[30] To prevent invasive burn sepsis, the burn physician should be cognizant of the maximum period of therapeutic efficacy of the topical agent used. The infected burn requires aggressive topical therapy.[24] Also important is the time when the burn is evaluated, e.g., at initial assessment, daily assessment, preoperative assessment, during surgery, after an autograft, or during the rehabilitative phase. Shallow burns may be treated by one method, while the full-thickness burn injury must be treated by another.

Despite all efforts, prevention of bacterial contamination of the burn wound is not possible. When the wound has been grossly contaminated by bacteria, careful attention must be paid to cleansing the patient as well as to the choice of an antimicrobial agent. Body hygiene plays a very important part of the management of the burn wound. Showering or bathing of the entire patient is indicated whenever the general condition of the patient is stable. Antimicrobial agents such as povidone-iodine (1 in 15 ppm) or sodium hypochlorite (425 or 850 μg/ml) are added to showering or bathing water.[55]

The small, shallow burn may be treated with ointment (e.g., Neosporin) or a variety of nonadhering dressings (e.g., Xeroform, Furacin, Adaptic, Vaseline gauze). Another alternative is the use of a synthetic dressing (e.g., Biobrane). When selecting a topical agent the physician must determine how often the wound should be evaluated. This depends on the dressing technique used and the reliability of the child's family. Occasionally, the small, shallow, partial-thickness burn may be treated with a variety of topical antimicrobials under nearly the same circumstances as a full-thickness burn injury.[35] This situation occurs in hospitalized burned patients, particularly if the patient has other deeper burns that require topical therapy.

Topical antimicrobials are applied prophylactically in all hospitalized burned patients.[24] In full-thickness burn wounds, the topical antimicrobial agent applied must have the ability to penetrate through the eschar without losing its efficacy.[56] Surface microbacterial cultures often give an inadequate impression of the bacterial population in the deeper tissue layers. Small biopsies of representative burn tissue[16] studied by histopathologic techniques and quantitative culture assay give a more accurate reflection of the potential for burn colonization or burn-wound invasion.[19] These techniques should be utilized serially in the areas of concern. Topical antimicrobial coverage must be coordinated with necessary surgical procedures such as releasing the constricting effect of the overlying dead tissue layer (escharotomy).[48] In addition one must be concerned with the complication of tetanus in the presence of the anaerobic environment and provide appropriate active or passive immunization.

If early excision of the burn wound is not elected and topical chemotherapy is the method of burn wound treatment, nonviable tissue must still be removed. Prior to the use of topical antibacterial agents, eschar separation occurred spontaneously between the 10th and 14th postburn days. This spontaneous separation was due to bacterial autolysis. Successful control of the bacterial population of the burn wound has resulted in prolonged adherence of the eschar. Therefore, it is necessary to remove necrotic tissue from the burn wound as soon as the tissue is clearly nonviable. Physical removal of nonviable tissue is an extremely important aspect of burn wound care and may take the form of daily surgical cleansing of the loosening eschar, intradermal debridement, full-thickness excision,[14] or enzymatic dissolution of the eschar.[62]

Consideration must be given to the local effects of the medications, and the systemic side effects of both topical and other prescribed agents[45, 46] are important. Pain on the application of topical agents mitigates their routine use, particularly on the superficial burn wound. Most of the topical antimicrobial agents are absorbed[43, 56] and may require metabolization before they can be excreted. The rate of absorption of a given agent, the blood or tissue levels achieved, and the side effects and toxicity to be expected should be known. Several topical agents containing silver nitrate may cause methemoglobinemia.[59] Other agents cause acid-base disturbances and electrolyte depletion.[45]

In addition to the topical agent and dressing technique, the effect on the patient's physical and occupational therapy program must be considered. These programs may play an important role as to which topical agent can be applied and which dressing technique used in conjunction with the overall wound care plan. Likewise the cost of topical agent and the dressings used as well as availability of and funds for numerous personnel must be considered. Adequate nutritional care is essential to ensure an optimal level of energy and protein for rebuilding the burn wound, for epithelialization, and for graft "take."[9, 21] Attention to optimal perfusion for wound healing and graft take and to the role that the topical antimicrobial agent plays in wound healing is important.

Superinfection will require a change in topical agent, a change in the wound debridement plan, and perhaps a change to systemic antibiotics. The culture results must be interpreted in light of the clinical situation. If the cultures repeatedly indicate an inordinately high bacterial density and a clinical situation consistent with the presence of significant wound sepsis, another topical agent should be used. The selection of the alternative topical agent should be based on whether unacceptably dense surface colonization has occurred or whether invasion of adjacent tissue is occurring.

If invasion is occurring, an agent known to be absorbed through the wound should be selected. Subescharotic abscesses must be promptly unroofed, and devitalized tissue and debris, which favor the proliferation of microorganisms, must be removed or excised.[30]

The administration of systemic antibiotics is required when invasive burn infection is suspected or diagnosed. In addition systemic antibiotics may be useful during periods when the burn is being grafted or when it is not evaluated on a daily basis. The unwanted side effects that broad-spectrum antibiotics have on the patient's intestinal surface microbial flora must be considered. For example, invasive candidiasis usually occurs as a direct consequence of intestinal overgrowth of *Candida albicans.*[18] Some investigators have advocated the administration of oral antifungal agents.[50] Rigid, aseptic control of venipuncture sites adjacent to or through the burn wound is mandatory[3] with aggressive management of pyogenic thrombophlebitis, a well-known complication of prolonged venous cannulation.[42]

Since even the best topical therapeutic regimen will not eradicate the bacteria within the burn wound, control of the wound flora is merely a way of buying time that must be spent in a vigorous attempt to convert the open, dirty burn wound to a closed, clean one. This must be accomplished in a reasonable period of time, or the bacterial proliferation will escape effective control, and burn wound sepsis will supervene despite all our efforts. Thus closure of the burn wound should begin as soon as possible.[14] Topical therapy must be modified and tailored to meet the criteria of an aggressive burn wound closure plan and not vice versa.

TOPICAL AGENTS

This section discusses the topical agents currently in use and is not intended to be an all-inclusive presentation.

Since none of the agents is always successful, it may be necessary to substitute a different one on all or part of the burn wounds at some time or stage of treatment. The use of topical agents is initiated by the usual burn-wound protocol and modified by serial, frequent (at least daily), clinical observations augmented by quantitative culture data and laboratory studies as well as the operative status of burn wound closure.

Unless a strong sulfa allergy history or other contraindication exists, treatment begins with silver sulfadiazine applied on a single layer of fine mesh gauze, held in place with a net dressing (see Fig 9–1).[61] Signs or symptoms of burn-wound infection, increasing quantitative bacteriologic cultures or cultures greater than 100,000 organisms per gram of burn eschar (at junction of viable tissue), or histological evidence of invasion of subjacent viable tissue may prompt a change in the topical agent, usually to mafenide.

Mafenide is used on well-circumscribed electrical burns and already heavily colonized burns that present late to the burn center. The open technique is used with this topical agent (Fig 9–2).

Nitrofurazone is used over fresh grafts (including meshed grafts), on persons who are allergic to sulfa drugs or in whom a rash develops during the use of silver sulfadiazine and/or mafenide, when the wounds are nearly closed, and on small burns that are treated by the closed technique (e.g., shallow, partial-

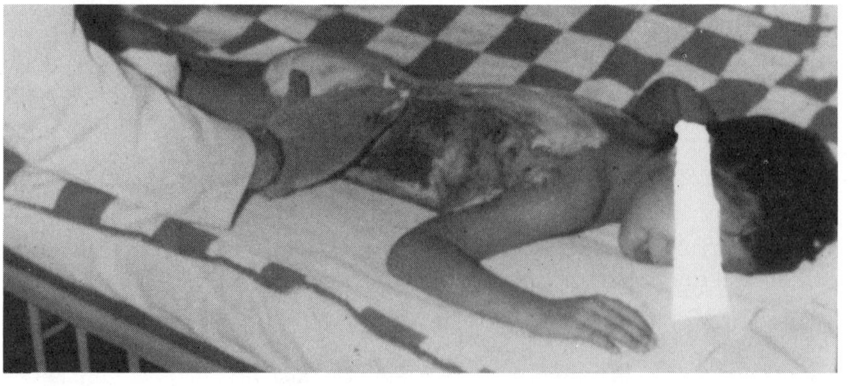

FIG 9–2.
Mafenide cream is applied using the open technique to the burn on the back of a child. (Photograph courtesy of Jerry M. Shuck, M.D.)

thickness hand burn). Occasionally, silver sulfadiazine and nitrofurazone are alternated as recommended by McCauley.[29]

Povidone-iodine is reserved for the wound that is soft and difficult to excise tangentially. The desiccating effect of this agent applied for 24 hours prior to operation has been useful. Silver nitrate solution (0.5%) is not used often because of logistic problems, the staining of personnel, equipment, clothing, and facilities, the special expertise needed to "read" the burn wound, and fluid and electrolyte problems, but it is a useful agent to have in the armamentarium.

Gentamicin is rarely used except on patients with superinfected wounds and strong sulfa allergies. Neosporin and bacitracin are used on shallow, partial-thickness burns of the face. Scarlet red is used on donor sites as is Xeroform and Biobrane. Familiarity with all the topical agents currently used and a protocol for their logical use on any burned patient is essential.

Short descriptions of silver sulfadiazine, mafenide, nitrofurazone, povidone-iodine, gentamicin, cerium nitrate-silver sulfadiazine, 0.5% silver nitrate, and scarlet red follow. Additional information should be obtained from the package insert data for each specific topical agent.

Silver Sulfadiazine

Silver sulfadiazine has been widely used during the past several years. It is formed by reacting silver nitrate with sodium sulfadiazine compounded in a water-soluble cream base in a 1% concentration. This concentration was arbitrarily selected because it contains approximately the same amount of silver as does 0.5% silver nitrate (30 mEq/L). Sulfadiazine is a well-known competitive inhibitor of para-aminobenzoic acid. The antimicrobial effect of silver is through multiple sites of action. Silver sulfadiazine probably acts primarily on bacterial cell walls inducing visible ultrastructural changes. Bacterial DNA replication may be impaired due to silver binding in that molecule.

The in vitro antimicrobial spectrum of silver sulfadiazine includes *Staphylococcus aureus, Enterobacteriaceae, Escherichia coli,* and *Candida albicans.* A 1% concentration provides amounts of the agent well above those necessary in vitro to inhibit the growth of sensitive microorganisms. Used prophylactically, silver sulfadiazine may delay wound colonization by gram-negative bacilli for 10 to 14 days in extensive burns, after which the wounds nearly invariably become colonized in moderate density.

Silver sulfadiazine cream should be applied liberally to the wound. The area on which the topical agent is used can either be left open or covered with a dressing. The semiclosed method uses fine mesh gauze impregnated with silver sulfadiazine, which is prepared in the surgical central supply or pharmacy, placed in sterile covered stainless steel boats, and transported to the burn treatment room as needed. The dressing is applied on patients one-layer or at most two-layers thick and held in place with an elastic net.[61] The child's burn wounds can be covered quickly following showering or tubbing. Eighteen-inch square sheets of impregnated fine mesh gauze can be used to cover back torso, front torso, and each leg and foot, while half sheets will encompass each arm. Precut elastic net is used to hold the impregnated gauze in place. Such use is fast, efficient, and cost-effective. The additional advantages of the semiclosed technique are the guaranteed close approximation of the drug to the burn wound, the smaller total quantity of drug required because the topical agent is not easily rubbed off, and the conformity and stability of the dressing.

The dressings are removed and the child's wounds are cleansed in a shower device or tub every 12 hours. The dressings are reapplied. If the wounds are draining considerably, they may require dressing every 8 hours to replenish the topical agent that is washed away. Because of the intense personnel commitments required when silver sulfadiazine-impregnated dressings are changed, less frequent dressing changes have been used with this agent with no apparent loss in efficacy.[35]

Cutaneous sensitivity reactions to silver sulfadiazine occur in 4% to 8% of patients but are rarely severe enough to warrant withdrawal of the agent, particularly in children. Better wound hygiene will usually suffice in the treatment of such sensitivities. If not, a temporary change in topical agent may be necessary. Exposure of the cream to direct sunlight results in the oxidation of silver to a metallic gray color, but the cream does not stain linen or skin. When silver sulfadiazine is applied to dermal burns, it combines with wound exudate to form a proteinaceous gel several millimeters thick on the surface of the wounds. This "peel" should be removed and can be separated easily in sheets after a few days.

Even in extensive burns, significant or persistent toxic effects related to silver sulfadiazine are rare because of its poor absorption, a factor that has undoubtedly contributed to its popularity. Some absorption of sulfadiazine does occur. Blood levels are 1.5 to 4 mg/dl. depending on the size of the burn and the interval postinjury. Crystalluria, a well-known toxic effect of sulfonamides, is rare. Transient leukopenia typically occurs around the fourth or fifth day of application of silver sulfadiazine in about 5% of patients.[17] The leukopenia is ordinarily in the low-normal range but inappropriate to the magnitude of the associated injury. The leukopenia usually spontaneously remits despite the continued use of the drug. If it doesn't or if the absolute white blood cell count drops below 2,000/cu mm, the topical agent is changed, at least temporarily. The clinical significance of the leukopenia is unknown but probably does not correlate with septic episodes.

When the wound size exceeds 60% of body surface area (BSA), treatment failure is frequent. Gram-negative bacilli, particularly Enterobacteriaceae, can become highly resistant to sulfadiazine as a result of its protracted use. The mortality rate attending the use of silver sulfadiazine roughly parallels that observed using 0.5% silver nitrate solution.[34] Several patterns of antibiotic resistance have occurred as the result of interspecies transfer of resistant plasmids, especially from *Enterobacter* species, a phenomenon almost certainly due to the selection pressure exerted by the protracted use of silver sulfadiazine.[5]

Mafenide Acetate

Mafenide is a methylated sulfonamide available commercially as a 10% preparation in a water-miscible, hygroscopic cream base. Mafenide is not significantly bound by protein or inactivated by wound exudates. Mafenide should be used to control invasive burn wound infections, especially when they are relatively localized (e.g., electrical), and burns caused by organisms sensitive to the drug. This agent should not be used as the first-line, prophylactic, topical agent. It should be reserved for infections that require rapid penetration of the eschar for control and when other topical antimicrobials have failed. The agent should be used for as brief a period as possible and withdrawn promptly when there is evidence of significant systemic toxic effects. Careful monitoring of acid-base balance and pulmonary function are essential.[30]

Mafenide has a large spectrum of activity against both the common gram-negative burn-wound pathogens (e.g., *Pseudomonas aeruginosa*) and the gram-positive pathogens, including clostridia. It has little antifungal activity.

Mortality rates decrease significantly in patients with burns of up to approximately 60% of BSA. Deaths from burn wound sepsis, especially those caused by *Pseudomonas aeruginosa*, are infrequent. The mortality from its routine use is equivalent to that observed with 0.5% silver nitrate or silver sulfadiazine. However, superinfection, especially by antibiotic-resistant *Providencia stuartii*[8] and fungal superinfections occur with some frequency when the drug is used routinely.

Additional toxic effects have been reported.[35]

Mafenide is applied using the open technique (see Fig 12–2). It causes pain on application to partially burned areas, probably because of its high osmolarity. Another of its undesirable effects is inhibition of spontaneous epithelial regeneration. Both the retardation in epithelialization and absorption of the drug are exacerbated by closed dressing techniques. Therefore, such techniques are contraindicated, but the semiclosed technique can be used provided the fine mesh gauze is kept at *only* one layer. The advantages of this technique are the same as described above.

Mafenide is readily absorbed from burn wounds, so rapidly in fact that therapeutic wound concentrations cannot be maintained unless the agent is reapplied at 12-hour intervals. The drug is deaminated to its acidic paracarboxy metabolite and excreted primarily by the kidneys. Mafenide is a strong carbonic anhydrase inhibitor whose application to large wounds promptly results in the alkalinization of the urine. This combination of acid-loading and impairment of renal bicarbonate conservation predictably leads to metabolic acidosis, which is compensated for by hyperventilation. Tachypnea, with a sustained increase in minute ventilation (up to 50 L/minute) is a result. Static compliance of the lung falls.[35] This compensatory respiratory response regularly occurs with the use of topical mafenide and often restricts the use of mafenide in children. Respiratory failure or pneumonia ultimately occurs in significant numbers of patients unless the drug is discontinued. Deaths from pulmonary failure related to the toxicity of the drug are comparatively common. Patients with preexisting respiratory insufficiency (e.g., inhalation injury) should be monitored very carefully.

Nitrofurazone

Nitrofurazone (Furacin), 2-([5-nitro-2-furanyl]methylene)hydrazinecarboxamide, has a more limited role in burn-wound care. The antimicrobial is inactivated by the protein drainage of the wound. The resultant base provides a nonstick dressing provided the agent is not completely washed away from the dressing. The topical agent is applied using the semiclosed method and reapplied once each day. It may also be used over allografts, xenografts, and autografts as well as over partial-thickness burns. When used for these indications, the wound is dressed with an occlusive dressing and allowed to remain intact for up to 4 days without clinical observation. This stipulates that the wound have a low potential for infection, particularly with *Streptococcus* and *Staphylococcus*. If grafts are occluded, perioperative gram-positive antibiotic coverage is useful, but careful assessment for local wound drainage or odor and systemic signs of infection is required.

The rash complication rate is thought to be less than 4%. Rare reports of lethal hypersensitivity reactions to this drug exist, but other studies have reported no untoward reaction when nitrofurazone was alternated with silver sulfadiazine.[29] The local bacterial control was excellent under this protocol.

Povidone-Iodine

Povidone-iodine is a complex of polyvinylpyrrolidone and iodine with a long record of clinical efficacy as an antiseptic for use on normal skin (e.g., surgical scrubs) and mucous membranes. It is compounded for topical use in a water-miscible cream base with 1% iodine content. It has a wide antimicrobial spectrum, but protein binding of iodine in the open wounds may result in a diminished in vivo antimicrobial effect.

The agent can be used with both the open and semiclosed techniques. Patients frequently complain of pain not unlike that with mafenide. This may be due to the strongly acidic (pH 2.43) cream or to other side effects. Studies show rapid absorption and extraordinarily high blood-iodine content. Lethal metabolic acidosis attributed to povidone-iodine renal toxicity has been reported and includes a case in which the patient had a relatively small burn of 35% of BSA.[43]

Gentamicin Sulfate

Gentamicin is a bactericidal, aminoglycoside antibiotic available for topical use as a 0.1% cream or ointment. Gentamicin is used systemically in the treatment of gram-negative infections, especially those caused by *Pseudomonas*.

The drug is readily absorbed when applied topically to open wounds. Gentamicin is useful for invasive infection. It should be applied for brief periods to the smallest possible areas. Blood levels of the drug should be carefully monitored since ototoxic or nephrotoxic effects may occur with the use of this agent. Superinfection with resistant bacterial strains will quickly occur with its protracted topical use.

Cerium Nitrate-Silver Sulfadiazine

Silver sulfadiazine is modified by adding 100 gm/dl aqueous solution of cerium nitrate so that the final concentration of cerium is 2.2% (0.05M) and the sulfadiazine is thus diluted to slightly less than 1%. In vitro experiments indicated that the minimal bactericidal concentration of ionic silver could be reduced approximately threefold by the presence in the medium of ionic cerium in concentrations less than that required for a bactericidal effect due to cerium alone. Cerium was selected from among the lanthanides, all of which have antimicrobial activity in vitro, because it is readily available, has low toxicity, and is poorly absorbed from open wounds, primarily because of the insolubility of its phosphate and protein salts.

Gram-negative bacilli are rarely present on cerium-treated wounds, but gram-positive bacteria, particularly *Staphylococcus aureus*, are not as effectively suppressed as when either silver nitrate or silver sulfadiazine has been used.[30] The thin cream can be applied topically and covered with dressings except to face and genitalia.

Blood cerium levels in patients with major burns treated for many weeks with the cerium nitrate-silver sulfadiazine are less than 10 mg/dl. Two of 300 patients treated with the agent have evidenced transient methemoglobinemia due to bacterial reduction of nitrate and subsequent absorption, but no other toxic effect attributable to cerium has been demonstrated.[30]

Treatment failures have been few and septic deaths from any cause have occurred only in elderly patients and those with massive (>80% of BSA) injuries.[30] The mortality rate was very low even in large burn wounds of 50% to 80%.[12] Bowser et al.[4] were not able to show efficacy over and above that of silver sulfadiazine in a prospective study. Nevertheless, this combination may prove to be an effective and safe prophylactic topical agent for extensive burns.

Silver Nitrate Solution (0.5%)

Moyer et al.[38, 39] reintroduced 0.5% silver nitrate solution as a topical agent for the treatment of burns in 1965. Properly used, it is an effective prophylactic agent for burns of less than 50% total surface area. It is not widely used clinically anymore because it leaves black stains and has a somewhat limited scope of efficacy. In addition, the cost of dressings and of manpower to appropriately care for these dressings, as well as to clean the linen, walls, and floors, is prohibitive compared to other methods of topical therapy. Moreover, the mineral leaching by the hypotonic solution requires additional monitoring and therapy. Hyponatremia can occur rapidly, particularly in infants with extensive burns. The treatment spectrum includes common bacterial and fungal burn wound pathogens. *Staphylococcus aureus* is recoverable from 30% to 50% of wounds, but its density is generally low and staphylococcal bacteremia is uncommon. Fungal superinfections are rare unless concomitant administration of systemic antibiotics is intense and prolonged. The emergence of silver-resistant organisms is uncommon, probably because silver inhibits growth by several mechanisms, rather than acting at a single locus on the bacterium.[30]

Silver nitrate solution is applied to thick cotton dressings (40-ply) held in place by bias-cut stockinette in a closed technique. These dressings must be wetted every 2 hours to ensure a constant source of silver ions at the wound surface, to prevent the wound from drying, which increases the concentration of silver ions to injurious levels (>2%), and to minimize evaporative water loss and its attendant caloric requirement.[54] Silver nitrate does not cause appreciable pain on open wounds. Necessary removal of crusts of silver salts that tend to accumulate on uninjured or newly healed skin is tedious. Special skills are required to be able to "read" the burn wound and determine inflammation of the burn wound at an early stage. Since there is little absorption of silver through the eschar, the surface must be tended scrupulously before each application of the dressing. The dressings should be applied immediately after the burn injury before the wound is colonized, and silver nitrate solution should not be used for the treatment of true invasive burn wound sepsis.

Minimal absorption of silver occurs through open wounds because of the insolubility of its chloride and other biologically important salts that precipitate on the wound. Plasma silver levels are low, rarely exceeding 200 mg/dl. Most absorbed silver is excreted through the liver and kidney, the remainder being incorporated by reticuloendothelial cells where it causes no known abnormalities. Argyria does not occur with the topical use of silver nitrate, but care should be taken in patients with facial burns to avoid persistent wetting of the conjunctiva with silver nitrate solution, as permanent discoloration of the conjunctiva can result. Silver is essentially nonallergenic.

Distilled or deionized water must be used as a solvent for silver nitrate solution (29.4 mEq of silver per liter) to avoid the precipitation of the silver by chloride and other anions. When this hypotonic solution is kept in contact with open wounds, leaching of plasma sodium, potassium, and other electrolytes occurs regularly (350 mEq or more of sodium per square meter of wound surface area can be lost daily into the dressings). Oral or intravenous supplementation with as much as 20 to 30 gm of sodium chloride daily is necessary in patients with extensive injuries. Plasma and urine sodium and potassium content must be monitored carefully to gauge the necessary replacement therapy accurately. Diarrhea can occur from the large enteral salt supplements.

Many gram-negative bacteria can reduce nitrate to nitrite. Absorption of nitrite through the wound results occasionally in methemoglobinemia. This diagnosis should be entertained if the skin or wounds acquire a slate-gray or blue color, and/or the blood is brown despite a normal partial pressure of oxygen. The diagnosis is confirmed by determining the percentage of methemoglobin in the blood. Withdrawal of the silver nitrate solution is the recommended treatment in mild or moderate cases. Intravenous administration of reducing agents such as methylene blue or ascorbic acid will lower the methemoglobin concentration quickly in severe cases.

Treatment failure is common when burn size exceeds 60% of BSA. Silver nitrate may delay colonization for only a few days when wound size exceeds 70% of BSA. No reports of decreasing clinical efficacy with its protracted use have appeared.

Scarlet Red

Scarlet red is an azo dye used in 5% concentration (ortho-tolylazo-ortho-tolylazo-β-naphthol), soluble in lanolin, olive oil, and petrolatum that provides a low wound pH, which is not conducive to bacterial growth. This drug finds limited use on donor sites and partial-thickness burn wounds. It is applied in a single layer. Multiple layers tend to trap exudate and lead to infections beneath the dressings. It is painless on application, but many patients complain of pain in a donor site treated with scarlet red, probably because of desiccation and the stiff, unyielding dressing formed when blood or exudate combines with the dressing and drys. Therefore, the recommended use is on a shallow wound that has excellent hemostasis.

Some studies have shown accelerated epithelial growth compared to other topical agents. One disadvantage is that tanning, which is inevitable with repeated use of this dressing, may make serial evaluation of the wound for inflammation difficult. In addition, the dye stains the clothing and bedding as well as the personnel and thus has earned a reputation similar to that of 0.5% silver nitrate. Studies using high concentrations on rodents have shown the development of lesions that look like squamous cell neoplasms, but similar occurrences on burned patients are exceedingly rare.

SUMMARY

Topical antimicrobial agents are the first line of defense against infections in burn wounds. They should be used on all children with significant burn injuries and in those at risk because of inhalation injury or associated injury or illness, or in very young patients with lesser burns. Burn wound colonization must be delayed for as long as possible and burn wound sepsis prevented.

The topical agents currently available all have shortcomings, and some have considerable toxic effects. It is essential that the burn physician and other members of the burn team be able to recognize topical treatment failure promptly. An appropriate alternative agent must be substituted and aggressive wound care debridement instituted. Systemic antibiotics should be used sparingly, but are often necessary to treat burn wound sepsis or pulmonary or other concomitant infections, especially in patients with major injuries. The overall treatment program should minimize the chances of wound microbial contamination. Appropriate physical, metabolic, and nutritional supportive treatment is essential.

We must not lose sight of the fact that the best topical, therapeutic agent will not eradicate the bacteria within the burn wound. The control that the topical antimicrobials provide is merely a way of providing enough time to close the burn wound. If aggressive wound closure is not pursued, or graft failures allow the burn wound to remain open, bacterial proliferation of the burn wound will escape effective topical control, and burn wound sepsis will supervene despite all our best efforts. It behooves us to use the topical antimicrobial armamentarium wisely and in perspective with the overall wound care plan.

REFERENCES

1. Babb JR, et al: Topical chemoprophylaxis: Trials with silver phosphate chlorhexidine, silver sulphadiazine and povidone-iodine preparations. *Burns* 1977; 3:65–71.
2. Ballin JC: Evaluation of a new topical agent for burn therapy. *JAMA* 1974; 230:1184–1185.
3. Bolasny BL, Shepard GH, Scott HW: The hazards of intravenous polyethylene catheters in surgical patients. *Surg Gynecol Obstet* 1974; 130:1184–1185.
4. Bowser, BH, Caldwell FT, Cone JB, et al: A prospective analysis of silver sulfadiazine with and without cerium nitrate as a topical agent in the treatment of severely burned children. *J Trauma* 1981; 21:558–563.
5. Bridges K, Lowbury EJL: Drug resistance in relation to use of silver sulphadiazine cream in a burns unit. *J Clin Pathol* 1977; 30:160–164.
6. Butcher HR Jr, Margraf HW, Gravens DL: The treatment of large cutaneous burns with silver creams. *J Trauma* 1969; 9:359–376.
7. Cesany P: Clinical experience with povidone-iodine (Betadine) in the treatment of burns and as an adjunct in plastic surgery. *Pharmatherapeutica* 1977; 1:514–521.
8. Curreri PW, et al: *Providencia stuartii* sepsis: A new challenge in the treatment of thermal injury. *Ann Surg* 1973; 177:133–138.
9. Davies MRO: Intravenous and oral feeding after burns. *S Afr Med J* 1976; 50:1673–1675.
10. Feller I, Archambeault C: Thirds solution, in Feller I, Archambeault C: *Nursing the Burned*

Patient. Ann Arbor, Michigan Institute for Burn Medicine. Braun-Brumfield, Inc, 1973, p. 135.
11. Fox CL Jr: Silver sulfadiazine—a new topical therapy for *Pseudomonas* in burns: Therapy of *Pseudomonas* infection in burns. *Arch Surg* 1968; 96:184–188.
12. Fox CL Jr, Monafo WW Jr, Ayvazian VH, et al: Topical chemotherapy for burns using cerium salts and silver sulfadiazine. *Surg Gynecol Obstet* 1977; 144:668–672.
13. Haynes BW Jr: Burn therapy: A current appraisal. *Surg Annu* 1971; 3:125–147.
14. Heimbach D, Engrav LH: *Surgical Management of the Burn Wound*. New York, Raven Press, 1984.
15. Hummel RP, MacMillan BG, Altemeier WA: Topical and systemic antibacterial agents in the treatment of burns. *Ann Surg* 1970; 172:370–384.
16. Inancsi W, Wachtel TL: An operative technique for quantitative burn wound biopsy. Presented at the 15th Annual Meeting of the American Burn Association, New Orleans, March 1983.
17. Kiker RG, et al: A controlled study of the effects of silver sulfadiazine on white blood cell counts in burned children. *J Trauma* 1977; 17:835–836.
18. Krause W, Metheis H, Wulf K: Fungaemia and funguria after oral administration of *Candida albicans*. *Lancet* 1969; 1:598–599.
19. Krizek TJ, Robson MC: Evolution of quantitative bacteriology in wound management. *Am J Surg* 1975; 130:579–584.
20. Kucan JO, Robson M: Care of the burned ear, in Wachtel TL, Frank DH (eds): *Burns of the Head and Neck*. Philadelphia, WB Saunders Co, 1984, pp 75–88.
21. Lennard ES, et al: Association in burn patients of improved antibacterial defense with nutritional support by the oral route. *Burns* 1975; 1:98–107.
22. Lindberg RB, et al: The successful control of burn wound sepsis. *J Trauma* 1965; 5:601–616.
23. Lindberg RB, Moncrief JA, Mason AD: Control of experimental and clinical burn wound sepsis by topical application of sulfamylon compounds. *Ann NY Acad Sci* 1968; 150:950–960.
24. Lowbury EJL: Recent studies in the control of burn infection. *Burns* 1975; 2:26–32.
25. Lowbury EJL, et al: Alternative forms of local treatment for burns. *Lancet* 1971; 2:1111.
26. Lowbury EJL, et al: Topical chemoprophylaxis with silver sulphadiazine and silver nitrate chlorhexidine creams: Emergence of sulphonamide-resistant gram-negative bacilli. *Br Med J* 1976; 1:493–496.
27. MacMillan BG: Ecology of bacteria colonizing the burned patient given topical and systemic gentamicin therapy: A five-year study. *J Infect Dis* 1971; 124:278–286.
28. MacMillan BG, Hill EO, Altemeier WA: Use of topical silver nitrate, mafenide, and gentamicin in the burn patient: A comparative study. *Arch Surg* 1967; 95:472–481.
29. McCauley RL, et al: Silver sulfadiazine-nitrofurazone in the treatment of major burns. *J Burn Care Rehabil* 1984; 5:384–387.
30. Monafo WW, Avyazaian VH: Topical therapy. *Surg Clin North Am* 1978; 58:1157–1171.
31. Moncrief JA: Topical therapy of the burn wound: Present status. *Clin Pharmacol Ther* 1969; 10:439–448.
32. Moncrief JA: The development of topical therapy. *J Trauma* 1971; 11:906–910.
33. Moncrief JA: Medical progress: Burns. *N Engl J Med* 1973; 288:444–454.
34. Moncrief JA: Topical antibacterial therapy of the burn wound. *Clin Plast Surg* 1974; 1:563–576.
35. Moncrief JA: Topical therapy for control of bacteria in the burn wound. *World J Surg* 1978; 2:151–165.
36. Moncrief JA: Topical antibacterial treatment of the burn wound, in Artz CA, Moncrief JA, Pruitt BA Jr (eds): *Burns*. Philadelphia, WB Saunders Co, 1979, pp 250–267.
37. Moncrief JA, et al: Use of topical antibacterial therapy in the treatment of the burn wound. *Arch Surg* 1960; 92:558–565.
38. Moyer CA, et al: Treatment of large human burns with 0.5% silver nitrate solution. *Arch Surg* 1965; 90:812–867.
39. Moyer CA, Monafo WW: Effectiveness of dilute aqueous silver nitrate in the treatment of major burns. *Arch Surg* 1965; 921:200–210.
40. Nathan P, Holder IA, MacMillan BG: Burn wounds, microbiology, local host defenses and current therapy. *CRC Crit Rev Clin Lab Sci* 1973; 4:61–100.
41. Ollstein RN, et al: Alternate case study of topical sulfamylon and silver sulphadiazine in burns. *Plast Reconstr Surg* 1971; 48:311–317.
42. O'Neill JA, et al; Suppurative thrombophebitis—a lethal complication of intravenous therapy. *J Trauma* 1968; 8:256–267.
43. Pietsch J, Meakins JL: Complications of povidone-iodine absorption in topically treated burn patients. *Lancet* 1976; 1:280–282.
44. Polk HC, Monafo WW, Moyer CA: Human burn survival study of the efficacy of 0.5%

aqueous silver nitrate. *Arch Surg* 1969; 98:262–265.
45. Polk HC, Tessler RH: Sodium transit across burn wounds treated with silver nitrate solutions (0.5%). *Ann NY Acad Sci* 1968; 150:682–684.
46. Prince HN, et al: Drug resistance studies with topical antiseptics. *J Pharm Sci* 1978; 67:1629–1635.
47. Pruitt BA Jr: Use of Sulfamylon in burned patients, in Lynch JB, Lewis SR (eds): Symposium on the Treatment of Burns. St. Louis, CV Mosby Co, 1973, pp 117–122.
48. Pruitt BA, Jr, Dowling JA, Moncrief JA; Escharotomy in early burn care. *Arch Surg* 1968; 96:502–507.
49. Pruitt BA Jr, O'Neill JA Jr, Moncrief JA, et al: Successful control of burn wound sepsis. *JAMA* 1968; 203:1054–1056.
50. Richardson GI, et al: Fungal infection in burn patients: Results of using 5-fluorocytosine (flucytosine). *Burns* 1975; 1:113–118.
51. Robson MC, Kucan JO: The burn wound, in Wachtel TL, Kahn V, Frank HA (eds): *Current Topics in Burn Care.* Rockville Md, Aspen Systems Corp 1983, pp 55–63.
52. Rode HP, et al: An experimental evaluation of the germicidal efficacy of three topical antimicrobial agents in burns. *Prog Pediatr Surg* 1981; 14:189–208.
53. Shuck JM, Moncrief JA: Safeguards in the use of topical mafenide (Sulfamylon) in burn patients. *Am J Surg* 1969; 118:864–810.
54. Shuck JM, Moncrief JA, Monafo WW: The management of burns: I. General considerations and the Sulfamylon method. II. The silver nitrate method. *Curr Probl Surg* 1969; 6:3–65.
55. Smith RF, et al: Effects of sodium hypochlorite on the microbial flora of burns and normal skin. *J Trauma* 1974; 14:938–944.
56. Sefanides M: In vitro penetration of topical antiseptics through eschar of burn patients. *Ann Surg* 1976; 183:358–364.
57. Stone HH: Wound care with topical gentamicin, in Polk HC Jr, Stone HH (eds): *Contemporary Burn Management.* Boston, Little, Brown & Co, 1971, pp 203–216.
58. Teplitz C: The pathological burns and the fundamentals of burn wound sepsis, in Artz CP, Moncrief JA, Pruitt BA Jr (eds): *Burns.* Philadelphia, WB Saunders Co, 1979, pp 45–94.
59. Ternberg JI, Luce E: Methemoglobinemia: A complication of the silver nitrate treatment of burns. *Surgery* 1968; 63:328–330.
60. Wachtel TL: Care of the burn wound, in Wachtel TL, Frank DH (eds): *Burns of the Head and Neck.* Philadelphia, WB Saunders Co, 1984, pp 56–63.
61. Wachtel TL, et al: A semiclosed method of burn wound dressing. *J Burn Care Rehabil* 1984; 5:158–162.
62. Wachtel TL, Parks SN, Dimick AR: Early enzymatic debridement and grafting of burned hands: Evaluating the Travase fast-graft method for deep dermal burns. *J Burn Care Rehabil* 1983; 4:325–330.
63. Wallace AB: The exposure treatment of burns. *Lancet* 1951; 1:501–504.

10 / Nutrition and Metabolism

WILEY W. SOUBA, M.D., Sc.D.
BETH A. SCHINDLER, R.D., M.S.
HUGO F. CARVAJAL, M.D.

No group of surgical patients has benefited more from the advances in nutritional support than the burn patient. As recently as 15 years ago, many individuals with thermal injuries died from malnutrition, sepsis, and multiple-system organ failure because enteral and parenteral feedings were not possible or were inadequate. Today, a substantial number of adult and pediatric patients survive major burn injuries and complications such as sepsis. Virtually all burn patients may now receive nutritional support due to three recent developments: (1) the technique of central venous cannulation and infusion of hypertonic nutrient solutions into the superior vena cava, (2) the development of specific, enteral formula diets that can be taken orally or by feeding tube, and (3) the availability of fat emulsions for safe intravenous administration. In addition, growing knowledge of the alterations in intermediary metabolism and metabolic regulation that accompany severe injury has improved the nutritional-metabolic care provided to burn patients.

Extensive burn injury initiates the most marked alterations in body metabolism that can be associated with any illness observed in contemporary society. The persistent tachycardia, tachypnea, hyperpyrexia, and marked body wasting of the burned patient reflect the heightened metabolic activity and accelerated body catabolism that characterizes the metabolic response to injury. In the burned child, this profound catabolism is responsible for the malnutrition that rapidly develops when nutritional support is not provided (Fig 10–1). Moreover, burned children are frequently anorexic, confined to bed, and rarely take adequate calories spontaneously from a food tray. Frequent surgical procedures require that the patient receive nothing by mouth, and gastrointestinal complications often limit the use of the enteral route for feeding purposes. Hence, the provision of adequate nutrients in the form of parenteral and/or enteral feeding is essential.

This chapter will review the metabolic alterations that occur in patients sustaining thermal injuries. Methods to assess the nutritional needs of the pediatric burn patient will be provided along with the current knowledge of the nutritional requirements of these individuals. The basis for selecting the safest and most efficacious route of nutrient administration will also be discussed.

METABOLIC RESPONSE TO THERMAL INJURY

The majority of studies on the metabolic response to burn injury have focused on adult patients. However, most of the physiologic responses in children are similar, and hence a review of the neuroendocrine responses to thermal injury provides a basis for the nutritional-metabolic care provided to these individuals.

General Overview and Time Course

Thermal injury is followed by a well-described pattern of physiological responses.[34] The events are generally related to the sever-

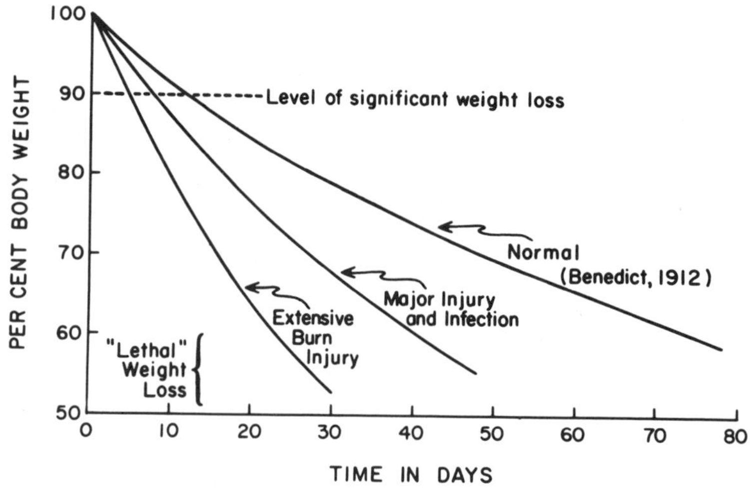

FIG 10–1.
Extensive burn injury accelerates weight loss and requires vigorous nutritional support. (From Souba WW, Bessey PQ: Nutritional support of the trauma patient. *Infect Surg* 1984; 3:727–736. Used by permission.)

ity of the burn injury, such that the greater the extent of the burn, the more pronounced the specific response. Burn injuries greater than 50% usually elicit a maximal physiologic response.

Cuthbertson[18] first described the time course for many of the posttraumatic responses. Two distinct time periods were identified: an early "ebb" and subsequent "flow phase." The ebb or shock phase in burn patients is usually relatively brief in duration (24 to 48 hours) and occurs immediately following the thermal injury. Initially, blood pessure, cardiac output, body temperature, and oxygen consumption are reduced. These events are associated with hypovolemia, hypoperfusion, and lactic acidosis due to the tremendous fluid losses that characterize the immediate postburn period. Retention of large quantities of sodium and water may occur during the process of fluid resuscitation, and dramatic increases in body weight, which may rise 20% above preinjury level, are not uncommon. During recovery, the edema fluid reenters the vascular compartment, and the sodium and water that were retained are slowly excreted by the kidneys. Although sodium and water retention may occur in patients with minor nonthermal injuries, the magnitude of these events are much less dramatic. Following adequate resuscitation, the "ebb" phase gives way to more accelerated responses. The "flow phase" is characterized by hypermetabolism, increased cardiac output, increased urinary nitrogen losses, altered glucose metabolism, and accelerated tissue catabolism.

Physiologic Responses to Burn Injury

Endocrine changes and their metabolic consequences

One of the earliest consequences of major injury is a rise in circulating cortisol, which occurs in response to a release of adrenocorticotropic hormone (ACTH) from the anterior pituitary gland.[67] Activation of the pituitary gland occurs when afferent nervous signals from the burn wound reach the hypothalamus to initiate the stress response. The rise in ACTH stimulates the adrenal cortex, which elaborates cortisol. This hormone may remain elevated for several weeks, especially if the burn wound is large and ungrafted. Cortisol exerts profound effects on tissue catabolism and results in mobilization of amino acids from skeletal muscle; these provide substrates for wound healing and serve as precursors for the hepatic synthesis of acute-phase proteins or new glucose. Associated with the activation of the adrenal cortex is stimulation of the adrenal medulla via the sympathetic nervous system with elaboration of epinephrine. This circulating neurotransmitter plays an important role in maintaining cardiovascular integrity during the ebb phase, but may also elicit metabolic responses if the augmented secretion rate continues over a prolonged period of time. In addition to increased circulating levels of epinephrine, norepinephrine rises during and following major burn injury. Excitement, pain, fear, and hypovolemia, which accompany the injury, are potent stimulators of the sympathetic nervous system. A major role of the catecholamine system is the stimulation of hepatic glycogenolysis and gluconeogenesis in concert with the production of glucagon and glucocorticoids.[34]

The neuroendocrine responses to injury also modify renal mechanisms involved in salt and water excretion.[34] Alterations in serum osmolality and tonicity of body fluids secondary to the trauma stress stimulate the secretion of aldosterone and antidiuretic hormone (ADH). Aldosterone is a potent stimulator of renal sodium retention, while ADH stimulates renal tubular water reabsorption. Although the neural and humoral mediators that result from tissue trauma may stimulate aldosterone release, afferent signals from volume receptors appear to be the major stimuli for these hormonal adjustments.

The ability to excrete a water load after major injury is reduced.[34] If kidney function is maintained, the burn-injured patient will concentrate the urine to 1 to 2 ml of water per milliosmole of solute excreted. This corresponds to a urine osmolality of 500 to 1,000 mOsm/L, even in the presence of adequate hydration. Hence, weight gain secondary to salt and water retention is a usual occurrence following burn injury. Edema occurs to a varying extent in all wounds, and this accumulation is proportional to the extent of burn injury. Administration of lactated Ringer's solution during resuscitation replaces the volume lost, and the excess fluid redistributes in the interstitial space. This "third-spaced" fluid will eventually return to the circulation as the wound edema subsides and diuresis commences.

Burn injury also alters the normal response of the endocrine pancreas. In general, the insulin/glucagon ratio is diminished. This response may be related to increased sympathetic activity or the rise in levels of circulating epinephrine, which is known to suppress insulin release. The rise in glucagon and fall in insulin serve as potent signals to accelerate hepatic glucose production, and in combination with other hormones (epinephrine and glucocorticoids), glucogenesis is maintained.

In summary, hormonal alterations that occur following injury are thought to orchestrate physiologic and biochemical changes that benefit the host. During the ebb phase, salt and water conservation support the circulating blood volume. Augmented hepatic glucose production provides essential fuel for the nervous system, red and white blood cells, and the healing wound. Skeletal muscle proteolysis provides amino acid precursors for gluconeogenesis and hepatic protein synthesis. Postoperative lipolysis provides abundant quantities of free fatty acids, which are utilized as a principal energy source. Current techniques of postinjury care minimize but do not eliminate these responses.

CHARACTERISTICS OF THE FLOW PHASE OF THE INJURY RESPONSE

HYPERMETABOLISM.—Hypermetabolism is defined as an increase in basal metabolic rate (BMR) above that predicted on the basis of age, sex, and body size. Metabolic rate is usually determined by measuring the exchange of respiratory gases and calculating heat production from oxygen consumption and carbon dioxide production. The degree of hypermetabolism is generally related to the severity of the burn injury.[7] Patients with severe injury (>50% of total body surface area [BSA]) demonstrate resting metabolic rates that may reach twice the basal levels. Rates of heat production in burned patients are often contrasted with those in postoperative patients, who rarely increase their BMR by more than 10% to 15% following surgical intervention.

Concomitant with the development of hypermetabolism, the burn patient usually develops a 1° to 2° C elevation in body temperature.[57] This posttraumatic fever is a well-recognized component of the injury response and represents an upward shift in the thermal regulatory set point of the brain. In general this febrile response is not marked, and the patient remains asymptomatic.

Increased oxygen consumption is a generalized response to injury; all tissues of the body seem to participate in this response.[7] In addition to injury severity, oxygen consumption is related to cardiac output. On a regional level, however, a disassociation exists between oxygen consumption and blood flow in certain cardiovascular beds. When comparing hemodynamic and metabolic events in burned and unburned lower extremities, oxygen consumption is similar in the two extremities, but blood flow to the injured limb is three to four times greater than in the non-injured leg. The increased blood flow is directed to the surface injury, not to the deep, underlying muscle. Thus, the wound is found to be an important regulator of regional events. In this case, it results in increased blood flow in apparent support of regenerative processes occurring in the wound that do not require oxygen. The kidney also increases consumption of oxygen. Renal blood flow, however, is variable and depends more on solute load and blood volume than oxidative requirements. Splanchnic blood flow is increased in rough proportion to increased regional oxygen consumption. Increased splanchnic flow and increased flow to the wound account for the major portion of the increased cardiac output following injury.

Visceral oxygen consumption increases markedly with thermal injury, while peripheral oxygen uptake remains a fixed percentage of total aerobic metabolism. Hence, burn hypermetabolism appears to be a generalized systemic response involving the entire body.[7] Consequently, the general increase in body heat production appears to be distributed in a relatively normal fashion, i.e., two thirds of the heat being produced in the visceral tissues and one third in the extremities. The heat produced in the burn patient is primarily a result of fat oxidation, and the major portion of the heat produced is the result of biochemical inefficiency. Some increase in mechanical work occurs in thermally injured patients because of the increased respiratory and cardiac activity, but this accounts for a minor portion of the total heat produced. Similarly, transport work may be slightly increased. However, synthetic work is clearly the major identifiable requirement for extra energy; the thermally injured patient produces new glucose, acute-phase proteins, albumin, and leukocytes, which are needed in the healing of a large surface wound. The increased energy required for protein synthesis may account for the major quantity of energy utilized for synthetic purposes. The relative contribution of all these synthetic processes to the production of body heat is unknown at this time.

The extra heat given off by these relatively inefficient metabolic processes in the burned child is sufficient to raise body temperature despite accelerated rates of heat loss across the surface wound. Because of increased rates of blood flow through the wound, body heat is channeled to the injured surface where it raises local temperature above that of the uninjured skin. This increased wound temperature serves to accelerate wound healing. Because rates of superficial blood flow are high, and heat is brought from visceral tissues to the wound, wound temperature is elevated above that of the unburned skin. If the cooling effect that is brought about by evaporation of water is considered, the influence of increased superficial blood flow in monitoring an elevated wound temperature is even more impressive. This increase in wound temperature supports cell proliferation and accelerates wound healing. However, the increased heat production imposes a metabolic cost to the patient and results in accelerated tissue catabolism and disruption of body mass. The increased energy demands must be met by a vigorous feeding program if the complications of catabolism and weight loss are to be avoided and the accelerated thermogenic mechanisms supported.

It was once thought that the increase in metabolic rate in injured persons, especially in those with burns, was a response to increased evaporative heat loss from the wound. This hypothesis was supported by the finding that raising ambient temperature reduced in part the hypermetabolic response following burn injury. However, even in very warm environments, burn patients remained hypermetabolic, and their body temperatures remained elevated. Burned children and other injured patients are internally warm, not externally cold, and have elevated core and mean skin temperatures. Furthermore, when allowed to select the ambient temperature of comfort, burn and injured patients invariably choose ambient temperatures higher than those of uninjured controls. These observations imply that injury resets upward the central thermostat located in the hypothalamus. Increased body temperature is associated with an increase in metabolic rate (temperature coefficient or Q_{10} effect). However, the increased oxygen consumption associated with increased body temperature only accounts for approximately 30% of the increase in heat production observed following injury. Increased metabolic rates seen following trauma are primary effects of the injury. They can be aggravated by cold exposure, pain, anxiety, other treatment-related factors, and complications, particularly associated infection.

ALTERED GLUCOSE METABOLISM.—Hyperglycemia is commonly seen following thermal injury, and at least during the ebb phase, the elevation of fasting blood glucose levels generally parallels the severity of the burn injury. Insulin levels are generally low, and glucose production is only slightly accelerated. During the flow phase insulin concentrations in the blood are normal or elevated, however, the hyperglycemia persists. This observation suggests an alteration in the relationship between insulin sensitivity and glucose disposal. Hepatic glucose production is increased, and the accelerated gluconeogenesis tends generally to be related to the extent of the injury. Studies on burn patients report that much of the new glucose generated by the liver arises from three carbon precursors (lactate, pyruvate, amino acids, and glycerol) released from peripheral tissues. The liver has generally been considered the central organ in gluconeogenesis. The accelerated gluconeogenesis characteristic of burn patients is mediated in large part by the glucocorticoid hormones that activate the enzymes of gluconeogenesis. However, recent work suggests that the gut and liver interact in a cooperative fashion in the synthesis of new glucose.[60] Administration of dexamethasone to dogs has revealed that the gut switches to an organ of net glucose release during glucocorticoid administration.[59, 60] Simultaneously, the uptake of gut glutamine, which serves as an alternate fuel, is accelerated and the glutamine carbons utilized for the synthesis of glucose. Gut alanine release is also increased, and this key gluconeogenic precursor can be consumed by the liver and utilized to support gluconeogenesis.

Wilmore and associates[68] measured substrate exchange across injured and uninjured extremities of severely burned patients to determine which peripheral tissues are utilized as large quantities of glucose are produced. Net glucose flux across uninjured extremities was low. This finding suggests that fat, not glucose, was the primary fuel for resting skeletal muscle in the postabsorptive state. However, glucose uptake across the burned extremity increased. In addition, the injured extremity released large quantities of lactate, which accounted for as much as 80% of the glucose consumed. This is consistent with our knowledge of the biochemistry of highly specialized cells of the wound and inflammatory tissue (fibroblasts, macrophages, and leukocytes) which undergo anaerobic metabolism and demonstrate a large capacity for lactate production. Additional measurements of blood flow and substrate concentration across the kidney and brain further characterize the glucose disposal and resting metabolism in burned patients. The glucose consumed by the central nervous system in the burn patient is approximately normal, whereas the rate of glucose consumed by the kidney may be as high as twice normal. Only a small fraction of the glucose is taken up by resting skeletal muscle, and the remainder is consumed by the wound. The wound converts most of the glucose to lactate, and the latter is recycled by the liver in the Cori cycle.

These alterations in glucose metabolism have a profound impact on the handling of the exogenously administered glucose contained in enteral or parenteral feedings. Thermally injured patients, like other trauma patients, are unable to dispose of intravenously administered glucose to the same degree that normal controls are. The quantity of insulin elaborated by patients with thermal injuries is significantly greater than controls if these rising insulin concentrations fail to increase glucose clearance in injured patients. Other studies have demonstrated failure to suppress hepatic glucose production in injured patients during glucose loading or insulin infusion. Wolfe et al.[74] using tracer methodology, found that endogenous suppression was only 73% of the infused glucose load in burned children. Glucose infusion at the rate used by Wolfe et al.[74] completely suppressed glucose production in normal volunteers. Direct measurements demonstrate that liver and skeletal muscle are tissues that are markedly resistant. Moreover, lipolysis is not reduced in trauma patients following glucose administration. For example, insulin-mediated forearm glucose uptake is markedly diminished in normal individuals following 2 hours of epinephrine infusion, and similarly, 3 days of glucocorticoid administration will decrease skeletal muscle glucose consumption.

ALTERATIONS IN PROTEIN METABOLISM.— Extensive urinary nitrogen losses occur in all patients suffering major thermal injuries.[69] Because of the magnitude of these losses and the progressive wasting of skeletal muscle mass that ensues, it has been established that the nitrogen losses result from a generalized breakdown of muscle protein. The unburned extremity demonstrates profound proteolysis as does the injured extremity. Like other systemic responses to thermal injury, the loss of nitrogen following burn injuries relates not only to the extent of the burn, but also to the preexisting nutritional status of the individual, the age of the patient, and, in part, the size of the muscle mass.

While nitrogen balance studies demonstrate marked negative nitrogen balance following burn injury, these studies reflect only net nitrogen catabolism and not the absolute rate of nitrogen breakdown in various tissues. In normal volunteers, nitrogen equilibrium is maintained by a careful balance between rates of protein synthesis and rates of degradation. Negative nitrogen balance will occur if the breakdown rate increases and protein synthesis remains the same, or if the breakdown rate remains the same and the rate of synthesis decreases.

That skeletal muscle is the origin of the urine nitrogen following extensive injury was initially suggested by Cuthbertson[17] in patients with long-bone fractures. Further evidence of net skeletal muscle breakdown has been demonstrated by quantifying the loss of amino acids from extremities of severely burned patients. Aulick and Wilmore[6] used plethysmographic techniques to measure leg blood flow and simultaneously determined arterial and femoral venous amino acid concentrations in burn patients. They found a threefold to fourfold increase in amino acid flux from the extremities of injured patients compared with normal volunteers. Alanine efflux was the most significantly elevated of the amino acids measured, however, glutamine was not measured. The increase in alanine from the legs of severely burned patients was generally related to the extent of the injury and the oxygen consumption of the burn patient but was not related to the size of the limb injury or to leg blood flow. Accelerated rates of α-aminonitrogen release from the limbs of these patients appeared to be a generalized catabolic effect of injury rather than a response to local inflammatory or metabolic events that may have occurred in the burned extremity.

While it is now recognized that amino acids are released from muscle in accelerated amounts following all kinds of injury, only recently has it been appreciated that the composition of amino acids efflux does not reflect the composition of muscle protein. Alanine and glutamine comprised 50% to 60% of the amino acids released, whereas each makes up only about 6% of muscle protein[51] (Fig 10–2). The branch-chain amino acids, on the other hand, make up approximately 6% of the released amino acids that constitute nearly 15% of muscle protein. Goldberg et al.[43] have proposed that the branch-chain amino acids serve as amino donors for α-ketoglutarate, yielding the corresponding branch-chain keto-acids and glutamate. The keto-acids can be converted to tricarboxylic acid cycle intermediates in skeletal muscle or can be exported via the bloodstream. Glutamate can serve as a precursor for glutamine synthesis or as an amino donor for alanine synthesis. These coupled reactions can explain the biosynthesis and increased release of alanine and glutamine as well as the diminished release of branch-chain amino acids. Oxidation of branch-chain amino acids by skeletal muscle is accelerated following injury, and skeletal muscle glutamine and alanine release is increased (or accelerated). Glutamine is consumed by the kidney where it is utilized for ammoniagenesis and contributes to acid-base homeostasis. This effect can be augmented in the dog by the administration of glucocorticoids. In addition, glutamine is taken up by the gastrointestinal tract and serves as an oxidative fuel.[72] The enterocytes convert glutamine primarily to ammonia and alanine, and these two substances are released into the portal blood. The ammonia is removed by the liver and converted to urea or glutamine,

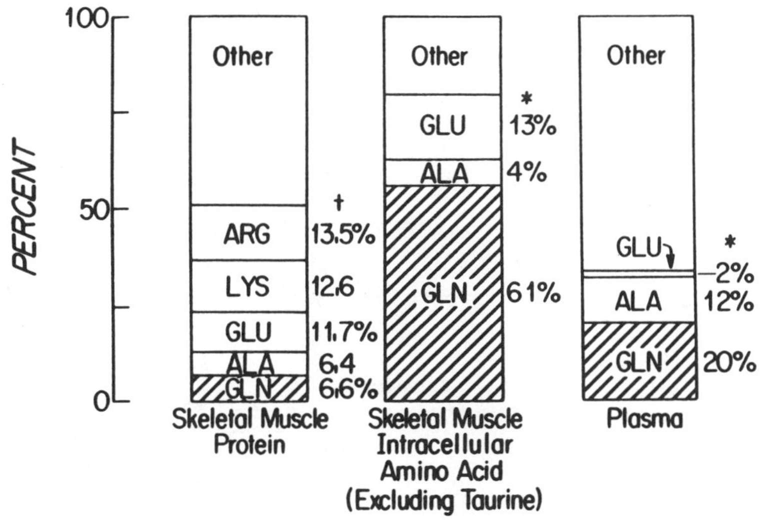

FIG 10–2.
Amino acid composition of normal man. ALA = alanine; ARG = arginine; GLN = glutamine; GLU = glutamate; LYS = lysine. Asterisk indicates data from Bergstrom J, Furst P, Noree LO, et al: Intracellular free amino acid concentration in human muscle tissue. *J Appl Physiol* 1974; 36:693. Dagger indicates data from Kominz DR, Hough A, Symonds P, et al: The amino acid composition of actin, myosin, tropomyosin, and the meromyosins. *Arch Biochem Biophys* 1954; 50:148. (From Souba WW, et al: *J Parenter Enteral Nutr* 1985; 9:608–617. Used by permission.)

while the alanine is removed by the liver and serves as a gluconeogenic precursor (Fig 10–3). Following experimental injury glutamine consumption by the bowel and the kidney is accelerated, and this appears to be mediated in part by the increased elaboration of glucocorticoids.[59] Hence, glutamine and alanine are the most important compounds that participate in the transfer of nitrogen from skeletal muscle to visceral organs. However, the metabolic handling of glutamine and alanine favor disposal of their nitrogens in the form of urea and ammonia and these latter components are excreted by the kidney (Fig 10–4).

FAT METABOLISM.—To support hypermetabolism, increased gluconeogenesis and interorgan substrate flux, stored triglycerides are mobilized and oxidized at an accelerated rate. Studies in burn patients as well as other injured patients have demonstrated that the respiratory quotient is approximately 0.7 to 0.75, suggesting that fat is the principal fuel oxidized. If unfed, severely injured patients rapidly deplete their fat and protein stores. Such malnutrition increases susceptibility to added stress of hemorrhage, surgery, and infection and may contribute to organ system failure, sepsis, and death. Hence, vigorous nutritional support using enteral or combined enteral-parenteral feeding during this catabolic phase of trauma is essential to reduce body waste and produce caloric equilibrium and weight stabilization. Fat emulsions that are isotonic and contain 1 to 2 calories/ml, may be administered by a peripheral vein to avoid the many hazards associated with central venous infusions.

STAGE OF SURGICAL CONVALESCENCE

The period of catabolism initiated by injury is characterized by inadequate nutrition and alteration of the hormonal environment, and it has been termed the "adrenergic-corticoid phase.[67] This is followed by the onset of anabolism, which occurs at a variable time in the patient's convalescence. In general, in the absence of complications, this phase starts when the burn wound has been adequately grafted. This turning point from catabolism to anabolism is referred to as the "corticoid-withdrawal

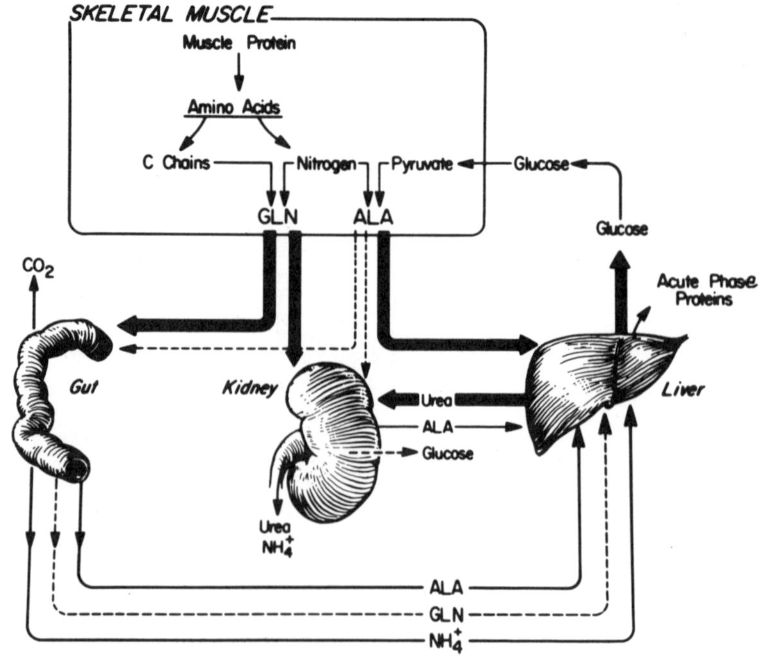

FIG 10–3.
Diagram indicating the interorgan exchange of glutamine (GLN), alanine (ALA), and ammonia (NH_4^+). C = carbon. (From Souba WW, et al: *J Parenter Enteral Nutr* 1985; 9:608–617. Used by permission.)

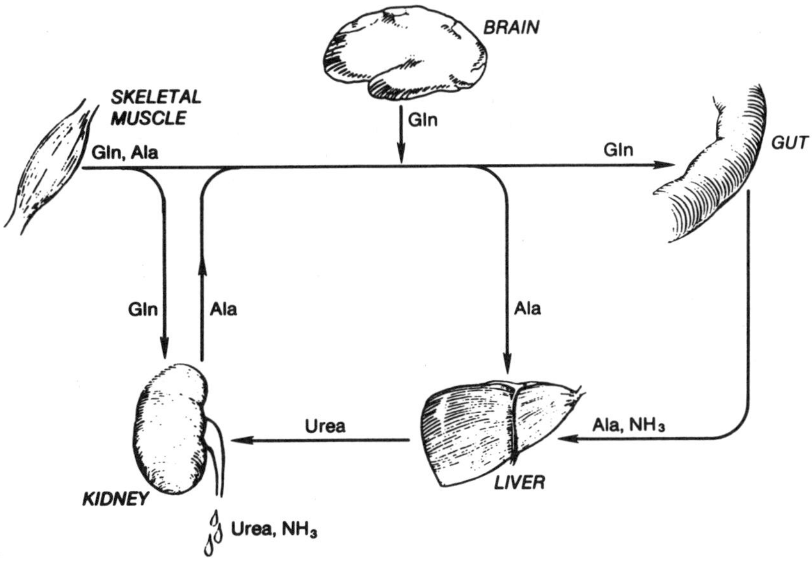

FIG 10–4.
Diagram illustrating the interorgan exchange of glutamine (GLN), alanine (ALA), and ammonia (NH_3)

phase" as it is characterized by positive nitrogen balance and weight gain.[34] Increased protein synthesis results from sustained enteral feedings. This synthesis is related to return of lean body mass and muscular strength. The positive nitrogen balance is usually in the range of 2 to 4 gm of nitrogen per day in the average adult, representing a gain of 60 to 120 gm of lean tissue daily. The total amount of nitrogen ultimately gained will equal the amount lost, but the rate of gain will be a much slower process than the rate of initial loss. The fourth and final phase of convalescence is one of late anabolism, the hallmark of which is a much slower weight gain.[67] During this period, the patient is in nitrogen equilibrium but in positive carbon balance, which results from the deposition of body fat.

FEEDING THE BURNED PATIENT

Although burn injury may affect persons of all ages, young, healthy, and productive individuals are the most commonly injured. Optimal care of these burned patients is often intensive and prolonged, and survival is followed by years of rehabilitation. Nutritional support of the burn patient is a major component of overall care and the focus of this section.

Determination of Nutritional Requirements

Most patients sustaining burn injury are well nourished before insult. However, in the absence of vigorous nutritional support, the profound catabolism associated with major thermal injury leads to malnutrition and its consequences. In general, nutritional support should commence following successful resuscitation and when the flow phase of injury has begun. The final goal in determining nutritional requirements should be to determine (1) the energy the patient requires, (2) the amount of nitrogen associated with protein accretion, and (3) the safe and effective level of the nutrients to be administered.

The total energy requirement of the burned patient represents the sum of several contributing factors including the BMR, the specific dynamic action (SDA) of ingested food substances, the energy expenditure due to activity, and the effect of the burn injury itself.[67] A normal child's BMR can be estimated from height and weight and with appropriate corrections for age and sex. Metabolic rate measurement in the burn patient is often referred to as resting metabolic expenditure (RME) and describes the energy needed by the patient, which includes energy required for basal metabolism plus energy required for eating and physical activity. Nomograms and equations that take into account the patient's degree of metabolic stress are available and predict RME with fairly good accuracy.

Burn patients have metabolic rates that are as high as twice predicted normal values and hence will require vigorous nutritional support. With adequate nitrogen and caloric intake; these patients will frequently gain some weight. It is important to remember that initially weight gain is usually due to water and/or fat deposition and that accretion of lean body mass only occurs when the burn wound has been covered and infection controlled.

Estimating energy requirements with reasonable accuracy is usually possible in most burn patients. Thus, actual measurements of metabolic expenditures are seldom necessary. However, in the research setting, a variety of techniques to measure oxygen consumption and carbon dioxide production are available, and from these measurements, metabolic rate can be easily calculated.

Once energy needs have been estimated or measured, nitrogen requirements can be determined. The primary factors that influence nitrogen balance include the quantity of nitrogen in the diet, the patient's metabolic rate, and the quantity and source of nonprotein energy that a patient receives. The impact of carbohydrate on nitrogen retention during a hypermetabolic disease process appears to be greater than the effect of equal calories of fat.[58] Protein utilization is relatively inefficient in the hypermetabolic burn patient and at the same time catabolism is marked. Therefore, significantly more dietary protein is required to combat the profound catabolism associated with burn injuries. Duke et al.[21] have shown that in such hypermetabolic patients, protein contributes 15% to 20% of total energy expenditure, which makes the optimal calories/nitrogen ratio for achieving maximal nitrogen retention about 150:1. This is the appropriate ratio used in standard central vein hyperalimentation solutions at the present time. Providing more nitrogen may improve nitrogen balance, but caution must be taken bacause such a large protein load may cause a rise in blood urea nitrogen (BUN) levels and may be undesirable in patients with compromised renal function or hepatic dysfunction.

Estimation of calorie requirements in children

The hypermetabolism associated with burn injury generally subsides when the majority of the wounds are grafted or healed.[52, 62] Until then, muscle proteolysis remains accelerated. That is, the body continues to provide precursors to the visceral organs for gluconeogenesis and the synthesis of acute-phase proteins. In children, the endogenous energy stores are limited, and hence these patients are at substantial risk of becoming severely malnourished. Aggressive nutritional support is essential to prevent the consequences of malnutrition.

Various formulas for estimating the caloric requirements of burned children have been utilized.[16, 48, 63] Hildreth and Carvajal[28] allow for both maintenance and burn injury requirements in their formula and use total body surface and body surface burned as the basis for the calculations. *Caloric requirements of the burned child* are estimated as follows:

1,800 kcal/sq m of *body surface* per day (maintenance requirements)
plus
2,200 kcal/sq m of body surface *burned* per day (extra calories required as a result of the injury).

The estimate of maintenance kilocalorie requirements is obtained from the recommended dietary allowances[15] for normal children and is expressed in terms of BSA rather than age or weight. The estimate of kilocalorie requirements for the burn injury takes into account the heat loss associated with predicted fluid losses occurring from evaporation and exudation from the burn wound. Such fluid losses are proportional to the size of the burn wound and occur at a rate of approximately 3,750 ml/sq m of BSA burned per day.[12] For every milliliter of fluid lost, 0.57 kcal are needed to maintain body temperature.[45] This formula allows the health care team to design a dietary program that should minimize depletion of energy and protein reserves and simultaneously promote weight gain and anabolism. In the clinical setting (52 severely burned children), Hildreth and Carvajal[28] demonstrated that adherence to the formula resulted in an average weight gain of 6% (n = 40), while those with insufficient caloric intake (n = 12) lost weight (Fig 10–5).

Every effort should be made to minimize energy demands by reducing external stresses. Pain, anxiety, fear, and cold stimulate the release of catecholamines[50, 66, 71] and raise energy requirements. Narcotics and tranquilizers should be utilized to reduce anxiety and pain.[39] External heating devices can be used to control cold stress. When operative procedures, tubbing, and dressing changes are necessary, attention should be given to maintaining a warm environment.

DETERMINATION OF PROTEIN REQUIREMENTS

It has been recognized that burned individuals require greater than normal protein intake to achieve positive nitrogen balance, which is necessary to heal the wound and replenish protein. Protein requirements are elevated as a result of accelerated tissue catab-

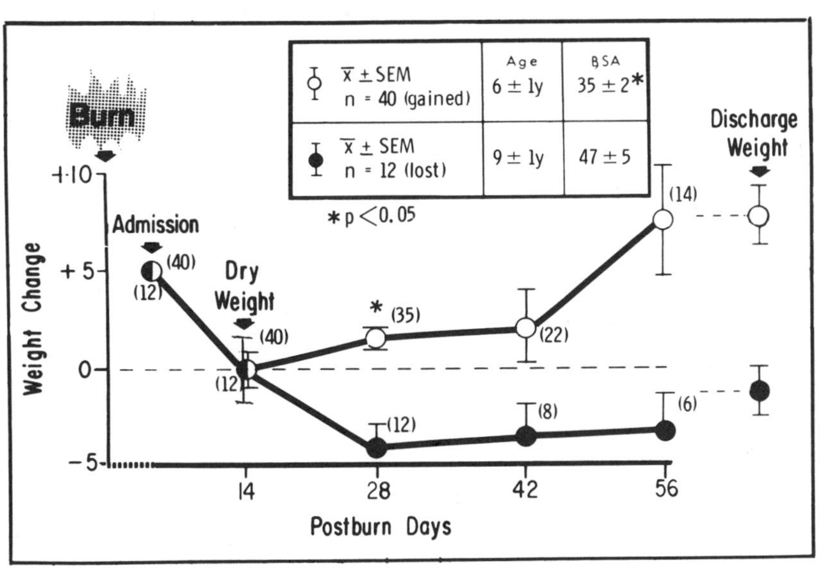

FIG 10–5.
Dry (14 days postinjury) and discharge weights of 52 severely burned children, prospectively monitored from the time of admission, regarding daily caloric intake. All patients with daily caloric intakes equal to or in excess of the formula predictions gained weight (n = 40), while those who failed to achieve the desired intake (n = 12) incurred a 3% to 4% weight loss. (From Hildreth M, Carvajal HF: Caloric requirements in burned children: A simple formula to estimate daily caloric requirements. *J Burn Care Rehabil* 1982; 3:78–80. Used by permission.)

olism, but the rate of protein synthesis is also increased.[33, 74] When protein intake is not sufficient to meet the needs of the patient, somatic muscle and visceral proteins become depleted. Alexander et al.[1] demonstrated that severely burned children on enteral diets containing more than 20% of the calories as high-quality protein, milk-whey protein supplement, had a better survival rate and fewer septic episodes than patients on other dietary regimens. Higher serum levels of total protein, transferrin, C3, and immunoglobulin G (IgG) were also observed (Table 10–1).

Although Alexander's data would favor the use of high protein concentrations for enteral nutrition of burned victims, the animal studies of Dominioni et al.[20] suggest that certain limits should not be surpassed. Using the guinea pig 30% burn model, these authors compared enteral diets containing 20%, 30%, and 40% of the calories as protein. They observed that the total liver protein content and serum albumin levels were maintained and that a 100% survival rate was attained in the group receiving 20% of their calories as protein. The use of 30% of the calories as protein resulted in a reduction in the amount of fat infiltration of the liver, but protein concentrations of greater than 40% of the calories increased liver fat deposition, induced diarrhea, and increased mortality. Thus, based on this information and our own clinical experience, we advocate that no more than 20% to 30% of the caloric requirements be provided in the form of high-quality protein.

VITAMIN AND MINERAL REQUIREMENTS

The optimal vitamin and mineral requirements of the child remain to be determined because experimental and clinical data are incomplete. Individual nutrient requirements are dependent, in part, on preburn status and the extent of injury.

The vitamins thiamine, riboflavin, niacin, and vitamin B_6 are components of essential enzymes and co-enzymes needed to metabolize carbohydrate, fat, and protein.[15] Accordingly, requirements for these vitamins will increase as energy requirements increase. However, such guidelines for other vitamins are not available. Animal studies suggest that deficiencies in vitamins A and D, ascorbic acid, thiamine, riboflavin, pyridoxine, niacin, pantothenic acid, and folic acid reduce host resistance to infection. Intakes necessary to prevent or treat deficiencies of the vitamins in stressed humans have not been established. Vitamin A supplementation in rats has been shown to stimulate fibroplasia consistent with

TABLE 10–1.
Aggressive Protein Feeding in Burned Children*

	CONTROL	HIGH PROTEIN	*P*
% Weight change from preburn weight (av)	−2.24 ± 1.7	4.01 ± 1.64	<.009
Av highest daily temperature (°F)	102.3 ± 0.1	101.8 ± 0.1	<.0001
Volume red blood cells transfused (ml/sq m/day)	92 ± 10	52 ± 7	<.0009
Nitrogen balance (gm/dl)	7.3 ± 0.7	9.0 ± 0.7	<.08
Total serum protein (gm/dl)	5.5 ± 0.1	6.3 ± 0.2	<.0002
Albumin (gm/dl)	2.93 ± 0.08	2.95 ± 0.08	Not significant
Transferrin (mg/dl)	200 ± 10	283 ± 18	<.0001
C3 (mg/dl)	1,371 ± 55	1,585 ± 64	<.01
IgG (mg/dl)	805 ± 52	975 ± 56	<.03

*Adapted from Alexander JW, MacMillan BG, Stinnett JD, et al: Beneficial effects of aggressive protein feeding in severely burned children. *Ann Surg* 1980, 192:505–516.

wound repair,[27] increase the strength of a healing skin incision,[54] and accelerate wound healing.[8, 61] Ascorbic acid is essential for the hydroxylation of lysine during collagen synthesis;[42, 49] however, dosages necessary for wound healing are unknown.[64] Levenson et al.[37] and Lund et al.[38] noted a diminished circulating level of vitamin C and a decreased tissue ascorbic acid concentration in seriously burned patients. The extent of the abnormalities paralleled the severity of the burn. Likewise, guinea pigs with third-degree burns involving 30% of their total BSA had impaired healing that was reversed by ascorbic acid supplementation. Thus, it was suggested that the diet of these patients be supplemented with approximately 1 gm of ascorbic acid per square meter per day.

While administration of vitamins in excess of the recommended dietary allowances (Tables 10–2 and 10–3) may be justified in burned children, some vitamins, particularly fat-soluble vitamins, are toxic in large quantities. In addition, some water-soluble

TABLE 10–2.
Estimated Safe and Adequate Daily Dietary Intakes of Selected Vitamins and Minerals*

	VITAMINS†			
	AGE, YR	VITAMIN K, μG	BIOTIN, μG	PANTOTHENIC ACID, MG
Infants	0–0.5	12	35	2
	0.5–1	10–20	50	3
Children	1–3	15–30	65	3
and	4–6	20–40	85	3–4
adolescents	7–10	30–60	120	4–5
	11+	50–100	100–200	4–7

		TRACE ELEMENTS‡					
	AGE, YR	COPPER, MG	MANGANESE, MG	FLUROIDE, MG	CHROMIUM, MG	SELENIUM, MG	MOLYBDENUM, MG
Infants	0–0.5	0.5–0.7	0.5–0.7	0.1–0.5	0.01–0.04	0.01–0.04	0.03–0.06
	0.5–1	0.7–1.0	0.7–1.0	0.2–1.0	0.02–0.06	0.02–0.06	0.04–0.08
Children	1–3	1.0–1.5	1.0–1.5	0.5–1.5	0.02–0.08	0.02–0.08	0.05–0.1
and	4–6	1.5–2.0	1.5–2.0	1.0–2.5	0.03–0.12	0.03–0.12	0.06–0.15
adolescents	7–10	2.0–2.5	2.0–3.0	1.5–2.5	0.05–0.2	0.05–0.2	0.10–0.3
	11+	2.0–3.0	2.5–5.0	1.5–2.5	0.05–0.2	0.05–0.2	0.15–0.5

		ELECTROLYTES		
	AGE, YR	SODIUM, MG	POTASSIUM, MG	CHLORIDE, MG
Infants	0–0.5	115–350	350–925	275–700
	0.5–1	250–750	425–1275	400–1200
Children	1–3	325–975	550–1650	500–1500
and	4–6	450–1350	775–2325	700–2100
adolescents	7–10	600–1800	1000–3000	925–2775
	11+	900–2700	1525–4575	1400–4200

*Adapted from Committee on Dietary Allowances. *Recommended Dietary Allowances,* ed 9. National Academy of Sciences.
†Because there is less information on which to base allowances, these figures are not given in the main table of *Recommended Dietary Allowances* and are provided here in the form of ranges of recommended intakes.
‡Since the toxic levels of many trace elements may be only several times usual intakes, the upper levels for the trace elements given in this table should not be habitually exceeded.

TABLE 10–3.

Recommended Dietary Allowances: Designed for the Maintenance of Good Nutrition of Practically All Healthy People in the United States*

		FAT-SOLUBLE VITAMINS			WATER-SOLUBLE VITAMINS							MINERALS					
	AGE, YR	VITAMIN A, μG RE†	VITAMIN D,‡ μG	VITAMIN E, mg α-TE§	VITAMIN C, MG	THIAMINE, MG	RIBOFLAVIN, MG	NIACIN, MG NE‖	VITAMIN B-6, MG	FOLACIN¶ μG	VITAMIN B-12,# μG	CALCIUM, MG	PHOSPHORUS, MG	MAGNESIUM, MG	IRON, MG	ZINC, MG	IODINE, μG
Infants	0.0–≤0.5	420	10	3	35	0.3	0.4	6	0.3	30	0.5	360	240	50	10	3	40
	0.5–1.0	400	10	4	35	0.5	0.6	8	0.6	45	1.5	540	360	70	15	5	50
Children	1–3	400	10	5	45	0.7	0.8	9	0.9	100	2.0	800	800	150	15	10	70
	4–6	500	10	6	45	0.9	1.0	11	1.3	200	2.5	800	800	200	10	10	90
	7–10	700	10	7	45	1.2	1.4	16	1.6	300	3.0	800	800	250	10	10	120
Males	11–14	1000	10	8	50	1.4	1.6	18	1.8	400	3.0	1200	1200	350	18	15	150
	15–18	1000	10	10	60	1.4	1.7	18	2.0	400	3.0	1200	1200	400	18	15	150
Females	11–14	800	10	8	50	1.1	1.3	15	1.8	400	3.0	1200	1200	300	18	15	150
	15–18	800	10	8	60	1.1	1.3	14	2.0	400	3.0	1200	1200	300	18	15	150

* Adapted from Food and Nutrition Board, National Research Council: Recommended Dietary Allowance. Washington DC, National Academy of Sciences, 1980.
† RE indicates retinol equivalents. 1 retinol equivalent = 1 μg retinol or 6 μg β-carotene.
‡ Vitamin D as cholecalciferol. 10 μg cholecalciferol = 400 International Units (IU) of vitamin D.
§ α-TE indicates α-tocopherol equivalents. 1 mg/day of α-tocopherol = 1 α-TE.
‖ NE indicates 1 NE (niacin equivalent) is equal to 1 mg of niacin or 60 mg of dietary tryptophan.
¶ Folacin indicates allowances refer to dietary sources as determined by Lactobacillus casei assay after treatment with enzymes (conjugates) to make polyglutamyl forms of the vitamin available to the test organism.
# The recommended dietary allowances for vitamin B_{12} in infants is based on average concentration of the vitamin in human milk. The allowances after weaning are based on energy intake (as recommended by the American Academy of Pediatrics) and consideration of other factors, such as intestine absorption.

vitamins have been shown to produce adverse effects when taken in excessive amounts.[5, 9, 19, 26, 29, 65, 73]

The minerals that are known to be important in human nutrition can be classified into two categories: (1) those that are present in large quantities (sodium, potassium, calcium, magnesium, and phosphorus), and (2) those present in only trace amounts (iron, zinc, copper, iodine, selenium, fluoride, manganese, and chromium). Precise mineral requirements in burned patients remain to be determined, and further research is needed to establish guidelines for supplementation.

Sodium and potassium are discussed under fluid and electrolyte requirements. Phosphorus levels may decline in patients with extensive burns during the "corticoid-withdrawal" phase of injury when there is a large excretion of salt and water, which can cause a sizable loss of phosphorus. Simultaneously, during the anabolic phase, the phosphorus is taken up by cells that may contribute to the development of hypophosphatemia. The consequences of severe hypophosphatemia include red blood cell dysfunction, leukocyte dysfunction, central nervous system dysfunction, and rhabdomyolysis.[35] Nonetheless, correction of hypophosphatemia must be cautious since the administration of phosphorus salts may result in hyperphosphatemia, deposition of calcium phospate resulting in hypocalcemia, and hyperkalemia. Milk contains 1 gm each of phosphorus and calcium and is a safe alternative for those patients who can tolerate milk feedings. Zinc deficiencies have been associated with impaired cellular immunity, poor wound healing, impaired protein synthesis, anorexia, and altered taste and smell.[4, 22, 25, 46, 47, 53] Zinc requirements may be increased in the burned patient, and supplementation may enhance hepatic protein synthesis and improve wound healing. However, there are no controlled studies in humans that evaluate the efficacy or dosage of zinc supplements in burned patients. Impaired cellular immunity has also been reported in children suffering from iron deficiency anemia.[13, 40] Copper deficiency can lead to leukopenia, skeletal demineralization, anemia, and neutropenia.[39] Chromium deficiency has been associated with glucose intolerance in a patient receiving total parenteral nutrition.[31] Recommended allowances and safe levels of intake for minerals (see Table 10–3) and trace minerals (see Table 10–2) for normal individuals have been recommended by the National Academy of Sciences[15] for enteral intake, and guidelines for parenteral use have been established by the American Medical Association[3] (Table 10–4).

Until more information is gathered regarding the administration of vitamins and minerals in the burned child, supplementation should not greatly exceed the established guidelines for healthy individuals, unless a deficiency is documented.

Goals of Nutritional Support

Nutritional therapy should be directed toward achieving specific goals. Depending on the patient's status, these goals should be as follows:

1. To identify the metabolic and nutritional needs of the child
2. To reduce net nitrogen losses and promote protein repletion
3. To provide adequate fuels and an effective method of delivery
4. To assess the effectiveness of the nutritional program
5. To diminish the rate of weight loss and body protein breakdown
6. To maintain body weight and protein stores
7. To increase body weight and protein mass (anabolism)

These objectives must be integrated into the overall patient care plan and should receive special consideration whenever fluid restriction, organ failure (kidney, lung, liver), septicemia, mechanical ventilation, or any other supportive therapy limits the physician's ability to provide optimal nutritional support. Anabolism and positive nitrogen balance are dif-

TABLE 10–4.
Suggested Daily Intravenous Intake of Essential Trace Elements*

	PEDIATRIC PATIENTS, μg/kg†	STABLE ADULT	ADULT IN ACUTE CATABOLIC STATE‡	STABLE ADULT WITH INTESTINAL LOSSES‡
Zinc	300§ 100 ‖	2.5–4.0 mg	Additional 2.0 mg	Add 12.2 mg/L small bowel fluid lost; 17.1 mg/kg of stool or ileostomy output¶
Copper	20	0.5–1.5 mg		
Chronium	0.14–0.2	10–15 gm		20 μg#
Manganese	2–10	0.15–0.8 mg		

* Adapted from American Medical Association, Department of Foods and Nutrition: Guidelines for essential trace element preparation for parenteral use. *JAMA* 1979, 241:2051–2054.
† Limited data are available for infants weighing less than 1,500 gm. Their requirements may be more than the recommendations because of their low body reserves and increased requirements for growth.
‡ Frequent monitoring of blood levels in these patients is essential to provide dosage.
§ Premature infants (weight less than 1,500 gm) up to 3 kg of body weight. Thereafter, the recommendations for full-term infants apply.
‖ Full-term infants and children up to 5 years old. Thereafter, the recommendations for adults apply, up to a maximum dosage of 4 mg/day.
¶ Values derived by mathematical fitting of balance data from a 71-patient-week study in 24 patients.
\# Mean from balance study.

ficult, if not impossible, to achieve in the critically ill, hypermetabolic burn patient, but the provision of adequate calories and protein will often lessen if not match the profound catabolism seen in this group of patients. When the disease process has been resolved, protein synthesis will occur, and muscle mass will return to its preillness level. The burn patient who is able to walk and use the various muscle groups will frequently achieve positive nitrogen balance and anabolism during periods of refeeding. Spontaneous conversion from a catabolic to an anabolic state is usually not observed in severely burned patients until burn closure with autograft has been accomplished, unless supernormal diets are administered. Thus, if wound closure is not promptly achieved after development of suitable granulation tissue, an increased requirement for exogenous calories is likely to exist for many weeks following burn injuries.

Delivery Technique and Available Diets

While the usual hospital diet is easy to prepare, nutritious, and capable of providing adequate amounts of calories, proteins, and vitamins, the burned child rarely consumes significant quantities of food. These patients are often anorexic, occasionally have a nasogastric or an endotracheal tube in place, and/or a nonfunctional gastrointestinal tract. Thus, alternative forms of feeding must be considered. The most frequent approach to the problem is to provide between-meal nutritional supplements and encourage a good working relationship between the dietitian, the nurse, and the patient.

ENTERAL TUBE FEEDINGS

The cornerstone of nutritional management is providing enough exogenous calories and nitrogen to prevent prolonged catabolism. Whenever possible, the gastrointestinal route should be utilized since nutrients are better utilized, and it is safer and less expensive than the parenteral route. The actual caloric requirements depend not only on the size of the injury and BSA but also on the depth of the burn and presence or absence of associated complications. Estimates of daily energy expenditure have been discussed earlier.

Soft and small nasogastric tubes are available and well tolerated by burn patients, and a variety of tube-feeding formulas are now available (Table 10–5). More recently diets have been tailor-made for patients with renal or hepatic insufficiency. Carbohydrates are the major source of energy in nearly all enteral formulas, and their content will determine their relative sweetness and osmolality. Feeding should initially progress slowly with half- or full-strength solutions, and as soon as the gastrointestinal tract adapts to the liquid diet, the quantity and strength should be advanced rapidly. When using nasogastric tubes, it is important to evaluate residual volume at each feeding to prevent gastric dilation and vomiting. Nasogastric tube feeding may be done by intermittent bolus or continuous administration.

The initial feedings are provided as homogenized cow's milk or an equivalent formula. Unless a history of allergy or intolerance exists, milk provides a palatable, familiar formula, which contains the recommended 20% of the calories as protein. Slow advancement of the volume delivered can minimize the effects of dose-related lactose intolerance. In the presence of milk intolerance or allergy, an isotonic, soy-based, lactose-free formula can be utilized. Cow's milk should not be fed to infants during their first year of life because of its association with occult gastointestinal bleeding, iron deficiency anemia, and cow's milk allergy.[2, 44] An infant formula supplement with a protein module (Table 10–6) can be formulated for children less than 1 year of age.

Cow's milk (20 kcal/oz) can be mixed with a formula of higher caloric concentration when a more concentrated source of kilocalories is needed to meet estimated requirements without exceeding fluid needs. In our experience, enteral formulas are best tolerated when caloric concentrations are advanced slowly up to a maximum of 27 kcal/oz. Greater caloric concentrations are usually poorly tolerated, and small gains are frequently offset by bouts of abdominal distention, vomiting, and diarrhea.

For patients who will not voluntarily take oral feedings, milk or formula feedings can be provided using a feeding tube and infusion pump set to deliver the calculated fluid allowance.[45] Feedings are usually given on a continuous basis to minimize the likelihood of vomiting, aspiration of stomach contents, or diarrhea. In children, who are more sensitive to an osmolar load, the feeding tip should remain in the stomach, and the head of the bed should be elevated to protect against aspiration. The rate of infusion should be gradually increased every 4 to 6 hours until the estimated requirements are achieved. Simultaneously, the rate of intravenous infusion is decreased so the calculated hourly fluid requirements are met but not exceeded.

Preoperative, perioperative, and postoperative periods for burn scrubs, debridement, and grafting require periods of fasting. Therefore, the nutritional demands of the burned child are not met during these periods. To help meet the protein demands during these fasting periods, the child is administered intravenous protein either as 5% albumin or as fresh-frozen plasma. Intravenous protein is administered until the diet program can be resumed.

A standard high-calorie, high-protein diet can be initiated as the pediatric burn patient demonstrates the ability to consume solid foods. Fluids should be restricted to the prescribed milk or formula. A high-calorie, high-protein diet is given in addition to the calculated nutrient requirements provided by the milk or formula to allow for "catch-up" nutrient uptake needed to compensate for fasting periods associated with operative procedures. Once a patient demonstrates the ability to consume an adequate diet and has achieved a positive caloric balance, the child can be weaned from the nasogastric feeding tube.

PERIPHERAL VEIN INFUSIONS

Glucose, amino acid solutions, and fat emulsions can be safely infused through peripheral veins, but they must be nearly iso-

TABLE 10–5.
Enteral Formulas

PRODUCT	MANUFACTURER	KCAL PER ML KCAL/ML	PROTEIN, %	FAT, %	CARBOHYDRATE, %	NA+, mEQ/L	K+, mEQ/L	OSMOLALITY, (mOSm/KG/ H_2O)	DESCRIPTION
Cow's milk	Not manufactured*	0.65	20	51	29	21	39	. . .	3.7% fat
Similac	Ross†	0.68	9	48	43	10	21	290	Standard infant formula contains lactose
Enfamil	Mead Johnson‡	0.68	9	50	41	9	17	300	Standard infant formula contains lactose
Isomil	Ross†	0.68	11	49	40	14	24	250	Milk-free, soy protein isolate infant formula
Prosobee	Mead Johnson‡	0.68	12	48	40	12	20	200	Milk-free, soy protein Isolate infant formula
Ensure	Ross†	1.06	14	31.5	54.5	37	40	450	Nutritionally complete
Sustacal	Mead Johnson§	1.00	24	21.0	55.	41	54	620	Nutritionally complete
Ensure Plus	Ross†	1.50	15	32.0	53	50	59.5	600	High-calorie nutritionally complete
Sustacal HC	MJ§	1.50	16	34	50	36	38	600	High-calorie, nutritionally complete
Osmolite	Ross†	1.06	14	31	55	24	26	300	Isotonic, nutritionally complete
Isocal	MJ§	1.06	13	37	50	53	34	300	Isotonic, nutritionally complete
Entrition	Biosearch§	1.00	14	31.5	54.5	30.5	30.7	300	Isotonic, nutritionally complete
Osmolite NH	Ross†	1.06	17	30	53	40.5	40	310	High nitrogen, isotonic, isotonic nutritionally complete
Isotein HN	Sandoz ‖	1.19	23	25	52	29.5	22	300	High-nitrogen, isotonic; fat: 25% medium-chain triglycerides (MCT), 75% soy fat
Isocal HCN*	MJ§	2.00	15	45	40	35	43	690	High-calorie, high-nitrogen, fat: 30% MCT, 70% soy fat
Magnacal	Biosearch¶	2.00	14	36	50	43.5	32	590	High-calorie nutritionally complete

Travasorb MCT	Travenol#	2.00	20	30	50	30	89	590	High-calorie, nutritionally complete; fat: 80% MCT, 20% sunflower
Two Cal HN	Ross†	2.00	17	40	43	43	59	750	High-calorie, high-nitrogen, liquid lactose free
Traumacal	MJ§	1.50	22	40	38	51	36	490	High-nitrogen, high-branch chain amino acid, nutritionally complete
Stresstein	Sandoz ‖	1.20	23	20	57	28	28	910	High-nitrogen, high-branch chain amino acid, nutritionally complete
Vivonex HN	Norwich Eaton**	1.00	18	1	81.5	23	30	810	High-nitrogen, chemically defined diet
Vital HN	Ross†	1.00	17	9	74	20	34	460	High-nitrogen, partially hydrolyzed diet, nutritionally complete

* *Agriculture Handbook*, no. 8–1. Washington, DC, United States Department of Agriculture, Agricultural Research Service, 1976.
† *Product Handbook*. Columbus, Ohio, Ross Laboratories, 1985.
‡ *Pediatric Products Handbook*. Evansville, Ind, Mead Johnson Nutritional Division, 1984.
§ *Enteral Nutrition Management System Product Handbook*. Evansville, Ind, Mead Johnson Nutritional Division, 1985.
‖ *Source Chart*. Minneapolis, Sandoz Nutrition, 1985.
¶ Biosearch Medical Products Inc, Somerville, NJ 1985.
# Travasorb Enteral Nutrition Diets, Travenol Laboratories Inc, Nutrition and Flow Control Division, Deerfield, Ill, 1983.
**Norwich Eaton Pharmaceuticals Inc, Procter and Gamble Co, Norwich, NY, 1984.

TABLE 10–6.
Protein Modules

PRODUCT	MANUFACTURER	CALORIES PER GM	PROTEIN PER GM	SOURCE OF PROTEIN
Casec	Mead Johnson*	3.7	0.88	Calcium caseinate
Propac	Organon†	4.0	0.75	Whey protein concentrate
Pro-Mix-R.D.P.	Navaco‡	3.6	0.84	Whey protein concentrate
Pro Mod	Ross§	5.6	1.0	Whey protein concentrate
Nutrisource Protein	Sandoz ‖	4.0	0.75	Lactalbumin, egg white solids
Nutrisource Amino Acids	Sandoz ‖	3.9	1.0	Free amino acids (AA)
Nutrisource AA-HBC	Sandoz ‖	3.8	1.0	Free amino acids-44% AA branched-chain

* *Enteral Nutrition Management System Product Handbook.* Evansville, Ind, Mead Johnson 1985.
† Organon Nutritional Products, Organon Inc, West Orange, NJ, 1982.
‡ Mavaco Laboratories, Division of Lifetime Industries, McAllen, Tex, 1985.
§ Ross Laboratories, Columbus, Ohio, 1986.
‖ *Source Chart.* Minneapolis, Sandoz Nutrition, 1985.

tonic to avoid peripheral vein sclerosis. Therefore, the amount of calories administered via this route are limited. In general, peripheral vein solutions do not provide adequate calories and nitrogen in and of themselves and hence do not promote anabolism. Their use is limited to burn patients who are minimally hypermetabolic and to those with no evidence of organ system dysfunction. Occasionally the additional calories provided via the peripheral vein, in conjunction with those taken orally, will be adequate to support or allow anabolism to occur. Unlike central vein solutions, antibiotics and other medications, as well as blood and blood products, may be infused through the same intravenous catheter, but the venotomy site should be changed every other day if possible.

Intravenous fat emulsion is an efficient fuel source in that it provides more than twice the energy per unit weight (9 kcal/gm) than does either carbohydrate or protein. Fat emulsion particles are cleared from the bloodstream in much the same way as chilomicrons after fatty meals are ingested. Whereas the body can synthesize most long-chain fatty acids, linoleic acid cannot be synthesized and therefore is an essential nutrient. Essential fatty acid deficiency can be prevented in burn patients by supplying 5% to 10% of daily caloric requirements as essential fatty acids. Complications from fat emulsions are limited to phlebitis, minor disorders of platelet adhesiveness, febrile reactions, hypertriglyceridemia, and abnormalities of pulmonary function. A 10% fat emulsion provides 1.1 kcal/ml, and a 20% emulsion provides 2 kcal/ml. Although this represents a high calorie density, the low osmolality of these solutions makes delivery by the peripheral vein safe and practical.

Assessment of Nutritional Status

Indicators of nutritional status must be assessed and monitored routinely to ensure adequate nutritional therapy is provided to combat the catabolic effects of injury and the associated effects of surgical procedures and sepsis.

NUTRITION HISTORY

Dietary and social history should include usual food intake, food allergies, cultural or religious preferences, and chewing and swallowing difficulties. Such information frequently gives clues to the type of nutritional problems that may be encountered during treatment and recovery. The history can play an important part in the approaches used to improve nutritional status through the use of accustomed and preferred foods and the identification of factors that might interfere with the nutritional support plan.

NUTRIENT INTAKE ANALYSIS

Nutrient intake should be measured daily to assess the adequacy of the diet in meeting the estimated nutritional caloric requirements (Fig 10–6). Intake should include all nutrients received via enteral and parenteral routes and oral diet. Graphs can be utilized to depict the sources and quantity of protein and carbohydrate received (see Fig 10–6). Daily monitoring may identify nutritional deficits before weight and laboratory values reveal such depletions. In addition, the dietitian may discover the need to implement an alternative means of nutrient delivery.

ANTHROPOMETRY

Admission height and weight measurements of a burned child should be charted to determine appropriateness for age. Such screening may reveal a deficit in the preinjury nutritional status. Anthropometric measurements may prove a useful method of following body composition during convalescence from the burn injury.

Weight monitoring during the hospital course provides a means of assessing the adequacy of nutritional support. In the burned child, weight loss may indicate an inadequate nutritional support regimen, but also may be secondary to fluid losses, massive surgical debridement, amputations, and/or the changing of bulky dressings. A weight loss of greater than 10% of the preburn weight is often associated with complications,[14, 32, 39, 41] and death often results when acute weight loss exceeds 30% of preinjury levels. The endogenous caloric reserves of a child are limited due to small body size, therefore, weight loss should not be allowed to exceed 5% of the estimated dry weight in children with a burn injury. A daily weight graph provides a visible means of monitoring weight status and preventing weight deficits of greater than 5%. Whenever possible, this should be correlated to actual caloric intake (see Fig 10–5).

CONFIRMATORY LABORATORY TESTS

Biochemical data can be used to identify visceral protein deficiencies. Concentrations of circulating serum proteins are commonly used as indicators of visceral protein status. Visceral proteins are essential for host defense, wound healing, substrate transport, oncotic pressure, and enzyme functions.[30] Serial measurements of these proteins provide an objective means of determining adequacy and response to nutritional support. In the burned child, deficits of serum protein concentrations occur rapidly as a result of nitrogen losses through the wound and altered protein metabolism.[56, 66] Repletion of these proteins occurs when energy and protein demands are satisfied, and adequate substrate supply is provided. Circulating proteins commonly used to indicate visceral protein status include serum albumin, transferrin, retinol-binding protein, and thyroxin-binding prealbumin. Serum albumin has a relatively long half-life, which makes it a poor marker for monitoring acute changes. In addition, levels of serum albumin rise when supplemental infusions of intravenous albumin are given to maintain intravascular volume. Thus, it may be difficult to accurately correlate changes in serum albumin with nutritional support. Serum retinol-binding protein and thyroxin-binding prealbumin have half-lives of 10 hours and 2 days, and therefore changes in their serum concentrations rapidly reflect changes in nutritional status; unfortunately, circulating levels may be a reflection of acute metabolic response to the stress of injury as well as malnutrition. Serum transferrin may be the most valuable and reliable indicator of visceral protein status due to its relatively short half-life of 8 to 10 days, and serum

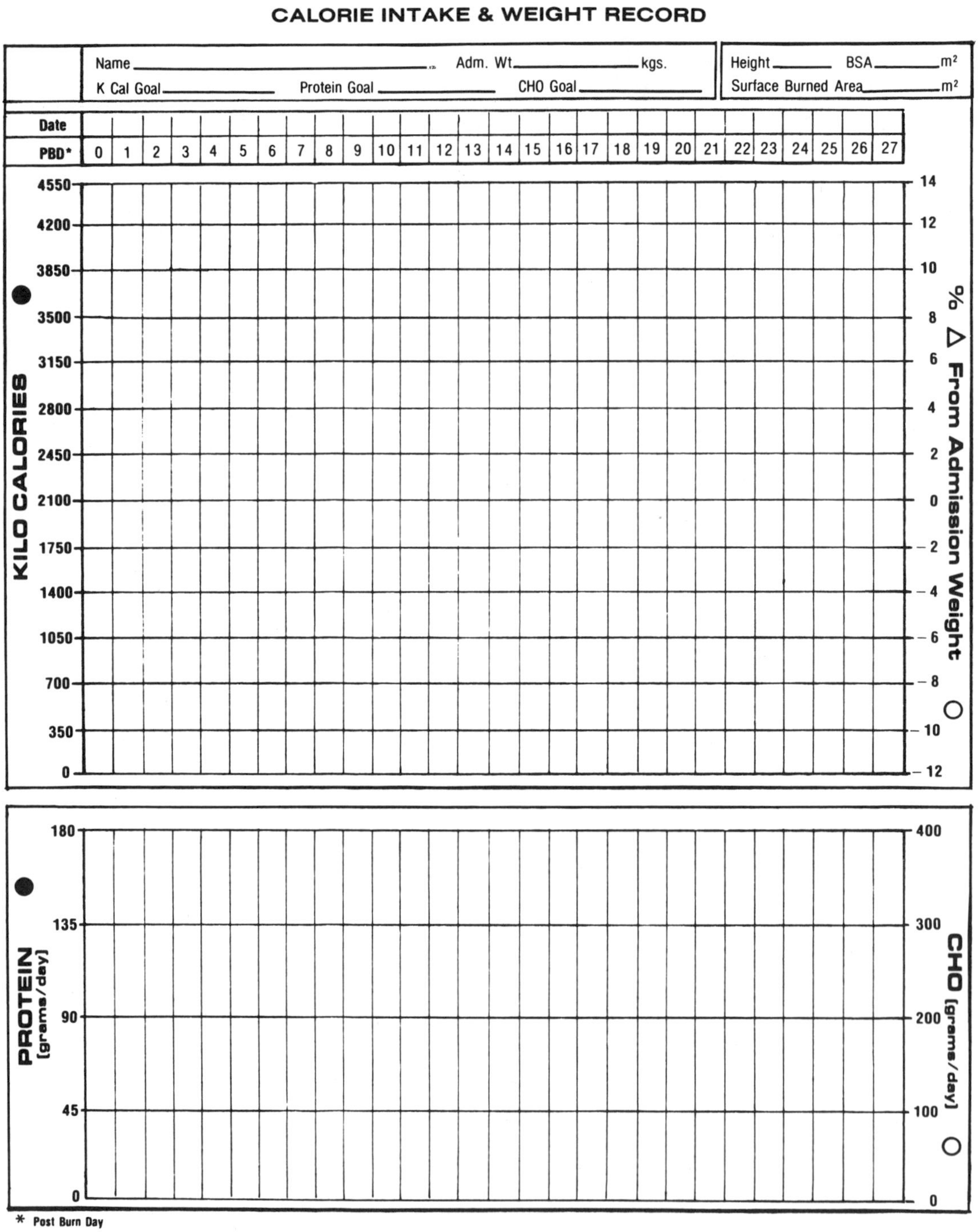

FIG 10–6.
Caloric intake and weight record.

transferrin values are independent of albumin infusions.[14] In addition, Jensen et al.[32] found low serum transferrin concentrations significantly correlated with subsequent incidences of infections and complications in 74 adult burn patients, indicating a relationship between visceral protein status and immunocompetence. Transferrin values should be obtained routinely every 10 to 14 days to monitor response to nutritional therapies. Hydration status affects the measurement of all the circulating proteins and therefore, should be considered when interpreting laboratory results.

NITROGEN BALANCE MEASUREMENTS

The body protein mass is in constant turnover as cells are catabolized and replaced by newly synthesized cells. Nitrogen balance estimations are used to reflect the overall rates of body protein synthesis and breakdown. The following formula is commonly employed:

$$\text{Nitrogen balance} = \text{nitrogen in} - \text{nitrogen out}$$

Intake of nitrogen is generally in the form of ingested protein or infused amino acids administered intravenously. Losses of nitrogen occur primarily in urine, stool, and skin. A reasonable estimation of urine urea nitrogen can be obtained from a 24 hour urine collection. A constant number of 2 to 4 is added to cover other nitrogen losses. One gram of nitrogen is equivalent to 6.25 gm of protein. Therefore, a negative nitrogen balance of negative 8.2 gm of nitrogen represents a protein loss of 51.2 gm.[23] The healthy individual is in nitrogen equilibrium since intake equals losses. However, catabolic disorders, such as major burn injury, accelerate nitrogen losses, and these stressed patients may exhibit profound negative nitrogen balance (see Fig 10–1). Burn exudate represents another source of significant nitrogen loss.[56] Therefore, a standard correction factor for nonurea nitrogen would not be valid. Bell et al.[10] developed a model for predicting total urinary nitrogen (TUN) from urinary urea nitrogen (UUN) and observable characteristics of burned adult and pediatric patients. The loss of urinary nitrogen is estimated from the following equation and is appropriate only for the acute phase after injury:

$$\text{TUN} = 0.2840 + 0.9084 \log \text{UNN} + 0.002319 \ \% \ \text{burn} + 0.002146 \ \text{age}$$

Based on this predicted value, fecal nitrogen loss (1 gm/day),[55] and wound nitrogen loss (10% open wound = 0.02 gm of nitrogen per kilogram per day; 11% to 30% open wound = 0.05 gm of nitrogen per kilogram per day; 31% open wound = 0.12 gm of nitrogen per kilogram per day),[33] the nitrogen balance (nitrogen input minus nitrogen output) can be estimated:

$$\begin{aligned}\text{Nitrogen balance} = {} & \text{total dietary nitrogen (gm/24 hr)} \\ & - \text{TUN (gm/24 hr)} \\ & + \text{fecal nitrogen loss (gm/24 hr)} \\ & + \text{wound nitrogen loss (gm/24 hr)}\end{aligned}$$

If the patient sustains a large increase in BUN over the 24-hour period when the urine is collected, an adjustment factor, which will correct the nitrogen balance for the excess urea in blood, may need to be included. Although the measurement is not an absolute determination of nitrogen balance, when used in conjunction with other measures of nutritional status, it may provide an effective measure of determining the effectiveness of nutritional therapy.

REFERENCES

1. Alexander JW, MacMillan BG, Stinnett JD, et al: Beneficial effects of aggressive protein feeding in severely burned children. *Ann Surg* 1980; 192:505–516.
2. American Academy of Pediatrics, Committee on Nutrition: The use of whole cow's milk in infancy. *Pediatrics* 1983; 72:253.
3. American Medical Association, Department of Foods and Nutrition: Guidelines for essential

trace element preparations for parenteral use. *JAMA* 1979; 241:2051–2054.
4. Arakawa T, Tamura T, Igarashi Y, et al: Zinc deficiency in two infants during total parenteral alimentation for diarrhea. *Am J Clin Nutr* 1976; 29:197–204.
5. Ascorbic acid: Immunological effects and hazards (editorial). *Lancet* 1979; 1:308.
6. Aulick LH, Wilmore DW: Increased peripheral amino acids release following burn injury. *Surgery* 1979; 85:560.
7. Aulick LH, Wilmore DW: Hypermetabolism in trauma, in Girardier L, Stock MJ (eds): *Mammalian Thermogenesis*. London, Chapman and Hall, 1983, pp 259–304.
8. Barbul A, Thysen B, Rettura G, et al: White cell involvement in the inflammatory, wound-healing, and immune actions of vitamin A. *J Parenter Enteral Nutr* 1978; 2:129–138.
9. Barness LA: Safety considerations with high ascorbic acid dosage. *Ann NY Acad Sci* 1975; 258:523–527.
10. Bell SJ, Molnar JA, Krasker WS: Prediction of total urinary nitrogen from urea nitrogen for burned patients. *J Am Diet Assoc* 1985; 85:1100–1104.
11. Bergstrom J, Furst P, Noree LO, et al: Intracellular free amino acid concentration in human muscle tissue. *J Appl Physiol* 1974; 36:693.
12. Carvajal HF: A physiologic approach to fluid therapy in severely burned children. *Surg Gynecol Obstet* 1980; 150:379–384.
13. Chandra RK: Iron and immunocompetence. *Nutr Rev* 1976; 34:129–132.
14. Cohn KH, Blackburn GL: Nutritional assessment: Clinical and biometric measurements of hospital patients at risk. *J Med Assoc Ga* 1982; 71:27–35.
15. Committee on Dietary Allowances: *Recommended Dietary Allowances*, ed 9. Washington, DC, National Academy of Science, 1980.
16. Curreri PW: Nutritional replacement modalities. *J Trauma* 1979; 19(suppl 11): 906–908.
17. Cuthbertson DP: The disturbance of metabolism produced by bony and nonbony injury, with notes on certain abnormal conditions of bone. *Biochem J* 1930; 24:1244.
18. Cuthbertson DP: Observations on the disturbance of metabolism produced by injury to the limbs. *Q J Med* 1932; 25:233–246.
19. DiPalma JR, Ritchie DM: Vitamin toxicity. *Annu Rev Pharmacol Toxicol* 1977; 17:133–148.
20. Dominioni L, Orrawin T, Cheng-Hui F, et al: Enteral feeding in burn hypermetabolism: Nutritional and metabolic effects of different levels of caloric and protein intake. *J Parentr Enteral Nutr* 1985; 9:269–279.
21. Duke JH, Jorgensen SB, Broell J, et al: Contribution of protein to caloric expenditure following injury. *Surgery* 1970; 68:168.
22. Fosmire GJ, Sandstead HH: Effects of zinc deficiency on compositional development and protein synthesis in liver, heart, and kidney of suckling rats. *Proc Soc Exp Biol Med* 1977; 154:351–355.
23. Grant A, DeHoog S: *Nutritional Assessment and Support*, ed 3. Seattle, Grant & DeHoog, 1985;
24. Hegsted DM: Balance studies. *J Nutr* 1976; 106:307.
25. Henkin RI, Patten BM, Re PK, et al: A syndrome of acute zinc loss. *Arch Neurol* 1975; 32:745–754.
26. Herbert V, Jacob E: Destruction of vitamin B_{12} by ascorbic acid. *JAMA* 1974; 230:241–242.
27. Herrmann JB, Woodward SC: Stimulation of fibroplasia by vitamin A. *Surg Forum* 1969; 20:500–501.
28. Hildreth M, Carvajal HF: Caloric requirements in burned children: A simple formula to estimate daily caloric requirements. *J Burn Care Rehabil* 1982; 3:78–80.
29. Hughes RE: Nonscorbutic effects of vitamin C: Biochemical aspects. *Proc R Soc Med* 1977; 70:86–89.
30. Jeejeebhoy KN: Protein nutrition in clinical practice. *Br Med Bull* 1981, 37:11–17.
31. Jeejeebhoy KN, Chu RC, Marliss EB, et al: Chromium deficiency, glucose intolerance, and neuropathy reversed by chronium supplementation in a patient receiving long-term total parenteral nutrition. *Am J Clin Nutr* 1977; 30:531–538.
32. Jensen JG, Long JM, Dudrick SJ, et al: Nutritional assessment indications of post-burn complications *J Am Diet Assoc* 1985; 85:68–72.
33. Kien CL, Young VR, Rohrbaugh DK, et al: Increased rates of whole body protein synthesis and breakdown in children recovering from burns. *Ann Surg* 1978; 187:383–391.
34. Kinney JM, Felig P: The metabolic response to injury and infection, in DeGroot LJ (ed): *Endocrinology*. New York, Grune & Stratton, 1979, vol 3, pp 1963–1986.
35. Knochel JP: The pathophysiology and clinical characteristics of severe hypophosphatemia. *Arch Intern Med* 1977; 137:203–220.
36. Kominz DR, Hough A, Symonds P, et al: The amino acid composition of actin, myosin, tropomyosin, and the meromyosins. *Arch Biochem Biophys* 1951; 50:48.
37. Levenson SM, Green RW, Taylor FHL, et al:

Ascorbic acid, riboflavin, thiamine, and nicotinic acid in relation to severe injury, hemorrhage, and infection in the human. *Ann Surg* 1946; 124:840–856.

38. Lund CC, Levenson SM, Green RW, et al: Ascorbic acid, thiamine, riboflavin, and nicotinic acid in relation to acute burns in man. *Arch Surg* 1947; 55:557–583.
39. Luterman A, Adams M, Curreri PW: Nutritional management of the burned patient. *Crit Care Q* 1984; 34:42.
40. MacDougall LG, Anderson R, McNab GM, et al: Immune response in iron deficiency. *J Pediatr* 1975; 86:833–843.
41. Mason AD: Weight loss in burned patients. *J Trauma* 1979; 19:902–903.
42. Mussini E, Hutton JJ, Udenfriend S: Collagen proline hydroxylase in wound healing, granuloma formation, scurvy, and growth. *Science* 1967; 157:927–929.
43. Odessey R, Goldberg AF: Origin and possible significance of alanine production by skeletal muscle. *J Biol Chem* 1974; 249:7623–7629.
44. Oski FA: Is bovine milk a health hazard? *Pediatrics* 1985; (suppl)75:182–186.
45. Parks DH, Carvajal HF, Larson DL: Management of burns. *Surg Clin North Am* 1977; 57:875–894.
46. Pekarek RS, Powanda MC: Protein synthesis in zinc-deficient vats during tularemia. *J Nutr* 1976; 106:905–912.
47. Pekarek RS, Sandstead HH, Jacob RA, et al: Abnormal cellular immune responses during acquired zinc deficiency. *Am J Clin Nutr* 1979; 32:1466–1471.
48. Pleban WE: Nutritional support of burned patients: Bridgeport Hospital Burn Unit. *Conn Med* 1979; 43:767–768.
49. Prockop DJ, Guzman NA: Collagen diseases and biosynthesis of collagen. *Hosp Pract* 1977; 12:61–68.
50. Pruitt BA: Metabolic changes and nutrition in burns patients. *Ann Chir Plast* 1979; 24:21–25.
51. Ruderman NB: Muscle amino acid metabolism and gluconeogenesis. *Annu Rev Med* 1975; 26:245–258.
52. Rudowski WJ: The treatment of burns—summing up. *Burns* 1978; 4:67–71.
53. Sandstead HH, Lanier VC, Shepard GH, et al: Zinc and wound healing: Effects of zinc deficiency and zinc supplementation. *Am J Clin Nutr* 1970; 23:514–519.
54. Seifter E, Crawley LV, Rettura G, et al. Influence of vitamin A on wound healing in rats with femoral fracture. *Ann Surg* 1975; 181:836–841.
55. Serog P, et al: Energy and nitrogen balances in 24 severely burned patients receiving four isocaloric diets of about 10 MJ/m^2/day (2,392 kcals/m^2/day). *Burns* 1983; 9:422–427.
56. Soroff HS, Pearson E, Artz CP: An estimation of the nitrogen requirements for equilibrium in burn patients. *Surg Gynecol Obstet* 1961; 112:159–172.
57. Souba WW, Bessey PQ: Nutritional support of the trauma patient. *Infect Surg* 1984; 3:727–738.
58. Souba WW, Long JM III, Dudrick SJ: Energy intake and stress as determinants of nitrogen excretion in rats. *Surg Forum* 1978; 29:76–77.
59. Souba WW, Smith RJ, Wilmore DW: Effect of glucocorticoids on glutamine metabolism in visceral organs. *Metabolism* 1985; 34(5):450–456.
60. Souba WW, Wilmore DW: Gut-liver interaction during accelerated gluconeogenesis. *Arch Surg* 1985; 120:66–70.
61. Stratford F, Seifter E, Rettura G, et al: Impaired wound healing due to cyclophosphamide alleviated by supplemental vitamin A. *Surg Forum* 1980; 31:224–225.
62. Suarez A, Hess D, Hunt J: Early tangential excision of a deep dermal with immediate mesh homograft coverage. *J Burn Care Rehabil* 1980, 1:36.
63. Sutherland AB, Batchelor ADR: Nitrogen balance in burned children. *Ann NY Acad Sci* 1968; 150:700–710.
64. Vitamin C, disease and surgical trauma. *Br Med J* 1979; 1:437.
65. Vitamin C toxicity. *Nutr Rev* 1976; 34:236–237.
66. Wilmore DW: Nutrition and metabolism following thermal injury. *Clin Plast Surg* 1974; 1:603–619.
67. Wilmore DW: *The Metabolic Management of the Critically Ill.* New York, Plenum Medical Book Co, 1977.
68. Wilmore DW, Aulick LH, Mason AD Jr, et al: The influence of the burn wound on local and systemic responses to injury. *Ann Surg* 1977; 186:444.
69. Wilmore DW, Aulick LH, Pruitt BA Jr: Metabolism during the hypermetabolic phase of thermal injury, in Rob C (ed): *Advances in Surgery*. Chicago, Year Book Medical Publishers, 1978, p 193.
70. Wilmore DW, Goodwin CW, Aulick LH, et al: Effect of injury and infection on visceral metabolism and circulation. *Ann Surg* 1980; 192:491.
71. Wilmore DW, Long JM, Mason AD, et al: Catecholamines: Mediator of hypermetabolic

response to thermal injury. *Ann Surg* 1974; 180:653–669.

72. Windmueller HG: Glutamine utilization by the small intestine. *Adv Enzymol* 1982; 53:201–237.
73. Winter SL, Boyer JL: Hepatic toxicity from large doses of vitamin B_3 (nicotinamide). *New Engl J Med* 1973; 289:1180–1182.
74. Wolfe RR, Goodenough RD, Burke JF, et al: Response of protein and ureakinetics in burn patients to different levels of protein intake. *Ann Surg* 1983; 197:163–171.

SECTION IV

SURGERY

11 / Anesthetic Considerations

STEPHEN M. LARSON, D.M.D.

Anesthetic management of patients with burn injury dates back to early Egyptian medico-religious instruction. Various forms of topical therapy included combinations of onions and salt; yolk of eggs, oil of roses, and turpentine; and fine linen soaked in saffron pomade.[11] The latter remedy apparently gave reasonable pain relief and accomplished covering of the burned tissue. In 1836, burn wounds were painted with vinegar until pain was relieved. Opium or opium and wine were also administered for relief of pain.

Anesthetics were first used for burn management in 1900 when chloroform was administered to reduce the pain of dressing change. In 1922 topical administration of tannic acid gained recognition for relief of pain, and in 1944 morphine was advocated for pain relief in doses of up to 130 mg given intramuscularly for patients in shock.[11] At about the same time, short-acting barbiturates, nitrous oxide/oxygen/ether, and/or cyclopropane were incorporated into burn-dressing therapy to achieve pain relief and more rapid recovery. Unfortunately, the administration of full general anesthesia to these patients led to prolonged preoperative and postoperative starvation, which slowed healing and impaired the patient's general condition. In 1959 Visser and Tarrow[16] described the repeated use of halothane as an anesthetic for burn-dressing changes. No evidence of liver damage was observed. This was followed by the reported use of neuroleptanesthesia, and in 1970 ketamine, administered either intramuscularly or intravenously, was found to be satisfactory for burn surgery.

Pharmacologic advances and expanding knowledge of the pathophysiology of burn injury can provide better pain control and safer anesthesia leading to a reduction in mortality and morbidity.

PATHOPHYSIOLOGY

The immediate postburn period is associated with decreases in cardiac output of up to 50% of normal resting values.[3, 6] The vascular compartment becomes permeable to both proteins and crystalloid, and as a result of the reduction in venous return and stroke volume, cardiac output will continue to diminish. Despite rapid fluid resuscitation, cardiac output remains depressed until after the initial 24-hour resuscitation period when the circulatory system becomes hyperdynamic with increases in blood pressure, heart rate, and cardiac output (about two times normal). A myocardial depressant factor causing a decrease in myocardial contractility may be involved, and intraoperative toxemia or sepsis may also initiate circulatory instability or collapse as a result of the rapid entry into the circulation of bacterial emboli or toxic products[9, 17]

Edema occurs not only in burned tissue, but in nonburned tissue, particularly in the severely burned patient. Pulmonary edema is often seen in the postburn phase after fluid resuscitation rather than during the resuscitation phase. Respiratory tract injury from the inhalation of smoke and incomplete combustion products may cause a plethora of alterations in pulmonary mechanics and gas exchange. Also, evidence is accumulating of pulmonary alterations resulting from massive cutaneous burns without direct pulmonary injury.[2a]

Hypertension is an additional problem, occurring presumably as a result of elevated plasma catecholamines and/or activation of the renin/angiotensin system, and may require treatment with antihypertensive drugs. The patients with the greatest risk for development of hypertension are boys younger than 10 years.[14]

Renal function may be adversely affected as a result of the decrease in cardiac output and increase in renal vascular resistance.[6] Reductions in renal blood flow and urine production may be secondary to the release of catecholamines, andiuretic hormone (ADH), renin, and angiotensin. Studies suggest that the ADH response is stress-induced and results in the production of ADH levels beyond the physiologic range for antidiuretic effect. These studies support findings that ADH has a potential role as a vasoconstrictor.[10]

Obstruction of renal tubules by large amounts of myoglobin and hemoglobin released particularly following electrical injury may also adversely affect renal function.

Liver function may be altered by changes in perfusion states in the early resuscitation phase. Early elevations in serum glutamic oxaloacetic transaminase (SGOT) and decreased activity of detoxifying enzymes affect drug metabolism,[7] so drugs may need to be given in reduced dosages.

ANESTHETIC PREOPERATIVE ASSESSMENT

Preoperative discussion with the surgeon regarding the extent of planned surgery, positional changes of the patient, and anticipated problems with temperature maintenance will help to formulate an intraoperative plan for smoothly coordinated management and facilitate patient care. This evaluation of the burned child will then enable the anesthesiologist to plan a rational anesthetic course and hopefully circumvent intraoperative problems.

Airway Analysis

In the newborn and infant the cricoid is approximately 6.0 mm in diameter.[15] Phillips[12] notes that the mean anteroposterior diameter in the cricoid lumen increases by 0.5 mm/year to 12.5 mm at the age of 12 years. Also, the area enclosed by the infant glottis is about 14 sq mm when full cord abduction exists, and edema of only 1 mm will reduce glottis size by 65%.[12] Consequently, minimal edema formation may produce severe airway compromise.

Access to the airway must be defined preoperatively. In the presence of inhalation burns, or with burns to the face and head, laryngeal/pharyngeal/glottic edema is common, and the probability of airway closure during anesthetic induction is high. Edema of the face and neck may necessitate emergent endotracheal or nasotracheal intubation to protect the airway from edematous obstruction. Later, edema of the face and neck may also lead to difficulty in applying a mask or in ventilation as anesthesia is introduced.

Perioral and cervical burn eschar can present a major problem with opening the mouth and extending the neck. An analysis of the extent of mouth opening (distance between incisor teeth) and mechanism of restrictions as well as ability to extend and hyperextend the neck and head must be recorded in the acutely burned patient. Later, heavy scar contracture tissue in the neck may restrict the mobility necessary for laryngoscopy and intubation.

Hematological and Biochemical Considerations

The hemoglobin/hematocrit should be greater than 10 gm/30%. Results of a recent biochemical screen and blood gas/acid-base analysis must be obtained. Electrolyte and acid-base stability reflecting adequate state of hydration must be assured preoperatively. An oncotic pressure greater than 15 mm Hg is also expected.

ANESTHETIC PREOPERATIVE MEDICATION

Sedation deserves tailoring to the individual patient. In children with extensive burns or airway compromise, depressant narcotics or potent sedatives are generally contraindicated. If the child is receiving small, repeated doses of narcotics already, one should consider the continuance of the drug as a preoperative medication. Otherwise, further sedation via the intravenous (IV) route in a controlled environment is reserved for the operating room.

Older children with smaller burn injuries may benefit from small doses of narcotics or sedatives prior to transport to the operating room. In children less than 1 year old, preoperative medicines are rarely administered before their arrival in the operating room. Intramuscular morphine sulfate (0.1 mg/kg of body weight) or diazepam (0.1 mg/kg of body weight) may be administered orally with a small amount of water. Other drugs are given as needed IV with induction of anesthesia.

As in any preoperative situation, reassurance to the child along with a familiar smiling face may be the best medicine to help allay fear in the operating room.

TRANSPORTATION TO THE OPERATING ROOM

In the critically burned patient, needs during transport to the operating room may include protection of the airway, either by controlled ventilation through endotracheal tube, Ambu bag, and oxygen, or by spontaneous ventilation and accompaniment by appropriate professional personnel. The temperature should be maintained by keeping the patient covered and bringing him to a warm room after transport. Integrity of the IV line, if previously instituted, should be maintained by drip or infusion pump during transport.

OPERATIVE ANESTHESIA

Compassionate and comforting conversation during transfer to the operating room table must be maintained and the child's dignity preserved by retaining linens. A stuffed toy is to be encouraged!

Intravenous Access

Intravenous access can be extremely difficult in children, especially when extremities are burned. All attempts should be made to establish at least one 18- to 20-gauge peripheral IV line for rapid fluid or blood infusion. If the child arrives in the operating room with a working IV line, induction of anesthesia is accomplished through this, and a second IV line is sought following peripheral vasodilation produced by inhalation anesthetics.

Choices for IV sites include large veins of the hand and the saphenous vein at the ankle. The antecubital veins, femoral veins, or neck veins are used, or a venous cutdown is performed only when necessary. Invasive monitors such as central venous lines or intra-arterial lines are used only when specifically indicated because morbidity may outweigh their usefulness.

Monitoring

Intraoperative monitors must operate continuously and be versatile since the position of the patient is often changed or areas of the skin are scrubbed or grafted serially.

Blood pressure can be obtained by conventional blood-pressure cuff and stethoscope, but a more accurate and versatile monitor is a noninvasive ultrasound blood pressure monitor (Dinamapp), which can measure blood pressure from different extremity sites and has multiple-size cuffs.

The electrocardiogram (ECG) can be obtained through standard ECG adhesive pads, which may have to be repositioned or changed periodically due to inadequate contact or a wet field. Another alternative is the "butterfly" ECG single-adhesive pad, which can be applied to the back or chest. This is especially useful when few position changes are expected. Alternatively, extensively burned patients may require subcutaneous needle electrodes or metal skin staples with alligator clip adapters for electrical conduction since few dry or intact areas of skin may exist for adhesive pads to be effective.

Heart/breath sounds and temperature can be continuously monitored by the precordial stethoscope and earpiece with skin temperature probe, or if the patient is intubated, by either a 12 or 18 F esophageal stethoscope-temperature probe.

Anesthesia Induction

Induction of anesthesia can be accomplished in many ways. Airway control is, however, the first consideration in the plan for induction. The patient with facial and neck burns or contractures, which leave the patient with limitation of mouth opening or restriction to neck mobility, requires an alternate route of anesthetic induction.

In our practice, three situations are commonly considered:

1. For short, uninvolved procedures that do not require position changes or involve extensive blood loss, ketamine may be used. A small induction dose of 1 to 2 mg/kg of body weight administered intramuscularly will allow some degree of patient control with spontaneous respiration until IV access can be made. Then, additional doses of IV ketamine up to 1 mg/kg may be administered to achieve analgesia and surgical anesthesia. This can be supplemented with low concentrations of nitrous oxide and oxygen to provide a "smoother" anesthetic.

2. Long, complex procedures are best managed with a mask-inhalation anesthetic, followed by endotracheal intubation and maintenance with a potent inhalation anesthetic agent.

3. Patients with problem airways may require nasal or oral fiberoptic bronchoscopy and intubation, laryngoscopy when awake, or preintubation neck release with local anesthesia. In our experience, fiberoptic bronchoscopy has been a safe and effective method of achieving airway control. A small-diameter, flexible fiberoptic bronchoscope will have an average external diameter of 3.5 to 3.9 mm (Fig 11–1) and will accommodate a no. 4.0 endotracheal tube. A no. 4.5 endotracheal tube is needed to allow the patient to breathe spontaneously around the bronchoscope (Fig 11–2). Small doses of IV sedatives (e.g., dilute diazepam [Valium], 0.5-mg increments plus fentanyl, 5 to 10 μgm increments) and topical anesthesia (cocaine, diluted 1% to 2% solution) administered according to body weight are necessary to manage the awake pediatric patient for this procedure. An alternative is fiberoptic intubation over a ventilating mask or oral fiberoptic bronchoscopy after induction of anesthesia (Figs 11–3 and 11–4). The anesthesia may be induced and maintained with a potent inhalation anesthetic, such as halothane, so spontaneous ventilation can be maintained.

Anesthetic induction is predominantly carried out with halothane, nitrous oxide, and oxygen. The child breathes spontaneously, or ventilation is assisted until the trachea is intubated. Enflurane and isoflurane are also acceptable agents for induction and anesthetic maintenance in the few patients with suspected hepatic problems. Tracheal intubation should be done with care following observation of pharyngeal and laryngeal structures. Since edema in this area is common, endotracheal tube size should be selected according to existing conditions. The intubation should be atraumatic and tube placement easy and without resistance. A slight "leak" of air should exist at peak inspiratory pressures of 20 to 22 cm H_2O. Uncuffed endotracheal tubes and similar testing for "leak" of air at

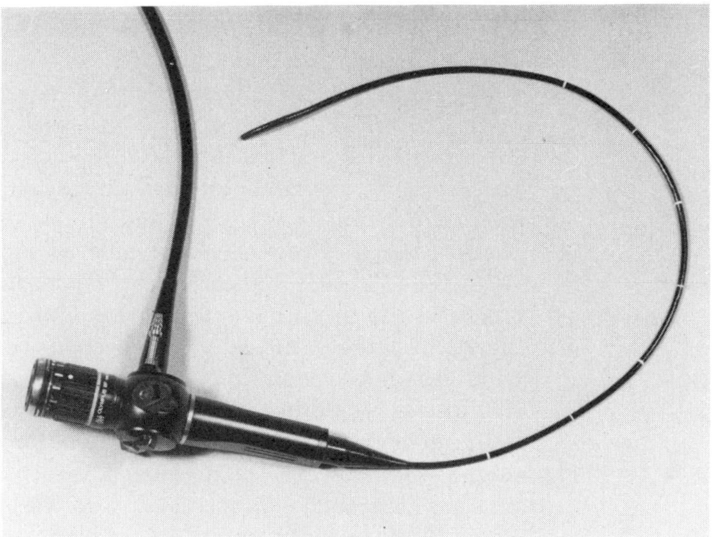

FIG 11–1.
Olympus small diameter fiberoptic bronchoscope (3.7 mm external diameter).

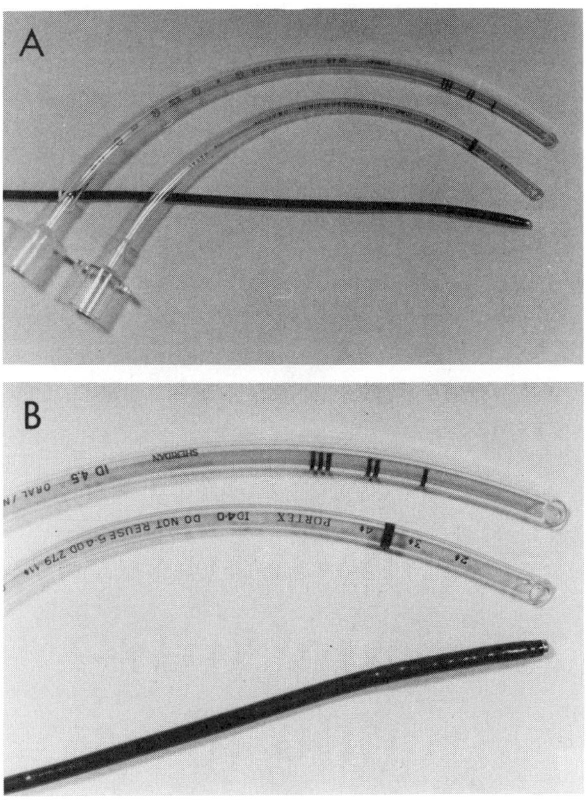

FIG 11–2.
A, small diameter fiberoptic bronchoscope with no. 4.0 and no. 4.5 uncuffed endotracheal tubes. **B,** close-up of no. 4.0 and 4.5 cuffed endotracheal tubes.

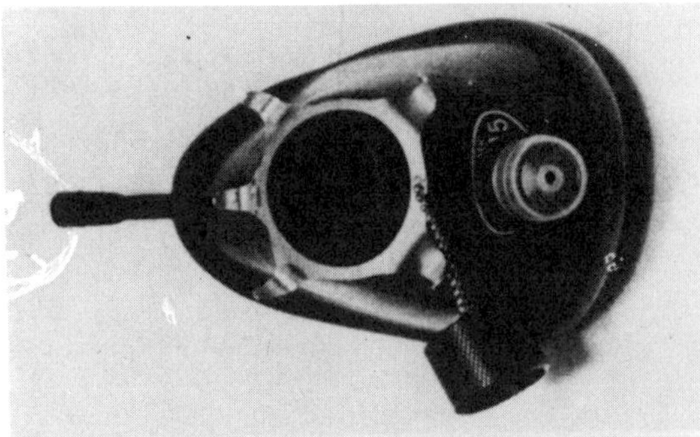

FIG 11–3.
Patil-Syracuse ventilating mask with front access sleeve. (AINCA Anesthesia Associates, Inc.)

peak inspiratory pressures are recommended in children 1 to 9 years old.

ANESTHETIC DRUGS

Inhalation Agents

Anesthetic agents suggested for anesthetic maintenance include ketamine, potent inhalation anesthetics (halothane,[2] enflurane, isoflurane), or neuroleptanesthetics with narcotics, nitrous oxide, and oxygen. Multiple halothane anesthetics in burned patients have not been associated with hepatotoxic response.[1, 7] Operative time, patient position, cardiovascular stability, and pain determine specific agent use. For moderate to lengthy procedures, a combination of inhalation anesthesia and narcotics (small doses of either fentanyl or morphine) has been useful in providing stable control of blood pressure and heart rate, both during the procedure and during the awakening and recovery phases.

Muscle Relaxants

Depolarizing muscle relaxants present specific risks in the burned patient. Succinylcholine-induced hyperkalemia[13] and cardiac arrest have been described in patients with thermal injury. In the 1969 study by Schaner et al.[13] a pattern of potassium ion elevation began 30 seconds after succinylcholine administration. Peak levels were reached at 5 minutes. A gradual decline to baseline levels occurred within 15 minutes. Electrocardiographic changes were not consistently diagnostic until serum potassium ion levels reached 8 mEq/L. Because of their availability, nondepolarizing muscle relaxants, such as pancuronium, vecuronium, and atracurium, are used for muscle relaxation and intubation of the trachea. Doses required may be elevated.[4, 5, 8] Studies indicated a 2.5-fold increase in the mean dose of pancuronium required in acutely burned children compared with the dose required in control children (Fig 11–5). In addition, a good correlation existed between dose required and size of burn (Fig 11–6). However, a prolonged recovery time, which did not correlate with dose, acuteness of burn injury, or size of burn, existed. Clinically, similar doses of vecuronium and pancuronium appeared to be required, although this has not been substantiated.

FLUID AND BLOOD REPLACEMENT

Fluid losses must be calculated and fluids replaced according to the number of hours the child has been given nothing by mouth (NPO) and to the hourly fluid requirements

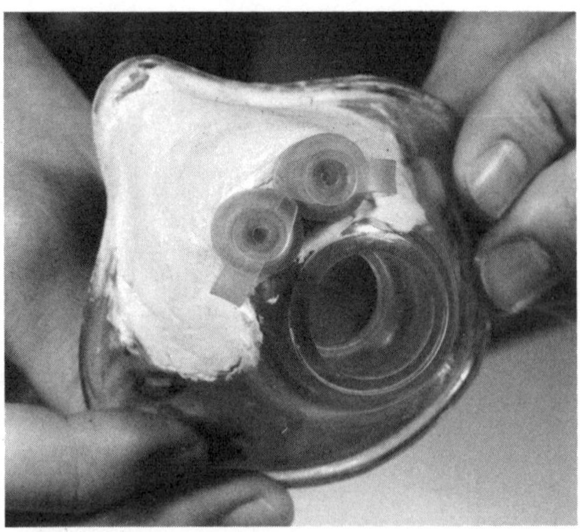

FIG 11–4.
Ventilating mask. (Photograph courtesy of Dr. B. Leiman, Department of Anesthesiology, University of Texas Medical School at Houston.)

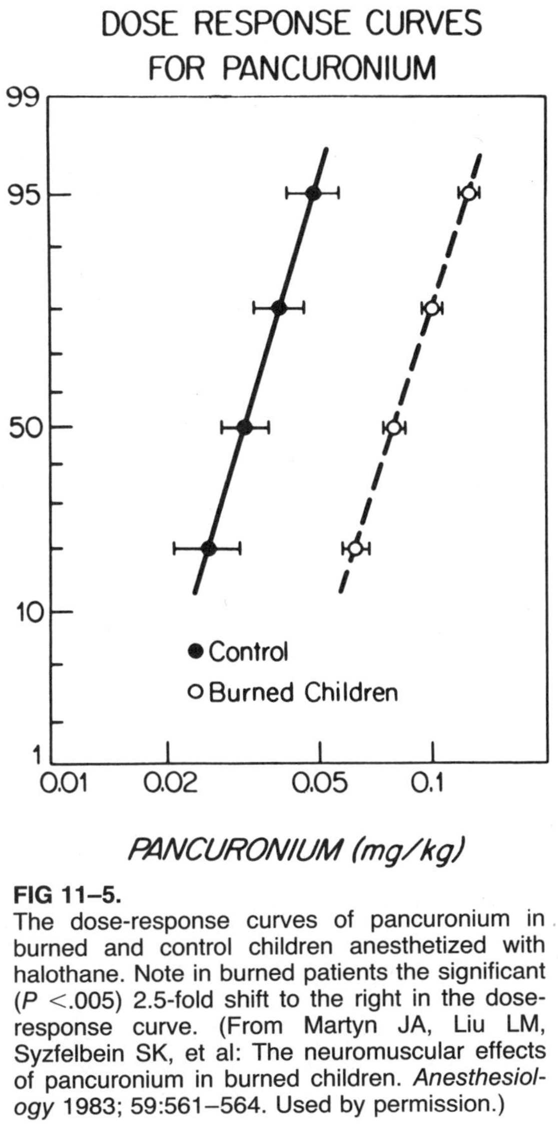

FIG 11–5.
The dose-response curves of pancuronium in burned and control children anesthetized with halothane. Note in burned patients the significant ($P <.005$) 2.5-fold shift to the right in the dose-response curve. (From Martyn JA, Liu LM, Syzfelbein SK, et al: The neuromuscular effects of pancuronium in burned children. *Anesthesiology* 1983; 59:561–564. Used by permission.)

during the surgical procedure. If continuous IV infusion was administered the night before surgery, the hourly rate of fluid infused must be checked. When an overnight IV line has not been in place, the correct number of NPO hours should be ascertained and fluid volume replaced after the IV infusion is started in the operating room. Replacement of half this volume is given in the first intraoperative hour and the second half given in the next hour.

Severe hypotension is commonly seen in dehydrated or hypovolemic children when an inhalation anesthetic, especially halothane, has been used. Therefore, IV placement and fluid replacement in the induction phase of anesthesia have a high priority. Five percent dextrose in lactated Ringer's solution is an acceptable replacement fluid for NPO deficits if there is no existing electrolyte imbalance or preoperative hyperkalemia. Following NPO deficit restoration, maintenance fluids with crystalloid should be administered hourly using lactated Ringer's solution at a rate of 4 to 6 ml/kg/hr. This rate is adjusted to maintain urine output at 1 ml/kg of body weight/hr.

Children with anemic states (hemoglobin, 10 gm/dl or less) or expected to lose significant quantities of blood during the procedure may benefit from presurgical transfusion with packed red blood cells. Recommended transfusion volumes are 5 to 10 cc of warmed, packed red blood cells per kilogram of body weight. This approach may help to avoid hypotension and hypovolemia in the early stages of the operative procedure. Thereafter, blood is replaced cubic centimeter for cubic centimeter of estimated blood loss by using hematocrit readings.

In children with adequate blood volume, blood loss is closely monitored and replaced as indicated. Samples can be obtained through sterile capillary tubes on the operative field and the volume of red blood cells determined by hematocrit centrifuge in the operating room. This technique allows the anesthesiologist to follow trends in blood loss and replacement since accurate estimates of blood loss are difficult to obtain during surgical excision and grafting. As the blood loss approaches 10% to 15% of the estimated blood volume, fresh-frozen plasma or albumin solution should be transfused to approximately half of replaced red blood cell volume. Other blood products are given if hemodynamic changes occur or clotting dysfunction is suspected.

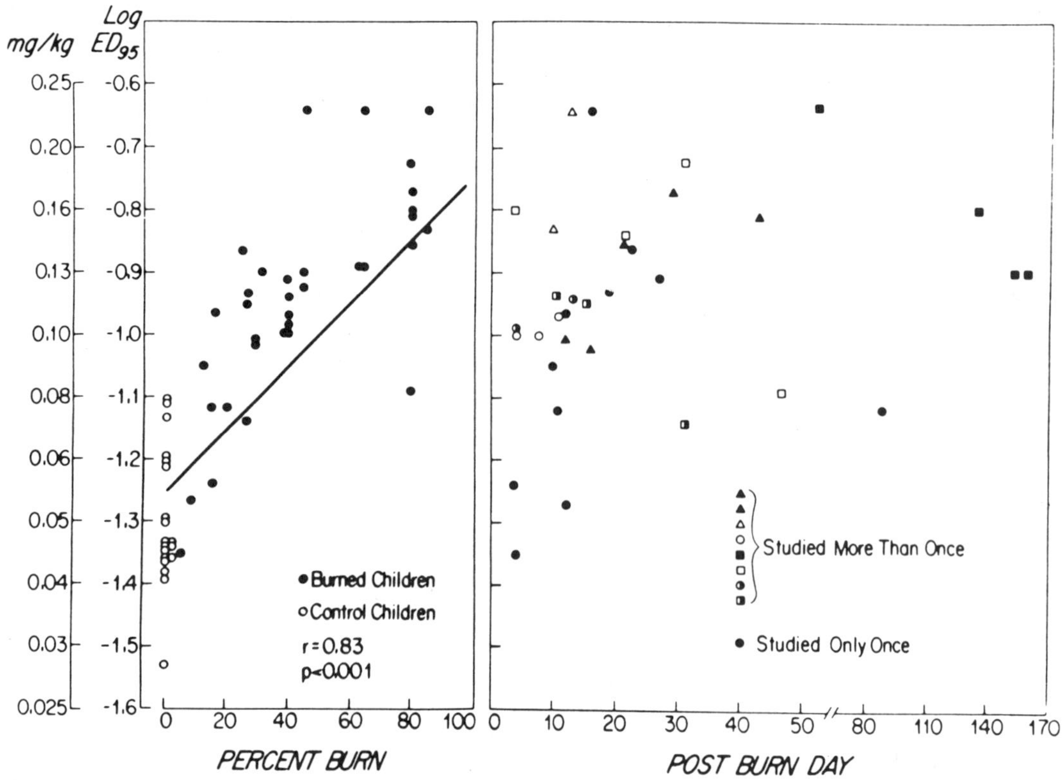

FIG 11–6.
The correlation between log dose of 95% twitch depression and magnitude of burn. Note the significant correlation between dose and magnitude of burn. Dose = mg/kg of pancuronium, ED = effective dose. (From Martyn JA, Liu LM, Szyfelbein SK, et al: The neuromuscular effects of pancuronium in burned children. *Anesthesiology* 1983; 59:561–564. Used by permission.)

TEMPERATURE

Intraoperatively, body temperature may be difficult to maintain. Methods of warming and preventing heat loss include use of a warming blanket on the operating room table, a warming humidifier to heat oxygen and anesthetic gases and overhead radiant heat lamps or a heat shield; increasing the ambient air temperature of the operating room to approximately 85° F; use of warm sterile sheets to cover exposed surface areas; and warming infused fluids and blood.

POSTANESTHETIC RECOVERY PERIOD

Concerns for the burned child in the recovery phase are similar to those of the operative phase. Adequacy of a patent airway and oxygenation must be assessed during awakening so increased demands of metabolism can be met. Massive fluid and blood replacement can cause further soft tissue or pulmonary edema, which needs to be recognized and treated early with appropriate therapy. Those patients who have had airway problems preoperatively, have undergone extensive blood loss and replacement, or have shown signs of early generalized edema formation should retain their endotracheal tubes for a period of time during recovery. Consideration should be made for overnight retention of the endotracheal tube with either spontaneous ventilation or controlled ventilation based on respiratory parameters or arterial blood gas analysis.

Body temperature must also be maintained during recovery, but heat loss is minimal since exposed areas are covered with dressings and bandages. Recovery of heat lost during the operative phase can be accomplished with blankets and an overhead warming unit, although heat recovery usually takes several hours.

Blood loss through oozing wounds needs continuous assessment and replacement. If the postsurgical hematocrit level is satisfactory (range, 36% to 40%), allowance can be made for wound blood loss. In this case, stabilization of blood loss and circulating blood volume occur during the hours following surgery. By checking evening and first postoperative-day hematocrit readings, one may find results of 32% to 34%, so additional transfusions are not required.

Systemic bacteremia indicating sepsis should be recognized in the recovery period. Tachypnea, hyperthermia, an increase in pulse rate, and a decrease in blood pressure are all signs of septicemia. Septicemia results during the major excision of infected wounds when toxic products of infection "shower" the circulation. Support resuscitation when indicated should be instituted to stabilize the patient during antibiotic therapy in cases of acute sepsis.

Potent analgesics should be given in appropriate doses to relieve pain without embarrassment to the airway or respiration. Discharge from the recovery room should take place when all changes of the recovery phase have stabilized. The patient should be awake and free of pain, and all vital signs should be stable.

Acknowledgment

The author wishes to express his appreciation to Stanley Deutsch, M.D., for his contributions in producing this manuscript.

REFERENCES

1. deCampo T, Aldrete JA: The anesthetic management of the severely burned patient. *Intensive Care Med* 1981; 7:55–62.
2. Gronert GA, Scharen PJ, Gunter RC: Multiple halothane anesthesia in the burn patient. *JAMA* 1968; 105:878–880.
2a. Hudson LD: Causes of the respiratory distress syndrome: Clinical recognition. *Clin Chest Med* 1982; 3:195.
3. Krishna G, Haselby KA, Rao CC, et al: The pediatric patient, in Stoelting RK, Dierdorf SF (eds): Anesthesia and Co-existing Disease. New York, Churchill Livingstone, Inc, 1983, pp 741–810.
4. Martyn JA, Liu LM, Szyfelbein SK, et al: The neuromuscular effects of pancuronium in burned children. *Anesthesiology* 1983, 59:561–564.
5. Martyn JA, Goudsouzian NG, Matteo RS, et al: Metocurine requirements and plasma concentrations in burned pediatric patients. *Br J Anaesth* 1983, 55:263–268.
6. Martyn JA, Snider MT, Szyfelbein SK, et al: Right ventricular dysfunction in acute thermal injury. *Ann Surg* 1980; 191:330–335.
7. Martyn JA, Szyfelbein SK: Pathophysiology and management of burn trauma in children. *Semin Anesth* 1984, 3:75–87.
8. Martyn JA, Szyfelbein SK, Ali HH, et al: Increased D-tubocurarine requirement following major thermal injury. *Anesthesiology* 1980, 52:352–355.
9. Moncrief JA: Effect of various fluid regimens and pharmacologic agents on the circulatory hemodynamics of the immediate postburn period. *Ann Surg* 1966; 164:723–752.
10. Morgan RJ, Martyn JAJ, Philbin DM: Water metabolism and antidiuretic hormone response following thermal injury. *J Trauma* 1982; 20:468–472.
11. Murray JF: The history of analgesia in burns. *Postgrad Med J* 1972; 48:124–127.
12. Phillips KR: Tracheostomy in children. *Ear Nose Throat J* 1979; 58:66–78.
13. Schaner PJ, Brown RL, Kirksey TD, et al: Succinylcholine-induced hyperkalemia in burned patients. *Anesth Analg* 1969; 48:764–770.
14. Stoelting RK, Dierdorf SF: The pediatric patient: Thermal (burn) injury, in Stoelting RK, Dierdorf SF (eds): *Anesthesia and Co-existing Disease*. New York, Churchill Livingstone Inc, 1983, p 396.
15. Tucher G: The infant larynx: Direct laryngoscopic observations. *JAMA* 1932; 99:1899–1902.
16. Visser ER, Tarrow AB: Fluothane for multiple burn dressing anesthetics. *Anesth Analg* 1959; 38:301–305.
17. Wilson RD: Anesthesia and the burned child. *Int Anesthesiol Clin* 1975; 13:103–217.

12 / The Surgical Management of Burns

DONALD H. PARKS, M.D.
DAVID J. WAINWRIGHT, M.D., F.R.C.S.(C.)

Early aggressive surgical management of the burn wound in selected thermally injured children is practiced in many burn centers. Advantages of this approach include decreased morbidity by decreasing the time interval from the acute injury until definitive wound closure, improved mortality, and shortened hospital stay.

Prerequisites for surgical intervention, particularly in patients with massive burns, must be established and include a team of specially trained personnel, definitive organization of the surgical team, and the availability of an adequately equipped facility.

HISTORY

Early attempts at the surgical management of the burn wound were reported by Wells in 1929, Young in 1942, and Cope in 1947.[15] MacMillan and Artz[14] reported in 1957 successful excisions of 25% or more of the total body surface area (TBSA) and Haynes,[6] in 1969, reported good results in burns of 15% or less when excision to the fascia was performed in 30 patients. Milestones were reached in 1968 when Janzekovic[11] described tangential excision and in 1975 when Burke et al.[1] reported on excision and autografting with immunosuppresion and homografting in 11 children. The Chinese experience[3] in early excision in massively burned patients has been dramatic, and more recently Herndon and Parks[7] have reported on success in management of burns greater than 80% of TBSA with early surgical excisional techniques. Gallico et al.[5] have reported on successful early excision and permanent coverage with autologous cultured human epithelium.

PREREQUISITES FOR SURGICAL MANAGEMENT

Personnel

Surgical intervention in the management of extensively burned children requires the availability of experienced surgeons, pediatricians, pediatric anesthesiologists, nurses, and other skilled support staff. The burned child presents a unique challenge to the surgical team, and only personnel skilled in the management of burn wounds in children should direct and monitor their care.

Facility

A fully equipped pediatric intensive care unit or pediatric burn unit must be available with the appropriate pediatric monitors, ventilators, and other equipment that may be required in the perioperative period. Although invasive monitoring is not routinely used, such devices should be available, particularly for critically ill children undergoing massive surgical excision.

The operating suite must be capable of being warmed efficiently and quickly (85° F), and full state-of-the-art monitoring capability must be present. In infants, an Ohio table is ideal. All surgical technical equipment must be preselected and available immediately so no anesthesia time is wasted.

Patient Factors

The patient's preoperative state of hydration should show evidence of adequate fluid resuscitation. A corrected hemoglobin level of greater than 10 gm/dl, albumin greater than 2.0 gm/dl or colloid oncotic pressure (COP) greater than 15 is recommended.

Adequate blood for transfusion must be available, and in extensive excisions, transfusable blood to total one half the patient's total blood volume should be available in the operating room, with blood warmers being mandatory. Vascular (venous) access must be assured with a catheter at least 20 gauge or larger. In many cases, a Foley catheter is inserted.

In the author's experience, the presence of concomitant inhalation injury is a contraindication to general anesthesia except under very specific circumstances.

Informed consent must be assured and obtained in writing from parents or legal guardians.

SURGICAL EXCISION PROCEDURES

Surgical procedures are classified as:

1. Tangential excision
2. Tangential débridement
3. Excision to fascia
   A. Small local third-degree burns
   B. Burn wound sepsis
   C. Massive burns

Tangential Excision

The concept of tangential excision was first expressed by Janzekovic[11] in 1968 and further elucidated by Jackson in classic articles in 1969 and 1972.[9, 10]

Tangential excision may be defined as excision of the necrotic surface of a burn wound and autogenous skin grafting when deep, partial skin loss or whole skin loss does not involve fat. Based on the vascular anatomy of burned skin, deep skin loss results in a superficial zone of necrosis or irreversible tissue loss surrounded by a zone of capillary stasis, which extends to the subdermal plexus of blood vessels. Despite this depth of injury, if subdermal veins are not thrombosed, then a skin graft will take on the deepest dermal tissue following excision of the zone of necrosis and part of the zone of stasis.[10] Failure to graft immediately or provide a physiological covering will result in irreversible necrosis of all dermis with microcirculatory thrombosis and, thus, full-thickness skin loss with eschar formation.

The diagnosis of the deep second-degree burn is based on appearance by excluding tissues in which frank charring, exposed fat, or thrombosed vessels are evident in the dead tissue. The damaged skin should be anesthetic but relatively soft to touch. A common appearance is of a relatively soft tissue surface that is bright red or bright red with a central whitish discoloration and with general preservation of the normal skin contours. That is, no depression of the burned area as seen in dehydration of third-degree burns should exist.

Tangential excision is usually performed 2 to 5 days postburn, usually after hemodynamic stabilization, and before bacterial colonization has occurred.

TECHNIQUE

Tangential excision (Figs 12–1 to 12–6) is performed with the patient under general anesthesia with blood available in the operating room and without perioperative antibiotics unless there is clinical evidence of established infection, such as *Streptococcus* cellulitis. In the latter case, parenteral penicillin is recommended and surgery generally delayed.

If a decision to carry out tangential excision is made immediately, then only a dry dressing on the wound is advised. Creams that tend to soften the burned tissues and render

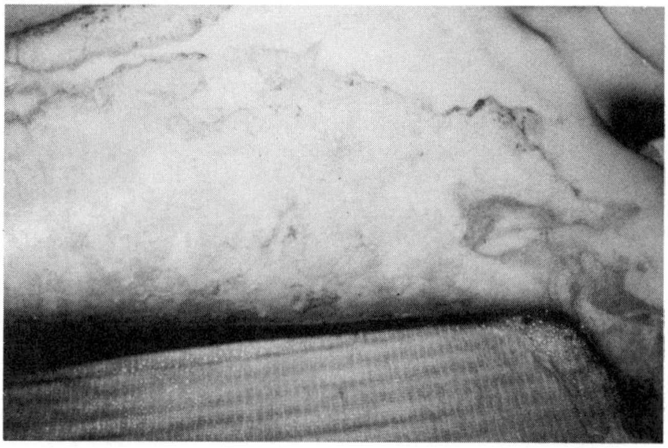

FIG 12–1.
Deep second-degree flame burn in a 10-year-old child.

them less amenable to the shaving technique should be avoided.

The use of a pneumatic tourniquet with partial exsanguination is recommended for burns of the extremities. Although the characteristic pinpoint bleeding pattern defining the appropriate depth of excision is obscured, with experience, this layer can be recognized and successfully grafted. Some surgeons have recommended the use of fluorescein prior to tourniquet inflation, but this has not been practiced in our center.

Thin slices of dead tissue approximately 8 to 12/1,000-in. thick are excised using a small hand dermatome, preferably the Weck or Goulian knife, and countertraction is applied to facilitate the slicing action. Care must be taken not to lacerate normal adjacent skin, and various contortions may be necessary to properly expose the burn surface for excision. Hemostasis is obtained by constant pressure, preferably with green towels and elastic wraps (Ace bandage wraps), while split-thickness skin grafts (STSGs) are harvested. At least 20 minutes should pass before the initial towel application is removed following tourniquet deflation.

STSGs are obtained using a Brown air-driven dermatome or Padgett dermatome, and a thickness of 8/1,000 in. is preferred. Meshing of the grafts in a 1.5:1 ratio has generally been carried out except in functional areas, such as the hands or face or over joints. The application of an unexpanded mesh graft appears to facilitate graft "take" and prevent hematoma or seroma formation.

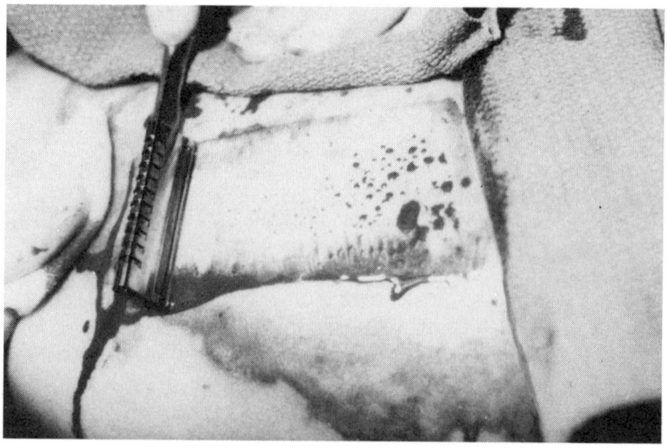

FIG 12–2.
Tangentially excising a deep second-degree burn wound with a Weck knife until pinpoint bleeding pattern is identified. Care is taken not to lacerate uninvolved skin. Tension is applied proximally and distally to facilitate excision.

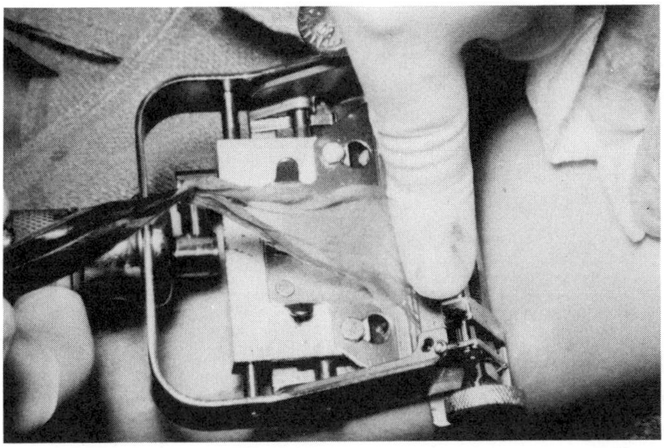

FIG 12–3.
Harvesting an 8/1,000-in. split-thickness skin graft with an air-driven dermatome.

Grafts are applied to the hemostatic, freshly excised wound, and a layer of N-Terface and fishnet gauze (e.g., Surginet) is used without any other methods for graft fixation. Staples or sutures are to be discouraged as methods of fixation.

Variations on the method may include the use of splints or plaster casts or skeletal suspension for stabilization of tissues during the early phases of graft take.[12]

The fresh grafts are then left undisturbed for 3 to 5 days and extremity elevation is assured. Aggressive occupational and physical therapy is usually indicated 7 to 10 days postgrafting. Generally, grafts are left exposed to the air following the first dressing change, and a mild lubricating lotion is applied.

RESULTS

Accurate excision over areas less than 20% of TBSA with immediate thin STSG in the early postburn period has been extremely successful. Tangential excision of burned hands has yielded particularly excellent results.[8] Decreased healing time, shortened hospital stay, and decreased hypertrophic scar formation are recognized advantages.

Tangential Debridement

Tangential debridement implies a surgical technique of removing slices of eschar in the presence of unequivocal full-thickness injury to expose subcutaneous fat or deeper structures. The goal is to eradicate necrotic tissue

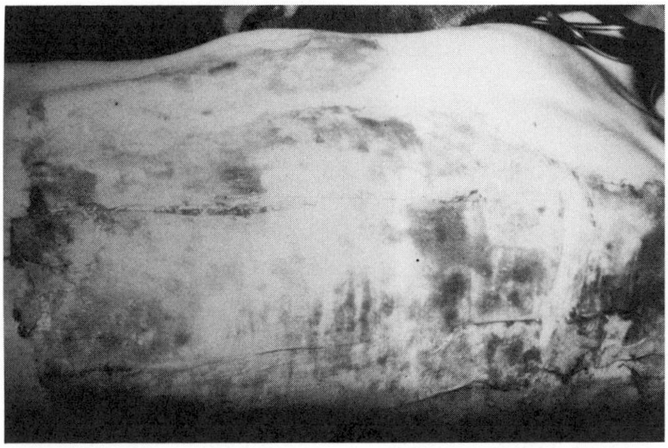

FIG 12–4.
Sheets of split-thickness skin graft applied to the excised surface once hemostasis is assured.

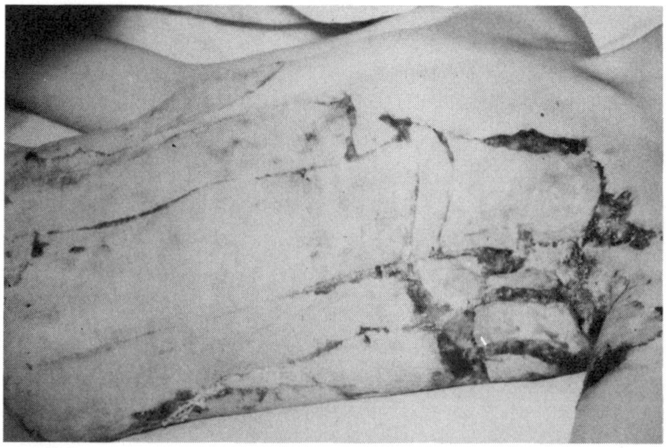

FIG 12–5.
Graft is adherent 10 days postburn; some decrusting and application of skin moisturizer indicated.

as quickly as possible to allow immediate autograft or the development of healthy granulation tissue to successfully accept autografts.

Tangential debridement is initially performed on the second to fifth postburn day and then every 5 to 10 days thereafter until all dead tissue has been eradicated. It is the most common procedure performed in our burn center.

TECHNIQUE

Tangential debridement (Figs 12–7 to 12–11) is performed under general anesthesia; antibiotics are not indicated unless an established infection is present. Pneumatic tourniquet use is encouraged where possible; otherwise hemostasis is achieved with electrocautery and sustained pressure using towels and elastic wraps or applying manual pressure.

The debridement is performed with a Weck, Goulian or Cobbett knife, by sequentially removing slices of dead tissue until healthy-appearing viable tissues are exposed. The extent of debridement is limited to 20% of the TBSA in most patients.

Once hemostasis has been obtained and exposure of a healthy base assured, then autografts, approximately 8/1,000-in. thick, meshed in a 1.5:1 ratio, are harvested and applied. Alternatively, immediate grafting may not be advised because of uncertainty of complete removal of devitalized tissues. Either porcine xenograft or a topical antimicrobial, usually silver sulfadiazine impregnated into a fine mesh gauze, rolled gauze, and elastic wraps are applied.

If xenograft is used, daily inspection is mandatory to identify purulent material or

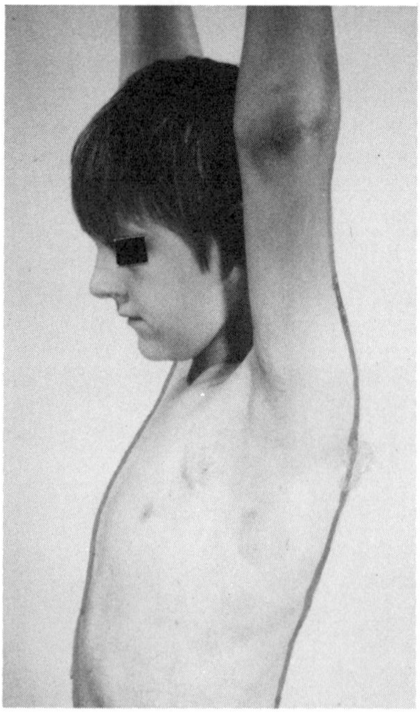

FIG 12–6.
Six months postburn with a few scattered areas of hypertrophic scar at the graft intersection and permanent pigment and textural alterations.

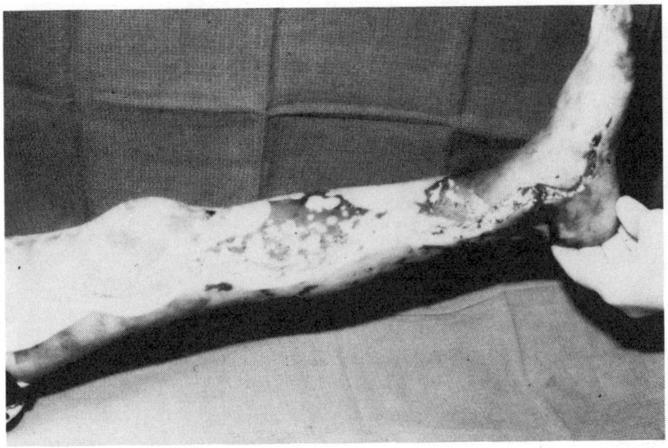

FIG 12–7.
Extensive third-degree burn of the left lower extremity in a 14-year-old boy. Note the escharotomy.

further necrosis of subcutaneous tissue. Removal and further surgical debridement may be indicated in such circumstances. Xenograft provides an excellent test of a recipient bed in terms of ultimate acceptance of autograft. If there is evidence of xenograft vascularization, then the xenograft is removed in the operating room and immediately replaced with an autograft, usually with a very high degree of success.

Tangentially debrided wounds dressed with topical antimicrobial agents are managed by daily hydrotherapy and redressed with topical silver sulfadiazine. Daily inspection is mandatory to identify further or residual tissue necrosis, and subsequent tangential debridements or general wound debridement in the operating room may be indicated until a completely viable bed has been obtained and autografting can be performed successfully. A 2- to 3-week delay usually exists between initial tangential debridement and grafting if grafting with the application of topical antimicrobials is performed. This delay may prevent necrosis of salvageable subcutaneous tissues and may also improve the ultimate take of autografts.

Fresh or preserved homograft skin also provides an excellent temporary wound cover and will take if that result is desired. Unfortunately, homograft tends to be somewhat difficult to obtain and is expensive to process and store.

Autografts, once applied, are retained with-

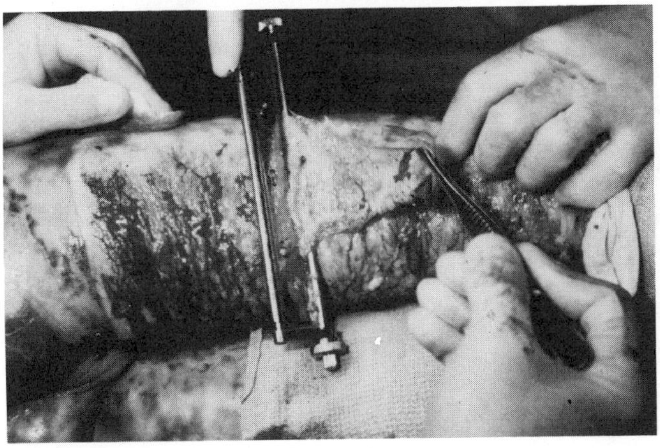

FIG 12–8.
Tangential debridement with a dermatome knife on the sixth postburn day. Note the full-thickness excision with exposure of subcutaneous fat. Once hemostasis is obtained, the wound is dressed with a topical antimicrobial agent.

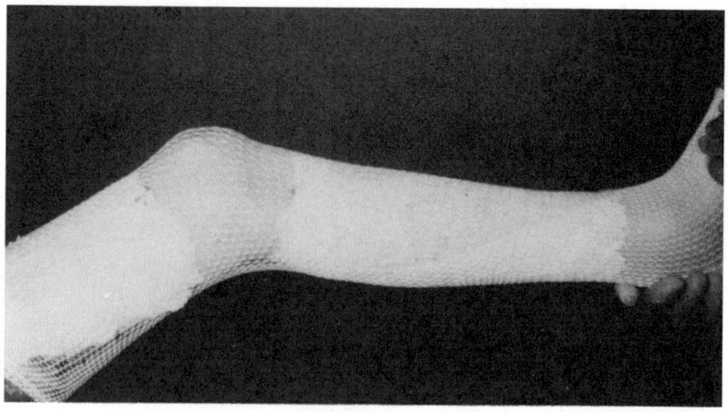

FIG 12–9.
Burn wound prepared by daily hydrotherapy and application of topical silver sulfadiazine fine mesh gauze and elastic net dressing.

out suture or staples but with N-Terface gauze and elastic netting. Autografts are exposed in approximately 3 days, and thereafter usually left exposed and treated with a mild lubricating lotion or cream.

RESULTS

If subcutaneous fat or granulation tissues are judged correctly or prepared with the use of xenograft or homograft, then excellent graft take results. Ideally, very early granulations provide the recipient bed for the split-thickness autografts. Prior to application, the most superficial granulation tissue should be debrided using a blunt instrument such as scalpel handle or forceps.

The major advantage of tangential debridement is salvage of subcutaneous tissue and thus preservation of body contours as compared to an excision to fascia. Later, reconstruction may be facilitated by preservation of subcutaneous fat or in many cases avoided entirely by preserving soft tissue and mobility.

The major disadvantage of tangential debridement is the increased risk of sepsis because a wound has been left open over a prolonged period of time. Careful wound management, strict nutritional support, and a dedicated team can overcome this disadvantage. Hospital stay may also be slightly prolonged until healthy granulation tissue has formed.

Excision to Fascia

Excision to fascia is indicated when (1) small local third-degree burns, (2) burn wound sepsis, or (3) massive burns exist.

SMALL LOCAL THIRD-DEGREE BURNS

Many patients present with well-demarcated, deep, third-degree burn wounds (Figs

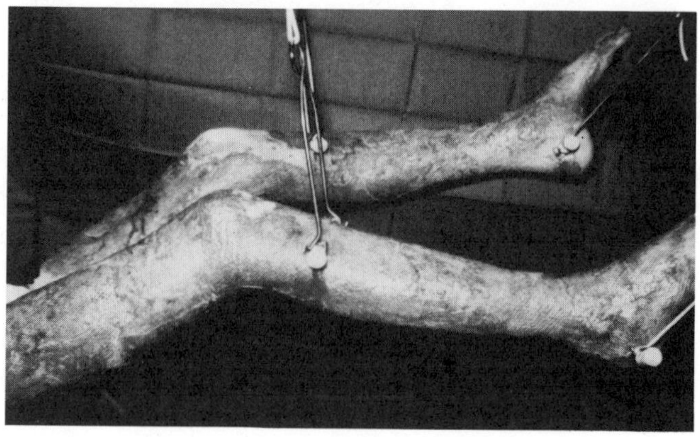

FIG 12–10.
Autograft, meshed in a 1.5:1 ratio, applied to healthy granulations at 3 1/2 weeks postburn. Note skeletal suspension for elevation positioning and graft care.

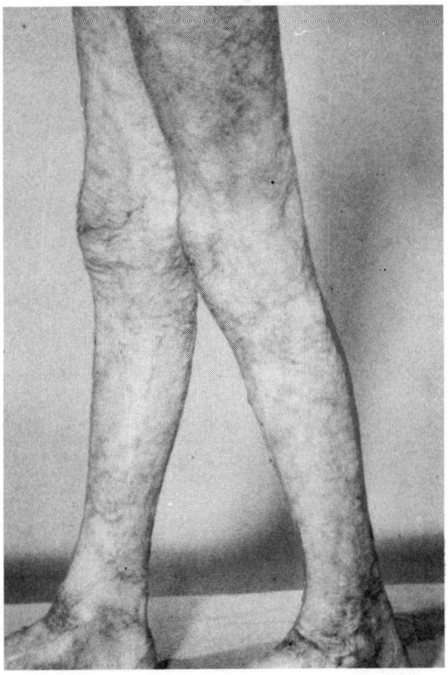

FIG 12–11.
Ten months postburn. Extensive irregular hypertrophic scarring, but excellent function and conservation of soft tissue contours based on residual subcutaneous fat.

12–12 to 12–15) such as those from hot presses, hot mufflers, or electrical arc or contact sources. The wound often appears depressed and grayish white, or is actually charred. Many of these types of injury are not extensive but are locally very deep; thus, early excision to the fascia is appropriate to accelerate wound closure.

Burn wound sepsis

Sepsis (Fig 12–16) is the major cause of death in hospitalized burn victims, and a major source of these septic episodes is the wound itself. The concept of burn wound sepsis was established in 1964 by Teplitz and colleagues,[20] who defined burn-wound sepsis as the presence in the wound of actively proliferating microorganisms that exceed 10^5 per gram of burn wound tissue and actively invade subjacent unburned tissue.

A study was designed to evaluate the feasibility and effectiveness of surgical management of the affected wound in the presence of burn wound sepsis.[17] Twenty-two nonpaired burned children, including 15 males and 7 females ranging in age from 9 months to 15 years (mean, 7.6 years), were identified as exhibiting burn wound sepsis. The surface area of the burn ranged from 33% to 91% with a mean burned area of 56.5% of the TBSA and a mean third-degree burned surface area of 37.1%. The parameters used to identify the presence of burn wound sepsis included (1) gross wound changes, (2) quantitative microbiology, and (3) qualitative microbiology.

When changes suggesting infection were noted in the wound, a biopsy in the suspi-

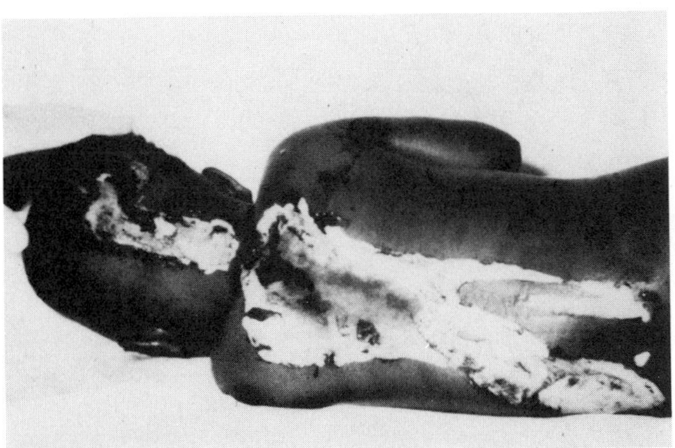

FIG 12–12.
A 3-year-old black girl with deep second- and third-degree muffler contact burn.

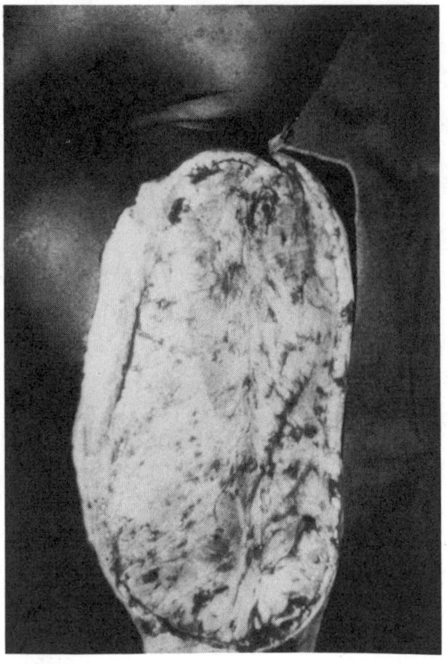

FIG 12–13.
Exposed fascia following formal excision on third postburn day.

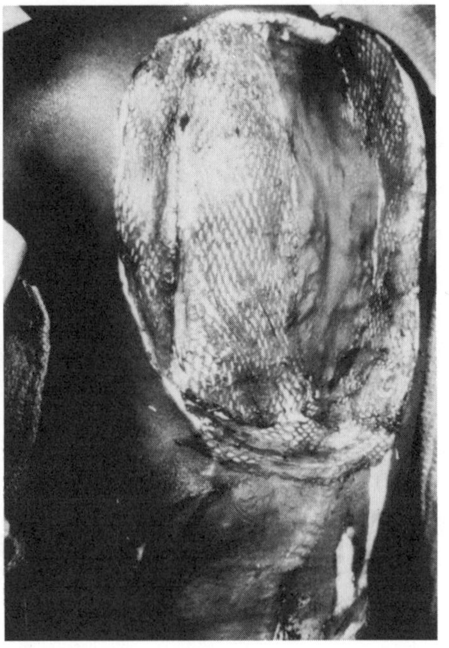

FIG 12–14.
Meshed and sheet split-thickness skin graft applied to freshly exposed fascial surface. Note tangentially excised and grafted cephalad zone (right side of figure).

cious area was performed and the tissue submitted for quantitative and qualitative microbiologic analysis. In most cases the qualitative report was available within 4 to 6 hours. Other patients had wound changes diagnostic of burn wound sepsis, and biopsy material was submitted at the time of the surgical management.

Appropriate measures for medical management of sepsis were invoked in all patients, and surgical excision was carried out under ketamine anesthesia even though some of these patients demonstrated signs and symptoms of severe systemic illness.

The surgical management consisted of ei-

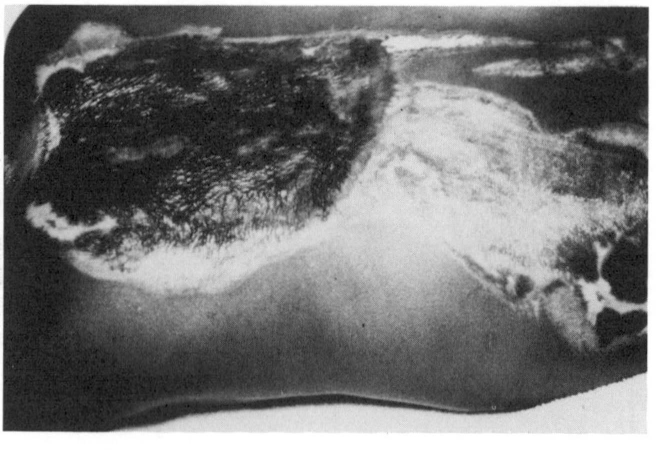

FIG 12–15.
Healed but cosmetically compromised excisional area 6 months postinjury.

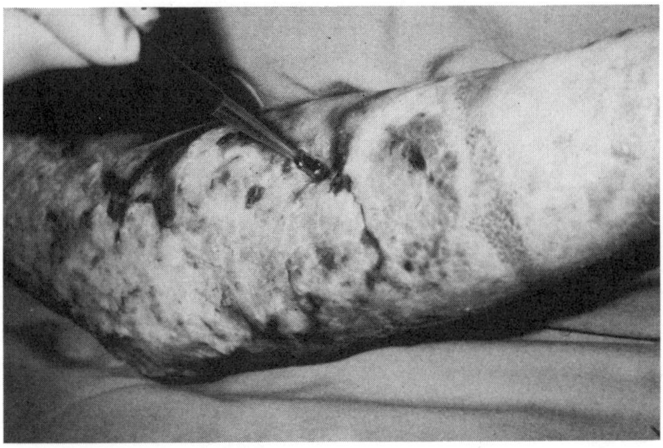

FIG 12–16.
Five mm punch biopsy from discolored, moist burn wound suspect for burn wound sepsis. Biopsy will be submitted for qualitative and quantitative microbiology.

ther excision to fascia or tangential debridement in the group with a surgically excised area ranging from 3% to 32% of the TBSA and blood loss averaging less than 20 ml/kg of body weight or approximately 25% of the total blood volume. Eleven of the 22 patients had positive blood cultures during the 48 hours before surgery, whereas blood cultures obtained during the 72 hours postoperatively in 17 patients revealed only one positive culture. No intraoperative deaths occurred but three children died at 2, 5, and 56 days, respectively, producing an overall mortality of 14%. Based on literature available at the time, this represented significant improvement in survival rates. The feasibility and effectiveness of surgical management in the presence of burn wound sepsis was thus confirmed.

Massive Burns

Early surgical intervention in the care of massively burned children (>60% of TBSA)[3] has contributed significantly to improved prognosis. A major factor in survival of such critically burned children appears to be early removal of eschar and wound closure with either skin substitutes or autograft. Because the availability of skin for autograft is limited, mortality is high and current research to develop skin substitutes is aggressive. Recent reports[2] of early massive wound excision and the application of a bilaminar membrane consisting of cross-linked bovine collagen glycosaminoglycan and an epidermal portion made of polysiloxane have been published. This collagen latticework provides a structure allowing for rapid capillary and fibroblastic ingrowth, producing neodermis after several days. The polysiloxane sheet is ultimately removed and epithelium produced by skin culture techniques is then applied to the neodermis.[3] This technique holds great promise for the future.

The author's approach in children with third-degree burns covering greater than 60% of TBSA is initial excision to fascia of an appropriate area, usually the anterior trunk (15% of TBSA), immediate harvest of all available autograft, and application of the autograft in the meshed conformation to the excised area.

At approximately 3- to 5-day intervals thereafter, burn surface areas of 10% to 15% are sequentially tangentially debrided in preparation for autografting once donor sites again become available. Intensive wound care, nutritional support, and patient monitoring is required during this multiple surgical process.

Several approaches have been described in treating massively burned children. Early extensive excision of burn wounds to fascia with coverage by cadaver skin has recently been compared with serial debridement and grafting and essentially no major differences in survival noted.[7] Other factors to be considered, though, must include functional, esthetic, and psychological outcome and require a great deal more work to define the most effective means of managing the burn wound.

TECHNIQUE

The surgical techniques for massive burns are seen in Figures 12–17 to 12–21. Intensive preplanning involving the surgeon, anesthesiologist, and others is essential. An area of eschar approximately 15% of TBSA is marked out for excision. The cutting cautery is used to incise the marked margins of the excision and the cold knife used to separate the specimen from the fascial surface. It is imperative that skilled assistants be available to coagulate vessels as the vessels coming through the fascia are exposed. Additionally, pressure is applied with towels on freshly exposed fascia as excision proceeds.

Once the specimen has been completely excised, saline-moistened towels are applied and attention is directed toward harvesting of all available skin for autograft. The appropriate dermatome is used with a setting of approximately 8/1,000 in., and if the scalp is used as a donor site, approximately 150 to 200 ml of saline is injected into the scalp to present a surface more amenable to graft harvesting. Hemostasis is obtained by applying pressure with towels, and scarlet red dressing is placed on the donor site and, in the case of the scalp, reinforced with cotton and elastic bandage wraps. All donor sites on the extremities are wrapped with elastic wraps for a period of 6 hours to ensure hemostasis beneath the scarlet red dressing. Subsequent donor site treatment is exposure and drying.

Once the grafts have been meshed in a 1.5:1 ratio, they are applied to the exposed fascial surface and a layer of N-Terface is placed over the grafts.

All grafts are exposed in 72 hours. All other unexcised areas are dressed daily with silver sulfadiazine dressings after cleansing with chlorhexidine gluconate (Hibiclens).

RESULTS

Fascia provides an excellent surface if grafted immediately with a split-thickness autograft. Little indication exists, however, for excision to fascia in routine burn care, since the ultimate cosmetic result is generally poor. In the case of small, local third-degree wounds, early wound closure and short hospital stay is realized, whereas in burn wound sepsis, improved survival occurs. In the author's experience, the early excision to fascia in the massively burned patient improved chances of survival by quickly decreasing the extent of burn wound.

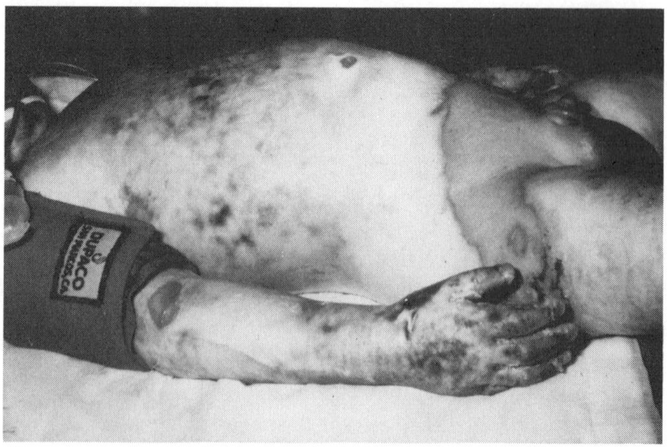

FIG 12–17.
Three-year-old male who sustained flame burn to 82% of TBSA. Prepared for surgical excision on the fourth postburn day.

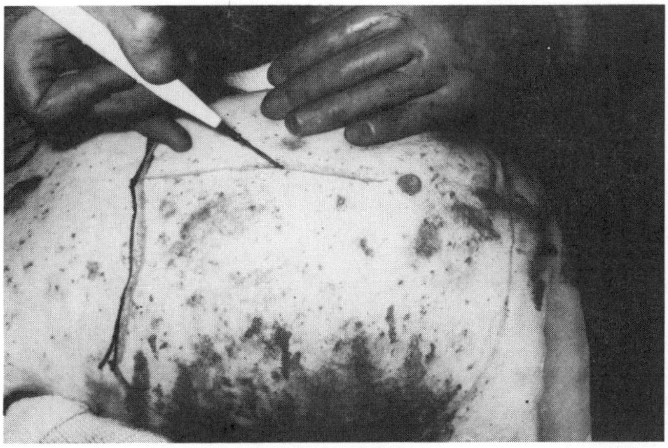

FIG 12–18.
Excisional site delineated over thoracoabdominal area. Note cautery knife excising eschar to the level of the fascia.

SPECIAL SURGICAL INDICATIONS IN BURNED CHILDREN

Tracheostomy

There are few indications for tracheostomy in acutely burned children. The major indication in early burn management is upper airway obstruction, which may be due to edema, a foreign body, or laryngeal trauma such that an endotracheal tube cannot be passed. The potential for upper airway obstruction should be recognized early, particularly following inhalation injury, so an appropriate endotracheal tube can be passed before onset of obstructive upper airway, oral, or facial edema. Tracheostomy is indicated in late burn management to (1) control secretions, (2) improve ventilator mechanics in children requiring long-term ventilator assistance, or (3) provide long-term intubation.

The preferred method of airway access is by nasotracheal intubation with careful monitoring and control of cuff pressures, strict hygiene, and secure fixation of the tube, avoiding destructive pressure to soft tissue, particularly that of the external nares.

Serious risks to tracheostomy include injury to adjacent vascular, neurologic, digestive, and pulmonary structures, as well as late complications such as hemorrhage, tracheoesophageal fistula formation, subglottic stenosis, and infection. Patients with burns about the upper chest and neck are particularly at risk for infection due to the risk of wound-lung autoinfection.[4] Prolonged intubation of

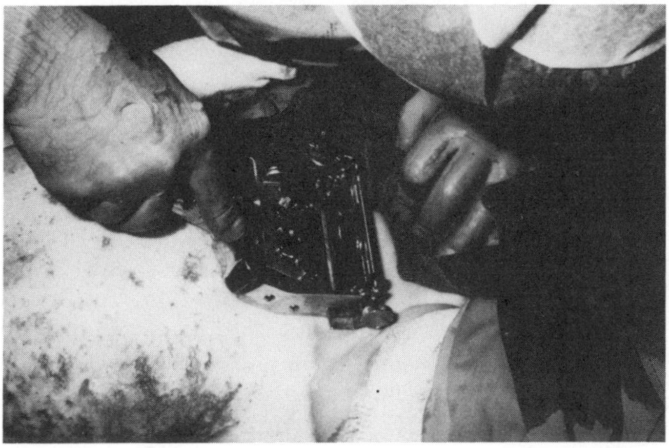

FIG 12–19.
Harvest of all available autograft at completion of excision to fascia.

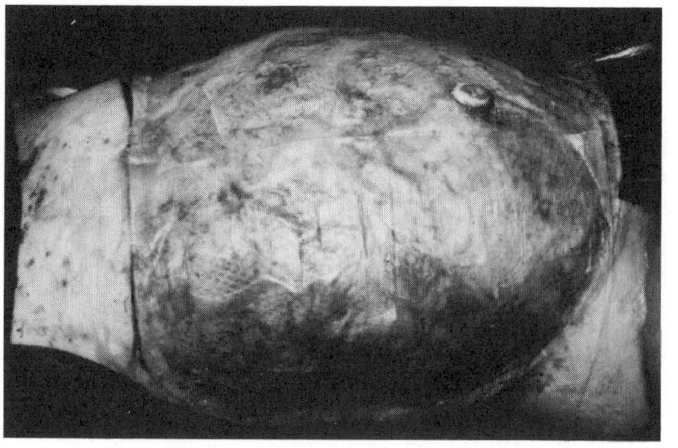

FIG 12–20.
Thin split-thickness skin graft meshed 1.5:1 and applied to freshly excised fascial surface. No graft fixation is indicated but a single sheet of interface is placed over grafts for 5 days.

up to 4 to 6 weeks has been tolerated with minimum complications. The general trend is toward this approach.[13]

Anatomical considerations

At birth the trachea is approximately 4 to 5 mm in diameter. The glottis in the infant is approximately 14 sq mm; 1 mm of edema reduces this area to 5 sq mm, which is a 65% reduction in the size of the glottis. The risks of delayed intubation, then, are underscored.[18] The proximity of vital structures to the small trachea, particularly in the infant, emphasizes the complexity in performing tracheostomy and the requirement for experience, surgical skill, and great care.

Technique

Tracheostomy (Figs 12–22 and 12–23) in burned children is usually carried out under general anesthesia following parenteral premedication with a drying agent and tranquilizer. Venous access must be established and principles of anesthesia in burned children applied (see Chapter 11).

The neck is slightly extended and appropriate preparation and draping carried out. We tend to leave the face completely open, with all draping confined to the upper chest and caudad portion of the body.

A short transverse incision, one finger's

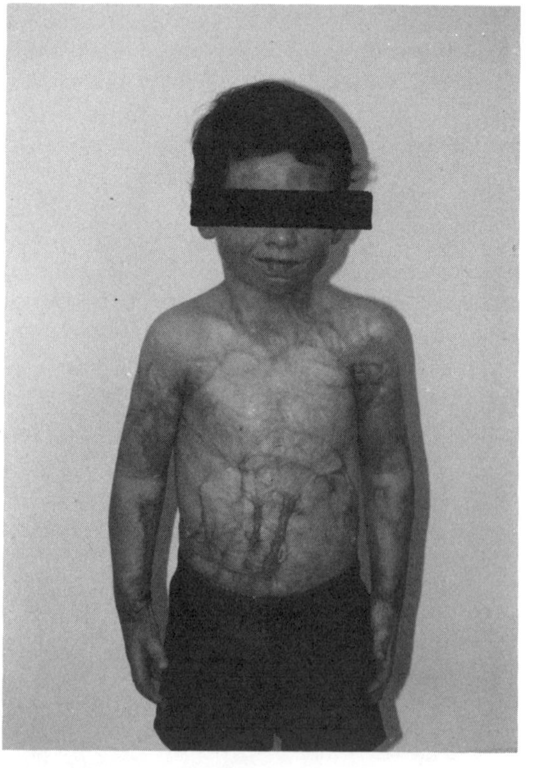

FIG 12–21.
Result at 3 years. After a series of tangential debridements and grafting procedures, wound closure was obtained and a relatively uncomplicated postburn course was experienced.

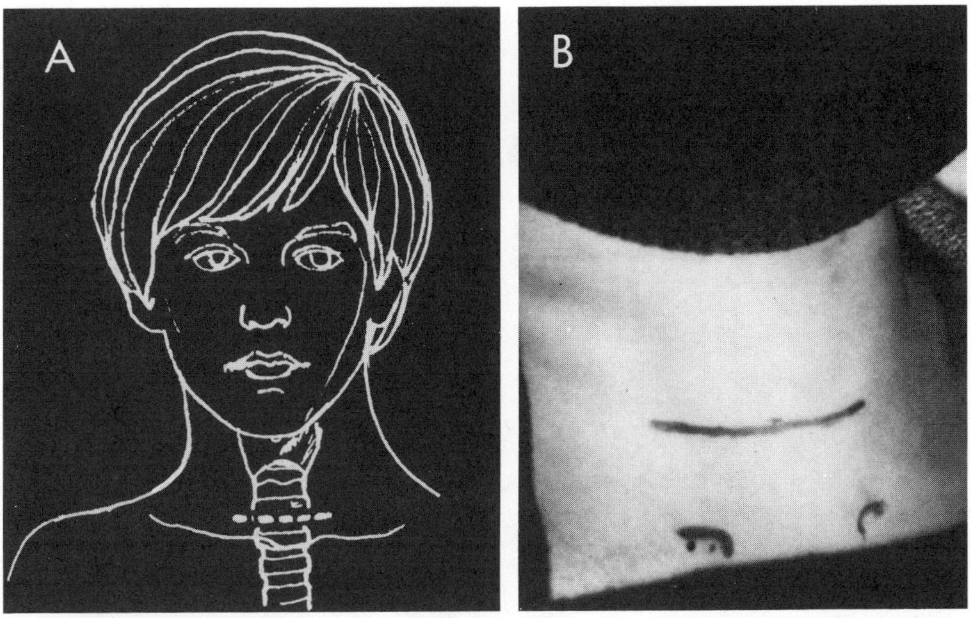

FIG 12–22.
A and **B,** incision marked for tracheostomy 1 cm above suprasternal notch in transverse orientation.

breadth above the suprasternal notch, is marked and the anatomic midline defined. The incision is carried through skin and subcutaneous tissues.

Using scissors, pretracheal tissues are gently separated and sequentially retracted from the midline until the thyroid isthmus or tracheal fascia is identified. The thyroid isthmus is generally retracted superiorly, the trachea visualized directly, and adherent fascia divided until the tracheal rings are clearly identified.

The tracheal midline is carefully marked and a 3–0 silk suture placed through the tracheal wall just above the second tracheal ring and passed caudad and retrieved outside the trachea just below the third tracheal ring on either side of the midline. These silk sutures are then retained with a hemostat and retracted laterally.

The trachea is vertically incised with a no. 11 scalpel blade to include the second and third tracheal rings immediately between the retracting silk sutures. This then secures the airway and if a nasal tracheal or endotracheal tube is present, it is removed at this time, and the correct size Shiley Silastic tracheostomy catheter with adapter is inserted. The tracheostomy incision is closed at its lateral extremes in a layered fashion and the catheter secured with supplied cervical straps. Proper placement is assured by direct vision and auscultation of the chest.

Subsequent tracheal site care requires daily cleansing of the skin with hydrogen peroxide or saline applied with cotton swabs. The securing straps should only be changed in the presence of personnel skilled in catheter replacement. It is not necessary to change the catheter frequently; however, if a catheter change is indicated, then it is preferable to wait 3 to 5 days after tracheostomy to avoid soft tissue collapse and loss of the tract during the changing interval.

TRACHEOSTOMY IN THE PRESENCE OF CERVICAL BURNS

The presence of thermal cutaneous burns at the tracheostomy incision site increases risks

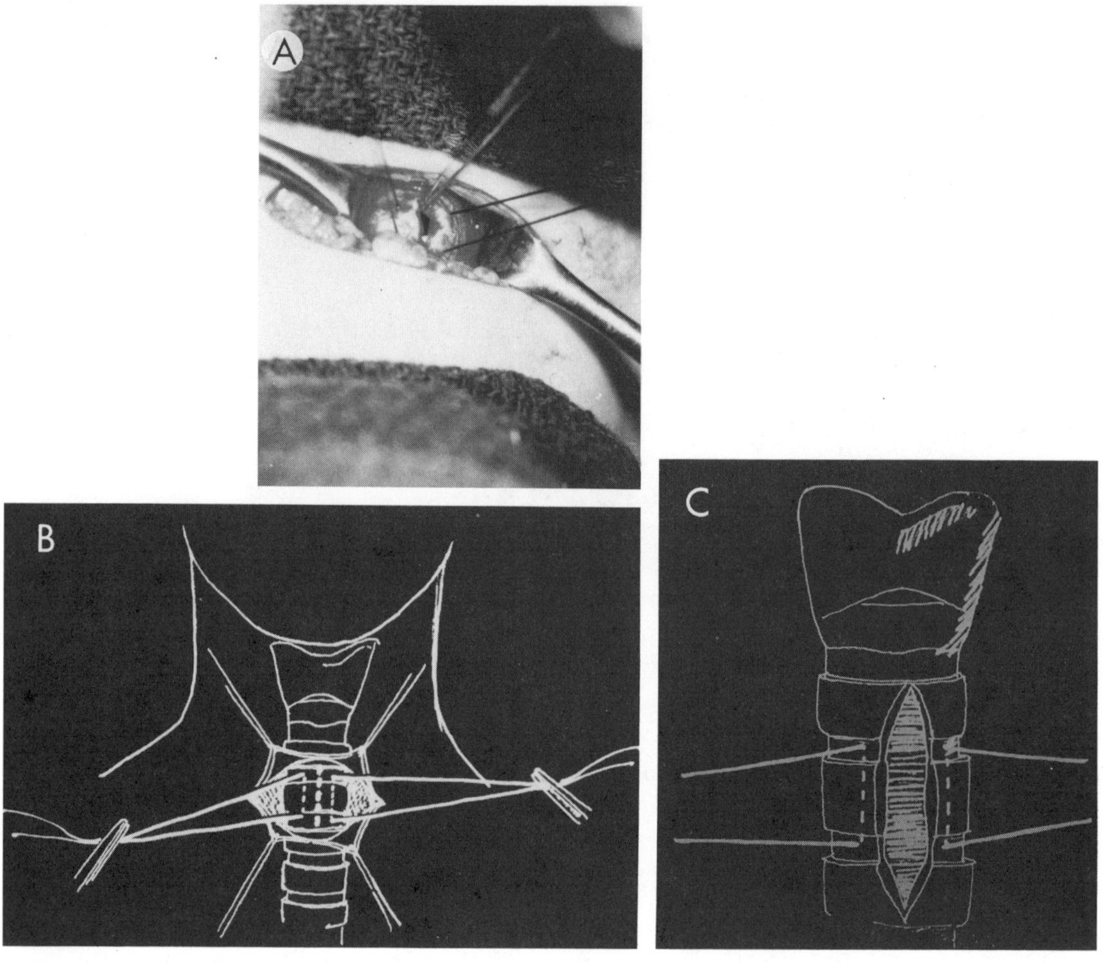

FIG 12–23.
A–C, trachea isolated with two silk sutures vertically on either side of the midline. Vertical incision at approximately the level of rings 1 and 2. Sutures retained for 7 to 10 days.

of contamination of the respiratory tract, especially the trachea and lungs. Consequently, a tangential excision or excision with immediate skin grafting should be carried out at the time of insertion of the tracheostomy tube. Although an extensive excision is not necessary, certainly local debridement and grafting can provide for decreased morbidity in the event of long-term cannulation by providing an adjacent clean, healed wound.

Suppurative Thrombophlebitis

The complication of suppurative thrombophlebitis has been reported in 4% of burned patients and generally results from (1) poor technique with cannula insertion, (2) inadequate local catheter care, and (3) prolonged catheterization at the same site.[19] Factors commonly encountered include insertion of the catheter in the emergency situation through burn tissue and without proper procedure being followed or in septic patients with few peripheral venous access sites and, thus, prolonged single-site catheterization.

Careful aseptic technique in the insertion of vascular-access catheters, close monitoring of the access sites, frequent catheter changes, and carefully monitored insertion-site hygiene can prevent the vast majority of such occurrences.

The diagnosis of suppurative thrombophlebitis is based on signs and symptoms, which include the following:

1. Local pain and discomfort
2. Fever of unknown origin
3. Tenderness along the course of a vein and associated with other signs of inflammation
4. Persistent, positive blood culture
5. Palpation of the vein and expression of purulent material from the catheter insertion site

In most cases, the treatment of suppurative thrombophlebitis is surgical.

TECHNIQUE

The anatomical course of the affected vein must be reviewed. A lazy-S incision over the affected blood vessel is made; the vessel is identified and carefully freed; tributaries are ligated; and the extirpation is extended until a normal or thin-walled vascular structure is encountered (Figs 12–24 and 12–25). Ligating the vessels with absorbable sutures such as Vicryl and packing the wound open are preferred. The wound may then be allowed to granulate and heal by secondary intent, or a delayed primary closure may be indicated if control of the suppurative process is confirmed.

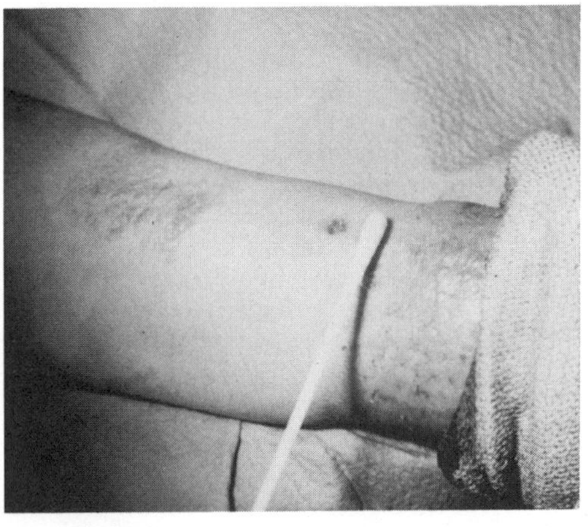

FIG 12–24.
Old IV site exuding pus. Culture is obtained.

Suppurative Perichondritis

Chondritis is a serious deforming infection primarily affecting the ear and nasal alae of the burned patient. Perichondritis is usually associated with adjacent soft tissue burns or pressure necrosis, bacterial contamination, and exposure of cartilage. The most common site is the ear; the association of cutaneous burn, inflammation with marked edema, and exquisite tenderness with purulent drainage confirms the diagnosis of chondritis in the ear.

Preventive measures include the application of topical antimicrobial agents, avoidance of pressure on the ear (such as by pillows or ill-devised dressings), and careful cleansing of the ear. Once chondritis is established, however, surgery is required for control of the painful aggressive disfiguring process.

TECHNIQUE

Debridement of established chondritis usually requires general anesthesia and often must be done on an emergency basis because of the aggressiveness of the process.

Necrotic debris should be thoroughly debrided and additional incisions, if indicated, made directly over affected areas. Involved cartilage that has not gone on to dissolution usually appears a dull yellowish color and should be completely excised. The excision should be carried until normal, thin, slightly bluish, normal cartilage is encountered.

Ideally, all exposed cartilagenous margins should be protected by advancing adjacent soft tissue if possible, and occasionally nonabsorbable sutures such as polypropylene (Prolene) are used to assure soft-tissue coverage of potentially exposed cartilage following debridement. A molded soft dressing is subsequently applied over a liberal application of topical ointment, such as gentamicin. Strict follow-up by daily wound inspection and palpation of the ear is necessary, since recurrence is quite common.

In our experience, excision of the involved cartilage is the treatment of choice. Other

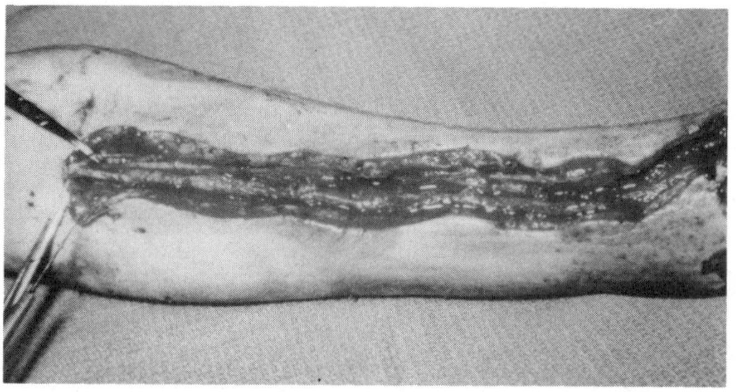

FIG 12–25.
Excision of forearm vein. Wound will be packed open and closed secondarily.

methods of conservative or nonsurgical treatment have generally not been successful.

REFERENCES

1. Burke JF, May JW Jr, Albright N, et al: Temporary skin transplantation and immunosuppression for extensive burns. *N Engl J Med* 1974, 290:269–271.
2. Burke JF, Yannas IV: Successful use of a physiologically acceptable artificial skin in the treatment of extensive burn injury. *Ann Surg* 1981; 194:413–428.
3. Chih-chun Y, Tsi-siang S, Wei-shia X: A Chinese concept of treatment of extensive third-degree burns. *Plast Resconstr Surg* 1982; 70:238–252.
4. Eckhauser FE, Billote J, Burke JF, et al: Tracheostomy complicating massive burn injury: A plea for conservatism. *Am J Surg* 1974; 127:418–423.
5. Gallico GG III, O'Conner NE, Compton CC, et al: Permanent coverage of large burn wounds with autologous cultured human epithelium. *N Engl J Med* 1984; 311:448–451.
6. Haynes BW Jr: Early excision and grafting in third-degree burns. *Ann Surg* 1969; 169:736–747.
7. Herndon DN, Parks DH: Comparison of serial debridment and autografting and early massive excision with cadaver skin overlay in the treatment of large burns in children. *J Trauma* 1986; 26:149–152.
8. Hunt JL, Sato R, Baxter CR: Early tangential excision and immediate mesh autografting of deep dermal hand burns. *Ann Surg* 1979; 189:147–151.
9. Jackson DM: Second thoughts on the burn wound. *J Trauma* 1969; 9:839–862.
10. Jackson DM, Stone PA: Tangential excision and grafting of burns: The method and a report of 50 consecutive cases. *Br J Plast Surg* 1972; 25:416–426.
11. Janzekovic Z: in Derganc M (ed): *Present Clinical Aspects of Burns: A Symposium.* Maribor, Yugoslavia 1968, pp 99–112, 215–230.
12. Larson DL, Abston S, Dobrkovsky M, et al: Use of skeletal suspension in grafting burned patients, in Lynch JB, Lewis SR (eds): *Symposium on the Treatment of Burns.* St. Louis, CV Mosby Co, 1979, pp 160–166.
13. Lewis FR, Schiobohm RM, Thomas AN: Prevention of complications from prolonged tracheal intubation. *Am J Surg* 1978; 135:452–457.
14. MacMillan BG, Artz CP: A planned evaluation of early excision of more than twenty-five percent of the body surface in burns. *Surg Forum* 1957; 7:88–93.
15. MacMillan BG: Primary excision, in *Practical Approaches to Burn Management.* Flint Laboratories, 1977
16. Parks DH, Carvajal HF, Larson DI: Management of burns. *Surg Clin North Am* 1977; 57:875–894.
17. Parks DH, Linares HA, Thomson PD: Surgical management of burn wound sepsis. *Surg Gynecol Obstet* 1981; 153:374–376.
18. Phillips KR: Tracheostomy in children. *Ear Nose Throat J* 1979; 58:401–407.
19. Pruitt BA Jr, Stein *JM*, Foley FD: Intravenous therapy in burn patients: Suppurative thrombophlebitis and other life-threatening complications. *Arch Surg* 1970; 100:399–404.
20. Teplitz C, Davis D, Mason AD, Jr, et al: Pseudomonas burn wound sepsis - I. Pathogenesis of experimental pseudomonas burn wound sepsis. *J Surg Res* 1964; 4:200–216.

13 / Skin Banking: Homograft and Amnion

PHILIP D. THOMSON, PH.D.
JAI K. PRASAD, M.D.
IRVING FELLER, M.D.

HOMOGRAFT

History

The ancient Chinese and Indian physicians were performing grafts and flaps for the repair of skin defects before the time of Christ.[1, 2] Homografts from living donors were reported as early as 1869 in France,[3] but the first recorded account of cadaveric homograft involved the treatment of a 10-year-old boy who had a lightning injury by using the skin of a suicide victim.[4] In that same year, 1881, Schede[5] reported homografts taken from amputations and fresh cadavers within 12 hours of death. The use of homografts to repair skin injuries has led to the development of technologies to preserve this living organ for use long after donor death. Carrel[6] is credited with the first attempts at preservation by refrigeration in 1912. His technique involved the use of petroleum jelly gauze to prevent drying of the skin at 4°C. By 1944, Strumia and Hodge[7] were initiating experimentation with preservation by freezing. After 1944, lyophilization became accepted as a method of storing skin.[8] As early as 1952, Dogo[9] reported that skin could be stored at 3°C for up to 22 days if acquired before 16 hours after death of the donor. In 1952, Allgower and Blocker[10] reported on viability of skin stored in a buffered saline, antibiotic, and plasma medium. During their experimentations on the immunobiology of grafting, Billingham and Medawar[11] reported the freezing and drying of mammalian skin. By 1966, the science of cryobiology for organ preservation was solidly established. Growing homograft cells in vitro to provide sheets of viable graft was being technically developed in the 1970s, and this, with the reported loss of human leukocyte antigen (HLA),[12] may prove to be an important step in developing new techniques for wound repair.

Procurement

One of the more difficult aspects of skin banking may be the education of the public to the need of homograft skin for burn treatment. Skin donation does not enjoy the publicity given to the solid organs and may be forgotten by those asking permission to harvest organs, if permission is not requested by burn unit or skin bank personnel. At times of grief, the mental picture arising from the request to donate skin may be overwhelming to family members left with the burden of donation. Living wills, drivers licenses, and other such documents will aid in notifying the family about the intentions of the deceased.

Before consent is obtained, care should be taken to assure that the potential donor meets the guidelines established for organ donation. The American Association of Tissue Banks guidelines[13] are provided in Table 13–1 as a reference. Care should be taken when obtaining permission for skin graft donation. Often

TABLE 13–1.
American Association of Tissue Banks Donor Selection Criteria*

1. The initial screening of a potential donor should include:
   A. History and physical
   B. White blood cell count and differential
   C. Screen for *Treponema pallidum*, Australian antigen, and AIDS
   D. Liver function tests
   E. Microbiology and cause of death
2. Potential donors below the age of 14 or over the age of 73 should be evaluated on an individual basis.
3. Donors should have no disease that, in the best current medical judgment, could be transmitted to and harm the recipient of the transplanted skin. These include: infectious disease, malignant disease, neurological degenerative disease, and disease of unknown etiology.

*From the American Association of Tissue Banks, Arlington, Va, 1987. Used by permission.

the family will be concerned about disfigurement, and all questions should be answered carefully. Consent forms should always specifically state skin harvest. Not all individuals understand that the skin is an organ; therefore, consent that asks for *any organ* may be misleading and result in unfortunate misunderstandings. Legal counseling should be obtained when initiating a skin bank, as laws vary from state to state concerning consent. In some states telephone consent may be used, which is most convenient for expediting skin harvest.

In our hospital, the admitting office is aware of donor criteria and notifies the skin bank or burn service of all deaths that may result in potential donations. The use of a paging service gives procurement personnel the greatest freedom. When a potential donor is identified, a call to the patient unit (intensive care unit, emergency room, etc.) will quickly determine if consent has been obtained or if the topic of organ donation has been discussed with the family. In most cases, the attending physician is consulted and may be the person who wants to approach the family with the request for organ donation. The attending physician often has a better understanding of the family and their feelings toward organ donation. It has been our experience that successful organ procurement is best done by one person asking for needed organs at one time.

Once consent is obtained, it is important that the body be refrigerated as quickly as possible. The ability to achieve this goal will depend on the family, their religious background, and the work load, i.e., the personnel ratio of the unit where the donor expired.

When the donor has been removed to the morgue, skin should be harvested within 18 hours of death.[14] It is our policy to harvest all homografts within 12 hours of death as our banking program demands highly viable skin cells.

All skin removal is done in the morgue under aseptic conditions. This reduces costs, does not waste operating room resources, and is more convenient for skin-bank personnel.

For skin harvesting, the donor is placed supine, the body is prepared by washing with iodophor-impregnated textured surgical sponges, and hair is removed by shaving. Once thoroughly washed, the body is sponged with 10% povidone-iodine. This iodine preparation is removed by a detergent solution containing 25% sodium alkyl sulfate (Duponol), which is prepared by our pharmacy. The body is then sponged with 70% isopropyl alcohol, which is allowed to stand for 3 minutes. The alcohol is removed by flooding the body with sterile water. The donor areas are draped with sterile linen and iodine and alcohol applied again. After the areas to be harvested are rinsed, they are wiped with sterile, light mineral oil to facilitate dermatome movement.

Skin is harvested using a motor-driven Brown dermatome. An air-driven motor is acceptable, but allows less portability. The motor drive for our dermatome is housed in a stainless steel cart, which holds all of the equipment and supplies necessary for skin removal. This portable system is ideal for use within our hospital and is adapted to fit into two steel suitcases for use outside our hospital. Dermatome settings of 5 cm width and 0.381 mm (15/1,000 in.) depth are ideal for our purposes. Skin is harvested by body areas beginning with the legs, then proceeding to the arms and trunk. When completed anteriorally, the body is turned prone, prepared, and the remainder of the skin harvested. Skin is never harvested from face, neck, hands, or feet. Table 13–2 shows the number of skin donors and number of square feet per donor obtained by our skin bank over the past 5 years. A recent survey of skin banks in the United States shows the national average to be 5.67 sq ft per donor.

Immediately after harvest, the skin is placed in sterile bottles containing skin-bank fluid, which is prepared in our pharmacy laboratory. This fluid is 80% balanced salt solution and 20% human plasma with 0.005 gm of gentamicin sulfate per 100/ml. The balanced salt solution is similar to Hanks' solution, except that only half of the calcium chloride is added, which makes the solution compatible with preserved plasma. Another skin-bank fluid that may be substituted is described by Netzer.[15]

Monitoring

The ideal homograft product should be both viable and free from microbial contamination. Viability testing has included the uptake of radio-labeled metabolites,[14, 16] enzymatic digestion,[17] oxygen consumption,[9] dye exclusion,[18] and grafting of human homograft onto athymic mice.[19] A review of 100 years of skin viability testing has been published by Jensen,[20] for those who wish to delve more deeply into the subject. The ultimate test is the result obtained; however, May[21] warns that graft "take" may be an unreliable measure of skin viability. Although claims that viability decreases at the rate of 10% to 20% per day,[14] our skin bank has successfully maintained skin at 4° C for up to 30 days. This skin, if harvested before 12 hours after death and properly handled, will maintain sufficient vascular integrity and cell viability to become pink and stabilized on suitable recipient beds within 72 hours of transplantation.

The need for homograft to be free of pathogenic microorganisms when used for the treatment of burns is obvious. May[22] produced a list of microorganisms that he found contaminating 100 skin donors when the skin was tested by specific body areas. In his study, staphylococcal species were the predominant organisms (60%), followed in order by *Aspergillus* (8.6%) and *Propionibacterium* (4.9%). The staphylococci were randomly distributed over the body, whereas *Aspergillus* was restricted to the buttocks, thighs, and chest. *Propionibacterium* was found only on the back. Our skin bank does not culture by body surface area but does culture a representative section of each square foot of skin harvested. Each sample of skin is placed in thioglycolate broth and incubated at 37° C for 48 hours. Results from the last 60 donors tested for microbial growth are shown in Table 13–3. The incidence of staphylococcal species in homograft correlates with that shown by May,[22] but no explanation is available for the difference seen in the incidence of *Propionibacterium*. Six of the donors (10%) failed to show any microbial growth in the original cultures. After 48 hours in the skin-bank solution, skin harvested from only three donors was deemed unfit for patient use because of microbial overgrowth. Heck and

TABLE 13–2.
University of Michigan Skin Bank Activity, 1982–1986

	1982	1983	1984	1985	1986
No. of donors	18	17	32	28	21
Skin per donor, sq ft	6.1	7.2	7.7	7.1	8.9
Patients receiving homograft	67	51	62	65	61
Homograft used, sq ft	128.0	143.8	189.3	190.0	186.0

TABLE 13–3.
Microbial Contamination of Cadaveric Homograft From 60 Donors at the University of Michigan Skin Bank

MICROORGANISMS	NO. OF DONORS CONTAMINATED	% CONTAMINATION
Staphylococcus sp.	32	53.3
Propionibacterium sp.	27	45.0
Diphtheroids	7	11.6
Candida sp.	4	6.6
Streptococcus sp.	4	6.6
Peptococcus/ Peptostreptococcus sp.	4	6.6
Clostridium sp.	1	1.6
Pseudomonas sp.	1	1.6
Escherichia coli	1	1.6
Bacillus sp.	1	1.6

colleagues[23] have reported a series of 362 donors in which 51 (14%) grew pathogenic organisms including *Escherichia coli* (22), *Clostridium* (6), Klebsiella (4), yeast (3), and *Proteus* (3).

Banking

As previously stated, it has been our policy to keep fresh homograft in our skin-bank fluid for periods of time up to 30 days. Usually, the supply is depleted before the end of that time. If, however, the supply is not depleted, skin is banked by step-down freezing. This process has been previously well documented[11, 24, 25] and requires additional expenditures. The skin is placed in fresh skin-bank fluid to which a cryopreservative (15% v/v glycerol) is added and then is refrigerated overnight at 4° C. The skin is placed between two pieces of sterile nylon netting and placed in a 5.5 × 9-in., heat-sealable pouch. These pouches are frozen in vapor-phase liquid nitrogen at 1° C/minute to −90° C in a flat format using a Cryo-Med 100 freezing system. It has been determined that flat-format cryopreservation is superior to rolled-format freezing for storage over long periods.[24] In side-by-side comparison trials, we have shown that cryopreserved skin, frozen for up to 6 months, is equal in quality and graft take to our fresh homograft (unpublished observations). We have been satisfied with the clinical results of homograft stored in this manner for periods exceeding 12 months.

Although glycerol is the accepted standard as a cryopreservative,[11] the use of other agents such as dimethyl sulfoxide has been reported.[2] When bringing skin from the temperature of liquid nitrogen (−196° C), many techniques have been explored including the use of microwaves.[26] The American Association of Tissue Banks recommends thawing skin at 37° to 42° C,[14] and an extensive study has revealed that 42° C water is superior for flat-format, controlled-rate frozen skin.[24]

Homograft Use

Homograft skin is maintained on the wound for prolonged periods of time due to the immunosuppression of the burned patient.[27] Burke has reported prolonged take of homograft in 11 children with 70% or greater body surface area burns after treatment with antithymocyte globulin.[28] Reports of homograft persisting on the wound for as long as 2 months without intentional immunosuppression of the patient have been made.[29, 30]

Homograft may be used alone on the wound or used with autograft in the alternate-strip method made popular by Jackson.[31]

Variations of this method such as the intermingled grafting reported by Yang, et al.[32] and mesh autografting with mesh homograft overlay reported by Alexander et al.[33] have been used.

We individualize the patients by size of burn, depth of burn, age of the patient, and past medical history. In larger burns, excision of the wound is initiated early with homograft as the choice for wound coverage. As homografts begin to be accepted by the patient, autografting is initiated, and the two techniques are alternated or used in conjunction until the wound is covered. Autografts then replace homografts, and in the final stages of acute care, only autografting is done (Fig 13–1).

In 1979, 19 skin banks reported 868 donors in the United States.[34] Five years later, only 1,046 donors were reported from 26 skin banks in a similar survey.[35]

Although it is difficult to separate pediatric use of cadaveric homograft from use by all other age groups, some data are available. The National Burn Information Exchange (NBIE)[36] provided the homograft data shown in Table 13–4. Only 8 of the 60 hospitals in the NBIE data base reported homograft use in pediatric patients with no full-thickness injury, whereas 28 hospitals reported using homograft in pediatric burns with some full-thickness component. It should be noted that only three of the reporting hospitals in this study group had a registered skin bank. This fact may account for the greater use of xenograft for wound coverage. Although included in the NBIE data shown, data from a 2-year period (1983–1984) at our burn center show that only one pediatric patient who had no full-thickness burn was treated with homograft. In that same 2-year period, 11 children who had some full-thickness burn were treated with homograft.

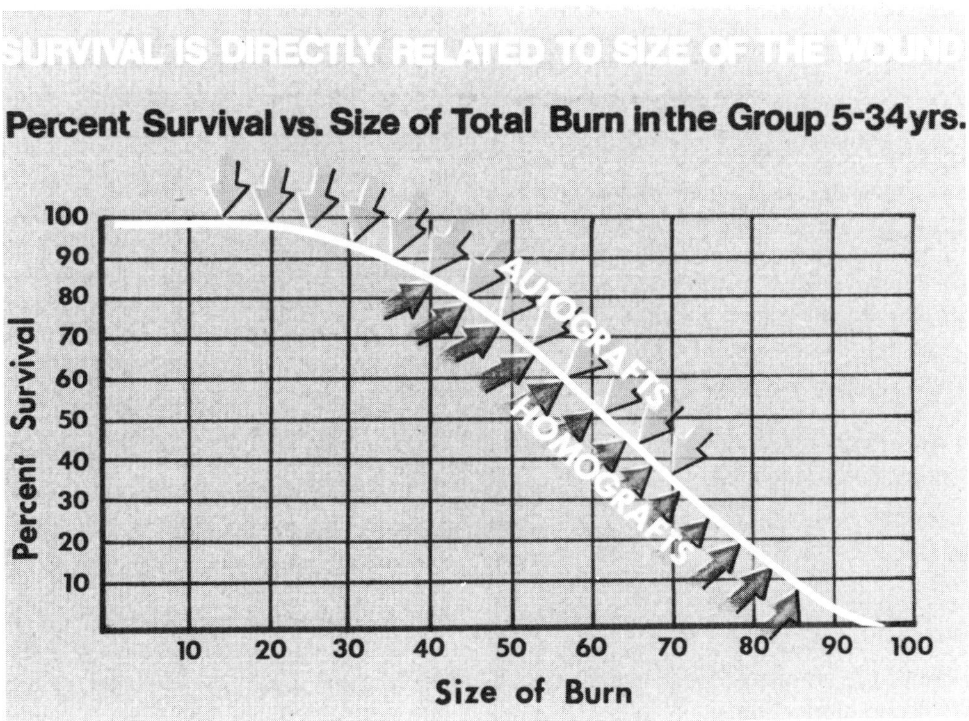

FIG 13–1.
Homograft and autograft use. Size of burn is percent of body surface area. (From Feller I, Jones CA: *Teaching Basic Burn Care.* National Institute for Burn Medicine, 1975. Used by permission.)

TABLE 13–4.

National Burn Information Exchange (NBIE) Data From 60 Reporting Hospitals, 1979–1984: Homograft vs. Xenograft Use in Burn Patients Less Than 16 Years of Age

	NO. OF PATIENTS	NO. OF PATIENTS WITH AUTOGRAFTS	NO. OF PATIENTS WITH HOMOGRAFT	NO. OF PATIENTS WITH XENOGRAFT
Patients with no full-thickness burns	5,287	181	10	115
Patients with some full-thickness burns	3,693	3,107	165	258

Use of other burn-wound coverings such as amnion or synthetic materials may account for the low-use rate of homograft in partial-thickness burns in some centers.[37, 38] It has been projected that homograft demand exceeds the supply by as much as 1,950 sq ft.[35] This supply/demand difference may account for the fact that homograft is not used in all full-thickness injuries of significant size.

AMNION

History

In 1910, William Thornton, a medical student under Dr. J. S. Davis at Johns Hopkins, is credited with the idea of using amnion for the treatment of skin defects.[39] The historical background for the use of this epithelial membrane for the treatment of burns begins with the work of Sabella[40] in 1912 and has been chronicled in other recent works.[37, 41, 42]

Procurement and Banking

Amnion is readily obtainable and depends on numbers of deliveries in the obstetric department for its availability. Once obtained, it may be processed for use in many different ways. The most common and popular ways reported in this country are the use of 0.025% sodium hypochlorite solution[41] and the use of povidone-iodine in saline (1:4) reported by Walker.[42]

Use

A review of data from the NBIE and their 60 reporting hospitals from 24 states gives some insight to the use of amnion for the treatment of pediatric burns. Table 13–5 shows that 43 pediatric patients under 16 years of age who had no full-thickness injury were treated with amnion in five of the reporting hospitals. In the group of 5,287 injuries with no full-thickness component reported from all hospitals, 16 were treated with synthetic grafts and 13 with some other skin covering. In this patient population, xenograft remains the most-used burn wound covering (see Table 13–4). In 3,693 pediatric patients with some full-thickness wound, 44 were treated with amnion, 40 with synthetic graft, and 21 with some other skin covering (see Table 13–5). Again, xenograft was the most-used covering with 258 patients reported in that group (see Table 13–4).

Walker[43] reported preparing 15,000 pieces of amnion for patient use at one hospital; these preparations accounted for use of amnion by at least 50 physicians. In a group of pediatric patients described in 1977, he reported a comparison of amnion-treated (n = 37) to nitrofurazone-treated (n = 73) patients, with both partial- and full-thickness wounds. No difference was noted in wound healing, but the amnion-treated group was more comfortable, more mobile, and required

TABLE 13–5.
National Burn Information Exchange (NBIE) Data From 60 Reporting Hospitals, 1979–1984: Amnion vs. Synthetic and Other Skin-Covering Use in Burn Patients Less Than 16 Years of Age

	NO. OF PATIENTS	NO. OF PATIENTS WITH AMNION	NO. OF PATIENTS WITH SYNTHETIC GRAFT	NO. OF PATIENTS WITH OTHER COVERING
Patients with no full-thickness burns	5,287	43	16	13
Patients with some full-thickness burns	3,693	44	40	21

fewer dressing changes.[43] Also, length of hospital stay was shorter for the amnion-treated group.

Piserchia and Akenzua[44] reported ten children ranging in age from 7 months to 11 years who had average partial-thickness burns of 24% of body surface area and who were treated with amnion. Only one of them developed a wound infection *(Pseudomonas)*, and when compared to nonbiological antimicrobial dressing (Sofratulle) controls, the amnion-treated group had shorter hospitalization (31 days, compared to 56 days).

Rahamut[45] has shown good results in children treated as outpatients; healing of superficial burns under amnion occurred in 7 to 10 days. In a 6-month trial against silver sulfadiazine, it was concluded that amnion was the cheaper dressing.

Our findings in a group of 18 pediatric patients ranging in age from 17 months to 14 years (mean, 11 years), having partial-thickness wounds of 4% to 49% body surface area (mean, 16.5%), and treated with amnion were similar to those of Rohamut.[45] When compared to wound healing in controls matched for age and burn size and treated with silver sulfadiazine, wound healing was faster in the amnion group (4 to 7 days; mean, 6.5 days) compared to 1 to 25 days; mean, 8.5 days. Although subjective, relief from pain was more often expressed by those patients dressed with amnion. Once amnion was adherent to the wound, daily care consisted of washing the surface of the amnion; no other dressings were required. Two patients in the antimicrobial cream group had wounds significantly populated with bacteria, whereas the amnion group had no wound infections.

SUMMARY

Homograft banking provides a temporary physiologic skin cover for severely burned patients with significant full-thickness injury until they can undergo autografting. A skin bank maintained by the burn center is a practical, financially feasible method of maintaining a supply of skin homografts. Likewise, amnion provides an ideal dressing for partial-thickness burns and can be procured, stored, and dispensed from the same skin bank.

REFERENCES

1. Rogers BO: Guide and bibliography for research into the skin homograft problem. *Plast Reconstr Surg* 1951; 7:169.
2. Traaholt L, Eskeland G: Skin banking in the treatment of burns: A practical approach to the processing and storing of allografts. *Ann Chir Gynaecol* 1980; 69:213.
3. Reverdin JL: Greffe epidermique. *Bull Soc Chir (Paris)* 1869; 493:511.
4. Girdner JH: Skin grafting with grafts taken from the dead subject. *Med Rec* 1881, 20:119.
5. Schede: VII Vereins Chronik: Arztlicher verein zu Hamburg. Sitzung von 25 Januar 1881. *Dtsch Med Wochenschr* 1881, 7:352.

6. Carrel A: The preservation of tissue and its applications in surgery. *JAMA* 1912; 59:523.
7. Strumia MM, Hodge CC: Frozen skin grafts. *Ann Surg* 1944; 120:431.
8. Hyatt GW, Turner TC, Bassett CAL: New methods of preserving skin, bone, and blood vessels. *Naval Med Newsletter* 1951; 18.
9. Dogo G: Survival and utilization of cadaver skin. *Plast Reconstr Surg* 1952; 10:10.
10. Allgower M, Blocker TG: Viability of skin in relation to various methods of storage. *Texas Rep Biol Med* 1952; 10:1–21.
11. Billingham RE, Medawar PB: The freezing, drying, and storage of mammalian skin. *J Exp Biol* 1952; 29:454.
12. Hefton JM, Madden MR, Finkelstein JL, et al: Grafting of burn patients with allografts of cultured epidermal cells. *Lancet* 1983; 2:428.
13. Standards Committee of the Skin Council of the American Association of Tissue Banks. Guidelines for the banking of skin tissues: *Am Assoc Tissue Banks Newsletter* 1979; 3:5.
14. May SR, DeClement FA: Skin Banking: III. Cadaveric allograft skin viability. *J Burn Care Rehabil* 1981; 2:128.
15. Netzer OM: Skin Bank Fluid. *Am J Hosp Pharm* 1960; 17:28.
16. Praus R, Bohm F, Dvorak R: Skin cryopreservation: I. Incorporation of radioactive sulfate as a criterion of pigskin graft viability after freezing to −196° C in the presence of cryoprotectants. *Cryobiology* 1980; 17:125.
17. Chamness JT, Kayes J, Hershey FB, et al: Enzymatic activity of banked skin. *Surg Forum* 1955; 6:573.
18. Prows J, Nathan P: Evaluation of storage conditions for refrigerated rabbit skin. *Cryobiology* 1980; 17:125.
19. Cram AE, Domayer M, Shelby J: Human skin storage techniques: A study utilizing a nude mouse recipient. *J Trauma* 1983; 23:924.
20. Jensen HS: 1984. Skin viability studies in vitro. *Scand J Plast Reconstr Surg* 1984; 18:55.
21. May SR: Cryopreservation and clinical use of human allograft skin, in Asos, Sumida S (eds): *Low Temperature Medicine*. Tokyo, Asakura Publishing Co, Ltd, 1982.
22. May SR, DeClement FA: Skin banking: II. Low contamination cadaveric dermal allograft for temporary burn-wound coverage. *J Burn Care Rehabil* 1981; 2:64.
23. Heck E, Blood S, Baxter C: The importance of the bacterial flora in cadaveric homograft donor skin: Bacterial flora in cadaver homograft. *J Burn Care Rehabil* 1981; 2:212.
24. May SR, DeClement FA: Skin banking methodology: An evaluation of package format, cooling and warming rates, and storage efficiency. *Cryobiology* 1980; 17:33.
25. Cochrane T: The low-temperature storage of skin: A preliminary report. *Br J Plast Surg* 1968; 21:118.
26. Ninnemann JL, Fisher JC, Frank HA: Clinical skin banking: A simplified system of processing, storage, and retrieval of human allograft. *J Trauma* 1978; 18:723.
27. Fisher JC: Endogenous immunosuppression: An opportunity to facilitate burn-wound closure, in Ninnemann, JL (ed): *The Immune Consequences of Thermal Injury*. Baltimore, Williams & Wilkins Co, 1981, pp 252.
28. Burke JF, Quinby WC, Bondoc CC, et al: Immunosuppression and temporary skin transplantation in the treatment of massive third-degree burns. *Ann Surg* 1975; 192:183.
29. Hackett ME: Cadaver homografts. *Proc R Soc Med* 1971; 64:18.
30. Ninnemann JL, Fisher JC, Frank HA: Prolonged survival of human skin allografts following thermal injury. *Transplantation* 1978; 25:69.
31. Jackson D: A clinical study of the use of skin homografts for burns. *Br J Plast Surg* 1954; 7:26.
32. Yang CC, Shih TS, Chu TA, et al: The intermingled transplantation of auto- and homografts in severe burns. *Burns* 1980; 6:141.
33. Alexander JW, MacMillan BG, Law E, et al: Treatment of severe burns with widely meshed skin autograft and meshed skin allograft overlay. *J Trauma* 1981; 21:433.
34. May SR, DeClement FA: Skin banking: I. Procurement of transplantable cadaveric allograft skin for burn wound coverage. *J Burn Care Rehabil* 1981; 2:7.
35. Heinbokel HE, Simon MR, Jordan MH: Cadaver allograft skin—supply and demand. *Proc Am Burn Assoc* 1985; 17:87.
36. Unpublished data. Ann Arbor, Mich, National Burn Information Exchange, 1984.
37. Thomson PD, Parks DH: Amnion as a burn wound dressing, in Wise D (ed): *Burn Wound Coverings: I*. Boca Raton, Fla, CRC Press, 1984, p 47.
38. Woodroof EA: Biobrane, a biosynthetic skin prosthesis, in Wise D (ed): *Burn Wound Coverings: II*. Boca Raton, Fla, CRC Press, 1984, p 1.
39. Matthews RN, Faulk WP, Bennett JP: A review of the role of amniotic membranes in surgical practice. *Obstet Gynecol Annu* 1982; 11:31.
40. Sabella N: Use of fetal membranes in skin grafting. *Med Rec NY* 1913; 83:478.

41. Thomson PD, Parks DH: Monitoring, banking, and clinical use of amnion as a burn wound dressing. *Ann Plast Surg* 1981; 7:354.
42. Walker AB: Use of amniotic membranes for burn-wound coverage, in Wise D (ed): *Burn Wound Coverings: I.* Boca Raton, Fla, CRC Press, 1984, p 55.
43. Walker AB, Cooney DR, Allen JE: Use of fresh amnion as a burn dressing. *J Pediatr Surg* 1977; 12:391.
44. Piserchia NE, Akenzua GI: Amniotic membrane dressing for burns in children: A cheap method for treatment for developing countries. *Trop Geogr Med* 1981; 33:235.
45. Rahamut N: The place of amniotic membrane in the treatment of burns in children. *Aust Nurses J* 1982; 11:21.

14 / Burn Wound Coverings and Biologic Dressings

JOHN P. REMENSNYDER, M.D.

Over the past several years there has been a profusion of new materials designed to aid in burn wound closure. Some are designed to provide temporary closure, others permanent. Some are entirely synthetic, others are derived from biological sources, and others are combinations of synthetic and biologic materials. For the purposes of this discussion, the term *burn wound covering* will be used to denote materials, both synthetic and biologic, that are intended to aid in or gain wound closure, either by covering the initial burn wound or the tissue left by subsequent burn wound excision.

Burn wound coverings can be divided into two broad categories: (1) synthetic fabrications and (2) biologically derived materials (Table 14–1). A synthetically manufactured film was first used as a burn wound covering by Pickerell in 1942.[1] He intended for the film to provide a barrier to bacteria and protect the wound until it had healed itself. In general, most of the early attempts to fabricate coverings were intended to facilitate normal healing processes rather than to replace skin or any of its various functions. More recently, unilaminate films have been developed and designed to closely regulate water and gas transfer to achieve an optimal microenvironment for normal wound healing. Increasingly, bilaminated materials are being used in an attempt to simulate skin. The two layers are analogous to the epidermis and dermis of normal skin.[2, 3] Purely synthetic bilaminates made with woven velour wound-contacting layers coupled with moisture-retaining films provide wound closure for remarkably long periods of time following full-thickness burn excision.[4, 5] Bilamination is also employed in the fabrication of an open collagen/proteoglycan matrix bonded to a synthetic film used to guide the formation of a permanent neodermis in full-thickness defects.[6] To date, bilamination appears to be a critical feature of the more successful burn wound covering fabrications.

The four biologic tissues listed in Table 14–1 are in a category by themselves in their usefulness in covering burn wounds and replacing skin. As organized tissues, they possess certain properties, such as bacterial suppression, that do not exist in any of the fabricated biological synthetics. The bases for these properties are not well understood, but the properties clearly inhere only in organized tissues. Epidermal cell sheets grown in the laboratory are now valuable clinically in gaining permanent closure in excised burn wounds.[7] The desirable combination of a loose collagen matrix coupled with viable epidermal cells is currently under investigation in several laboratories, but has yet to be used clinically.

CHARACTERISTICS

Virtually all of the desirable functions of the various burn wound coverings can be traced to one or more of the following four characteristics or properties:

1. Vapor and gas permeability
2. Adherence

TABLE 14–1.
Categories of Burn Wound Coverings.*

SYNTHETICS
Homogenous and unilaminar
Preformed films
Spray-on films
Forms
Sponges
Gels
Compound and bilaminar
Foam/film
Polyurethane/film
Velour/film
BIOLOGICALS
Fabricated
Fibrin films
Collagen
Sheets
Sponges
Collagen/caprolactone laminate
Cultured epidermal cells
Collagen/epidermal cells
Tissues
Autograft
Allograft
Xenograft
Amnion

*Adapted from Davies JWL: Synthetic materials for covering burn wounds: Progress towards perfection: I. and II. *Burns* 1984; 10:94–108.

3. Bacterial inhibition
4. Vascularization and "take"

To further categorize the myriads of burn wound coverings, it is necessary to analyze the above *characteristics,* which confer their usefulness. With such characteristics firmly in mind, it will then be possible to provide a *functional classification* of the various coverings by enumerating those necessary functions each brings to the complex mechanism of burn wound healing.

Vapor and Gas Permeability

Water and oxygen transport are the critical factors in the usefulness of burn wound coverings, with carbon dioxide transport occupying a minor role. Normal skin "respires" or transports materials, though in humans and mammals such transport is greatly reduced compared to transport in amphibians (e.g., the frog), in which respiratory exchange largely occurs directly through the skin. Measurement of vapor transport through various burn wound coverings can be calculated from measurements of a vapor-pressure gradient of the air layer immediately above the test surface.[8] This method is more sensitive than traditional weight-loss types of measurements, but in either case, the results are expressed as weight of evaporative water loss per unit time per unit area. Problems in comparing vapor permeability of various materials stem from use of different methods of measurement and expression of the results in differing units. Oxygen transfer measurement methods tend to be more uniform if an oxygen sensor in a controlled environment is used on one side of the membrane and a known oxygen concentration exists on the other. Rigid control of humidity and temperature is essential in measuring both water and oxygen transfers across membranes.

Water and oxygen transfer across burn wound coverings depend on the functional goal of the particular covering in question. Many synthetic films have been designed to permit a so-called "optimal wound environment" over a partial-thickness burn or an excised wound to facilitate wound healing. The concept of optimal environment derives from experiments carried out by Winter in 1962.[9] He showed that in young pigs experimental partial-thickness skin wounds kept moist by polyethylene film coverings epithelialized twice as fast as those wounds left exposed to air. Hinman and Maibach[10] confirmed this observation in a series of human volunteer experiments. Both groups believed that the presence of a crust or scab in the exposed wounds inhibited epithelialization and that a moist environment prevented scab formation and hence favored epithelialization. These observations hold true as long as there are few or no bacteria in the experimental wounds.

In providing for an optimal wound environment, one seeks a membrane that permits enough water transfer out to prevent exudate buildup, but not so much as to dry out the wound. Good oxygen transfer maintains an oxygen-rich environment over the healing wound. Table 14–2 shows some representative figures for various unilaminate synthetic films: the first two films show moderate water-vapor transport and high oxygen transport, the next two show lower vapor transfer and lower oxygen transport. One might expect in the latter two that reduced oxygen tension and exudate buildup would be problems in their use. Polyurethane alone is very permeable to water but has the disadvantage of being unduly stiff in the pure state.

By contrast, when seeking a material to substitute for skin either temporarily or permanently, one looks for a more limited rate of water vapor transfer comparable to that of normal skin. Table 14–3 shows the water vapor transfer of one film, two bilaminates, two tissues, and an open wound. The entirely synthetic bilaminates show a relatively high rate of water transfer compared to normal skin, while the partially biologically derived bilaminate (collagen lattice/silicone) shows a low water transfer comparable to normal skin. Water transfer may be varied by changing the pore size of the mesh or the film thickness of the bilaminated material. Xenograft, interestingly, has a value in the midrange.

In summary, appropriate water and oxygen transfer are desirable properties of synthetic and biologic coverings, but that appropriate rates differ depending on the particular function that one seeks in a particular burn wound covering.

TABLE 14–2.
Water Vapor and Oxygen Transport Across Unilaminate Synthetic Films

UNILAMINATE SYNTHETIC FILM	H_2O TRANSFER, GM/SQ M/24 HR	O_2 TRANSFER, ML/SQ M/24 HR
Polyurethane acrylate	637	14,100
Polyurethane polyvinyl ether	668	11,400
Polyurethane polyvinyl acrylate	449	5,419
Polyurethane vinyl acrylate	363	2,848
Polyurethane	1,090	—

TABLE 14–3.
Water Vapor Transfer Across Synthetics and Tissues

SYNTHETIC OR TISSUE	H_2O TRANSFER, MG/SQ CM/HR
Polyurethane acrylate	2.7
Nylon velour/silicone	4.1
Collagen lattice/silicone	1.0–10.0
Normal skin	1.2
Xenograft	2.4
Open wound	30.0

Adherence

Close adherence of a burn wound covering to the wound bed is perhaps the single most important characteristic of a successful covering. Adherence depends on physical, chemical, and, possibly, electrochemical factors. Tavis and colleagues[11, 12] have exhaustively investigated adherence of synthetics and tissue grafts to wound beds using tensiometric techniques. They found that such adherence occurs in two phases. *Phase 1*, the primary or chemical adherence, is fibrin dependent, and hence factors promoting coagulation will increase adherence in this phase. Phase 1 adherence occurs as early as 5 hours after application to the wound bed, can be inhibited by heparin, and destroyed by fibrinolysins. *Phase 2* begins about 72 hours after application to the wound bed and is due to fibroblastic ingrowth into tissue grafts and subsequent vascularization of the tissue. Synthetics presenting a weave or mesh to the wound surface become adherent during phase 2 by the physical ingrowth and intermeshing by fibrous tissue from the wound bed. In addition to the chemical and physical dimensions of adherence, Bartlett and his group,[13] who have investigated the zeta (ζ) potential of wound coverings, point out that a net positive change on the surface of the material favors thrombogenesis and hence adherences.

Adherence to the wound bed represents a critical characteristic of burn wound coverings for the following reasons: (1) With a tightly adherent covering, bacteria can be reliably excluded from the wound, and at the same time loss of vital protein-rich body fluids can be prevented; (2) if the covering is not tightly adherent, fluid may accumulate beneath the covering, thus physically separating the material from the bed; the wound eventually becomes contaminated, local sepsis occurs, and the wound condition worsens; and (3) close adherence is critical to resist any mechanical shearing forces that would tend to dislodge the covering and hence destroy its potential advantages.

Table 14–4 shows the relative adherences of two types of tissue grafts and a synthetic bilaminate. Both tissue grafts show similar levels of adherence at 5 and 72 hours. The bilaminate shows somewhat less adherence early, but shows an increased adherence at 72 hours—a phenomenon directly traceable to the method of fabrication of the undersurface of the bilaminate, which has a varigated open weave surface designed to encourage interlacing with fibrous ingrowth producing a high degree of phase 2 bonding.

In summary, with good adherence properties, the woven or open-lattice group of bilaminates can prevent bacterial contamination of the burn or excised wound, but this group does not possess intrinsic bactericidal properties as do some of the organized tissue grafts.

TABLE 14–4.
Adherence of Burn Wound Coverings to Excised Wound Bed

	5 HR, GM/SQ CM	72 HR, GM/SQ CM
Xenograft	65	250
Allograft	68	232
Nylon/velour/silicone	50	324

Bacterial Inhibition

Organized tissue grafts possess inherent bacterial inhibiting properties of obvious benefit to the burn or excised wound. Eade,[14] in direct and simple experiments in 1958, showed that within a few hours of placing a split-thickness autograft or allograft on a contaminated experimental wound, cultures from material taken from beneath the graft did not yield any bacteria. Morris et al.[15] in 1966 extended these observations to humans who had allografts in chronic open wounds. The phenomenon of bacterial inhibition in the presence of a tissue graft seems to be an innate property of the graft itself, since bacterial suppression occurs long before the graft becomes vascularized and incorporated into the wound. The mechanism of this suppressive ability still remains unknown despite continuing investigation. It is clearly a property of *organized tissue,* such as autograft, allograft, or xenograft, but not of uniform layers of biologically derived material such as collagen sheets or sponges. It was from Eade's[14] original observations that we have developed the now familiar technique of repeated application and changing of allografts in contaminated wounds to reduce bacterial levels to a point low enough to permit effective autografting. Autografts are more effective in bacterial suppression than allografts, which in turn are more effective than xenografts.

Bacterial suppression by organized tissue grafts must not be confused with prevention of contamination by well-adherent coverings, either biologically derived or synthetic. Synthetics permeable to water can be used in conjunction with aqueous solutions of topical antibiotics, e.g., 5% mafenide (sulfamylon), to treat contaminated wounds with some success. Other materials have been modified to achieve a direct pharmacologic antibacterial effect, such as xenograft or collagen lattice impregnated with the silver ion.

Generally, bacterial suppression seems to be an intrinsic property of organized tissue grafts and can only be conferred on synthetic materials by additional pharmacologic means.

Vascularization and Take

The fourth characteristic essential to the success of certain burn wound coverings is the desirable possibility of the covering or graft becoming vascularized by the wound bed and firmly bound by fibrous tissue growth, permitting a so-called graft take. Forty-eight to 72 hours after a graft is placed on an excised wound, new blood vessels invade the graft and are followed by fibroblasts, which lay down a dense mass of collagen, which in turn joins the graft to the bed. With autogenous tissue, such a condition is permanent; with allografts or xenografts, a familiar, active form of rejection involving activated lymphocytes occurs in 9 to 14 days, and the graft is ultimately destroyed by ischemic necrosis.

All three forms of tissue grafts, autografts, allografts, and xenografts, can become vascularized and take either permanently or temporarily, during which time the wound is well protected from bacterial invasion and fluid loss. Amnion is a useful burn wound covering of familiar biologic derivation. If the amnionic side is presented to the wound, vascularization does not occur, and the benefits as a wound cover are very temporary and limited; if the chorionic side is presented to the wound, temporary vascularization will occur, providing a more secure and long-lasting wound cover. Certain of the coverings fabricated of a synthetic film bound to an open collagen lattice will undergo a special form of vascular ingrowth with progressive destruction of the collagen and replacement by host fibrous tissue, thereby creating an instructed autogenous neodermis.[6] The velour and knitted synthetics become adherent temporarily by a phase 2 type of collagenous entanglement of the underside of the membrane, but never become truly vascularized.

As in all forms of grafting and wound coverage, mechanical factors must be carefully controlled. Adherence to and stability of the wound bed along with absence of hematoma or fluid collection clearly favor vascular ingrowth or take. Fluid accumulation, physical separation of the graft from the bed, or a high degree of bacterial contamination will inhibit vascularization.

In summary, only organized tissues become truly incorporated into a wound by vascularization and take, and only autogenous tissue becomes permanently incorporated.

FUNCTIONAL CLASSIFICATION

Based on the above discussion of the four important characteristics, it is possible to reduce the myriad numbers of burn wound coverings to a relatively simple classification scheme based on intended function. Previous classifications have been based on the nature of the materials[2, 3] or the chronology of their appearance.[5] Classification according to function helps in the understanding of a very disparate group of materials and hopefully prevents the tendency to ascribe similar properties and benefits to all simply because they seem alike. Burn wound coverings are classified according to their ability to carry out the following general functions:

1. Permit normal healing
2. Suppress bacteria
3. Debride surfaces
4. Serve as skin temporarily
5. Serve as skin permanently

A given type of covering can perform more than one function for the wound and hence appear in more than one category. For example, allograft, xenograft, and amnion—the so-called biological dressings—occur in at least three functional categories. In the following sections, coverings in each functional category will be discussed using a knowledge of their basic characteristics.

Permit Normal Healing

Some coverings (Table 14–5) function solely to permit normal healing of a partial-

TABLE 14–5.
Burn Wound Coverings to Permit Normal Healing

Synthetic films
Synthetic bilaminates
Amnion
Allograft
Xenograft
Autograft

TABLE 14–6.
Burn Wound Coverings to Suppress Bacteria

Autograft
Allograft
Amnion
Xenograft (plus silver)
Synthetic bilaminates plus silver
Synthetic films plus antiseptic
Synthetic bilaminates plus antiseptic

thickness burn injury or even a donor site by creating an optimal wound environment. They prevent bacterial contamination or actively suppressing bacteria already present in the wound. Synthetic films and bilaminates, given proper membrane transport characteristics, provide a proper environment to allow normal wound healing to proceed at an optimal rate. Organized tissue coverings provide the same, in addition to actively inhibiting bacterial growth. All of the above materials are useful in treating limited partial-thickness injuries on an ambulatory basis, as well as more extensive injuries that require hospitalization.

Suppress Bacteria

This group of coverings specifically inhibits bacteria in an already contaminated burn wound. Bacterial suppression, as previously discussed, is an important characteristic of certain burn wound coverings, and this characteristic likewise serves as the basis for a functional class of burn wound coverings (Table 14–6). Active bacterial suppression is a property of organized, naturally occurring tissue grafts such as the first four listed in Table 14–6. To enhance this characteristic in xenografts, ionic silver has been impregnated into the material.[16] Likewise, any coverings containing substantial amounts of collagen will bind silver ions to the triple helical collagen polymer and demonstrate increased bacterial inhibition.[17] Synthetic materials permeable to aqueous solutions and capable of tight adherence to a wound can be used successfully in the contaminated burn wound if an effective antiseptic agent is applied constantly to the synthetic surface.[18]

Debride Wound Surfaces

Wounds with any amount of nonviable material adherent to the surface must be debrided of this debris to ensure healing of a partial-thickness injury or to prepare a wound for successful grafting. Many burn wound coverings, both new and old, perform this function on dirty, partially debrided wounds (Table 14–7). Organized tissue grafts are absent from the list, since they have essentially no debriding ability. Despite the fact that such tissue grafts possess bacterial suppression properties, they play no role in debriding and preparing the heavily contaminated wound with partially adherent eschar and copious amounts of exudate. To attempt to use allograft, xenograft, or amnion in such a situation is to waste good biologic dressings.

Conventional cotton-mesh dressings lead the list of coverings with debriding characteristics since they remain the best material for gentle "textile debridement" of the burn wound. By using fine mesh cotton gauze and

TABLE 14–7.
Burn Wound Coverings to Debride Surface

Conventional cotton dressings
Polyurethane sponge
Collagen sponge
Synthetic (nylon/polyethylene) bilaminate

a "wet-to-dry" technique in which the moistened gauze is left on for a period of time and then gently removed before completely dry, a wound can be gradually freed of nonviable material without interfering with epithelialization and other aspects of normal wound healing.

Certain of the sponges, polyurethane and collagen in particular, have excellent debriding properties. However, they must not be allowed to remain on for too long, since with tightly adherent coagulated protein or even fibrous ingrowth, removal will cause gross disruption of the wound. At the very least, leaving synthetic sponges on a wound too long can lead to undesirable exudate being trapped below the surface. Synthetic bilaminates, particularly those with a relatively open mesh on the wound surface, will effectively debride wounds, but cost may make their application an expensive method of wound debridement, particularly when cheaper, reliable methods exist.

Recently, two groups[19, 20] introduced a synthetic bilaminate that incorporates a gel or hydrocolloid to specifically prevent debriding action when changed. While in contact with the wound, the gel becomes hydrated and swells, permitting easy removal, protecting the wound, but not providing any debriding action.

Serve as Skin Temporarily

This group, which includes all those coverings designed to temporarily close an excised burn wound, have skin-like benefits of bacterial exclusion and fluid and protein retention (Table 14–8). Their use may be limited to a few days or for much longer. This group of materials is particularly useful after a large, full-thickness burn has been excised in a patient who has very limited donor sites, since the wounds can be covered temporarily and effectively until the patient's own donor skin becomes available.

Cadaver allograft remains the single most reliable burn wound covering available to provide temporary wound closure after full-thickness excision. Reliability and extensive experience have confirmed allograft as the standard against which all other temporary skin substitutes must be judged. With the establishment of thoroughly reliable skin-banking techniques and proper quality control, a constant supply of human allograft can be made available within any major center.[25] In recent years, investigation has turned to methods of improving the effectiveness of human allograft. Aldehyde treatment has been shown to increase the "shelf life" of allografts and diminish their antigenicity so early immune rejection is avoided and, hence, potential time of usefulness increased.[26, 27] Recent work demonstrates that treating allografts with ultraviolet radiation and glucocorticoids depresses the Langerhans' cells and markedly prolongs the period the allograft is useful.[28] A consistently reliable method of diminishing or eliminating allograft antigenicity and immune rejection will strikingly enhance the clinical usefulness of human allograft as temporary wound coverage.

TABLE 14–8.
Burn Wound Coverings to Serve as Skin Temporarily

Synthetic bilaminates
Nylon/polyethylene
Nylon-collagen/silicone
Amnion
Xenograft (intermingled)
Allograft

Certain of the synthetic bilaminates with an outer vapor barrier of either silicone or polyethylene can be very effective as temporary skin substitutes, especially when allograft is either unavailable or in short supply. Great care should be exercised before using such materials, since all devitalized tissue must be excised before using synthetic bilaminates to cover a wound. Also, their use is limited in the coverage of heavily contaminated surfaces, since rapid exudate buildup can negate their potential advantages. In an optimally excised, bacterially clean burn wound, temporary wound coverage using a nylon-collagen velour/silicone bilaminate has been achieved for up to 3 months.[21]

Amnion, if used carefully, can provide effective temporary wound coverage in excised full-thickness burn wounds and can be useful in open contaminated wounds.[22] However, due to its fragility, amnion must be applied with extra care to achieve smooth application, and equal care must be taken to provide reliable fixation to avoid any shearing forces at the graft-wound interface.

Xenograft alone has some usefulness as a temporary skin substitute in an excised burn wound.[23] Recently, reports from China have described the use of xenograft in providing temporary coverage, while small autografts intermingled in the xenograft became vascularized and then spread beneath the xenograft, gradually lifting it off as the wound became epithelialized with the patient's own autogenous skin.[24]

TABLE 14–9.
Desirable Characteristics of Permanent Skin Substitute

Desirable Characteristics of Permanent Skin Substitute
Rapid adherence
Appropriate water vapor transfer
Intact bacterial barrier
Nonantigenic
Nontoxic
Hemostatic
Bacterial suppressant
Encourages fibrous ingrowth and bond
Flexible and elastic
Durable
Ease of handling
No wound contraction
Compatible surface change
Low cost
Long shelf-life

TABLE 14–10.
Burn Wound Coverings to Serve as Skin Permanently

Burn Wound Coverings to Serve as Skin Permanently
Collagen matrix/silicone
Collagen matrix/epidermal cells
Cultured epidermal cells

Serve as Skin Permanently

Ultimately, the ideal burn wound covering would be a fabricated material that is immediately available "on the shelf" and which, when placed on an excised burn wound, would be incorporated rapidly and permanently replacing the basic functions of skin on a long-term basis. Several authors have discussed the ideal desirable characteristics of a permanent skin substitute. Table 14–9 represents a composite list of such characteristics.[4, 5, 6, 29] To date, these techniques are still in the experimental or testing stage but have shown rich promise for difficult clinical situations.

Table 14–10 lists three burn wound coverings that serve as skin permanently. The first material listed is the so-called "artificial skin" developed by Burke and associates.[6] This material is fabricated in a bilaminate fashion using a collagen lattice of carefully controlled pore size coated with a proteoglycan, which helps regulate degradation of the lattice by the wound bed. The collagen lattice is tightly bonded to a thin silicone membrane, which serves as a vapor and bacterial barrier. The theoretical goal of its use is the creation of a neodermis formed of autogenous host fibrous tissue from the wound bed as the collagen lattice is broken down. When the process is complete, in about 30 days, the silicone film is peeled off and replaced with a very thin autograft to provide the cells to form an epidermal layer. When the process is complete, a neodermis and epidermal cell layer are present, which satisfy the full-thickness requirements of an excised wound. Wounds covered in this manner show excellent durability and very little wound contraction. Disadvantages include the necessity for very smooth application on complex surfaces such as those presented by joints and the face, and the necessity for the final, very thin, autogenous skin graft.

Collagen lattices incorporating autologous epidermal cells, if feasible, would provide a ready-made material embodying both major skin components and would approach the ideal permanent substitute. Groups experimenting with this technique have reported some early success in small animal experimentation but are limited by the time required to grow the epidermal cell component and are hampered by compatibility between living epidermal cells and the inert collagen matrix.[6, 30]

The use of rapidly grown sheets of cultured epidermal cells for permanent burn wound coverage not only is feasible but these sheets can now be used in life-threatening burns to gain early and complete closure of the burn wound.[7] The success of this technique is attributed to the extensive research carried out by Green and co-workers,[31, 32, 33] who demonstrated the methodology for the rapid growth of large stable sheets of epidermal cells. In practice, a small biopsy (1 sq cm) of normal skin is taken from the burned patient on entry. This is trypsinized and dispersed on a layer of modified fibroblasts in a combined Eagle/Ham altered medium. By 3 weeks, a 10,000-fold expansion is achieved in the form of a 3 to 4 cell-layer thick confluent epidermal cell sheet, which is then backed with petrolatum gauze for ease of handling and application. Saline dressings are used since the silver ion appears to be toxic to the fragile cell layers. The cells appear to take much as a thin split-thickness skin graft and will show rapid spread, keratinization, and thickening by 12 to 14 days. By 4 weeks an organized basement membrane composed of type 1 collagen has formed.[34] The long-term durability is the equivalent of conventional split-thickness skin grafts. The major drawback of this technique appears to be that since no dermal structure is provided, the wounds tend to contract creating significant secondary reconstructive problems. Other limitations include the fact that the cultured cells work best on freshly excised wounds, cannot be used concomitantly with silver nitrate, and require a sophisticated laboratory dedicated to and experienced in growing epidermal cells. Despite these limitations, the use of rapidly cultured epidermal cells occupies a vital place among the techniques of reliable coverage of the extensively burned patient.

SUMMARY

The many varieties of burn wound coverings possess common critical characteristics of water and oxygen permeability, adherence, bacterial suppression, and vascularization. Based on these characteristics, burn wound

TABLE 14–11.
Burn Wound Coverings and Functions*

	FUNCTION				
BURN WOUND COVERING	PERMIT NORMAL HEALING	SUPPRESS BACTERIA	DEBRIDE WOUND SURFACE	SERVE AS TEMPORARY SKIN	SERVE AS PERMANENT SKIN
Conventional dressings	+		+		
Synthetic films	+				
Synthetic sponges			+		
Synthetic gels	+				
Synthetic bilaminates	+		+	+	
Synthetics and antiseptics	+	+			
Amnion	+	+		+	
Xenograft	+	+		+	
Allograft	+	+		+	
Autograft	+	+			+
"Artificial skin"	+				+
Cultured epidermal cells	+	+			+

*Plus sign indicates that burn wound covering perform function delineated in column heading.

coverings may be divided into five classes based on the following functions:

1. Permit normal healing
2. Suppress bacteria
3. Debride surfaces
4. Serve as skin temporarily
5. Serve as skin permanently

Table 14–11 lists the common burn wound coverings and their appropriateness or lack thereof in each of the five functional classes. As more burn wound coverings are developed, their usefulness and role can be evaluated against existing materials by keeping in mind their important characteristics and intended functions.

REFERENCES

1. Pickerell KL: A sulphonamide film for use as a surgical dressing. *Bull Johns Hopkins Hosp* 1942; 71:304.
2. Davies JWL: Synthetic materials for covering burn wounds: Progress towards perfection: I. Short-term dressing materials. *Burns* 1984; 10:94–103.
3. Davies JWL: Synthetic materials for covering burn wounds: Progress towards perfection: II. Longer-term substitutes for skin. *Burns* 1984; 10:104–108.
4. Tavis MJ, Thornton JW, Bartlett RH, et al: A new composite skin prosthesis. *Burns* 1981; 7:123–130.
5. Pruitt BA, Levine NS: Characteristics and uses of biologic dressings and skin substitutes. *Arch Surg* 1984; 119:312–322.
6. Burke JF, Yannas IV, Quinby WC Jr, et al: Successful use of a physiologically acceptable artificial skin in the treatment of extensive burn injury. *Ann Surg* 1981; 194:413–428.
7. Gallico GG, O'Connor NE, Compton CC, et al: Permanent coverage of large burn wounds with autologous cultured human epithelium. *N Engl J Med* 1984; 311:448–451.
8. Lamke LO, Nilsson GE, Reithner HL: The evaporative water loss from burns and water-vapor permeability of grafts and artificial membranes used in the treatment of burns. *Burns* 1977; 3:159–165.
9. Winter GD: Formation of the scab and the rate of epithelialization of superficial wounds in the skin of the young domestic pig. *Nature* 1962; 193:293.
10. Hinman CD, Maibach H: Effect of air exposure and occlusion on experimental human skin wounds. *Nature* 1963; 200:377–378.
11. Tavis MJ, Thornton JW, Harvey JH, et al: Adherence to de-epithelialized surfaces: a comparative study. *Surg Forum* 1974; 25:39.
12. Tavis MJ, Thornton JW, Harvey JH, et al: Graft adherence to de-epithelialized surfaces: A comparative study. *Ann Surg* 1976; 184:594.
13. Morykmas MJ, Thornton JW, Hess C, et al: Surface change of synthetic and biological skin substitutes: Effects on adherence, abstract 69. *Trans Am Burn Assoc* 1983.
14. Eade GG: The relationship between granulation tissue, bacteria and skin grafts in burned patients. *Plast Reconstr Surg* 1958; 22:42–55.
15. Morris PJ, Bondoc CC, Burke JF: The use of frequently changed skin allografts to promote healing in the nonhealing infected ulcer. *Surgery* 1966; 60:13–19.
16. May SF, DeClement FA: Clinical evaluation of silver-impregnated porcine xenograft, abstract 68. *Trans Am Burn Assoc* 1982; p 7.
17. Fox CL, Modak SM, Stanford W: Silver-treated graft materials for coverage of infected burn wounds. *Ann Chir Plast* 1979; 24:265–267.
18. Zachary L, Heggers JP, Robson MC, et al: The use of topical antimicrobials combined with Biobrane in burn wound infections. *J Trauma* 1982; 22:833–836.
19. Hermans MHE, Hermans RP: Preliminary report on the use of a new hydrocolloid dressing in the treatment of burns. *Burns* 1984; 11:125–129.
20. Golan J, Eldad A, Rudensky B, et al: A new temporary synthetic skin substitute. *Burns* 1985; 11:274–280.
21. Briggs SE: Personal communication, 1985.
22. Quinby WC Jr, Hoover HC, Scheflan M, et al: Clinical trials of amniotic membranes in burn wound care. *Plast Reconstr Surg* 1982; 70:711–716.
23. Frank DH, Wachtel T, Frank HA, et al: Comparison of Biobrane, porcine and human allograft as biological dressings for burn wounds. *J Burn Care Rehabil* 1983; 4:186–190.
24. Yue-Liang D, Shu-Sung P, De-Zhen W, et al: Clinical and histological observations on the application of intermingled auto- and porcine-skin heterografts in third-degree burns. *Burns* 1983; 9:381–386.
25. May SR, DeClement FA: Skin banking: I–IV. *J Burn Care Rehabil* 1981; 2:7–23, 64–76, 128–141, 184–193.
26. Schechter J: Prolonged retention of gluteraldehyde-treated skin allografts and xenografts. *Ann Surg* 1975; 182:699–704.
27. Piccolo N, Petro JA, Salisbury RE: Increased adherence time of porcine xenograft pre-

treated with a cross-linking agent, abstract 44. *Trans Am Burn Assoc* 1983; p 51.
28. Alsbjorn BE, Sorenson B: Grafting with epidermal Langerhans cell depressed cadaver split skin. *Burns* 1985; 11:259–263.
29. Bartlett RH: Skin substitutes. *J Trauma* 1981; 21(suppl):731–732.
30. Bell F, Buttle DJ, Ehrlich HP, et al: Living tissue formed in vitro and accepted as skin-equivalent tissue of full thickness. *Science* 1981; 211:1052.
31. Green H, Kehinde O, Thomas J: Growth of cultured human epidermal cells into multiple epithelia suitable for grafting. *Proc Natl Acad Sci* 1979; 76:5665–5668.
32. Rheinwald JG, Green H: Serial cultivation of strains of human epidermal keratinocytes: The formation of keratinizing colonies from single cells. *Cell* 1975; 6:331–344.
33. Banks-Schlegel S, Green H: Formation of epidermis by serially cultivated human epidermal cells transplanted as an epithelium to athymic mice. *Transplantation* 1980; 29:308–313.
34. Compton CC: Unpublished observations, 1986.

SECTION V

INFECTION AND IMMUNOLOGY

15 / Immunologic Considerations in the Burned Child*

EDWIN A. DEITCH, M.D.

Many therapeutic advances in the care of the burn patient have been made in the past decade, yet infection remains a common cause of morbidity and mortality after thermal injury. The exact cause of the increased susceptibility of the thermally injured patient to infection has not been definitely established. However, it appears that the combination of impaired local and systemic antibacterial host defenses plus loss of the skin barrier to bacteria are major factors responsible for the increased incidence of infections in burn patients. This is not surprising, since normal skin plays a major role in the protection of the host against a wide range of potentially pathogenic microorganisms by functioning as a living physical barrier to bacterial invasion. In man, the risk of cutaneous infection is increased when (1) the surface integrity of the skin has been destroyed; (2) the skin has become macerated; (3) the normal cutaneous bacterial flora has been disrupted; or (4) when local arterial, venous, or lymphatic flow is impeded. Since all of these and other local predisposing factors are present to some extent after a thermal injury, the burn wound serves as a portal of entry for invading bacteria. This failure of local immunity in combination with impaired systemic immunity sets the stage for life-threatening local and systemic infections.

This chapter summarizes current information on the effects of a thermal injury on local and systemic host-defense systems. Special emphasis is placed on the relationship between failure of these host defenses and infection. The first part of this chapter reviews the immunobiology of the host's antibacterial defense systems and provides a background for discussion of the results of current studies of the immune state of the burn patient.

BIOLOGY OF HOST-DEFENSE MECHANISMS

The primary role of the immune system is the preservation of the body's integrity against invading microorganisms. Since the presence of bacteria represents a potential threat to the body's homeostasis, the host has developed both local and systemic defense systems to protect itself against invading microorganisms. Conceptually, the body's antibacterial defenses can be divided into: (1) local defenses, including mechanical barriers, such as the skin or mucous membranes, and (2) components of the inflammatory response, as well as the humoral and cellular components of the systemic defense systems.

The terminology used to describe the body's systemic immune system can be confusing, since the specific immune response includes only the reaction of cells to a bacterium (antigen) to which they have been exposed. These reactions include: (1) antibody formation, (2) direct cell-mediated cytotoxicity, and (3) noncytotoxic cell-cell interactions. The host-defense systems that respond specifically to foreign antigens include the nonspe-

*This work was supported in part by NIH grant no. GM 30705.

cific or inflammatory host-defense system (Table 15–1). Since the nonspecific or inflammatory host-defense system does not require previous exposure to the bacteria (antigen) to be activated, it is the primary defense system of the nonimmune host.

Loss of the skin barrier to bacteria allows potential bacterial pathogens to colonize the burn eschar, which in turn potentiates the ability of these organisms to successfully invade the host's tissue. In this situation, the inflammatory response becomes a major host-defense mechanism. The inflammatory response alerts the host's immune system that the mechanical barriers have been breached while providing the scaffolding on which effector systems can function. The major elements initially contributing to this inflammatory response include the plasma proteins, mast cells, tissue macrophages, and systemically recruited neutrophils and monocytes.[98] The noncellular elements of the inflammatory response modify the local environment to limit the spread of invading bacteria, render the invading bacteria more susceptible to phagocytosis, and recruit phagocytic cells to the inflammatory focus. The major noncellular mediators involved in this phase of the inflammatory process are components of the coagulation and complement cascades, and the vasoactive amines. Initiation of the noncellular phase of the inflammatory response occurs through a process termed *contact activation*.[25] Contact activation describes the sequential phenomenon of a negatively charged surface, such as basement membrane, collagen, or endotoxin, activating the plasma coagulation system, which then turns on the fibrinolysin, kinin, and complement systems.[79] In the burn patient, contact activation probably occurs when unexposed endothelialized surfaces are exposed by the local thermal injury. These endothelialized surfaces initiate the inflammatory response by the contact activation of Hageman's factor, which triggers local vascular thrombosis, as well as the production of multiple other vascoactive substances.[49, 63]

TABLE 15–1.
Major Elements of the Nonspecific and Specific Host-Defense Systems

CELLULAR	HUMORAL
Nonspecific Host-Defense System	
Neutrophils	Alternate complement system
Reticuloendothelial system	Fibronectin
Blood monocytes	Coagulation/fibrinolytic
Tissue macrophages	
Specific Immune System	
B lymphocytes	Antibodies
T lymphocytes	Lymphokines
Macrophages	Monokines
Plasma cells	Classical component system

Once the tissue-injury recognition phase has been initiated, activated complement components (especially C3a, C5a) both amplify the local humoral response and recruit functional phagocytes from the systemic circulation (Fig 15–1). C3a and C5a are potent anaphylatoxins that cause local venous constriction and increase capillary permeability.[62] In addition, these complement fragments are biologically active chemoattractants and thus attract circulating neutrophils and monocytes to the inflammatory site.[98] The locally recruited phagocytes function in concert with the locally and systemically generated humoral factors to eradicate the invading bacterial pathogens. The most important effector cell recruited by the inflammatory response is the neutrophil.[87]

The neutrophil is the principal cellular component of the nonspecific system and once microorganisms have breached the local cutaneous defenses, circulating neutrophils rapidly migrate to the site of inflammation and eliminate the microorganisms through the process of bacterial phagocytosis and intracellular killing. A defect in any one of the successive steps of neutrophil function leading up to the ingestion and killing of invading bacteria has been associated with an increased susceptibility to infection. The major sequential steps required for successful neutrophil-mediated bactericidal activity are schematically illustrated in Figure 15–2. These steps

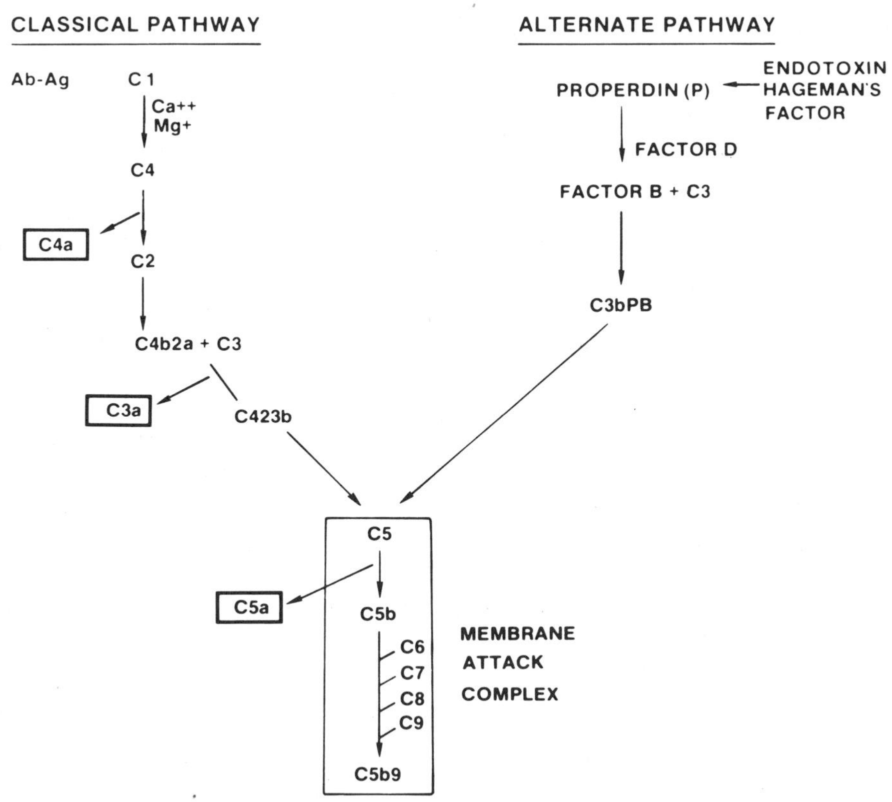

FIG 15–1.
The classical arm of the complement cascade is triggered by complement-binding antibodies (IgM, IgG) attached to the surface of an antigen (Ab-Ag). During activation of the classical arm of the complement cascade, the biologically active C4a and C3a fragments are generated. The alternate pathway can be activated in the absence of complement-binding antibodies by a variety of substances, including lipopolysaccharides, bacterial endotoxin, and Hageman's factor. Both systems converge at C5 and initiate the membrane-attack complex, which lyses the cell membrane of the target cell. During this terminal activation process, the complement fragment C5a, which functions as both an anaphylatoxin and a chemoattractant, is generated.

include adherence to the vascular endothelium at the site of inflammation (margination), migration through the vascular wall to the local site of bacterial invasion (chemotaxis), and, finally, the ingestion and killing of the invading bacteria. Each of these in vivo neutrophil functions can be measured in vitro, either directly or indirectly. The antibacterial action of the neutrophil is most effective in eradicating organisms that are present in tissues and in areas where the flow of blood is slow (e.g., pulmonary circulation) or has stopped altogether (e.g., site of inflammation). Blood-borne bacteria are not effectively cleared by circulating neutrophils since the flow of blood is too rapid in the systemic vasculature to allow sufficient contact time between neutrophil and bacteria for phagocytosis to occur. Circulating bacteria are primarily cleared from the blood by the fixed macrophages of the liver, spleen, and lymph nodes (reticuloendothelial system [RES]). The architecture of the RES is specifically developed for this function, since the RES organs consist of a sieve-like lattice of reticular fibers, and collagenous proteins to which the phagocytic cells

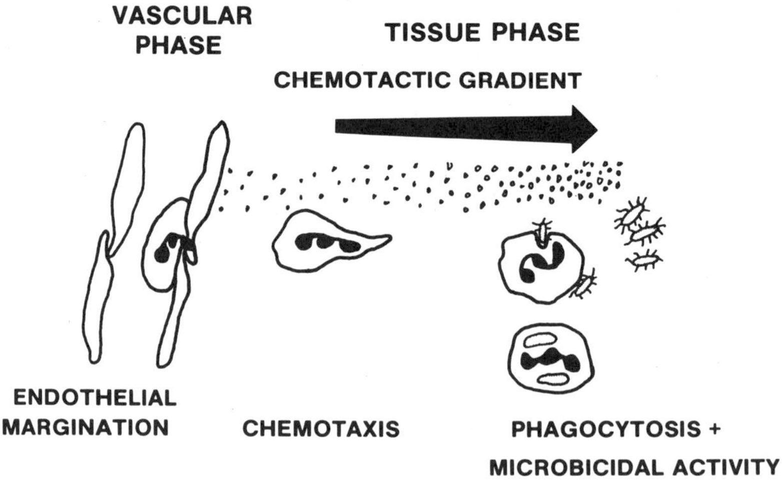

FIG 15–2.
Recruitment of circulating neutrophils to an inflammatory focus (nidus of bacteria) is mediated by the local generation of chemotatic factors. The circulating neutrophils sense these factors and respond by endothelial margination, migration through the vascular wall, and chemotaxis up the chemotactic gradient to the inflammatory focus. The activated neutrophils then phagocytize and kill the ingested bacteria.

are attached.[52] This anatomic arrangement ensures intimate contact between phagocytic cells and circulating bacteria and promotes the efficient phagocytosis and subsequent killing of bloodborne microorganisms by the fixed tissue macrophages.

The nonspecific humoral system assists the cellular system by coating invading bacteria with proteins that the phagocytes recognize through surface receptors (Fig 15–3). The coating of bacteria by humoral proteins is termed *opsonization* and the term *opsonin* refers to a protein that when bound to an antigen, increases the affinity of that antigen for a phagocytic cell. The major opsonin systems are composed of proteins of the classical and alternate complement systems, fibronectin, and antibody. Conceptually, opsonins can be viewed as links between the humoral and cellular elements of the nonspecific and the specific immune systems.

The specific immune system consists of macrophages, lymphocytes, plasma cells, and their humoral products (see Table 15–1). It is only recently, with the development of monoclonal antibodies, that the complex interactions between the cellular subpopulations of the immune system have begun to be understood on a cellular level. In contrast to the phylogenetically more primitive inflammatory host-defense system, the specific immune system responds specifically to antigenic sites on the surfaces of invading bacteria. This response is characterized by the production of antigen-specific antibodies formed against the invading organism. The antibody molecule is a bifunctional molecule which contains a constant region (Fc) that binds to the effector cell and a variable region (Fab2) that binds to the antigen. Antibodies serve as specific opsonins that increase the affinity of bacterial binding to neutrophils and fixed-tissue macrophages of the RES. In this way, the specific and nonspecific host-defense systems interact to defend the body against invading microorganisms. In addition, the presence of antibody bound to the surface of bacteria activates the classical component cascade (see Fig 15–1), by the binding of the first component of complement (C1q) to the Fc region of the antibody molecule. In fact, certain serum-sensitive strains of bacteria can be effectively killed by the antibody-mediated activation of complement in the absence of effector cells, such as neutrophils. For most antigens, the initial step in the induction of humoral immunity (antibody production) is the presentation of antigen by macrophages to helper thymus-dependent lymphocytes (T cells). Activation of the helper T cells results in the liberation of soluble mediators (lymphokines) that instruct B lymphocytes to proliferate and differentiate into antibody producing plasma cells. This process can be blocked or suppressed in many ways, such as by a failure of antigen presentation to the helper T cell, or by the activation of suppressor T cells or inhibitory macrophages (Fig 15-4).

Cell-mediated immunity includes a wide range of functions directly carried out by immune cells or their products, independent of antibody production. These functions include (1) the activation of macrophages to become more effective phagocytes; (2) the induction of null lymphocytes (killer [K] cells) that kill antibody-coated target cells; and (3) the production of cytotoxic T cells (natural killer [NK] cells) that kill foreign cells. The exact mechanisms controlling cell-mediated immunity are unclear. However, it appears that both macrophages and lymphocytes are composed of multiple subpopulations, some of which have either facilitory or inhibitory functions.

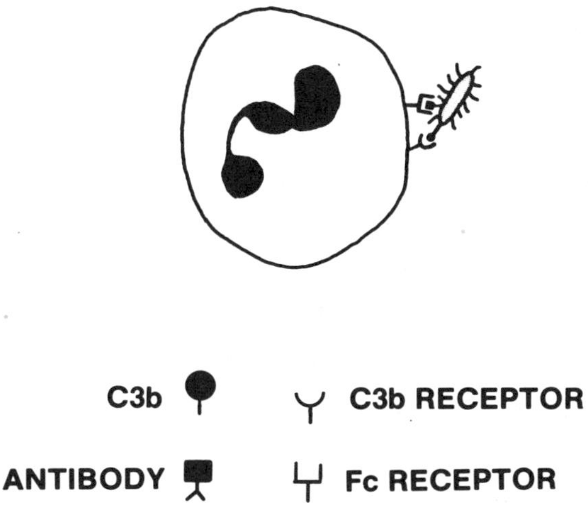

FIG 15–3.
Specific antibody and complement are the two major bacterial opsonin systems. Both antibody and the C3b component of complement serve as bridges, which physically connect the bacteria to the neutrophil, and thus facilitate the process of bacterial phagocytosis. Mechanistically, specific antibody binds to bacterial surface-membrane antigens via the variable (Fab) portion of the antibody molecule, while the constant (FcR) portion binds to surface receptors (Fc) of the neutrophil. In a similar fashion, exposed C3b bound to the bacterial surface joins the bacterium to the neutrophil by binding to the C3b neutrophil surface receptor.

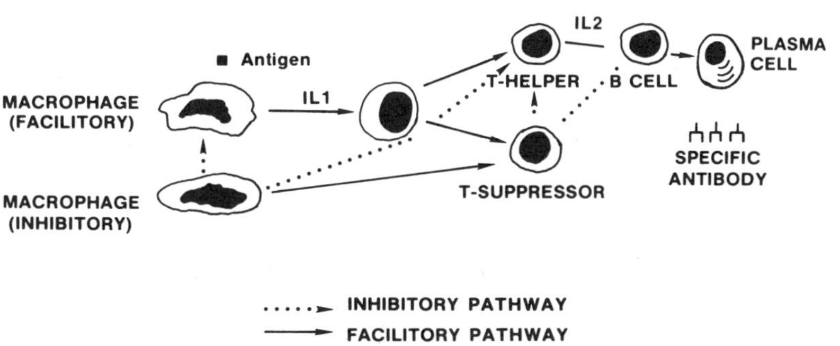

FIG 15–4.
In this schematic illustration of the major relationships between the various mononuclear cell subpopulations, solid lines indicate the pathways that increase the immune response, while broken lines designate pathways that down-regulate the immune response. Humoral factors (monokines and lymphokines) serve as the major messengers between the various cellular subpopulations. Two major humoral messengers are interleukin 1 (IL1) produced by facilitory macrophages and interleukin 2 (IL2) produced by helper T cells.

Evidence that T lymphocytes develop into different subpopulations specialized for certain functions was first presented by Kisielow et al.[64] in 1975. These investigators documented that postthymic mouse lymphocytes capable of exerting either helper or suppressor functions could be identified by the presence of Thy1 and Ly antigens on their cell surface. This work indicated that microscopically similar lymphocytes could be separated into functionally distinct subpopulations based on their surface antigenic phenotype. At present, when commercially available monoclonal antibodies are used, helper T cells can be distinguished from suppressor T cells,[88, 89] and both can be differentiated from B cells[48] (Table 15-2). Additionally, NK and K lymphocytes can be distinguished from other lymphocyte populations. Through studies which correlated cell surface receptors with biologic activity, we now know that when inhibitory macrophages or suppressor T cells are activated and their effects predominate, the immune response will be reduced. In contrast, increased activity of facilitory macrophages or helper T cells results in augmentation of the immune response. Under normal conditions, these mononuclear-cell subpopulations maintain immunologic homeostasis through the production of soluble products (lymphokines and monokines). Disruption of this normal immunologic balance can lead to autoimmune disease at one extreme or impaired resistance to infection on the other.

Full expression of host-defense mechanisms requires maturation of the specific immune system (T lymphocytes, B lymphocytes, and macrophages), as well as maturation of the cell lines and components concerned with the effector limb of immunity. These include the complement and properdin system, the RES, neutrophils, and mast cells. Increasing evidence has established that the normal human neonate is developmentally immature in many aspects of the specific immune and nonspecific inflammatory response.[78] For example, the newborn's capacity to produce antibodies differs both quantitatively and qualitatively from that of the adult. The serum of normal neonates contains approximately 10% of the normal adult level of IgM, adult levels of IgG due to placental transfer of maternal IgG, and no IgA. By age two years, serum-IgM concentrations have increased to normal levels, while adult concentrations of IgG are not reached until age four years to six years, and adult concentrations of IgA until puberty.[10, 21]

EFFECT OF THERMAL INJURY ON HOST-DEFENSE MECHANISMS

For many years it has been known that patients with thermal injuries develop multiple

TABLE 15–2.
Phenotypic Characterization of Functionally Distinct Lymphocytes*

LYMPHOCYTE POPULATION	HUMAN	MURINE
T cells	OKT3+, OKT11+	Thy 1+
T-helper/inducers	OKT4+, OKT8−	Lyt−1+
T-suppressor/cytotoxic	OKT4−, OKT8+	Lyt−2,3+
NK (natural killer)	FcR+, Ig−	Fcr+, Ig−
K cells	FcR+, Ig−	FcR+, Ig−
B cells	FcR+, Ia+, Ig+	FcR+, Ia+, Ig+

*Monoclonal antibodies of the OK series are used to identify human lymphocyte subpopulations, while the Thy(Ly) series are used to identify murine lymphocyte cell populations. FcR+ indicates that the surface receptor for the constant (Fc) region of the immunoglobulin molecule is present; Ig+, that the surface of the cell expresses immunoglobulin (Ig); Ig−, that immunoglobulin is not expressed on the cell surface; Ia+, that this Ia antigen is present on the surface of the cell.

defects of the immune system. These include alterations in immunoglobulin levels, changes in the concentration and activity of both the classical and alternative complement pathways, reduced levels of circulating plasma fibronectin, depressed serum opsonic activity, and impairment of the macrophages, lymphocytes, neutrophils, and the RES. Each of the host-defense systems will be described separately in the remainder of this chapter, but it is critical to keep in mind that these systems are activated in vivo simultaneously and function synergistically to prevent and control infection.

Local Immunity

A thermal injury, by destroying the skin barrier, allows the invasion of surface microorganisms into the viable subeschar tissues. Since the most common site of infection in septic burn patients is the burn wound, it appears that failure of local immunity may be an important predisposing factor to the development of infection in these burn patients. The opsonic activity of blister fluid from 18 burn patients was measured to determine whether changes in the bacterial flora of the burn wound may be related to changes in the local immune environment.[33] *Staphylococcus aureus* and *Pseudomonas aeruginosa* were chosen as test organisms, since they represent the most common species of microorganisms colonizing the burn wound. The results of this study indicate that blister fluid is as good an opsonin source for the killing of staphylococci by normal neutrophils as normal serum. However, the blister fluid does not adequately support either the phagocytosis or killing of pseudomonads by normal neutrophils. The fact that burn blister fluid has impaired opsonic activity for *P. aeruginosa,* but not for *S. aureus* indicates that a local humoral defect may be responsible, at least in part, for the high incidence of gram-negative organisms, especially pseudomonads, colonizing the burn wound after thermal injury. A series of repletion experiments indicated that the opsonic defect for *P. aeruginosa* is not due to the presence of inhibitors of opsonic or cellular activity, but to a lack of normal serum factor(s).[36] Further study of these specimens indicated that the opsinopathy is due to a local activation and consumption of complement components in the burn wound. However, the blister fluid could attract systemic phagocytes to the burn wound.[38] Of interest is the fact that blister fluid from 8 of 35 patients inhibited the mitogenic response of normal lymphocytes to the mitogen phytohemagglutinin (PHA).[44] The inhibition of normal lymphocyte activity by the suppressive blister-fluid specimens is not due to the presence of endotoxin in the blister-fluid specimens, but is associated with significantly elevated levels of C3 breakdown products compared to the nonsuppressive samples.[37] Thus, it appears that the local accumulation of C3 breakdown products in the blister fluid might down-regulate or suppress lymphocyte mitogenesis, as well as affect neutrophil function. Since lymphocytes, macrophages, and neutrophils express C3 receptors on their cell surfaces[103] and various fragments of C3 have been documented to modulate lymphocyte function,[106, 107] it is reasonable to speculate that complement components may modulate the local immune system.

The results of these studies strongly suggest that local biochemical changes in burn blister fluid may adversely affect local immunity and predispose the patient to burn wound sepsis. Since both neutrophil chemotaxis and random migration is depressed after thermal injury,[36, 51] the delayed arrival of neutrophils to the burn wound, in combination with impaired immune functions of the blister fluid, could result in uncontrolled local growth of microorganisms. Yet, whether the failure of local immunity would result ultimately in infection in a specific patient depends on many other factors, including the patient's overall immune state. Therefore, it is reasonable to conclude that a failure in local immunity may be necessary, but not always sufficient, for burn wound sepsis to occur.

Neutrophils

Because of the association between impaired neutrophil function and bacterial infections,[61] many investigators have measured neutrophil function in the burn patient. As illustrated in Figure 15–2, the successful eradication of invading bacteria requires several successive neutrophil responses, the failure of any of which could lead to an established bacterial infection. Decreased neutrophil chemotaxis frequently occurs after thermal injury,[39, 105] and the magnitude of the initial impairment in chemotaxis appears to be related directly to the magnitude of the injury. However, in spite of the relationship between impaired chemotaxis and thermal injury, there is conflicting evidence as to whether this chemotactic defect is prognostically important in identifying the patient at increased risk of becoming infected.[5, 55, 105] The etiologies of impaired neutrophil migration remain speculative, despite active investigation of this question. Controversy exists over whether the defect in chemotaxis is due to humoral suppressive factors,[43, 105] circulating toxins,[83, 95] or cellular deactivation by circulating complement factors.[99, 100] *Deactivation* is a term used to describe the phenomenon of in vivo activation of neutrophils leading to in vitro paralysis. In this phenomenon, neutrophils that have been exposed in vivo to chemoattractants, such as complement activation products, become relatively or absolutely refractory to subsequent stimuli in vitro. Evidence in support of this theory consists of the association of signs of in vivo neutrophil activation, such as neutrophil degranulation[32] and increased adherence[35] in the presence of decreased in vitro chemotactic activity. Additionally, evidence of in vivo neutrophil activation has been documented in neutrophils from trauma and anergic patients with abnormal in vitro neutrophil chemotactic responses.[24] To some extent, all of these mechanisms are probably operative in the burn patient.

No consistent defect in neutrophil bacterial phagocytosis after thermal injury has been documented,[5, 60] and in fact, several groups, including our own, have found phagocytosis to be increased in the burn patient.[5, 40] In contrast to neutrophil phagocytic activity, Alexander et al.[5, 6] documented in studies of burned, traumatized, and infected patients that a decrease in neutrophil bactericidal activity is associated with an increased risk of infection. This association of impaired neutrophil bactericidal activity with infection has been verified in a prospective study of 66 thermally injured patients.[40]

Although postburn impaired neutrophil bactericidal activity is associated with an increased risk of infection,[5, 40, 51, 86, 112] surprisingly little information is available on postburn neutrophil metabolism. A summary of the reported work on neutrophil metabolism after thermal injury indicates that spontaneous metabolic activity is increased as measured by nitroblue tetrazolium (NBT) reduction,[92] while stimulated metabolic activity is decreased as measured by the stimulated NBT test, oxygen consumption,[28, 54, 55] or chemoluminescence.[11] Whether the decreased stimulated oxygen consumption is due to impaired hexose monophosphate shunt activity, which is the major metabolic pathway in neutrophils, is unresolved.[56] Reports that serum from burn patients has impaired oxygen consumption activity in neutrophils has led some investigators to conclude that burn serum contains an inhibitor of neutrophil metabolism.[85] Yet, none of these published studies clearly explains the basis for the impaired microbicidal activity; it is not possible to determine the relevance of any of the reported metabolic changes to neutrophil bactericidal activity.

Reticuloendothelial System

The RES is an essential component of the nonspecific host-defense system. The RES clears circulating debris, such as aggregated protein, damaged cells, and fibrin from the bloodstream, in addition to removing bloodborne bacteria.[34] Efficient phagocytosis of these substances by the RES requires the presence of humoral factors, which coat the particles to promote their recognition, attachment, and ingestion by the fixed macrophages of the RES. During the last decade, it has become apparent that normal serum levels of the opsonin protein, fibronectin, are required for the RES to function optimally, and that the serum concentration of fibronectin is the limiting factor in RES reserve after trauma. The first direct human data on RES activity after thermal injury were published by Goldman et al.[50] in 1974. They found that plasma humoral recognition factor, an α_2-globulin, subsequently identified as fibronectin, was decreased after major burns in children, and that during septic episodes the protein levels decreased even further. Lanser et al.[69] in 1980, studied the effect of thermal injury on RES activity in 15 adult burn victims with a mean burn size of 40%. The RES activity was measured both by the liver-slice assay and by a direct immunoassay of fibronectin. Both fibronectin levels and RES activity were initially transiently depressed, but returned to normal within a few days. Both Lanser et al.[40] and others have documented that during septic episodes a secondary drop in fibronectin levels occurs and that this secondary drop in plasma fibronectin will identify patients at increased risk of sepsis. The exact cause of the initial depression in fibronectin appears to be due to its systemic consumption.[29, 72] The role of plasma fibronectin as an opsonin for nonbacterial debris is clear. Recent evidence suggests that fibronectin may also function as an opsonin for certain bacterial species such as *S. aureus*[67, 104] and that the combination of fibronectin depletion and complement inactivation results in a synergistic decrease in opsonic activity.[41]

The clinical consequences of impaired RES activity and depressed fibronectin levels may secondarily involve other organs, since during periods of RES depression the clearance of circulating debris and bacteria shifts from the liver to other organs, especially the lung. For example, after splenectomy in the rat, pulmonary localization of a test colloid increases 11-fold and remains elevated for at least 10 days.[23] Additionally, experimentally induced bacteremia during RES blockage increases the pulmonary clearance of bacteria and is associated with pulmonary margination and sequestration of circulating neutrophils.[68] Thus, RES blockage may ultimately result in pulmonary dysfunction due to the activation of neutrophils sequestered in the lungs.

Based on this information, it appears that impaired RES activity is associated with a decreased resistance to infection, as well as distant organ failure. Anecdotal reports of fibronectin repletion improving host resistance to infection and impaired organ function in injured or septic patients have been reported.[91, 94, 96] Although these reports are encouraging, controlled studies are needed to determine the exact clinical role of fibronectin replacement therapy in the therapeutic armamentarium of the burn therapist.

Humoral Defenses

Although many other humoral factors, in addition to fibronectin, are important in the control of bacterial infections, only two additional major opsonin systems present in biologic fluids will be discussed. These consist of the heat-stable immunoglobulins and the heat-labile complement components. In the nonimmune host, the alternate complement system is the major opsonin system and is activated by endotoxin, denatured serum proteins, or damaged cells in the absence of antibody.[57, 58] In the immune host, with high levels of specific antibody, complement plays an adjuvant role as a bacterial opsonin[65] (see Fig 15–1).

Serum opsonic activity has been studied extensively in patients with thermal injuries. These patients exhibit depressed serum opsonic activity for pseudomonads, *Escherichia coli*, and occasionally *S. aureus*.[7, 15, 16, 17] Impaired opsonic activity does not appear to be a reliable indicator of sepsis, since impaired opsonic activity has been observed during both septic[16, 19] and nonseptic periods.[4, 7] Impaired opsonic activity when present appears to be related to systemic activation and subsequent consumption of components of the alternate complement system. The defect in opsonic activity due to complement consumption is not limited to the thermally injured patient, but also occurs after trauma and in patients with gram-negative bacterial infections.[18, 47, 59] In addition to their systemic role as opsonins, these humoral factors are important locally, since complement components serve as local opsonins in the tissues, and one of the complement breakdown products, C5a, is a major chemoattractant for neutrophils (described in detail under section on local immunity). Although serum immunoglobulins levels are transiently decreased after thermal injury,[13, 16, 30] they return to normal quickly, and this acute hypoimmunoglobulinemia does not appear to be associated with an increased susceptibility to infection.[9] Thus, in general, serum immunoglobulin levels are not accurate indicators of sepsis or recovery in the burn patient.

Specific Immune System

Beginning with the observation that a burn victim may have delayed rejection of skin allografts, many studies have been performed to evaluate cell-mediated immunity in the burn patient. Although many investigators have measured cell-mediated immunity, either in vivo as skin test reactivity, or in vitro as lymphocyte blastogenic transformation, there is no consensus on whether cell-mediated immunity is normal,[81] increased,[31, 73] or decreased[27, 102, 108] after thermal injury. Furthermore, controversy exists over whether changes (when observed) in the in vitro lymphocyte response correlate prognostically with sepsis or death.[14, 27, 81, 109] The results of several groups of investigators,[27, 81] as well as our own,[42] indicate that changes in the patient's cellular in vitro response to the mitogen PHA do not correlate with sepsis development or death. These results are in conflict with others,[109] who reported that the magnitude of the depression in the in vitro lymphocyte response to PHA is less in surviving than nonsurviving patients. On careful examination of these reports, it appears that the differences in these studies are related to differences in patient care protocols, patient selection, methodology, and data analysis. For example, one major difference between our work and the work of Wolfe[109] is that these investigators do not utilize early excision and grafting in their patients. Instead they begin operating on their patients between the 20th and 25th postburn day; in contrast, we began operatively to excise and close the burn wound within the first postburn week. This difference in operative approach may be of significant biologic importance, since early excision of the burn wound in animals is associated with the restoration of thymic activity[46] and increased resistance to infection.[71]

A major potential weakness of all standardized in vitro assays is the fact that the assay may not accurately reflect the complex interactions that are occurring in vivo. Therefore, we measured the spontaneous blastogenic transformation (SBT) of our patient's lymphocytes immediately after they were harvested from the blood, as well as after 4 days in tissue culture containing the mitogen PHA.[42] By measuring both the unstimulated SBT and the stimulated PHA blastogenic response, we could correlate the level of the patients' intrinsic (in vivo) lymphocyte activity with the results of in vitro assays. The results of these studies documented that the patients' spontaneous (in vivo) SBT activity is increased, while the PHA stimulated activity is normal or decreased. Furthermore, in contrast to the PHA stimulated activity, the level of SBT activity accurately reflected the patient's clinical status, including the onset of sepsis. Our SBT results documenting an increased level of in vivo cellular activity, especially during sepsis, are consistent with a recent report indicating that lymphocytes from burn patients are spontaneously producing elevated levels of immunoglobulins.[97] Thus, it appears that impaired in vitro cell-mediated immunity is not due primarily to a defect in the ability of the cells to be activated.

Three major hypotheses have been proposed to explain the acquired defect in cell-mediated immunity that occurs after thermal injury. These hypotheses include: decreased numbers of helper T cells,[12] increased numbers of suppressor T cells,[14, 77, 80] and the presence of circulating humoral suppressor factors.[26, 83] The fact that, in our patients as well as others, the immunosuppressive capacity of patients serum does not consistently correlate with the levels of spontaneous or stimulated cellular activity[27, 42, 108] casts doubt on the thesis that circulating humoral factors are principally responsible for the observed changes in cell-mediated immunity. The selective activation of suppressor T cells to prevent an autoimmune type reaction against thermally modified dermis is an attractive hypothesis and is supported by the fact that the thermally injured patients produce autoantibodies against dermis.[1] However, other investigators have documented that suppressor cell activity is an early and transient phenomenon[74] and that when suppressor cell activity and PHA responses are measured simultaneously, the magnitude of the decrease in the PHA response cannot be completely accounted for by increased suppressor cells activity.[109]

Alternatively, the biological phenomenon known as antigenic competition[2] could explain the combination of increased spontaneous activity associated with a depressed stimulatory response. In antigenic competition, cells that have already been stimulated become relatively resistant to further stimulation. The hypothesis of in vivo stimulation leading to an impaired in vitro response is consistent with our findings using PHA as a probe, as well as with the work of others[97] who documented a similar phenomenon in immunoglobulin production after thermal injury. However, antigenic competition is a complicated process, relating to both the duration and level of the initial stimulant and thus is unlikely to be completely responsible for these findings.

Cellular exhaustion or down-regulation of helper T cells could also explain the association of increased spontaneous blastogenic activity and normal or decreased PHA stimulation. This possibility is supported by recent evidence documenting that interleukin 2 is decreased after thermal injury. Interleukin 2, a lymphokine (soluble-mediator) produced by helper T cells, is important in triggering the proliferation of activated T cells.[90, 110] Currently, it is not possible to say with certainty which of these alternatives, if any, occurs at the cellular level. However, a clear understanding of what occurs at the cellular level is critical for the development of rational therapeutic modalities to augment host resistance to infection.

Hypothesis of Immunologic Basis of Burn Wound Sepsis

The following hypothesis, illustrated in Figure 15–5, is an attempt to integrate the previously described immunological defects into a working model that explains the immunologic basis of the increased susceptibility of the burn patient to life-threatening infections originating from the burn wound. This proposed scenario is based primarily on the failure of the nonspecific host-defense system. However, dysfunction of the specific immune system is also important, since one of the major roles of the specific immune system is to amplify and focus the ability of the nonspecific host-defense system to control invading bacteria.

The combination of impaired neutrophil chemotaxis and opsonic activity of the burn blister fluid allows bacteria to colonize (contaminate) the burn eschar in sufficient numbers to invade and propagate in the viable subeschar tissues. If the invading bacteria are opsonized, phagocytized, and killed by local phagocytes in combination with the late-arriving neutrophils, the infection is controlled locally. However, if local bacterial control does

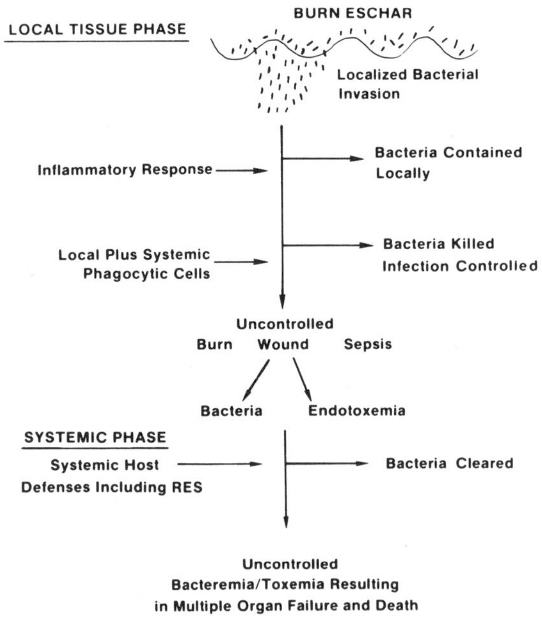

FIG 15–5.
Working model of the relationship between burn wound sepsis and the host's antibacterial defense systems.

not occur, due to impaired bactericidal activity of the locally recruited phagocytes, then the surviving bacteria will multiply, and the infection will extend into contiguous viable tissue. At some point, the level of bacteria in the tissue rises to the degree that bacteria enter the systemic circulation. The bloodborne bacteria are initially cleared by the RES. Eventually, the continued bactermia from the uncontrolled local infection results in RES overload, manifested as a secondary decrease in the level of plasma fibronectin. At this point, the clearance of circulating debris and bacteria shifts from the liver to other organs, especially the lung, contributing to pulmonary insufficiency and the development of multiple organ-system failure.

THERAPEUTIC OPTIONS

From the previous discussion, it is clear that a thermal injury is associated with profound changes in many components of the local and systemic antibacterial host defenses. Although the exact importance of each of the burn-induced immune defects to the host's ability to prevent and control bacterial invasion and sepsis is not known, it is reasonable to conclude that each component contributes in some fashion to the host's overall immunological reserve. Furthermore, since the susceptibility to bacterial infections is related not just to the bacterial pathogen, but also to the immune state of the host, therapeutic maneuvers must be directed not just towards the eradication of the invading microbial pathogen, but also toward mechanisms to bolster the host's resistance to infection.

Over the past decade the important relationship between malnutrition, impaired host defenses, and infection has been the focus of intensive investigative efforts. Today we know that the majority of the immunologic abnormalities that occur after a major thermal injury are similar to those associated with protein-calorie malnutrition (Table 15–3).[22, 76, 84, 111] The clinical importance of aggressive nutritional support in improving host defenses and improving survival is clearly documented by the results of a recent prospective study of aggressive nutritional support in burned children.[3] Since immunosuppressive factors have been identified in burned skin,[66, 95] as well as in the sera of burned patients,[20, 26, 109] attempts to improve host defenses by early excision of the burn wound have been carried out. Experimentally, early excision of the burn wound has been shown to reduce the catabolic response, restore immune competence,[46, 53] and increase the resistance of burned animals to infectious challenges.[71] Furthermore, evidence has accumulated indicating that the presence of necrotic tissue may result in the consumption of host-defense factors,[42, 59] as well as be a source of immune-depressant factors.[53, 95] Based on these studies and recent human data documenting that local immunity is impaired at the burn wound,[36] and that excision of the burn eschar improves the immune responsiveness of the burn patient,[101] it is not

TABLE 15–3.
General Trends in Systemic Host Defenses After Thermal Injury or During Malnutrition*

	BURN PATIENT		
	NONSEPTIC	SEPTIC PERIOD	MALNUTRITION
Cellular			
Neutrophil			
Chemotaxis	↓	↓	↓
Phagocytosis	N	N	↓
Bactericidal activity	N, ↓	↓	↓
Lymphocytes			
Endogenous (SBT)	↑	↑	—
Stimulated	N, ↓	N, ↓	N, ↓
Macrophages	↓	↓	↓
Humoral			
Complement	↓→N	↓	↓
Fibronectin	↓→N	↓	↓
Antibody	↓→N	N	N, ↓

*N indicates normal; ↑, increased; ↓, decreased; —, Not Done; → changes to.

surprising that early removal of the burn eschar may reduce the risk of sepsis in the burn patient. Thus, by combining early definitive surgery (to limit the period of stress and remove the burn eschar) with aggressive nutritional support (to improve systemic host defense), the burn surgeon may be able to effectively reduce the risk of infection in the patient with a major thermal injury.

Beginning with the experiments of Jenner in 1798 using cowpox as an immune adjuvant to prevent smallpox, many attempts have been made to bolster host defenses with vaccines, humoral and cellular immune components, as well as immunomodulators.[6, 8, 45, 94] Although this approach has had only limited clinical success, with a better understanding of the effects of burn trauma and infection on the immune system, improved patient resistance to infection by supporting the host's immune and inflammatory defense systems should be possible.

CONCLUSION

Despite the development of "new" and "improved" antimicrobial agents, sepsis remains a common cause of death in the burn patient. This fact is not surprising, since it is of little importance which organism is causing the infection if the patient's intrinsic antibacterial defenses cannot respond. Realization of the limitation of antibiotics has prompted many investigators to study the immune and inflammatory systems in patients sustaining thermal trauma, with the ultimate goal of improving host defenses and increasing survival.

In this chapter, the current literature on burn-induced changes in the local and systemic antibacterial defense systems has been reviewed, stressing human studies over animal experiments when human data were available. From this review, it is clear that thermal injuries are associated with multiple defects of the humoral and cellular components of both the nonspecific host-defense system and the specific immune system. However, no consensus has been reached on the prognostic and clinical significance of many of the described defects. This confusion is compounded by the fact that different laboratories employ different methodologies to measure a specific immune parameter in patients treated with different clinical regimens.

Of potentially greater significance is the fact that in many studies only one immunologic variable was measured. Since immune defects do not occur in isolation, it is difficult to determine whether a particular abnormality is a primary event of clinical importance or secondary to another unmeasured abnormality. We believe that the goals of future studies should be to clarify which immune defects or constellation of defects are due to the stress of the injury versus those that are associated with sepsis or death. This can be accomplished only by performing studies that measure multiple aspects of the defense systems simultaneously. This concept cannot be stressed too strongly, since in vivo the host-defense systems act synergistically to prevent and control infections. Only after the complex interrelationships between the various cellular and humoral components of the host-defense systems are fully understood will the researcher be able to develop specific immunomodulators, which the clinician will be able to use to safely reduce the risk of infection in the burn victim.

REFERENCES

1. Ablin RJ: Immunologic sequelae to thermal injury: I. Frequency and relationship of epithelial antibodies to extent of burn. *Clin Immunol Immunopathol* 1976; 5:195–207.
2. Adler FL: Competition of antigens. *Prog Allergy* 1964; 8:41.
3. Alexander JW, MacMillan BG, Stinnet JD, et al: Beneficial effects of aggressive protein feeding in severely burned children. *Ann Surg* 1980; 192:505–517.
4. Alexander JW, McClellan MA, Ogle CK, et al: Consumptive opsoninopathy: Possible pathogensis in lethal and opportunistic infections. *Ann Surg* 1976; 184:672–678.
5. Alexander JW, Ogle CK, Stinnet JD, et al: A sequential, prospective analysis of immunologic abnormalities in an infection following severe thermal injury. *Ann Surg* 1978; 188:809–816.
6. Alexander JW, Ogle CK, Stinnet JD, et al: Fresh frozen plasma vs. plasma protein derivative as adjunctive therapy for patients with massive burns. *J Trauma* 1979; 19:502–511.
7. Alexander JW, Ogle CK, White SM, et al: The relationship between host-defense variable and infection in severe thermal injury. *Burns* 1978; 5:248–254.
8. Alexander JW, Stinnet JD: Immunotherapeutic approaches to the treatment of infection in the surgical patients, in Simmons RL, Howard RJ (eds): *Surgical Infectious Diseases.* New York, Appleton-Century-Crofts, 1982, pp 417–428.
9. Alexander JW, Stinnet JD, Ogle CK, et al: A comparison of immunologic profiles and their influence on bacteremia in surgical patients with a high risk of infection. *Surgery* 1979; 86:94–104.
10. Allansmith M, McClellan BH, Butterworth M, et al: The development of immunoglobulin levels in man. *J Pediatr* 1968; 72:276–290.
11. Allen RC, Pruitt BA: Humoral-phagocyte axis of immune defense in burn patients. *Arch Surg* 1982; 117:133–140.
12. Antonacci AC, Reaves LE, et al: Flow cytometric analysis of lymphocyte subpopulations after thermal injury in human beings. *Surg Gynecol Obstet* 1984; 159:1–8.
13. Arturson G, Hogman CF, Johansson SG, et al: Changes in immunoglobulin levels in severely burned patients. *Lancet* 1969; 1:546–548.
14. Baker CC, Miller CL, Trunkey DD: Predicting fatal sepsis in burn patients. *J Trauma* 1979; 19:641–648.
15. Bjornson AB, Altemeier WA, Bjornson HS: Reduction in C3 conversion in patients with severe thermal injury. *J Trauma* 1976; 16:905–911.
16. Bjornson AB, Altemeier WA, Bjornson HS: Changes in humoral components of host-defense following burn trauma. *Ann Surg* 1977; 196:88–96.
17. Bjornson AB, Altemeier WA, Bjornson HS, et al: Host-defense against opportunist microorganisms following trauma. *Ann Surg* 1978; 188:93–101.
18. Bjornson AB, Altemeier WA, Bjornson HS: Host defense against opportunist microorganisms following trauma. II. Changes in complement and immunoglobulins in patients with abdominal trauma and in septic patients without trauma. *Ann Surg* 1978; 188:102–108.
19. Bjornson AB, Altemeier WA, Bjornson HS: The septic burned patient. A model for studying the role of complement and immunoglobulins in opsonization of opportunist microorganisms. *Ann Surg* 1979; 189:515–527.
20. Bjornson AB, Bjornson HS, Altemeier WA: Serum-mediated inhibition of polymorpho-

nuclear leukocyte function following burn injury. *Ann Surg* 1981; 194:568–575.

21. Buckley RH, Dees SC, O'Fallon WM: Serum immunoglobulins: I. Levels in normal children and in uncomplicated childhood allergy. *Pediatrics* 1968; 41:600–611.
22. Chandra RK: Nutrition, immunity, and infection: Present knowledge and future directions. *Lancet* 1983; 1:688–691.
23. Chaudry IH, Tabata Y, Schleck S, et al: The effect of splenectomy on reticuloendothelial function and survival following sepsis. *J Trauma* 1980; 20:649–656.
24. Christou NV, McLean APH, Meakins JL: Host defense in blunt trauma: Interrelationships of kinetics of energy and depressed neutrophil function, nutritional status, and sepsis. *J Trauma* 1980; 20:833–841.
25. Cochrane CG, Griffin JH: Molecular assembly in the contact phase of the Hageman factor system. *Am J Med* 1979; 67:657–664.
26. Constantian MB: Association of sepsis with an immunosuppressive polypeptide in the serum of burn patients. *Ann Surg* 1978; 188:209–215.
27. Constantian MB: Impaired reactivity of burn patient lymphocytes to PHA in autologous serum: Failure to improve responsiveness by washing in vitro. *J Surg Res* 1979; 27:84–92.
28. Curreri PW, Heck EL, Brown L, et al: Stimulated nitroblue tetrazolium test to assess neutrophil antibacterial function: Prediction of wound sepis in burned patients. *Surgery* 1973; 74:6–13.
29. Curreri PW, Wilterdink ME, Baxter CR: Characterization of elevated fibrin split products following thermal injury. *Ann Surg* 1975; 181:157–160.
30. Daniels JC, Larson DL, Abston S, et al: Serum protein profiles in thermal burns: I. Serum electrophoretic patterns, immunoglobulins, and transport proteins. *J Trauma* 1974; 14:137–152.
31. Daniels L, Lewis S, Ritzman S: Altered nucleic acid synthesis in lymphocytes from patients with thermal burns. *Surg Gynecol Obstet* 1980; 149:783–788.
32. Davis JM, Dineen P, Gallin JI: Neutrophil degranulation and abnormal chemotaxis after thermal injury. *J Immunol* 1980; 124:1467–1471.
33. Deitch EA: Opsonic activity of blister fluid from burn patients. *Infect Immun* 1983; 41:1184–1189.
34. Deitch EA: Review of the effect of stress and trauma on plasma fibronectin and the reticuloendothelial system. *J Burn Care Rehabil* 1983; 4:344–351.
35. Deitch EA: The relationship between thermal injury and neutrophil membrane functions as measured by chemotaxis, adherence, and spreading. *Burns* 1984; 10:264–270.
36. Deitch EA, Dobke M, Baxter CR: Failure of local immunity. A potential cause of burn wound sepsis. *Arch Surg* 1985; 120:78–84.
37. Deitch EA, Emmett M: Early protein alteration in blister fluid and serum associated with burn injury. *J Trauma* 1986; 26:34–39.
38. Deitch EA, Gelder F, McDonald JC: Biologic effect of blister fluid from thermal injuries on peripheral neutrophil chemotaxis. *J Trauma* 1982; 22:129–133.
39. Deitch EA, Gelder F, McDonald JC: Prognostic significance of abnormal neutrophil chemotaxis after thermal injury. *J Trauma* 1982; 22:199–204.
40. Deitch EA, Gelder F, McDonald JC: Sequential prospective analysis of the nonspecific host-defense system after thermal injury. *Arch Surg* 1984; 119:83–89.
41. Deitch EA, Gelder F, McDonald JC: The role of plasma fibronectin as a nonantibody noncomplement opsonin for *Staphyloccocus aureus*. *J Trauma* 1984; 24:208–213.
42. Deitch EA, Landry KN, McDonald JC: Postburn impaired cell-mediated immunity may not be due to lazy lymphocytes but to overwork. *Ann Surg* 1985; 201:793–802.
43. Deitch EA, McDonald JC: Influence of serum on impaired neutrophil chemotaxis after thermal injury. *J Surg Res* 1982; 33:251–257.
44. Deitch EA, Smith BJ: The effect of blister fluid from thermally injured patients on normal lymphocyte transformation. *J Trauma* 1983; 23:106–110.
45. Donati L, Larrazin A, Signorini M, et al: Preliminary clinical experiences with the use of immunomodulators in burns. *J Trauma* 1983; 23:816–831.
46. Echinard CE, Sajdel-Suklowska E, Burke PA, et al: The beneficial effect of early excision on clinical response and thymic activity after burn injury. *J Trauma* 1982; 22:560–565.
47. Fearon DT, Ruddy S, Schur PH, et al: Activation of the properdin pathway in patients with gram-negative bacteremia. *N Engl J Med* 1975; 292:937–940.
48. Gallin JI, Fauci AS (eds): Lymphoid cells, in *Advances in Host Defense Mechanisms.* New York, Raven Press, 1983, vol 2.
49. Ghebrehiwet B, Silverberg M, Kaplan AP:

Activation of the classical pathway of complement by Hageman Factor fragment (HFf). *J Exp Med* 1981; 153:665–676.

50. Goldman AS, Rudloff HB, McNamee R, et al: Deficiency of plasma humoral recognition factor activity following burn injury. *J. Reticuloendothelial Soc* 1974; 15:193–198.
51. Grogan JB, Miller RC: Impaired function of polymorphonuclear leukocytes in patients with burns and other trauma. *Surg Gynecol Obstet* 1973; 137:784–788.
52. Ham AW, Axelrad AA, Cormack DHH, (eds): *Blood Cell Formation and the Cellular Basis of Immune Response.* JB Lippincott, Co, Philadelphia, 1979, pp 355–364.
53. Hansbrough JF, Peterson V, Kortz E, et al: Postburn immunosuppression in an animal model: Monocyte dysfunction induced by burned tissue. *Surgery* 1983; 93:415–423.
54. Heck EL, Browne L, Curreri PW, et al: Evaluation of leukocyte function in burned individuals by in vitro oxygen consumption. *J Trauma* 1975; 15:486–489.
55. Heck E, Edgar MA, Hunt, JL, et al: A comparison of leukocyte function and burn mortality. *J Trauma* 1980; 20:75–77.
56. Heck EL, Edgar MA, Maste BS, et al: The role of NADH-NADPH oxidase activity in the leukocyte function of burned patients. *J Trauma* 1979; 19:49–51.
57. Heideman M: Complement activation in vitro induced by endotoxin and injured tissue. *J Surg Res* 1979; 26:670–673.
58. Heideman M: The effect of thermal injury on hemodynamic respiratory and hematologic variables in relation to complement activation. *J Trauma* 1979; 19:239–243.
59. Heideman M, Saravis C, Clowes GHA: Effect of nonviable tissue and abscesses on complement depletion and the development of bacteremia. *J Trauma* 1982; 22:527–532.
60. Howard RJ: Effect of burn injury, mechanical trauma, and operation on immune defenses. *Surg Clin North Am* 1979; 59:199–211.
61. Howard RJ: Host-defense against infection. *Curr Probl Surg* 1980; 17:267–317.
62. Hugli TE: Complement anaphylatoxins as plasma mediators, spasmogens and chemotaxins in Reisfeld RA, Mandy WJ (eds): *Current Topics in Molecular Immunology.* New York, Plenum Press, 1979, pp 255–279.
63. Kaplan AP: Initiation of the intrinsic coagulation and fibrinolytic pathways of man: The role of surfaces, Hageman Factor, prekallikrein, high-molecular weight kininogen and Factor XI. *Prog Hemost Thromb* 1978; 4:127–135.
64. Kisielow P, et al: Ly antigens as markers for functionally distinct subpopulations of thymus-derived lymphocytes of the mouse. *Nature* 1975; 253:219.
65. Klebanoff SJ, Clark RA: Phagocytosis, in Klebanoff SJ, Clark RA (eds). *The Neutrophil: Function and Clinical Disorders.* New York, North-Holland Publishing Co., 1980, pp 163–217.
66. Kremer B, Allgower M, et al: The present status of research in burn toxins. *Intensive Care Med* 1981; 7:77–81.
67. Lanser ME, Saba TM: Fibronectin as a cofactor necessary for optimal granulocyte phagocytosis of *Staphylococcus aureus. J Reticuloendothelial Soc* 1981; 30:415–424.
68. Lanser ME, Saba TM: Neutrophil-mediated lung localization of bacteria: A mechanism for pulmonary injury. *Surgery* 1981; 90:473–481.
69. Lanser ME, Saba TM, Scovill WA: Opsonic glycoprotein (plasma fibronectin) levels after burn injury. *Ann Surg* 1980; 192:776–782.
70. Lawler SD, Ukaejiojo EO, Reeves BR: Interaction of maternal and neonatal cells in mixed lymphocyte culture. *Lancet* 1975; 2:1185–1187.
71. Levine NS, Salisbury RE, Mason AD: The effect of early surgical excision and homografting on survival of burned rats and of intraperitoneally-infected burned rats. *Plast Reconstr Surg* 1975; 56:423–429.
72. Loegering BJ: Hemolysis following thermal injury and depression of reticuloendothelial system phagocytic function. *J Trauma* 1981; 21:130–134.
73. Mahler D, Batchelor JR: Phytohemagglutinin transformation of lymphocytes in burned patients. *Transplantation* 1971; 12:409–411.
74. McIrvine AJ, O'Mahoney JC, Saporoschetz I, et al: Use of monoclonal antibodies and functional assays to define the role of suppressor cells. *Ann Surg* 1982; 196:297–304.
75. Meakins JL, Christou NV, Shizhal HM, et al: Therapeutic approaches to anergy in surgical patients: Surgery and levamisole. *Ann Surg* 1978; 190:286–296.
76. Miller CL: Immunological assays as measurements of nutritional status: A review. *J Parenter Enteral Nut* 1978; 2:554–566.
77. Miller CL, Baker CC: Changes in lymphocyte activity after thermal injury: The role of suppressor cells. *J Clin Invest* 1979; 63:202–210.
78. Miller ME: Current topics in host defenses of the newborn. *Adv Pediatr* 1978; 29:59–95.
79. Morrison DC, Cochrane CG: Direct evidence for Hageman factor (Factor XII) acti-

vation by bacterial lipopolysaccharides (endotoxins). *J Exp Med* 1974; 140:797–811.

80. Munster AM, Lancet I: Posttraumatic immunosuppression is due to activation of suppressor T-cells. *Lancet* 1976; 1:1329.
81. Munster AM, Winchurch RA, Birmingham WJ et al: Longitudinal assay of lymphocyte responsiveness in patients with major burns. *Ann Surg* 1980; 192:772–775.
82. Ninnemann JL: Immunosuppression following thermal injury through B cell activation of suppressor T-cells. *J Trauma* 1980; 20:206–213.
83. Ninnemann JL, Fisher JC, Wachtel TL: Thermal injury-associated immunosuppression: Occurrence and in vitro blocking effect of post recovery system. *J Immunol* 1979; 122:1736–1741.
84. O'Mahony JB, McIrvine AJ, Palder SB, et al: The effect of short-term postoperative intravenous feeding upon cell-mediated immunity and serum suppressive activity in well-nourished patients. *Surg Gynecol Obstet* 1984; 159:27–32.
85. Pearson G, Nakamura M, Heck E, et al: Impaired oxygen consumption activity of neutrophils by inhibitor(s) in burn sera. *J Burn Care Rehabil* 1982; 208–211.
86. Ransjo U, Atrurson G, Hakansson L, et al: Some aspects of neutrophil granulocyte function in burn patients. *Burns* 1978; 5:255–259.
87. Rebuck JW, Crowley JH: A method of studying leukocyte function in vivo. *Ann NY Acad Sci* 1955; 59:757–807.
88. Reinherz EL, et al: Separation of functional subsets of human T-cells by a monoclonal antibody. *Proc Natl Acad Sci USA* 1979; 76:4061–4065.
89. Reinherz EL, Schlossman SF: Regulation of the immune response-inducer and suppressor T-lymphocyte subsets in human beings. *N Engl J Med* 1980; 303:370–373.
90. Robb JR: Interleukin 2: The molecule and its function. *Immunol Today* 1984; 5:203–209.
91. Robbins AC, Doran JE, Reese AC, et al: Clinical response to cold insoluble globulin replacement patient with sepsis and thermal injury. *Am J Surg* 1981; 142:636–638.
92. Roe EA, Jones RJ: The NBT test in burned patients. *Br J Exp Pathol* 1979; 60:167–170.
93. Rosenthal SR: Burn toxin and its competition. *Burns* 1982; 8:215–219.
94. Saba TM, Blumenstock FA, Scovill WA, et al: Cryoprecipitate reversal of opsonic 2-surface binding glycoprotein deficiency in septic surgical and trauma patients. *Science* 1978; 201:622–624.
95. Schonenberger GA, Burkhardt F, Kalberer F, et al.: Experimental evidence for a significant impairment of host defense for gram-negative organisms by a specific cutaneous toxin produced by severe burn injuries. *Surg Gynecol Obstet* 1975; 141:555–561.
96. Scovill WA, Annest SJ, Saba TM, et al.: Cardiovascular hemodynamics after opsonic α_2-surface binding glycoprotein therapy in injured patients. *Surgery* 1979; 86:284–293.
97. Shorr RM, Erschler WB, Gamelli RL: Immunoglobulin production in burned patients. *J Trauma* 1984; 24:319–322.
98. Solomkin JL, Simmons RL: Cellular and subcellular mediators of acute inflammation. *Surg Clin North Am* 1983; 63:225–243.
99. Solomkin JS, Jenkins MK, Nelson RD et al: Neutrophil dysfunction in sepsis: II. Evidence for the role of complement activation products in cellular deactivation. *Surgery* 1981; 90:319–327.
100. Solomkin JS, Nelson RD, Chenoweth DE et al: Regulation of neutrophil migratory function in burn injury by complement activation products. *Ann Surg* 1984; 200:742–746.
101. Stratta RJ, Saffle JR, Ninneman JL, et al: The effect of surgical trauma and grafting procedures on postburn lymphocyte suppression. *J Trauma* 1985; 25:46–52.
102. Sukhtankar AY, Sengupta SR: Cellular immunity in burns. *Burns* 1982; 8:168–171.
103. Sundsmo JS: The leukocyte complement system. *Fed Proc* 1982; 41:3094–3098.
104. Verbrugh HA, Peterson RK, Smith DE, et al: Human fibronectin binding to staphylococcal surface protein and its relative inefficiency in promoting phagocytosis by human polymorphonuclear leukocytes, monocytes, and alveolar macrophages. *Infect Immunol* 1981; 33:811–819.
105. Warden GD, Mason AD, Pruitt BA: Suppression of leukocyte chemotaxis in vitro by chemotherapeutic agents used in management of thermal injuries. *Ann Surg* 1975; 181:363–369.
106. Weigle WO, Morgan EL, Goodman MG, et al: Modulation of the immune response by anaphylatoxin in the microenvironment of the interacting cells. *Fed Proc* 1982; 41:3099–3103.
107. Weiler JM, Ballas ZK, Neddleman BW, et al: Complement fragments suppress lymphocyte immune response. *Immunol Today* 1982; 3:238–242.
108. Wolfe JN, O'Connor NE, Young AE, et al: Relative clinical importance of serum sup-

pressor substances and cellular suppression in major burns. *Surg Forum* 1980; 31:58–61.
109. Wolfe JN, Saporoschetz AB, Young AE, et al: Suppressive serum, suppressor lymphocytes, and death from burns. *Ann Surg* 1981; 193:513–520.
110. Wood J, Roderick M, O'Mahony J, et al: Inadequate interleukin-2 production: A fundamental immunological deficiency in patients with major burns. *Ann Surg* 1984; 200:311–320.
111. Wunder JA, Stinnet JD, Alexander JW: The effects of malnutrition on variables of host defense in the guinea pig. *Surgery* 1978; 84:542–550.
112. Yetgin S: Bactericidal function of neutrophils in burned patients. *Burns* 1979; 5:188–191.

16 / The Burn Wound: Microbiological Aspects

IAN ALAN HOLDER, Ph.D.

Infection is a major complication of burn injury and is responsible for between 50% to 75% of in-hospital deaths.[11] The moist, thermally coagulated burn wound, with its constantly replenished supply of diffusing serum nutrients and its warm surface temperature, provides an environment conducive to rapid microbial growth. As the local microbial growth increases, the potential for invasion of subjacent viable tissue and penetration into the circulation increases. Once the organisms gain access to the bloodstream, foci of infection far removed from the initial site of microbial colonization can be established, and their continued, uninterrupted growth may lead to a septic condition.

HISTORICAL PERSPECTIVE

The microorganisms that cause burn wound infections have changed over the years. To a large extent, these changes have been related to the advances made in the treatment of burn patients. The various organisms causing burn wound sepsis and mortality and their relationship to available antimicrobial therapy are presented graphically in Figure 16–1.

In the preantibiotic era, before accurate knowledge of the fluid and electrolyte requirements of burn patients were realized, burn victims died early as a result of hypovolemia and burn shock. Those patients who survived the acute burn-shock phase of their injury became infected by overt gram-positive bacterial pathogens, β-hemolytic *Streptococcus* and *Staphylococcus aureus*.[6, 32, 40, 53] With the exception of an occasional report of gram-negative bacteria causing infection in burn patients,[25, 35] these two gram-positive bacteria continued to be the most troublesome burn wound infections until the 1950s. During the latter 1940s and early 1950s, improvements in fluid therapy and the introduction of penicillin made their effects felt in the treatment of infections in burn patients. Burn patients no longer died as readily from acute burn shock, and infections with streptococci were successfully treated with penicillin. Initially, staphylococcal infections could be treated with penicillin as well, and those penicillin-resistant strains could be treated with broad-spectrum antibiotics, which were introduced soon after penicillin. Subsequently, these strains were treated with penicillinase-resistant penicillins.

A "new" burn patient evolved at this time—a patient who survived the early acute shock phase of thermal injury, whose gram-positive bacterial infections could be controlled with penicillin-class antibiotics, and who, though immunologically compromised, could be kept alive by technical advances in therapy and treatment. In this environment new infectious threats to the burn patient arose, i.e., the opportunistic gram-negative pathogens *Escherichia coli*, *Klebsiella-Enterobacter*, *Proteus* and, especially, *Pseudomonas aeruginosa*. In 1952, Jawetz[26] observed that "*Pseudomonas aeruginosa* was not a true common pathogen but behaved as an 'opportunist' causing true infections only under conditions of impaired host resistance." A 1957 study of

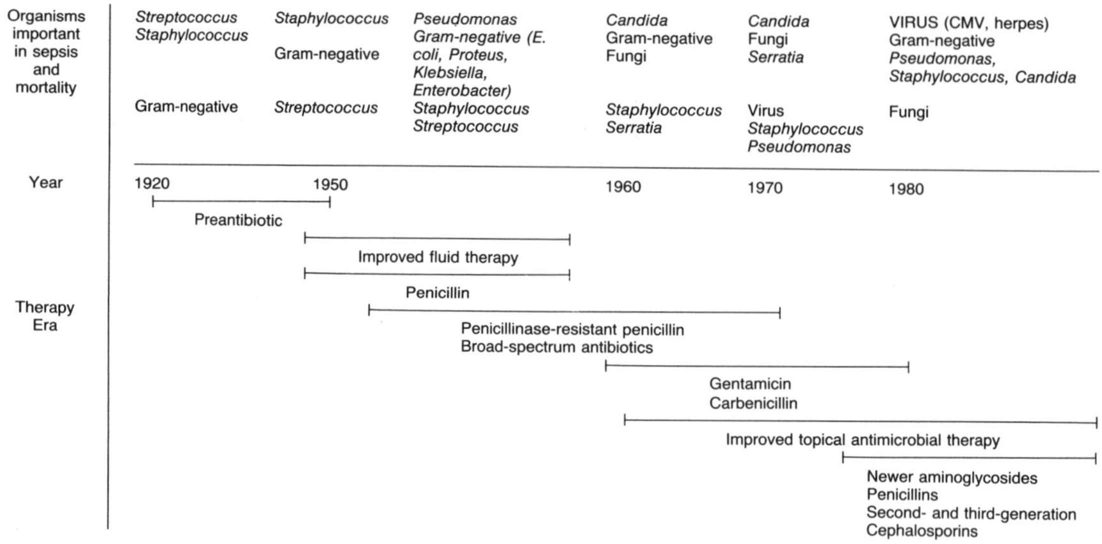

FIG 16–1.
Various organisms causing burn wound sepsis and mortality and their relationship to available antimicrobial therapy during different eras.

172 children and 103 adults with burns of 10% or more of the body surface revealed that *P. aeruginosa* infection was the major cause of death in patients surviving the initial 48 hours postinjury.[43] It was reported also that the continued use of prophylactic antibiotics favored earlier and more severe *Pseudomonas* sepsis[65] and that penicillin therapy given to patients with pulmonary burns played an important role in the selection of gram-negative infections among those patients.[69] With the introduction of newer antimicrobials and antibiotics for specific systemic and topical use for the treatment of *Pseudomonas* infections, reports of more infections and deaths from other gram-negative bacteria (*E. coli, Klebsiella-Enterobacter, Proteus mirabilis,* etc.) appeared.[5, 69] A high mortality from *Serratia marcescens* bacteremia in burn patients was also reported.[18]

The era of modern antimicrobial therapeutics resulted in additional changes. Not only was the list of genera of bacteria infecting the burn patient altered, but a set of circumstances was established that predisposed the burn patient to a new threat—infection by opportunistic fungi. Dennis et al.[8] called attention to *Candida* septicemia in severely traumatized patients, including burned patients. A study of burns in military personnel over a period of several years found that fungal infection was present in 25% of patients autopsied from 1960 to 1963, compared with 64% of autopsied cases from 1964 to 1967. The predominant organism isolated was *Candida*, but *Aspergillus*, *Mucor* and *Geotrichum* were also found.[3, 62] While *Candida albicans* caused the most severe systemic infections, *Candida tropicalis* and *Candida parapsilosis* were found to be causes of fungal sepsis and mortality in burn patients.[33, 42, 64] We have also recently isolated *Candida lusitaniae* from the blood of one of our patients. (The patient was treated with a course of amphotericin B therapy and recovered.)

In the past 25 years, reports of viral infections (herpes, cytomegalovirus [CMV] and adenovirus) have appeared in the literature, but their clinical significance remains to be elucidated.[28, 37, 67] For additional information on viral infections in burned children, see Chapter 17.

CONTEMPORARY MICROBIOLOGY

As is evident in Table 16–1, the types of microorganisms associated with burn infections are circumscribed. Few, if any, frank enteric, pulmonary, or sexually transmitted bacterial or fungal pathogens are included. *Staphylococcus aureus* is the most frequently isolated organism, followed by *P. aeruginosa*, enterococcus, and a variety of gram-negative opportunists. The isolation and identification of these organisms pose no real challenge to the microbiology laboratory. The figures in Table 16–1 reflect averages from a number of reporting institutions; it must be kept in mind, however, that each burn treatment facility is its own microcosm. While each institution may isolate organisms that would be found at any other burn unit, the microflora present at any one institution is influenced by treatment modalities used at that institution and by their choice of antibiotics. Therefore, when considering the microorganisms involved in burn infections, we must do so with the understanding that there are individual as well as institutional variations.

TABLE 16–1.

Distribution of 648 Microorganisms Recovered From Infected Burns (National Nosocomial Infection Study 1980–1982)

ORGANISMS	NO. RECOVERED	% OF TOTAL
Staphylococcus aureus	157	24.2
Pseudomonas aeruginosa	135	20.8
Enterococci	76	11.7
Escherichia coli	50	7.7
Enterobacter cloacae	50	7.7
Serratia marcescens	39	6.0
Klebsiella sp.	22	3.4
Staphylococcus epidermidis	19	2.9
Candida albicans	14	2.3
Proteus sp.	12	1.9
Nonenterococcal streptococci	12	1.9
Pseudomonas sp.	6	0.9
Anaerobes	6	0.9
Acinetobacter sp.	5	0.8
Aspergillus sp.	4	0.6
Candida (nonalbicans)	3	0.5
Providencia sp.	2	0.3
Other bacteria	28	4.3
Other fungi	8	1.2

At the Shriner's Burns Institute, Cincinnati, with the exception of S. *aureus*, the percentage of specific bacteria and fungi recovered from burn wounds was significantly reduced between the years 1964 to 1983 (Table 16–2). This reduction reflects improvements in patient management, advances in local wound care, and improved topical antimicrobial therapy. The percentage of pneumonias has declined over these years, but the percentages of urinary tract infection and septicemias have remained relatively constant (Table 16–3). Improved treatment, which allows patients with larger burns and, hence, greater immunologic compromise to survive for longer periods of time, would explain this apparent inconsistency.

From 1979 to 1983, the average percentages of septicemia caused by gram-positive bacteria, gram-negative bacteria, and fungi (*Candida* only) were 70, 13, and 13, respectively. Only one third of these cases were confirmed by positive blood culture. Therefore, most cases of septicemia are diagnosed on clinical grounds and treated on the basis of microorganisms most frequently on the burn wounds. Usually, a combination of an aminoglycoside and extended-range penicillin is used to give broadest bacterial coverage. If fungi are colonizing the burn wound, and culture results, e.g., stool or urine, indicate that they are in other sites as well, a course of amphotericin B treatment may be initiated. This has been a relatively successful approach to identifying and treating septic patients since septic deaths have been reduced by approximately one half between the periods 1964–1968 and 1979–1983 (Table 16–4). Table 16–2 shows that S. *aureus* is the most commonly isolated bacterium in burn infections. While gram-positive bacteria (mainly S. *aureus*) cause the highest percentage of septicemia in our hospital (average for the period 1979 to 1983, 70%), the data in Table 16–4 suggest that the antibiotics available to treat gram-positive bacterial sepsis provide a successful

TABLE 16–2.
Organisms Recovered From Burn Wounds of 1,752 Patients With Acute Burn Wound Sepsis (Shriners Burns Institute, Cincinnati Unit)

	1964–1968	1969–1973	1974–1978	1979–1983
No. of admissions	241	399	498	614
Organism, % recovered				
Staphylococcus aureus	78	66	77	77
β-hemolytic *Streptococcus*	17	7	5	6
Other *Streptococcus*	70	59	54	46
Pseudomonas aeruginosa	70	56	30	22
Klebsiella-Enterobacter	59	57	27	23
Escherichia coli	64	55	42	24
Proteus sp.	29	27	27	15
Other gram-negative	51	29	27	15
Candida sp.	68	61	34	13
Candida albicans	46	44	35	17

outcome most of the time. On the other hand, sepsis with gram-negative bacteria accounted for only 13% of total cases of septicemia but caused 84% of deaths due to sepsis. Of the gram-negative bacteria involved in deaths due to sepsis, the vast majority (66%) were caused by *P. aeruginosa*. These statistics reflect both the unique host-parasite interaction which occurs between the burned patient and *P. aeruginosa*,[21] as well as the genetic "plasticity" of *P. aeruginosa*, which allows it to develop mechanisms of resistance to a wide variety of new antibiotics and other antimicrobial agents.

In the past few years, invasive burn wound sepsis with high (86%) mortality has been reported to be caused by *Enterobacter cloacae*.[10, 49] In addition, outbreaks of, and overall increases in, infections caused by *Acinetobacter* have been found in some burn units.[15, 58] Experience has shown that enterococcal bacteremia from burn wounds is a bad prognostic sign in these patients.[60] These organisms may be among the new, emerging microbial threats to the burn patient in the decade of the 1980s.

TOPICAL ANTIMICROBIAL SUSCEPTIBILITY TESTING

The introduction in the mid-1960s of 0.5% silver-nitrate solution and mafenide acetate for topical use in controlling microbial growth heralded the modern era of topical treatment of burn wounds.[47, 48] Since that time a wide variety of topical antimicrobial agents, including gentamicin, nitrofurazone, silver sulfadiazine, and povidone-iodine have become available.[9, 12, 39] As each topical agent became available, it gained proponents who fre-

TABLE 16–3.
Infections Associated With Burns in 1,752 Acutely Burned Patients (Shriners Burns Institute, Cincinnati Unit)

	1964–1968	1969–1973	1974–1978	1979–1983
No. of admissions	241	399	498	614
Infection, no. (%)				
Septicemia	74 (31)	87 (22)	121 (24)	175 (29)
Pneumonia	38 (16)	38 (10)	53 (11)	55 (9)
Urinary tract infections	23 (10)	28 (7)	46 (9)	52 (9)

TABLE 16–4.
Death Due to Sepsis in 70 Patients (Shriners Burns Institute, Cincinnati Unit)*

	1964–1968	1969–1973	1974–1978	1979–1983	TOTAL
Deaths due to sepsis	25	17	14	14	70
Organism					
Staphylococcus aureus	3	1	5	2	11
Pseudomonas aeruginosa	21	5	5	8	39
Klebsiella-Enterobacter	1	2	1	—	4
Escherichia coli	—	1	—	1	5
Serratia sp.	—	—	—	1	1
Candida sp.	—	8	—	2	10

*From Holder I, Schwab M, Jackson L: Eighteen months of routine topical antimicrobial susceptibility testing of isolates from burn patients: Results and conclusions. *J Antimicrob Chemother* 1979; 5:455–463. Used by permission.

quently used such topicals exclusively for all burn wound treatment. However, studies that compared different agents showed that some were more effective against some microorganisms and less so against others.[39, 41] Furthermore, potential problems have been reported in the use of each agent, and none is uniformly effective.[20, 22, 27, 30, 31, 50, 59, 61] In addition, development of resistant microorganisms has been observed with the continued use of certain topicals including mafenide acetate, gentamicin, nitrofurazone, and silver sulfadiazine.[2, 16, 19, 22] The use of silver sulfadiazine and nitrofurazone on an alternate 8-hour basis has been recommended to obviate some of the problems just discussed.[40, 55] Despite this, most burn units still use one topical agent exclusively to treat all wounds on all patients, regardless of the type of microorganism(s) colonizing and possibly infecting the wound. The most commonly used topical agent today is silver sulfadiazine.

In 1978, an agar-well diffusion topical antimicrobial test assay was described.[50] According to this method, samples of various topical antimicrobials are placed in wells (cut with a sterile cork borer) in an agar plate. A tube of melted agar, cooled to 50°C, is inoculated with the test organism and is used to overlay the antimicrobial-containing plate, thus inoculating the plate and sealing the antimicrobials in the wells. After incubation at 37°C for 24 hours, the plate is read. A clear zone around the antimicrobial test well indicates that the test organism is susceptible to the topical agent, while the absence of any clear zone shows that the organism is resistant. An example of such an assay is shown in Figure 16–2. The results of these test assays were shown to correlate well with the effectiveness of the topical agent in clinical use. This assay system has been used routinely in our institution since 1978, and we have determined that a proportion of all bacterial strains tested are resistant to the action of one or more of the most commonly used topical antimicrobial agents (Table 16–5).[22] The assay system has been used to compare the activities of new topical antimicrobials with those already in current use.[20, 22] Results from such testing can inform the clinician as to which of the various topical agents that are available for clinical use should not be used (the infecting microorganism is resistant to their action). Testing also identifies the topical agent most likely to accomplish the intended goal. The use of the most appropriate topical antimicrobial to inhibit the growth of the specific microorganism colonizing each burn wound would restrict the overall usage of any one agent, thereby reducing the environmental pressure on the microflora to develop resistance to any one topical agent.

It seems incongruous that the burn sur-

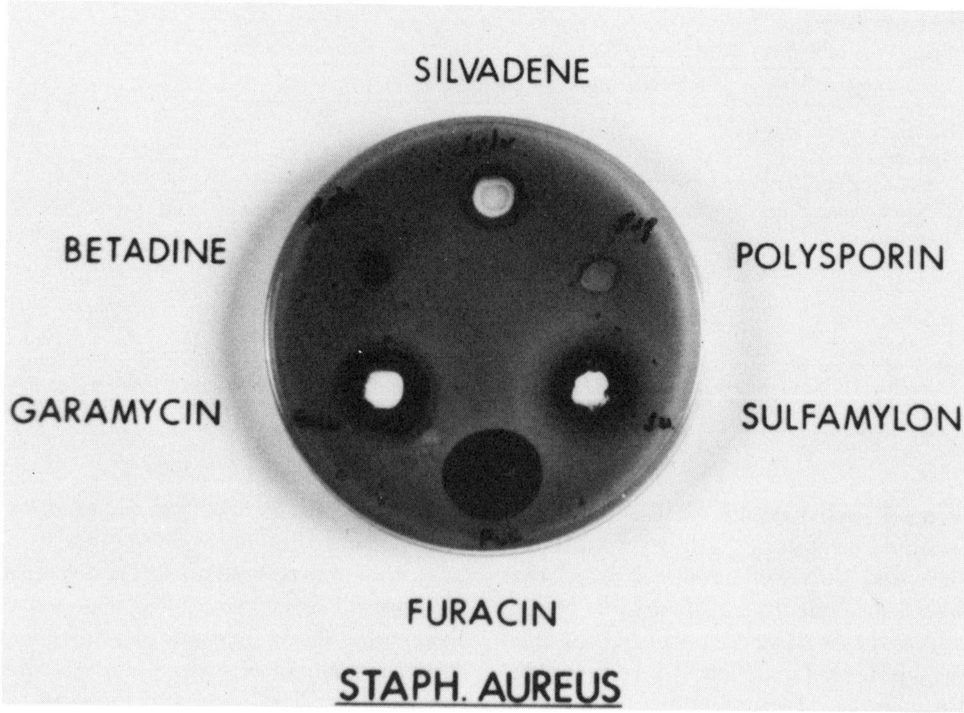

FIG 16–2.
Topical antibiotic sensitivity test assay of *S. aureus* against six topical antimicrobial agents. Clear zones around the antimicrobial-containing well (gentamicin sulfate [Garamycin], nitrofurazone [Furacin] and mafenide [Sulfamylon]) indicate that the test organism is susceptible to the action of the antimicrobial, whereas microbial growth up to the edge of the well (povidone-iodine [Betadine], silver sulfadiazine [Silvadene], and bacitracin zinc–polymyxin B sulfate [Polysporin]) indicates resistance.

geon, who insists on susceptibility testing to help in the decision as to the most appropriate parenteral antimicrobial agent to use for sepsis, should blindly use the one "house" topical antimicrobial agent when a method to make a more educated selection is available. This or similar methods may not be ideal, but they are better than the current "house" topical approach. While it is recognized that topical susceptibility testing may not be feasible at some institutions, whenever possible it should be used.

TO QUANTITATE OR NOT TO QUANTITATE?

The classical studies of Teplitz et al.[66] established the course of invasion of microorganisms from the burn eschar surface into adjacent or subjacent tissues, into deeper unburned tissues, and then into the circulation to cause burn wound sepsis. Their data showed that burn wound sepsis occurred only when eschar counts exceeded 10^5 microorganisms/gm of tissue, wet weight. Because of this, various methods to quantitate the number of microorganisms infecting burn wound tissue have been proposed. Brentano and Gravens[1] and Serafinska et al.[57] quantified sterile, saline-soaked gauze pads (gauze capillarity method) placed on the burn wound surface for varying periods of time. A moist-surface swab procedure was compared with the gauze capillarity method, and no difference was reported in the numbers of bacteria recovered.[13, 14] Using a surface-wash technique

TABLE 16–5.
Comparison of Susceptibility/Resistance Patterns When Various Topical Antimicrobial Agents Are Tested Against a Variety of Microorganisms

		TOPICAL AGENTS TESTED							
		NITROFURAZONE OINTMENT, %		SILVER SULFADIAZINE, %		MAFENIDE ACETATE, %		GENTAMICIN, %	
ORGANISMS	NO. OF ISOLATES TESTED	S*	R*	S	R	S	R	S	R
S. aureus	96	100	0	94.8	5.2	94.8	5.2	60.4	39.6
Enterococcus	32	68.8	31.2	65.6	34.4	100	0	93.8	6.2
P. aeruginosa	40	0	100	87.5	12.5	100	0	97.5	2.5
E. coli	25	100	0	92.0	8	56	44	100	0
Miscellaneous gram-negative organisms*	24	87.5	12.5	87.5	12.5	75	25	100	0

*S indicates susceptible, R, resistant, gram-negative organisms include *Proteus* sp., *Enterobacter* sp., and *Klebsiella* sp.

in a surgical wound infection model, McRipley and Whitney[46] found that surface wound counts reflected the dynamics of total wound counts as determined by homogenization of biopsied tissue. Others[56] reported that surface-wash procedures recovered 90% of the bacteria placed on a surgically induced surface wound and that homogenization of the infected tissue after the wash procedure recovered the additional 10% but that homogenization of the tissue without washing permitted only 60% recovery. The same authors showed that the moist-surface swab procedure recovered only 10% of the total bacteria present. On the other hand, a moist swab wound-surface quantitative culture method was used with success to follow the clinical efficacy of topical antimicrobial therapy.[50]

While a variety of other methods, including quantitative gram-stain and slide procedures[17, 71] and histologic evaluation of biopsies[29, 52] have been proposed, the most common quantitative wound culture method is biopsy.[34, 38, 39, 55] In these procedures, homogenization of the biopsied burned tissue precedes dilution and plate counting. A wide variety of homogenization apparatuses have been used, but in a recent evaluation of several types of homogenizers, Spengler et al.[63] recommended the Polytron tissue grinder. Whatever homogenization method is used, consistency and standardization of techniques is essential.

The necessity for, and reliability of, quantitative biopsies of burn wounds has come into question recently. Advances in management of the burn wound (aggressive debridement, early tangential excision, nutritional support, and patient-individualized topical antimicrobial therapy) have reduced the numbers of microorganisms in the burn wound and thus the necessity for quantitative assay.[24] We have not used quantitative culturing for a decade and do not feel that its elimination has had a negative impact on overall patient care or survival from infection. In addition to clinical-care improvements, which have reduced the importance of quantitative biopsy cultures, the reproducibility of these techniques has been questioned. While Volenec et al.[68] examined sequential, paired biopsy samples taken from three separate locations on each of four burn patients and found that skin biopsy was a reliable procedure for quantitating organisms, Woolfrey, et al.[70] used divided biopsy samples and observed that only 38% of paired quantitative results agreed within the same $\log_{10}$ units. Thus, even though the controversy lingers on, the questions that have been raised are based on sound experimental data and should be closely examined. The final decision, however, must await further studies on the subject. (For a full discussion on the subject, the reader is referred to the *Clinical Microbiology Newsletter* 1983; 5:51–52 and 1984; 6:21–23.)

CONCLUSIONS

The microorganisms of importance in causing burn wound infections have changed over the years. In most cases, the changes have occurred in relationship to technologic advances in overall patient care and antimicrobial therapy. These advances will continue, and new organisms will emerge as important pathogens to the burned patient. Because of this, no organism found in the patient's wounds or other tissues should be taken lightly. Such may represent a contaminant, but it may also presage an emerging burn wound pathogen. Furthermore, we must understand that while certain microorganisms are more likely to be associated with burn patients, each unit will generate its own flora, which will be modified by its own treatment and antibiotic policies. Thus, the latter must be considered whenever microbial control techniques are being evaluated.

Finally, an open mind must be kept to allow new ideas. The "use of only one topical antimicrobial" and the "we must do quantitative wound biopsy" dogma must be reevaluated in light of more current information. Whatever decisions are made in that regard must be based on current information, rather than traditional guidelines.

REFERENCES

1. Brentano L, Gravens DL: A method for the quantitation of bacteria in burn wounds. *Appl Microb* 1967; 15:670.
2. Bridges K, Lowbury EJ: Drug resistance in relation to use of silver sulfadiazine cream in a burns unit. *J Clin Pathol* 1977; 30:160–164.
3. Bruck HM, et al: Opportunistic fungal infection of the burn wound with phycomycetes and *Aspergillus*. *Arch Surg* 1972; 102:476.
4. Butcher H, Margraf H, Gravens D: The treatment of large cutaneous burns with silver creams. *J Trauma* 1969; 9:359.
5. Cason KS, Lowbury EJ: Mortality and infection in extensively burned patients treated with silver nitrate compresses. *Lancet* 1968; 1:651.
6. Cruickshank R: The bacterial infection of burns. *J Pathol* 1935; 41:367.
7. Davis B, Lilly H, Lowbury E: Gram-negative bacilli in burns. *J Clin Pathol* 1969; 22:634.
8. Dennis D, Peterson C, Fletcher W: *Candida* septicemia in the severely traumatized patient. *J Trauma* 1968; 8:177.
9. Fox J, Rappole B, Stanford W: Control of pseudomonas infections in burns by silver sulfadiazine. *Surg Gynecol Obstet* 1969; 128:1021–1026.
10. Gayle WE, et al: Resistant *E. cloacae* in a burn center: The ineffectiveness of silver sulfadiazine. *J Trauma* 1978; 13:317.
11. Gelfand JA: Infections in burn patients: A paradigm for cutaneous infections in the patient at risk. *Am J Med* 1984; 76(suppl): 158–165.
12. Georgiade N, Georgiade R, Garrett W: The use of new potent topical antibacterial agent for the control of infection in the burn wound. *Plast Reconstr Surg* 1967; 39:349–356.
13. Georgiade NG, Lucas MC, Osterhout S: A comparison of methods for quantitation of bacteria in burn wounds: II. Clinical evaluation. *Am J Clin Pathol* 1969; 3:40.
14. Georgiade NG, Lucas MC, Osterhout S: A comparison of methods for quantitation of bacteria in burn wounds. *Am J Clin Pathol* 1970; 5:40.
15. Green AR, Milling MAP: Infection with *Acinetobacter* in a burn unit. *Burns* 1983; 9:292–294.
16. Heggers JP, Robson MC: The emergence of silver sulfadiazine-resistant *Pseudomonas aeruginosa*. *Burns* 1978; 5:184–187.
17. Heggers JP, Robson MC, Doran ET: Quantitative assessment of bacterial contamination of open wounds by a slide technique. *Trans R Soc Trop Med Hyg* 1969; 63:532–534.
18. Henjyoji EY, et al: Bacteremia due to *Serratia marcescens*. *J Trauma* 1971; 11:417.
19. Holder IA: Gentamicin resistant *Pseudomonas aeruginosa* in a burns unit. *J Antimicrob Chemother* 1976; 2:309–311.
20. Holder IA: In vitro susceptibility of organisms isolated from burns to topical cotrimox-

azole. *J Antimicrob Chemother* 1981; 7:623–627.

21. Holder IA: The pathogenesis of infections owing to *Pseudomonas aeruginosa* using the burned mouse model: Experimental studies from the Shriner's Burns Institute, Cincinnati. *Can J Microbiol* 1985; 31:393–402.
22. Holder I, Schwab M, Jackson L: Eighteen months of routine topical antimicrobial susceptibility testing of isolates from burn patients: Results and conclusions. *J Antimicrob Chemother* 1979; 5:455–463.
23. Holder IA, Vanderpool L, Wesselmann J: Para-chloro-meta-xylenol (PCMX): A new, potential topical antimicrobial agent. *J Burn Care Rehabil* 1985; 6:58–61.
24. Horton RC, et al: Influence of early excision and closure, nutritional, topical, and systemic antibacterials on burn wound infection. *Bull Clin Rev Burn Injuries* 1984; 1:26–27.
25. Jackson D, Lowbury E, Topley E: *Pseudomonas pyocyanea* in burns: Its role as a pathogen, and the value of local polymyxin therapy. *Lancet* 1951; 2:137.
26. Jawetz E: Infections with *Pseudomonas aeruginosa* treated with polymyxin B. *Arch Intern Med* 1952; 89:90.
27. Jerrett F, Ellerbe S, Demling R: Acute leukopenia during topical burn therapy with silver sulfadiazine. *J Antimicrob Chemother* 1978; 136:818–819.
28. Kagan RJ, et al: Herpes simplex virus and cytomegalovirus infections in burned patients. *J Trauma* 1985; 25:40–45.
29. Kim SH, et al: Use of frozen section technique for burn wound biopsies: Comparison with standard rapid section techniques. Presented at the 15th Annual Meeting of the American Burn Association. New Orleans, La, 1983.
30. Koch AE, Burchall JJ: Reversal of the antimicrobial activity of trimethoprim by thymidine in commercially prepared media. *Appl Microb* 1971; 22:812–817.
31. Kulich MI, et al: Hyperosmolality in the burn patient: Analysis of an osmolal discrepancy. *J Trauma* 1979; 20:223–228.
32. Langhor J, Owen C, Cope O: Bacteriologic study of burn wounds. *Ann Surg* 1947; 125:452.
33. Law E, Holder I, MacMillan B: *Candida parapsilosis* fungemia in burned patients: Three case reports. *Burns* 1984; 10:203.
34. Lawrence JC, Lilly HA: A quantitative method for investigating the bacteriology of skin: Its application to burns. *Br J Exp Pathol* 1972; 53:550.
35. Liedberg N, Reiss E, Artz C: Infection in burns: III. Septicemia, a common cause of death. *Surg Gynecol Obstet* 1954; 99:151.
36. Lindberg RB et al: Hospital epidemics of *Pseudomonas aeruginosa* resistant to therapy in burn patients, abstract 13. Proceedings of the 7th Annual Meeting of the American Burn Association, Denver, Colo, 1975, p 45.
37. Linnemann CC, MacMillan BG: Viral infections in pediatric burn patients. *Am J Dis Child* 1981; 135:750–753.
38. Loebl EC, Marvin JA, Heck EL, et al: The use of quantitative biopsy cultures in bacteriologic monitoring of burn patients. *J Surg Res* 1974; 16:1–5.
39. Loebl EC, Marvin JA, Heck EL, et al: The method of quantitative burn-wound biopsy cultures and its routine use in the care of the burned patient. *Am J Clin Pathol* 1974; 61:20–24.

39a. Lowbury E, Oxon D, Jackson D: Local chemoprophylaxis for burns with gentamicin and other agents. *Lancet* 1968; 30:654–657.

40. Lynch JB, et al: Changing patterns of mortality in burns. *Plast Reconstr Surg* 1971; 48:329.
41. MacMillan BG: Ecology of bacteria colonizing the burned patient given topical and systemic gentamicin therapy: A five-year study. *J Infect Dis* 1971; 124:5278–5286.
42. MacMillan B, Law E, Holder I: Experience with *Candida* infections in the burn patient. *Arch Surg* 1972; 104:509.
43. Markley K, et al: Fatal pseudomonas septicemia in burned patients. *Ann Surg* 1957; 145:175.
44. McCauley RL, et al: Alternating therapy in major burns: Silver sulfadiazine vs. silver sulfadiazine-nitrofurazone. *J Burn Care Rehabil* 1984; 5:384–387.
45. McManus WF, et al: Burn wound infection. *J Trauma* 1981; 21:753–756.
46. McRipley RJ, Whitney RR: Characterization and quantitation of experimental surgical wound infections used to evaluate topical antibacterial agents. *Antimicrob Agents Chemother* 1976; 10:38–44.
47. Moncrief JA, et al: The use of a topical sulfonamide in the control of burn wound sepsis. *J Trauma* 1966; 6:407–415.
48. Moyer CA, et al: Treatment of large human burns with 0.5% silver nitrate solution. *Arch Surg* 1965; 90:812–867.
49. Munster AM: Treatment of invasive *Enterobacter cloacae* burn wound sepsis with topical nitrofurazone. *J Trauma* 1984; 24:524–525.
50. Nathan P, et al: A laboratory method for the

selection of topical agents to treat infected burn wounds. *Burns* 1978; 4:177–187.
51. Nathan P, Holder, I, MacMillan B: Burn wounds: Microbiology, local host defenses, and current therapy. *Crit Rev Clin Lab Sci* 1973; 4:61–100.
52. Neal GD, et al: Burn wound histologic cultures: A new technique for predicting burn wound sepsis. *J Burn Care Rehabil* 1981; 2:35–39.
53. Pack GT: The pathology of burns. *Arch Pathol* 1926; 1:767.
54. Robson M, Schaerf R, Krizek I: Evaluation of topical povidone-iodine ointment in experimental burn wound sepsis. *Plast Reconstr Surg* 1974; 54:328–334.
55. Robson MC, Heggers JP: Bacterial quantification of open wounds. *Milit Med* 1969; 134:19.
56. Saymen DG, et al: Control of surface wound infection: Skin versus synthetic grafts. *Appl Microb* 1972; 23:509–512.
57. Serafinska D, Bukowska D, Zietkiewicz W: Studies of bacterial growth on the granulating surface and the percentage of graft taking in burns. *Bull Pol Med Sci Hist* 1966; 9:131.
58. Sheretz RJ, Sullivan ML: An outbreak of infections with *Acinetobacter calcoaceticus* in burn patients: Contamination of patients' mattresses. *J Infect Dis* 1985; 151:252–258.
59. Shipley ER: Re-evaluation of furacin as a topical agent in the treatment of surface infections. *Am Surg* 1965; 31:238–241.
60. Shlaes DM, et al: Enterococcal bacteremia without endocarditis. *Arch Intern Med* 1981; 141:578–581.
61. Shuck JM, Moncrief JA: Safeguards in the use of topical mafenide (Sulfamylon) in burned patients. *Am J Surg* 1969; 118:864–870.
62. Spebar MJ, Walters MJ, Pruitt BA, Jr: Improved survival with aggressive surgical management of noncandidal fungal infections of the burn wound. *J Trauma* 1982; 33:867–868.
63. Spengler MD, Rodeheaver GJ, Edlich RF: Technical considerations in quantitative bacteriology. *J Burn Care Rehabil* 1982; 2:200–202.
64. Stieritz D, Law E, Holder I: Speciation and amphotericin B sensitivity studies on blood isolates of *Candida* from burned patients. *J Clin Pathol* 1973; 26:405.
65. Stone HH: Review of *Pseudomonas* sepsis in thermal burns. *Ann Surg* 1966; 163:297.
66. Teplitz C, et al: *Pseudomonas* burn wound sepsis: II. Hematogenous infection at the junction of the burn wound and the unburned hypodermis. *J Surg Res* 1964; 4:217.
67. Torstenson O, Meyer W, Quie P: Burn wound infection with viruses. *N Engl J Med* 1970; 282:1272.
68. Volenec FJ, et al: Burn wound biopsy bacterial quantitation: A statistical analysis. *Am J Surg* 1979; 138:697–698.
69. Wickman K: Studies on burns. XIV. Bacteriology. II. *Acta Chir Scand* 1970; suppl 408: 1–34.
70. Woolfrey B, Fox J, Quall C: An evaluation of burn wound quantitative microbiology: I. Quantitative eschar cultures. *Am J Clin Pathol* 1981; 75:532–537.
71. Woolfrey B, Fox J, Quall C: An evaluation of burn wound microbiology: The quantitative gram stain. *J Burn Care Rehabil* 1982; 3:171–175.

17 / Viral Infections in Children With Burns

STEVE KOHL, M.D.

The frequency and severity of infections due to bacteria and fungi in adults and children who have suffered burns is well recognized. This subject is reviewed in Chapter 16. In contrast, much less attention has been focused on the importance of viral infections in burn patients. Nevertheless, the picture that has evolved in the past 10 years clearly indicates that viral infections in burned children are surprisingly common and may be of life-threatening severity.

The many immunologic defects occurring during the acute and subacute period of burn trauma and therapy have been recently reviewed.[1] It is clearly beyond the scope of this chapter to delineate these defects. It is possible that defects in antibody levels, serum opsonic activity, cell-mediated immune responses, interferon production, and lymphocyte cytotoxicity may all contribute to decreased resistance to viral infections. We have recently demonstrated that in patients with severe burns, the ability of macrophages to destroy herpes simplex virus (HSV)–infected cells in the presence of antibody (antibody-dependent cellular cytotoxicity) was defective during the subacute period of recovery.[7] This is precisely the time the burn patient manifests viral infections.

The burn patient is uniquely susceptible to several viruses. These include cytomegalovirus (CMV), HSV, and varicella-zoster virus (VZV). Other viral infections that may occur with a higher frequency include Epstein-Barr virus (EBV) and adenoviruses. Due to the risk factor of blood transfusion, in the past, hepatitis B, and now non-A, non-B hepatitis is a problem in burn patients. Since hepatitis viruses are not unique to burn patients, and their disease manifestations are not atypical, they shall not be dealt with in this review.

HERPESVIRUSES

Clearly the viruses that cause the greatest problem in the burn patient are those belonging to the human herpesvirus group. Indeed, each of the large, enveloped DNA viruses in this group has been shown to occur with an unusual frequency. In the case of HSV, CMV, and VZV, they also may cause more severe illness than expected in the normal patient.

Cytomegalovirus

Cytomegalovirus has recently been implicated to cause asymptomatic and symptomatic infections quite often in burn patients. In several studies summarized in Table 17–1, the rate of CMV infection in burn patients is astoundingly high. Those studies[8, 10] that involved only children are concordant with the general trend of a 20% to 40% incidence of CMV infection as determined by either serologic response or viral excretion.

In children, the period of CMV infection is generally from 4 to 21 weeks after the burn,[8] with a mean of 8 to 13 weeks after the acute burn. The risk of CMV infection is higher in children with more severe burns. Thus, in pa-

TABLE 17–1.
Cytomegalovirus Infections in Burn Patients

CMV EXCRETION, NO. (%)	SEROLOGIC RESPONSE, NO. (%)	REFERENCE†
3/10 (30)	15/74 (20)	12
ND*	9/40 (22)	8 (retrospective)
7/24 (29)	6/24 (25)	8 (prospective)
18/33 (55)	13/33 (39)	10
ND	17/52 (33)	6

*ND indicates not determined.
†Study 8 was done in a retrospective and prospective fashion. Study 4 and 5 were only of pediatric patients. The patients in study 6 had at least 20% BSA burn.

tients with CMV infection, the average percentage of third-degree burn was 46% to 51% of the body surface area (BSA), compared to 22% to 36% in patients without CMV.[8] Alternatively, in those with third-degree burns over 30% of the BSA, 73% (16 of 22) shed CMV, compared to 18% (2 of 11) with third-degree burns less than 30% of the BSA.[10] Similarly, 54% (12 of 22) of patients with third-degree burns over 30% of the BSA had serologic responses to CMV as compared to 9% (1 of 11) with less severe burns.[10]

In a prospective study of children with burns,[8] two patterns of viral shedding existed. Several patients shed virus in the urine early (7 to 11 days after the burn), while another population shed virus later (2 to 4 months after the burn). The latter patients tended to excrete virus for several months.

Risk factors for CMV infection other than total burn area also included more frequent blood transfusion (13.4 vs. 5.8 in patients without CMV infection, $P < .01$) and more skin grafts (7.4 vs. 3.6, $P < .01$).[8] The majority of serologic responses in the children were changes from seronegativity to seropositivity, indicating primary disease.[8, 10] Some patients did demonstrate only titer rises, indicating reactivation of endogenous virus.[10] In older patients, as expected, the incidence of reactivation diseases (45%) was more common than primary disease (17%).[6]

Of the four children with late onset CMV diseases (all of whom were initially seronegative), 4 had unexplained fever, 3 hepatitis, and 3 lymphocytosis.[8] These patients tended not to manifest atypical lymphocytosis.[3] In a series of 150 patients from a burn center in Prague, Czechoslovakia, seven deaths were attributed to CMV infection.[13] The two patients presented were both adults. In a prospective pediatric series, 4 of 75 patients (5.5%) manifested clinically recognizable CMV infection.[8]

Thus, CMV is a particularly common problem in burn patients. The diagnosis can be established by serologic response and culture of urine, nasopharynx, and, perhaps, white blood cells. In the near future, nucleic-acid hybridization techniques will increase the speed and sensitivity of CMV diagnosis.

While there is currently no therapy for CMV, establishment of a diagnosis may permit discontinuation of unnecessary antimicrobial therapy. Studies of high-titer anti-CMV antisera are necessary in patients who are seronegative to attempt to prevent primary CMV infections. Attempts should be made to use either blood from CMV seronegative donors, or washed, frozen red blood cells, which will reduce the risk of transmission via transfusion to seronegative patients.[2]

Herpes Simplex Virus

Herpes simplex virus was probably the first virus associated with burns. Scott et al.[11] described an infant with a digital cigarette burn, which subsequently became infected with HSV. That the course of HSV in the burned patient may be unusually severe was documented by Foley et al.,[4] who reported six adults with HSV-infected burns.

The incidence of HSV infection in burn patients has been studied (Table 17–2). The two studies of children[8, 10] suggest a 12% to 27% incidence of HSV infection. As with CMV infection, more severe burns were associated with a higher risk of HSV infection. Patients with third-degree burns over 30% of the BSA had a higher incidence of serologic response (36%) than those with smaller burns (9%).[10] The mean time of serologic response was 4.8 weeks postburn. Thus in children and adults, the onset of HSV infection was earlier than CMV.[6, 8, 10] Many of the children reported were asymptomatic, while several had typical fever blisters in their mouths.

In contrast, severe, life-threatening illness has been reported due to HSV in burn patients. Foley et al.[4] described three deaths due to disseminated HSV among six patients. The typical illness begins with infection of the burn wound with vesicles and ulcers, which often appear atypical in nature. Only at the edge of the wound will the vesicles be more characteristic. The wounds often become hemorrhagic and necrotic or display focal erosions (Fig 17–1). These usually occur at healing partial-thickness injury.[4, 5] The patients, especially those with primary illness, are at risk of disseminated visceral disease[5] or generalized cutaneous eruption.[9] The viral infection may also convert a partial-thickness injury to a full-thickness injury. These areas are excellent sites for secondary bacterial infection.

Diagnosis is made by demonstration of viral inclusion bodies in the wound. While serologic response may be helpful, culture for HSV is rapid and specific. Antigen detection tests by fluorescent antibody or enzyme-linked assays will be available in the near future. Atypical areas of necrosis should be carefully studied by cytologic analysis of scraping or biopsy and culture.

Therapy for HSV in the immunocompromised host should include intravenous administration of acyclovir, 250 mg/sq m BSA (or 5 mg/kg) three times per day for 5 to 10 days, depending on clinical response.[14] Since these patients are at risk of dissemination, even apparently trivial disease should be treated rapidly.

Prevention may be aided by exogenous immunoglobulin, although to date there are no confirmatory results. Staff with active HSV must avoid these patients, and patients with HSV should be isolated.

Varicella-Zoster Virus

As HSV, VZV may secondarily infect burn wound sites. It would appear to be much less common. A retrospective study demonstrated a serologic response to VZV in 2 of 36 (5%) of children with burns.[8] These are two references to small epidemics of VZV infections in pediatric burn units.[4, 15] Lesions tend to occur both in areas of healing second-degree burn sites and donor graft sites. The vesicles may be very deep, extending into the dermis, and leaving punched-out lesions.[15] The infection may interfere with the "take" of skin grafts. While systemic complications have not been reported in the patients, it would seem

TABLE 17–2.
Herpes Simplex Virus Infection in Burn Patients

HSV EXCRETION, NO. (%)	SEROLOGIC RESPONSE, NO. (%)	REFERENCE
ND*	3/40 (8)	8 (retrospective)
3/24 (12)	6/24 (25)	8 (prospective)
2/15 (13)	9/33 (27)	10
ND	21/52 (40)	6

*ND indicates not determined.

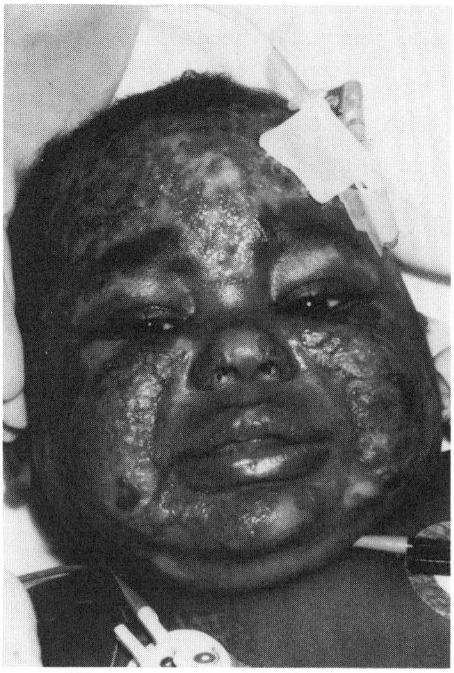

FIG 17–1.
Herpes simplex infection in a burned child. Note the vesicles and ulcers at the margin of the burn wound.

that treatment or prevention in this high-risk group is indicated.

Diagnosis is by cytologic analysis and culture, as for HSV. Treatment is also the same as for HSV, although the dose of acyclovir is 500 mg/sq m BSA (or 10 mg/kg) three times per day since VZV is less susceptible to acyclovir than HSV. Prevention of infection in burn patients inadvertently exposed to VZV would include administration of varicella-zoster immunoglobulin within 72 hours.

OTHER VIRUSES

The only other viruses demonstrated to occur with some regularity in children with burns were Epstein-Barr virus (3 of 40 [8%]) and adenovirus (3 of 24 [12%]). These were demonstrated by serologic response and were all asymptomatic.[8] In the same study, no hepatitis B conversion occurred.

SUMMARY

Thus, several viruses, especially those of the herpes group, cause frequent and severe infections in children with burns. Their diagnosis can facilitate discontinuation of inappropriate antibiotics and, in the case of HSV and VZV, initiation of appropriate antiviral therapy. Surveillance of severely burned patients for other viral infections, as rotavirus or parainfluenza virus, which are known to occur with increased frequency in immunosuppressed patients, may help explain their "pathogen-negative" infections.

REFERENCES

1. Bjornson AB, Bjornson HS: Theoretical interrelationships among immunologic and hematologic sequelae of thermal injury. *Rev Infect Dis* 1984; 6:704–707.
2. Brady MT, Milam JD, Anderson DC, et al: Use of deglycerolized red blood cells to prevent posttransfusion infection with cytomegalovirus in neonates. *J Infect Dis* 1984; 150:334–339.
3. Deepe GS, MacMillan BG, Linnemann CC Jr: Unexplained fever in burn patients due to cytomegalovirus infection. *JAMA* 1982; 248: 2299–2301.
4. Foley FD, Greenawald KA, Nash G, et al: Herpes virus infection in burned patients. *N Engl J Med* 1970; 282:652–656.
5. Garcia M, Edwards MS: Herpes simplex infection of burn wounds. *South Med J* 1981; 74:991–992.
6. Kagan RJ, Naragi S, Matsuda T, et al: Herpes simplex virus and cytomegalovirus infection in burned patients. *J Trauma* 1985; 25:40–45.
7. Kohl S, Ericsson CD: Cellular cytotoxicity to herpes simplex virus-infected cells of leukocytes from patients with serious burns. *Clin Immunol Immunopathol* 1982; 24:171–178.
8. Linnemann CC Jr, MacMillan BG: Viral infections in pediatric burn patients. *Am J Dis Child* 1981; 135:750–753.
9. Nishimura M, Maekawa M, Hino Y, et al: Kaposi's varicelliform eruption: Development in a patient with a healing second-degree burn. *Arch Dermatol* 1984; 120:799–800.
10. Pollard RB: Herpes simplex virus and cytomegalovirus in burned children, in *Programs and Abstracts of the 21st Interscience Conference on Antimicrobial Agents and Chemother-*

apy. Washington, DC, American Society for Microbiology, 1981, p 236.

11. Scott TFM, Coriell L, Blank H, et al: Some comments on herpetic infection in children with special emphasis on unusual clinical manifestations. *J Pediatr* 1952; 41:835–843.
12. Seeman J, Konigova R: Cytomegalovirus infection in severely burned patients. *Acta Chir Plast* 1976; 18:142–151.
13. Seeman J, Konigova R, Lysenkova I: Fatal outcome of cytomegalovirus infections in severe burns. *Acta Chir Plast* 1980; 22:166–170.
14. Tomford JW, Kumar ML, Franz NA, et al: Burn wound infection with herpes simplex. *Clin Res* 1984; 32:794A.
15. Weintraub WH, Randolph JF: A chickenpox epidemic in a pediatric burn unit. *Surgery* 1974; 76:990–994.

18 / Septicemia and Septic Shock

HUGO F. CARVAJAL, M.D.

Acute bacteremia, endotoxemia, and septic shock are common complications of severe burn injuries,[15, 17, 22, 23, 104] and despite major advances in burn care, infection remains the most common factor leading to death in burn patients.[3, 14, 51, 53, 62, 120] Gram-negative organisms are the most common offenders[15, 60, 62, 72, 105] (see also Chapter 16 "The Burn Wound—Microbiologic Aspects"). Infection can occur at any time following the injury, but it is most common during the second to third week after the burn.[53] It is also most likely in deep and extensive burns, and particularly frequent in immunocompromised patients,[11] patients with smoke inhalation, or patients with other major complications[86] (Table 18–1). Since flame burns are more extensive than scald burns, they are more commonly associated with sepsis (Table 18–2).

DIAGNOSIS

Early diagnosis of septicemia and institution of appropriate antibiotic therapy and other therapeutic measures are essential for survival. Unfortunately, the diagnosis of sepsis during the early phases is difficult to ascertain. There are no pathognomonic signs or symptoms of septicemia, and the burn injury itself, particularly when severe, leads to many alterations in body homeostasis, which significantly overlap with the signs, symptoms, and laboratory abnormalities that characterize the early response of the organism to burn sepsis.[6, 21, 87, 108] The larger the burn, the greater the risk of bacterial colonization and septicemia, but also the more likely the patient is to exhibit symptoms as a result of the injury. Thus, when the burned patient presents with mild to moderate symptoms, the physician is confronted with a diagnostic dilemma, sometimes delaying the diagnosis and treatment unduly or encouraging the premature institution of antibiotic therapy; the latter is often associated with selection of resistant bacterial strains, while the former usually leads to increased morbidity and mortality.[35, 52, 116]

The clinical signs and symptoms most commonly associated with septicemia in burned children are (1) altered sensorium, ranging from lethargy to confusion, delirium and coma; (2) gastrointestinal symptoms, such as diarrhea, vomiting, abdominal distention, and paralytic ileus; (3) changes in vital signs such as tachycardia, tachypnea/dyspnea, fever, hypothermia, and hypotension; (4) hemodynamic impairment, including peripheral vascular insufficiency (with cold, clammy, and cyanotic skin), cardiorespiratory insufficiency, oliguria, and/or polyuria; and (5) evidence of bacterial colonization of the burn wound with invasion of viable tissues.[15, 42, 63, 76, 91] Laboratory data that although not pathognomonic, would support the diagnosis of sepsis include (1) hypoxemia and alterations in acid-base balance, (2) leukopenia or leukocytosis, (3) thrombocytopenia with or without evidence of consumption coagulopathy, (4) abnormal chest roentgenograms, (5) positive blood, wound, or urine cultures, and (6) histologic evidence of bacterial invasion of viable tissue.[15, 60, 76]

During the early stages, the signs and symptoms of sepsis are subtle and nonspe-

TABLE 18–1.
Risk Factors for Septicemia/Endotoxemia in Burned Children*

	SEPTIC GROUP	NONSEPTIC	SIGNIFICANCE
Body surface area burned, % (SEM)†	60 (3)	23 (1)	$P < .001$
Third-degree burn, sq m (SEM)	0.5 (0.1)	0.07 (0.01)	$P < .001$
Burn to diagnosis, days (SEM)	26 (6)	—	Not applicable
Burn to diagnosis, range of days	2–112	—	Not applicable
Smoke inhalation, no. (%)	9/16 (56)	290/227 (13)	$P < .005$

*Adapted from Carvajal HF, Feinstein R, Traber DL: An objective method for early diagnosis of gram-negative septicemia in burned children. *J Trauma* 1981; 21:221–227.
†SEM = standard error of the mean.

cific.[48] However, as the disease progresses, florid symptomatology becomes evident.[3] The late stages present no real diagnostic challenge, and terminally, multiple organ failure is invariably present.[5, 95, 108, 109] Depending on the infecting organism, virulence, and inoculum, as well as the condition of the patient prior to infection, rapid progression from one stage to another takes place, and death is a common final event. Appropriate therapeutic interventions during the late stages of sepsis usually prolong life but do not always alter the outcome. Early institution of therapy, on the other hand, carries a much better prognosis and usually results in marked reductions in morbidity and mortality.[8, 10, 15, 16, 35, 107, 113]

Since the key to improved survival is early diagnosis, which requires frequent evaluation of the patient's condition, various monitoring and detection programs have been proposed.[15, 82] Serial blood cultures, for example, are often recommended, but the data thus generated have been disappointing.[14, 104–106] Transient episodes of bacteremia due to surgical manipulation of the wound or dressing changes usually resolve spontaneously and do not require therapy.[80, 93] However, their detection by blood culture creates a further dilemma. Likewise, contamination of the specimen at the time of collection often leads to unnecessary therapy and physician anxiety. If on the basis of the clinical symptoms septicemia is a serious consideration, the blood culture is invaluable for isolation of the organism and selection of appropriate antibiotics; but since a minimum of 24 to 48 hours is required for growth and identification of the organism, the diagnostic value of the blood culture is limited, even when meticulous attention to technique is undertaken.[60] Simultaneous duplicate blood cultures, obtained from separate sites and following careful cleansing of the skin, help to evaluate the risk of inadvertent contamination, but their value as a monitoring tool and early predictor of sepsis remains limited.

Negative blood cultures have been reported from patients with massive burn wound colonization and frank symptomatology,[15, 57] including cases in which invasion of

TABLE 18–2.
Septicemia in Burned Children by Burn Etiology*

	SEPTIC GROUP	NONSEPTIC	SIGNIFICANCE
Flame burns	15/16 (94%)	153/227 (67%)	$P < .005$
Scalds	1/16 (6%)	67/227 (30%)	$P < .005$

*Adapted from Carvajal HF, Feinstein R, Traber DL: An objective method for early diagnosis of gram-negative septicemia in burned children. *J Trauma* 1981; 21:221–227.

subjacent viable tissue was demonstrated and positive blood cultures have been found in the absence of burn sepsis.[76] The lack of correlation between blood cultures and wound cultures has been attributed to lymphatic spread of gram-negative bacilli from the burn wound[105, 106] and rapid uptake by the reticuloendothelial system of any small inoculum that may gain access to the bloodstream. Bacteriological assessment of the burn wound by surface culture or quantitative biopsy has similar drawbacks (see Chapter 16, "The Burn Wound: Microbiological Aspects"), and the lack of standard methodology continues to be a source of controversy.[37, 42, 43, 49, 69, 70, 84, 112]

Histologic demonstration of bacterial invasion into underlying viable tissue, as reported by Pruitt,[84, 86] Parks,[76] and Linares,[53] appears promising but requires further development. Collection of the biopsy samples remains a subjective approach that must be standardized before it gains widespread acceptance. Another drawback is that the method requires a pathology laboratory willing to process samples immediately and provide feedback to clinicians within a few hours.

For the individual patient already suspected of having gram-negative sepsis, the information derived from the biopsy (histologic and microbiologic data) can be valuable, particularly if it can be correlated with other clinical and laboratory findings (see Chapter 23, "Autopsy Findings in Burned Children").

Some of the risk factors for septicemia that have been identified in burned children include (1) flame burns, (2) extensive burns (>40% BSA), (3) full-thickness burns in *excess* of 0.5 sq m, (4) smoke inhalation, (5) immunologic incompetence,[3] and (6) poor nutritional state.[4, 15, 53] Thus, it seems appropriate that monitoring efforts for septicemia be concentrated on these high-risk populations; however, even in these patients early confirmation of the diagnosis remains a difficult task. Measurements of acute phase reactants, including α_1-antitrypsin, α_1-antichymotrypsin, C-reactive protein, orosomucoid, and haptoglobulin, as proposed by Moody et al.,[67] as well as serial determinations of plasma fibronectin[13] can be used to support the diagnosis of septicemia as well as to assess the effectiveness of therapy, but their diagnostic value in and of themselves is limited. The presence of red debris on Ficoll-Hypaque gradients, which has been reported to occur concomitantly with marked immunosuppression and prior to the development of sepsis, may be of value in selected patients to predict severe sepsis and minimize morbidity and mortality.[8]

AN ALGORITHM FOR MONITORING AND DIAGNOSIS OF BURN SEPSIS

In 1981, Carvajal et al.[15] reported the results of a prospective study in 243 burned children (burns ranging from 2% to 98% of their BSA) who were monitored at each nursing shift (three times per day) during their entire hospitalization for the presence and severity of eight signs and symptoms believed to be useful in the diagnosis of gram-negative septicemia (Fig 18–1). In addition, a battery of laboratory tests aimed at further defining the diagnosis of sepsis (Fig 18–2) were obtained whenever significant departures from the norm were observed. During the 26 months of study 16 patients (22 instances) whose clinical and laboratory findings suggested the diagnosis of gram-negative septicemia were identified. Using various multiple linear regression and linear discriminant function procedures, several possible models for early diagnosis of gram-negative septicemia were studied. The two most practical of these (models I and II), designed to yield a score less than 0 (negative range) for patients with septicemia and greater than 0 (positive range) for the nonseptic population, were selected. Model I (see below), composed only of the clinical variables (sensorium, respiratory rate, gastrointestinal (GI) symptoms, and appearance of the wounds), was developed taking into consideration the actual scores, their squared values, and pairwise cross product. Model II was similarly arrived at, using both

Variable	Numerical Score				Raw Score Per Nursing Shift			Corr. Fact.	Corrected Score		
	0	1	2	3	7-3	3-11	11-7		7-3	3-11	11-7
Sensorium	Alert	Lethargic	Confused Delireous	Semi-Coma				x 6			
G. I. Symptoms	None	Recurrent regurgitation or diarrhea	Vomiting	Significant Abnormal distention				x 8			
Appearance of wounds or grafts	Dry clean	Pale and Wet		Foul smelling soupy or purulent				x 5			
Persistent increase in respiratory rate (>4 hr.)	<40/ min.	40-50 min.	50-60/ min.	>60/min.				x 5			
Fever	<100° F	100°-102° F	102°- 103° F	>103° F				x 5			
Hypothermia >1 hr.	98°-100° F	98°- 97° F	97°- 98° F	<96° F				x 7			
Fall in Systolic Pressure	± 10%			>30%				x 8			
Persistent Oliguria (>4 hr.)	120/160/ ml/m^2/ 4 hr.	60-120 ml/ m^2 / 4 hr.	40-60 ml/ m^2 / 4 hr.	<40 ml/ m^2 / 4 hr.				x 6			
				TOTAL							

FIG 18–1.
Preliminary score sheet. (From Carvajal HF, Feinstein R, Traber DL, et al: An objective method for early diagnosis of gram-negative septicemia in burned children. *J Trauma* 1981; 21(3):221–227. Used by permission.)

the clinical and the laboratory variables. The determination of both models I and II involved first identifying several "best" subsets of the many variables considered using the maximum R^2 (R = coefficient of multiple correlation) approach.[39, 40, 68] The most reasonable of these "best" subsets were selected for further use (see the specific variables given in the two models below). Once the variables for each model were selected, their coefficients in the linear discriminant functions were determined for classification purposes. Model I had a coefficient of multiple correlation (R) of 0.75, and the overall model as well as each of the terms in the model were statistically significant ($P < .05$). Thus patients were classified as either septic or nonseptic. This classification was then compared to a more exhaustive retrospective clinical review that made use of data not available at the time of the computer-assisted classification. On this basis, model I was found to yield a 7% false positive rate and an 18% false negative rate, or a sensitivity of 82% and a specificity of 93% with *24 hours of anticipation*. The sensitivity and specificity for model II were 86% and 97%, respectively. The two models are described below:

Model I: y = 4.66 − 1.5 (score for sensorium) − 6.25 (score for respiratory rate) + 1.35 (score for respiratory rate^2) − 1.12 (GI symptoms score × score for wounds).

Model II: y = 8.1 − 18.45 (score for sensorium) + 3.24 (score for sensorium × score for wounds) − 2.02 (GI symptoms score × score for wounds) − 0.28 (score for

Variable	Numerical Score					Raw Score	Corr. Fact.	Corrected Score
	0	1	2	3	4			
White Blood Count	5-10,000	4 - 5000 or 10-12,000	3 - 4000 or 12-15,000	2 -3000 or 15-20,000	$<$2000 or $>$20,000		6	
Platelet Count	$>$200, 000	150 - 2000,000 per mm^3	100 - 150,000 per mm^3	50 - 100,000 per mm^3	$<$50,000 per mm^3		10	
paO_2	$>$90	80-89 mmHg	65-79 mmHg	50-64 mmHg	$<$ 50 mmHg		8	
Arterial Blood pH	7.35	7.35 - 7.30	7.3 - 7.2	7.2 - 7.1	$<$ 7.1		6	
Blood Culture	Neg.	positive (single org.)			2 cultures positive (single org.)		10	
Urine Culture	Neg.				Positive + LDH-5 $>$13 mU/ml		5	
Limulus Assay	Neg.		1 + Twice	2 + once or 1 + twice	3-4 + once or 2 + twice		10	
Skin Biopsy Culture	Neg.	Positive			10^5/gr (same org. as bld.cul.)		8	
DIC	Absent				present		10	
Chest x-Ray	Neg.			Focal Pneu-monia	Lobar or Diffuse Pneumonia		10	
					TOTAL			

FIG 18–2.
Laboratory data score sheet. (From Carvajal HF, Feinstein R, Traber DL, et al: An objective method for early diagnosis of gram-negative septicemia in burned children. *J Trauma* 1981; 21(3):221–227. Used by permission.)

wounds × score for temperature) − 0.78 (score for respiratory rate × score for temperature) − 1.25 (score for respiratory rate × score for platelet count) − 1.43 (score for respiratory rate × score for arterial oxygen pressure [Pa_{O_2}]).

The scoring chart derived from this study and currently used in our institution for monitoring and diagnosis of gram-negative sepsis in burned children is shown in Figure 18–3. A second study that prospectively compared the use of the above algorithm to the conventional methods for monitoring and diagnosis of septicemia in 395 burned children has been recently completed (Carvajal HF, unpublished data) (Table 18–3). In this study the patients were allocated to the study (computer algorithm) group or the control (conventional method) group using an envelope system that allowed stratification and matching of the patients in the two groups according to age, type of burn, and burn size. Judging from the preliminary analysis, the incidence of septicemia was slightly lower in the computer (12%) than in the conventional group (16%). Septic patients in the computer and conventional groups had mean burns averaging 57% and 55% of the total BSA respectively, and three patients in each group died of their injuries (see Table 18–3).

Even though no significant differences between groups were detected, it must be pointed out that the study was carried out at the Shriners' Burns Institute in Galveston, where the conventional method for diagnosis

Variable	Numerical Score					Raw Score Per Nursing Shift			Total Score (24 hrs.)
	0	1	2	3	4	7-3	3-11	11-7	
Change in Sensorium	Alert	Lethargic	Confused Delireous	Semi-Coma					
G. I. Symptoms	None	Recurrent regurgitation or diarrhea	Vomiting	Significant Abdominal Distention					
Appearance of wounds or Grafts	Dry clean	Pale and wet		Foul smelling soupy or purulent					
Persistent increase in respiratory rate (>4 hr.)	<40/ min.	40-50/ min.	50-60/ min.	>60/min.					
Fever	<100°F	100°-102°F	102°-103°F	>103°F					
Platelet Count	>200, 000	150- 200,000 per mm³	100- 150,000 per mm³	50- 100,000 per mm³	<50,000 per mm³				
paO_2	>90	80-89 mmHg	65-79 mmHg	50-64 mmHg	<50 mmHg				

FIG 18–3.
Scoring chart for continuous monitoring of gram-negative septicemia in burned children. (From Carvajal HF, Feinstein R, Traber DL: An objective method for early diagnosis of gram-negative septicemia in burned children. *J Trauma* 1981; 21:221–227. Used by permission.)

of sepsis (following our first study) was biased toward the use of the same variables for clinical diagnosis that were incorporated in the sepsis algorithm. Thus, the fact that no differences between groups were demonstrated actually represents a significant accomplishment that further validates the monitoring tool. In other words, the importance of this study did not lie in accomplishing an "earlier diagnosis of sepsis" in "highly specialized burn units" but in developing an accurate monitoring tool that would provide the inexperienced with the diagnostic skills of the experts.

By requiring and relying on the participation of nurses in the diagnostic process, the proposed system emphasizes the team approach to the patient and places some of the responsibility for detection of septicemia on

TABLE 18–3.
Prospective Use of the Sepsis Algorithm in a Pediatric Burn Facility*

	COMPUTER DIAGNOSIS	CONVENTIONAL DIAGNOSIS	TOTAL
Patients diagnosed with gram-negative septicemia	20/200	22/195	42/395
BSA burned ($\bar{x}$), %	55	57	56
No. of septic episodes	24	31	55
Length of stay, days (septic patients only)	76	92	84
Deaths	3	3	6

*Adapted from Carvajal HF, unpublished data, 1986.

the nurse. By virtue of being at the bedside for extended periods of time, nurses are ideally suited to monitor these patients, and any tool that would assist them in their task is likely to gain widespread acceptance.

Our present monitoring efforts in burned children make use of the two algorithms described above (models I and II), and the data are collected using the scoring chart depicted in Table 18–3. A model I sepsis score is calculated daily on every acutely burned patient. This is usually accomplished with a programmable calculator, but a computer is best suited to store, manipulate, and display the data in various ways. Any time that the model I daily score is in the negative range (less than 0), the possibility of septicemia is entertained, and arterial blood is obtained for pH and blood gas analysis and platelet count. As soon as the results of these tests are available (usually within an hour), a model II score is likewise calculated; if this score is also below 0, the possibility of gram-negative sepsis is assumed to be high and additional diagnostic tests (i.e., complete blood cell count [CBC], blood, urine and wound cultures, wound biopsy, chest x-ray, and plasma colloid osmotic pressure) are obtained. In most cases antibiotic therapy is begun while awaiting the results of confirmatory studies. In the event that the diagnosis of sepsis is confirmed, a full course of antibiotics is given, and once completed, sepsis monitoring is resumed.

In summary, the sepsis scores derived from the use of these tables should alert the burn team to the possibility of gram-negative sepsis, but documentation of the diagnosis and institution of therapy must still be individualized. In other words, the system should not be considered a substitute for comprehensive clinical evaluation of the patient. Users must also recognize that a minimum of three consecutive shift scores for each of the variables must be obtained before a presumptive diagnosis of gram-negative septicemia can be formulated. In addition, two important limitations must be recognized:

1. Even though the proposed methods allow one to make the diagnosis of gram-negative septicemia 24 hours earlier than conventional techniques, a 14% false negative rate remains a problem. Presumably, these patients can be diagnosed one day later with or without the use of the decision table.

2. Some of the conditions (variables) must be subjectively evaluated; hence the individual collecting the data must be trained according to well-defined criteria.

A word of caution concerns patients with gram-positive septicemia who are less likely to disclose changes in the appearance of the wounds, changes in sensorium, or GI symptoms, and thus could be missed by this monitoring instrument. The above limitations notwithstanding, implementation of this system should favorably affect the morbidity and mortality of burned patients whose greatest threat is infection with gram-negative endotoxin-producing organisms. In the first place, the diagnosis of septicemia could be made earlier. Second, involvement of nursing personnel in the diagnostic process is a highly desirable step. Third, the system can provide an organizational framework that would improve patient care, as well as the attitude of medical and nursing personnel.

STAPHYLOCOCCAL SEPSIS

Staphylococcus aureus is a common pathogen in most burn units and is responsible for a significant number of infections.[52, 104] Not all cases of *Staphylococcus* infections are associated with septicemia, but every infection has the potential to invade viable tissue and seed the bloodstream. Wound infection characterized by microabscesses, tissue necrosis, increased amounts of exudate, wound conversion, and graft loss are the most common presenting findings. Occasionally, pneumonia, empyema, tracheobronchitis, or kidney infection may be the first site of infection to be recognized. Intravenous (IV), intra-arterial, and central venous catheters are common sources of infection, and septicemia can develop before the origin of the infection is detected and the catheter removed. Cutdown entry sites for catheter placement must be inspected daily for discoloration, inflammation, and purulence. Even after the catheter is removed, infection at these sites may continue to seed the bloodstream and may go unrecognized.[87] Although *Staphylococcus aureus* and other gram-positive organisms may produce septicemia and multiple microabscesses in several organ systems, the signs and symptoms differ from gram-negative septicemia.

Unless the infection is in the upper or lower respiratory tract,[18] respiratory symptoms are late findings in *Staphylococcus* sepsis. Hypoxemia does not usually develop, and the adult respiratory distress syndrome is only rarely present; when it develops it is usually secondary to therapeutic interventions. Likewise, GI symptoms such as vomiting, abdominal distention, and paralytic ileus are notoriously absent from the presenting clinical picture. Changes in sensorium tend to develop late, and hemodynamic instability, including evidence of renal functional impairment, are uncommon. Thus, in general, the patient with staphylococcal septicemia presents with symptoms related to the site of infection; pneumonia, empyema, and pleural effusion can lead to respiratory failure, but only when the infection has spread throughout both lungs; bacterial endocarditis usually presents with spiking fevers, changing murmurs, and evidence of microembolization. The latter can result in central nervous system symptoms, signs of kidney embolization (such as hematuria and proteinuria), and evidence of liver involvement. However, organ failure is rare, except as a terminal event.

Although rare during the early stages, disseminated staphylococcal infections may occur in association with endotoxin-like symptomatology. This phenomenon is secondary to the absorption of endotoxin from the GI tract. The entry of the endotoxin is somehow favored by alterations in the GI tract mucosa induced by the gram-positive organisms.[22] This type of clinical picture including multiple organ failure is almost invariably present as a final event. In addition, the possibility of combined infections must be kept in mind, as they frequently occur in the severely burned child and provide justification for wide-spectrum antibiotic coverage until the responsible organism is properly identified.

The diagnosis of gram-positive infections is usually based on (1) clinical symptoms; (2) obvious evidence of infection by inspection of the wounds and IV sites; (3) auscultation and percussion of the chest for tracheobronchitis, pneumonia, and empyema; (4) auscultation of the heart for murmurs; (5) chest x-ray; (6) cultures of blood, exudative lesions, or boils; and (7) wound biopsy for microbiologic and histologic evidence of tissue invasion.

The clinical algorithm used for diagnosis of gram-negative infections may not be applicable to this type of infection and should not be relied on for this purpose.

TREATMENT

Regardless of the methods or mechanism by which the diagnosis of gram-negative septicemia is established, time is of essence and treatment must be instituted at once—usually before confirmatory evidence of infection is available. Rapid progression to death within a few hours of onset has been reported in burned patients, and survival is dependent on an early diagnosis and prompt institution of treatment.

The management of the septic patient is mainly supportive, with the primary therapeutic objective being to prevent, minimize, or counteract the effects of endotoxin, thereby buying time for the body to rid itself of the noxious agents. The supportive measures that must be simultaneously instituted are (1) antimicrobial therapy; (2) fluid, electrolyte, and protein replacement; (3) measures to optimize oxygen transport; (4) pharmacologic measures to ensure adequate circulation, combat acidosis, and stabilize lysosomal membranes; and (5) surgical intervention geared at removal of the source of infection.

Antimicrobial Therapy

Systemic wide-spectrum antibiotic therapy must be instituted without delay. This should be directed to eradication of the most common offenders (see Table 16–2, Chapter 16, "The Burn Wound: Microbiologic Aspects"). Proper selection of specific antibiotics is highly dependent on whether or not wound surface cultures or data from quantitative microbiology of the burn wound are already available.[42] If not available, therapy is initiated with an aminoglycoside, such as tobramycin or amikacin, and a penicillinase-resistant penicillin, such as methicillin or nafcillin, in full therapeutic doses. At institutions where methicillin-resistant *Staphylococcus aureus* is prevalent, vancomycin is commonly substituted.[46] If the patient is in shock, has evidence of multiple organ failure, or continues to deteriorate despite antibiotic therapy, a third antibiotic such as ticarcillin, an antipseudomonal penicillin, is added. Surveillance microbiologic data is useful to detect development of strains resistant to gentamicin or tobramycin[86] and may thus favor amikacin as the initial drug of choice. Third-generation cephalosporins with activity against gram-negative bacteria and excellent tissue penetration continue to emerge and offer promise for the future, but their use in burned children has been limited.

In general, the dose of aminoglycosides necessary to accomplish any given blood level is higher in children than in adults. This is related to increased water turnover and higher surface-to-weight ratios characteristic of young children as well as to increased clearance of the drug in the urine and burn exudate.[32] Thus the usual starting doses of tobramycin in children are between 6 to 9 mg/kg/day or 2 to 3 mg/kg/dose. The optimal dose, however, must be determined by repeated measurements of antibiotic blood levels[12] and if available, minimal inhibitory concentrations (MIC) and serum static levels.

Fluid, Electrolyte, and Protein Replacement

The basic defect in septic/endotoxic shock occurs at the cellular level. The cell fails to process or utilize oxygen as a result of a metabolic block, and energy production is limited. The net effect of this is a predominance of anaerobic metabolism with the consequent production of lactic acid and the development of a metabolic acidosis.[95, 115] The goal of therapy is to improve oxygen availability at the cellular level and optimize its uptake. Thus, improvement of arterial blood oxygenation and maintenance of adequate circulation (cardiac output) represent priorities of treatment. The effects of endotoxins, however, are multiple,[24] and the lung remains a primary target organ.[11] An important area on which the lipopolysaccharide exerts its damage is the alveolocapillary junction.[110] Platelets, leukocytes, and other formed elements aggregate and lyse, releasing mitochondrial enzymes[1, 11] in the pulmonary microcirculation. Pulmonary hypertension develops, and fluid escapes the intravascular space. In addition to increased hydrostatic pressure, vascular permeability is increased,[11] and protein and other high-molecular-weight substances gain access to the pulmonary interstitium and eventually the alveoli as well.[109] Pulmonary edema develops, and oxygen transport at the level of the alveolocapillary junction is impaired (diffusion defect). Edema also results in inactivation of pulmonary surfactant and a tendency toward alveolar collapse and development of atelectasis. Thus, a significant percentage of alveoli are perfused, but not ventilated (shunt effect), and venous blood returns to the left heart without being oxygenated in its passage through the lungs. The resulting hypoxemia further worsens oxygen uptake at the cellular level.

Excessive fluid losses at sites of inflammation, venular vasodilation, stasis, increased vascular permeability, vomiting, paralytic ileus, and occasionally diarrhea, usually lead to hypovolemia and decreased blood return to the heart. This is further accentuated by pulmonary hypertension[118, 119] and impaired myocardial contractility, with a consequent fall in cardiac output.[38, 108, 115]

While we favor the use of colloid-containing fluids for circulatory support, we recognize that careful physiologic monitoring at the bedside should determine the proper solution to utilize and the most appropriate time for each intervention.

The optimal goal for fluid therapy in the septic/endotoxic burn patient is restoration of circulatory function and tissue perfusion. This must be accomplished without overloading the circulation, fostering pulmonary edema, or worsening the respiratory failure. In other words, fluid administration must be accomplished at the least possible physiologic cost.

Certain principles must be stressed:

1. Evaluate the physiologic derangement and its consequences and balance them against possible complications of fluid therapy, i.e., if the blood pressure is reduced but is sufficient to maintain glomerular ultrafiltration, and urine continues to be produced, then circulatory hemodynamics are probably acceptable, particularly if the patient is not hypoxemic nor acidotic. Under these circumstances fluid therapy should be directed toward maintenance of a relatively compensated state, rather than correction of the total hemodynamic deficit. The latter may otherwise require excessive fluids, inotropic agents, and/or vasoconstrictive drugs, which may worsen fluid flux at the level of the pulmonary capillary and tend to enhance pulmonary edema.

2. Use only isotonic solutions, and in the least possible amounts. Hypotonic salt solutions have no place in the management of the hemodynamically unstable septic patient. Even isotonic salt solutions leave the vascular compartment within minutes and tend to expand the interstitial fluid space to a greater extent than the intravascular space.[111]

3. Use colloids (5% to 15% human serum albumin solution) to reduce fluid intake and maintain colloid osmotic pressure (COP) above 15 to 16 mm Hg.[103, 114]

4. Be satisfied with small gains in the right direction and avoid major therapeutic swings.

The most common physiologic derangement in the pediatric burn patient in whom septicemia develops is a normal or high cardiac output (CO) and a low systemic vascular resistance (SVR). This so-called hyperdynamic state of septic shock[50] is a manifestation of early sepsis and is usually associated with a good prognosis.

Progression of the endotoxic shock to the hypodynamic state, characterized by a low CO and high SVR, indicates failure of the normal compensatory mechanisms and a greater degree of metabolic and physiologic derangement (Fig 18–4). This late phase of

Septic Shock

Variable	Early	Late
C.O.	↑	↓
SVR	↓	↑
VO_2	↑↓	↓
CVP	↓	↑
PCWP	↓	↑
Urine output	↑	↓

FIG 18–4.
Cardiovascular hemodynamics during the early (hyperdynamic phase) and late (hypodynamic phase) of septic shock. Cardiac output, CO; systemic vascular resistance, SVR; oxygen consumption, VO_2; central venous pressure, CVP; pulmonary capillary wedge pressure, PCWP. (Adapted from Sayeed MM: Pulmonary cellular dysfunction in endotoxic shock: Metabolic and transport derangements. *Circ Shock* 1982; 9:335–355; Traber DL, Adair TH, Adams T: Hemodynamic consequences of endotoxemia in sheep. *Circ Shock* 1981; 8:551–561; Weil MH, Nishijima H: Cardiac output in bacterial shock. *Am J Med* 1978; 64:920.)

shock carries a poor prognosis and frequently culminates with the death of the patient.

Depending on the degree of arteriolar vasoconstriction, venular vasodilation (capacitance bed), the combined effect of these two variables on CO, and the blood pressure (derived from the product of CO and SVR), excessive fluid administration may not be necessary during the early phase. In most cases, isotonic fluids (5% dextrose in 0.9% sodium chloride or 5% dextrose in lactated Ringer's solution) at maintenance rates are sufficient to support the patient during this phase (Fig 18–5). However, if the colloid osmotic pressure (COP) is below 15 mm Hg, the blood pressure is low, or severe oliguria develops, colloids must be added to the resuscitation fluids. The effects of endotoxin on renal hemodynamics are depicted in Fig 18–6. Administration of a lethal dose of *Escherichia coli* endotoxin (1 mg/kg) to range sheep is usually associated with significant changes in renal hemodynamics that may or may not be preventable but are often reversible. The animal may become polyuric, oliguric, or completely anuric within a few hours of injection.[108] At this stage urine production cannot be relied on to assess the state of hydration, and fluid balance must be adjusted according to the difference between expected and actual urine production. A tendency toward high-output renal failure with a relatively fixed urine osmolality and a high urine output represents the most common clinical syndrome during the early phases. This concentration defect must be recognized early if hypernatremia and dehydration are to be avoided.

EXAMPLE.—Let us assume that prior to the development of septic shock, a 7-year-old child with a body surface area of 0.9 sq m and a 50% burn (BSA burn 0.45 sq m) was receiving fluids by mouth at a rate of 125 ml/hour. His blood pressure has now dropped to 80/60 mm Hg, and his urine output has decreased to 15 ml/hour for the last 2 hours. Analysis of arterial blood gases reveals a pH of 7.5, a partial pressure of CO_2 in arterial blood (Pa_{CO_2}) of 30 mm Hg, and a bicarbonate level of 22 mEq/L, and the Pa_{O_2} is 60 mm Hg.

In this example the patient is probably hyperdynamic, and the drop in blood pressure and urine output are probably secondary to a decrease in SVR. Effectively, the patient is hypovolemic, but tissue perfusion is probably adequate as there is no evidence of metabolic acidosis. Even though the urine output is decreased, the fact that urine continues to be produced indicates that glomerular ultrafiltration and thus capillary pressure has been

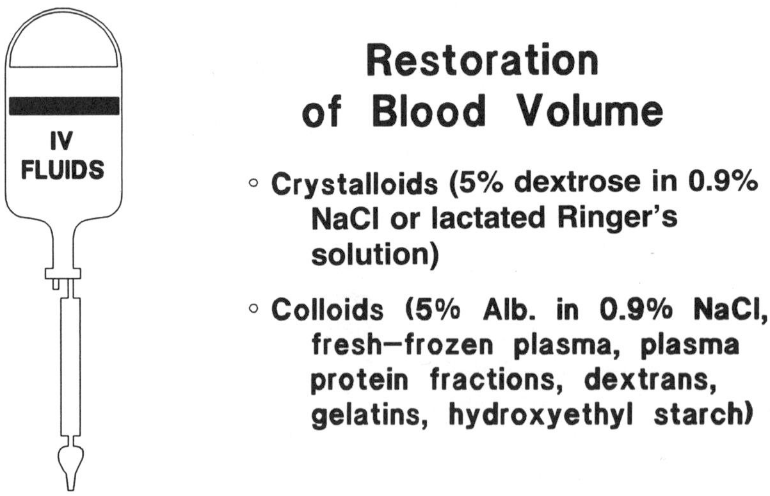

FIG 18–5.
Choice of resuscitation fluids in patients with septicemia and/or septic shock. Alb. indicates albumin.

Variable	Response		
	Immediate	Early (0-3 hours)	Late (3-6 hours)
Blood Pressure	↓ ↓	↓	↓
Cardiac Output	↓ ↓	→	↓
Heart Rate	→	↑	↑
Peripheral Resistance	↑ ↑	↓	↑
Blood pH	↓	↓	↓
Arterial paO_2	↓ ↓	↓↓	↓
Arterial pCO_2	↓	↓	↓↓
Base Excess	↓	↓↓	↓↓↓
Hematocrit	↑	↑	↑
Plasma Renin	↑	↑↑	↑
Urine Flow	↓ ↓	↓↓	↓↓
Urine OSM	↑	→	↓
Plasma OSM	↑	↑	↑
cH_2O	↑	↑ ↑	↑↑
$\frac{cOSM}{GFR} \times 100$	→	↓	↓
Serum Sodium	→	→	↑
Fractional Na Excretion	→	→	→
Serum Potassium	→	↓	↓
Fractional K Excretion	→	→	→
Serum Chloride	→	→	↑
Fractional cl Excretion	→	→	→
Renal Plasma Flow	↓ ↓	→	↓
GFR	↓ ↓	↓ ↓	↓↓
FF	→	→	→
PAH Extraction Ratio	↓	↓	↓↓
WBC	↓	↓	↓

FIG 18–6.
Hemodynamic and kidney function changes in experimental endotoxemia (sheep).

maintained, and kidney perfusion is at acceptable levels.

Thus, under these circumstances we would begin IV therapy with an isotonic solution of 5% dextrose in lactated Ringer's solution at a rate of 125 ml/hour (the same total fluid intake the patient was receiving), and except for antacids,[61] the patient receives nothing by mouth. If the COP is low we would add 5% albumin to the hydrating fluids and would maintain the rate of fluid administration unchanged until an increase in COP above 15 mm Hg is attained. If hypotension or oliguria worsens, serum lactic acid increases, or a metabolic acidosis develops, we would then add a vasoactive amine such as isoproterenol, dopamine, or dobutamine in full therapeutic doses until a blood pressure response is achieved.

If the condition of the patient continues to worsen, hemodynamic monitoring becomes mandatory, and a flow-directed, balloon-tipped Swan-Ganz catheter is then inserted. Heretofore, fluid administration, whether colloid or crystalloid, push or continuous infusion, is best guided by repeated measurements of cardiac index (CI), mean pulmonary artery pressure (MAP) and pulmonary capillary wedge pressure (PCWP), oxygen transport variables (O_2 availability, consumption, and extraction), SVR, pulmonary vascular resistance (PVR), stroke volume, and left ventricular stroke-work index (LVSWI). During this phase, pulmonary edema is a common complication, and excessive fluid administration must be avoided at all cost. Maintenance of COP-PCWP gradient to levels above 4 mm Hg has been shown to prevent or minimize edema formation in the lungs,[88] but such is not easily attainable (Fig 18–7). Albumin administration in concentrations of up to 15% may increase COP, but simultaneous effects upon left-heart filling pressures (pulmonary capillary wedge pressure [PCWP]), may negate any potential benefits from the rise in COP, and thus the need for continuous hemodynamic monitoring. An alternative to colloid administration would be to attempt a reduction of the hydrostatic pressure in the lung microvessels. Such would be indicated even though the pulmonary vascular pressures are in the normal range. Furthermore, this should be attempted with full realization that it may affect CO and systemic oxygen delivery. Nonetheless, the effects of progressive pulmonary edema are so devastating that reduction of the pulmonary hydrostatic pressure to the lowest possible value should be considered a major therapeutic objective.

Measures to Optimize Oxygen Transport

The Swan-Ganz catheter also allows for monitoring of pulmonary function, and particularly important variables to measure include (1) oxygen available (VQ), (2) oxygen consumption (VO_2), and (3) venous admixture

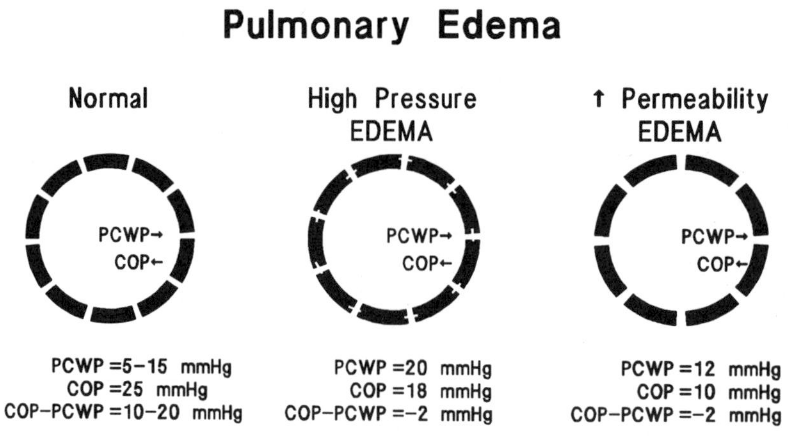

FIG 18–7.
COP-PCWP gradient under normal conditions, high pressure, and increased permeability pulmonary edema. (Adapted from Rackow EC, Fein IA, Leppo J: Colloid osmotic pressure as a prognostic indicator of pulmonary edema and mortality in the critically ill. *Chest* 1977; 72:709–713.)

(shunt effect) or perfusion in excess of ventilation (QS/QT).

A reduced oxygen consumption in the presence of adequate supply, the hallmark of septic shock, may indicate a metabolic block or failure of the cell to process oxygen, but it may also result from arteriovenous shunts that effectively "amputate" sick cells from the circulation, and available oxygen (VQ) is not utilized.[95] This represents a normal physiologic response to contracted intravascular volume. Under these circumstances, a bolus of crystalloid-colloid fluids for the purpose of rapidly-expanding the intravascular volume may reduce arteriovenous shunts and thus restore VO_2 to normal.[44, 101]

Estimation of the true or absolute shunt (anatomical and capillary shunts plus venous admixture) provides additional information to guide fluid therapy. Aggressive cardiopulmonary therapy, fluid restriction, and diuretics would be indicated if the absolute shunt exceeds 30% or progressive deterioration of the patient's condition so requires it.[100]

ADULT RESPIRATORY DISTRESS SYNDROME

Adult respiratory distress syndrome (ARDS) represents one of the most serious complications of gram-negative septicemia in burned patients and the major reason interventions aimed at improving oxygen transport are needed.[7, 89] Adult respiratory distress syndrome represents a conglomerate of signs, symptoms, and laboratory abnormalities associated with respiratory failure and multiple etiologies. Although not exclusive to burn injuries or sepsis, ARDS is frequently seen in association with gram-negative septicemia and is almost invariably present in all burned victims who die following an episode of sepsis.[53] In addition to septicemia, several risk factors exist that predispose burned patients to the development of ARDS. These include aspiration of gastric contents, multiple blood transfusions, smoke inhalation, prolonged ventilatory support, pneumonia, and extensive trauma.

Adult respiratory distress syndrome, also known as "shock lung," "posttraumatic pulmonary insufficiency," "wet lung," "respiratory lung," and "Da Nang lung," is characterized by increased vascular permeability, decreased lung compliance, and decreased functional residual capacity (FRC); in most patients, one can also demonstrate decreased lung volumes, increased alveoloarterial oxygen gradients, pulmonary shunting, formation of hyaline membranes, diffuse pulmonary infiltrates, and areas of consolidation and atelectasis on chest x-ray (see Fig 18–3). It is more common in adults, but ARDS can occur in children as well.[41] It represents the most severe insult and reaction of the lung, particularly the alveolocapillary interface, to a variety of noxious stimuli. Patients disclosing the full-blown syndrome require maximal ventilatory support with high forced inspiratory oxygen (FIO_2), high inspiratory pressures, high levels of positive end-expiratory pressure (PEEP), and, in most cases continuous invasive monitoring. Despite maximal efforts in this regard, careful attention to fluid balance, and maintenance of cardiac hemodynamics, progressive deterioration of lung function eventually leads to multiple organ failure, and death may occur.[80] In burned patients, ARDS has been reported during the immediate postburn period and following aspiration of gastric contents, but is more commonly associated with gram-negative septicemia and/or fluid overload, the former usually contributing to the latter.

Treatment remains largely supportive, with the main objectives being to reopen atelectatic alveoli, to improve pulmonary circulation, and to decrease intrapulmonary shunting. This usually requires continuous positive-pressure ventilation using a volume-cycled ventilator, high FIO_2s (0.5 to 1.0), and high levels of PEEP (10 to 20 cm H_2O). Low inspiratory flows and large tidal volumes usually improve intrapulmonary gas distribution and minimize dead-space ventilation and barotrauma. Distribution is further improved by creation of an inspiratory plateau.[54] Although a careful balance between risks and benefits must be considered in each patient before the decision for invasive monitoring is made, most burned children with sepsis who are receiving maximal ventilatory support and are requiring PEEP levels in excess of 12 to 15 cm H_2O are best managed by careful monitoring of cardiorespiratory variables, and repeated measurements of oxygen transport data with the Swan-Ganz catheter.[88] The goal of mechanical ventilation is to optimize oxygen transport (oxygen availability and oxygen consumption) without jeopardizing venous return or CO. Optimal PEEP levels must be sought. These can be defined as those that result in maximal reduction in intrapulmonary shunting without compromising left-ventricular stroke volumes. In most cases, the myocardium must be supported as well by cautious volume administration, inotropic support, or afterload reduction. These measures are usually necessary for the patient to tolerate the increase in PEEP that is required to maintain FRC at levels that assure adequate oxygenation.

The flow-directed, balloon-tipped catheter (Swan-Ganz) has been extensively used in both adults and children with ARDS with encouraging results.[83] In the burned child, however, the complication of central catheters are significantly higher,[59, 87, 93] and their risks may outweigh any potential benefits. On the other hand, treatment of the burned child with sepsis who has developed ARDS "blindly" (without the benefit of hemodynamic and oxygen-transport monitoring) is challenging, to say the least, and the results are often discouraging.

Pharmacologic Measures to Ensure Adequate Circulation, Combat Acidosis, and Stabilize Lysosomal Membranes

In addition to antibiotic therapy, various other pharmacologic agents are needed in the management of the patient with sepsis. Physicians must be thoroughly familiar with the effects of these drugs and the indications for their use[28] and must be prepared to carry out invasive monitoring to better assess the physiologic responses of the patient to the various therapeutic interventions.

VASOACTIVE AMINES

While in most cases volume expansion with isotonic electrolytes or colloid-containing solutions is sufficient to maintain blood pressure and cardiac hemodynamics, the early use of inotropic and vasopressor agents may prevent excessive fluid, electrolyte, and colloid administration. During the warm shock phase (hyperdynamic state), the CO is elevated and SVR is decreased; the blood pressure is maintained, and no evidence of circulatory insufficiency or lactic acidosis exists. However, as the condition of the patient worsens, the peripheral resistance progressively increases, and the CO falls. Decreased myocardial contractility and a drop in CO (unresponsive to volume administration) characterize the hypodynamic or cardiogenic shock phase.[44] Under these circumstances, fluid balance must be meticulously maintained, and inotropic support of the cardiac muscle becomes increasingly important. The salient effects of the drugs that have been shown to be useful in this regard are discussed below.

DOPAMINE.—Dopamine hydrochloride is a sympathomimetic amine that occurs naturally as intermediate precursor of norepinephrine and is widely used for the treatment of shock. The unique effects of dopamine compared to other catecholamines is that it dilates mesenteric and renal blood vessels through stimulation of dopaminergic receptors. Through this mechanism, dopamine increases renal blood flow (RBF), glomerular filtration (GFR), natriuresis, and urine production. This effect is seen at low pharmacologic doses in the range of 1 to 2 μg/kg/minute, which usually have little if any effect on the heart. Doses in the range of 5 to 10 μg/kg/minute also stimulate β-adrenergic receptors in the heart and increase CO, but usually do not increase heart rate or blood pressure.[25, 27] Doses greater than 10 to 15 μg/kg/minute stimulate α-adrenergic receptors to produce generalized vasoconstriction, which raises arterial blood pressure, but significantly decrease tissue perfusion and thus foster lactic acid production and metabolic acidosis. At doses greater than 20 μg/kg/minute, α-adrenergic-mediated vasoconstriction may reverse the dopaminergic vasodilatation of the mesenteric and renal vasculature, resulting in decreased blood flow to the kidney.[33]

Dopamine is indicated in the management of septic shock to improve myocardial contractility, CO, and renal blood flow.[27, 29, 55] In most cases doses in the range of 5 to 10 μg/kg/minute are sufficient to accomplish these goals. As the CO increases, a mild to moderate effect on blood pressure may be observed even at these relatively low doses. Thus, even though the blood pressure may remain below normal, RBF, GFR, and urine output are usually maintained at acceptable levels, and metabolic acidosis is prevented. A further drop in blood pressure, however, may not be tolerated and anuria, metabolic acidosis, and organ failure rapidly ensue. In the latter case, higher doses of dopamine (>10 to 15 μg/kg/minute) may be necessary to maintain blood pressure and flow to vital organs, but tissue perfusion suffers and metabolic acidosis may not be avoidable. For these reasons, we do not recommend the use of doses higher than 15 μg/kg/minute.

ISOPROTERENOL

Isoproterenol is the most active of the sympathomimetic amines that act almost exclusively on β-receptors. Isoproterenol has positive inotropic and chronotropic effects on the heart, but in contrast to dopamine, it lowers peripheral vascular resistance. This latter effect occurs primarily in skeletal muscle but also in the renal and mesenteric vascular beds, and the diastolic pressure usually falls. The increase in CO, secondary to an increased venous return, increased myocardial contractility, and an increase in heart rate, usually compensates for the fall in SVR; the systolic pressure may even increase, but the diastolic and mean arterial pressures are usually lowered. High doses (>0.15 μg/kg/minute) are more likely to result in hypotension.

In septic shock, isoproterenol usually increases renal blood flow and maintains urine production. Because of this, as well as because of its effects on peripheral vascular resistance, isoproterenol alone or in combination with dopamine is ideally suited for the treatment of the hypodynamic phase of septic shock. However, if significant hypotension has already developed, volume expanders, as well as the concomitant use of dopamine, is usually necessary to restore perfusion to vital organs. Although isoproterenol has not been demonstrated to have much effect on pulmonary vascular resistance, its relaxing effects upon bronchial smooth muscle is also advantageous for the treatment of ARDS.

DOBUTAMINE

Dobutamine is a drug with intermediate effects between dopamine and isoproterenol.[34, 78] It enhances the contractile force of the heart without increasing the heart rate and, in doses of 2.5 to 15 μg/kg/minute, increases the CO without much effect on peripheral vascular resistance and only minimal increases in heart rate.[116] Dobutamine has no effects on renal vasculature, but as it increases CO, it indirectly improves perfusion of the kidneys. Unless the patient is in shock, we routinely initiate therapy with isoproterenol in doses of 0.1 μg/kg/minute, and in the absence of metabolic acidosis or significant hypotension, we maintain the patient on a single drug for 24 to 48 hours. If the blood pressure cannot be maintained, additional fluid pushes may be administered, and dopamine is usually added to the regimen (10 to 15 μg/kg/minute). Once the patient is stabilized, replacement of the above drug combination with dobutamine may be a desirable end point before the weaning process is begun. While lactic acid measurement and analysis of arterial gases are adequate to monitor oxygen delivery and tissue perfusion, hemodynamic monitoring is better suited to guide drug therapy as well as other intervention, particularly when the patient has reached the hypodynamic or uncompensated shock phase.

Other drugs such as sodium nitroprusside,[9, 19, 65] tolazoline,[117] hydralazine,[2] and prostaglandins[66] may be indicated under specific circumstances and when other measures have failed to effect reversion of physiologic derangement.[44] In children sodium nitroprusside is the agent of choice, as its onset of action is rapid and its effects are of short duration.[58] In summary, patients with septic shock should be initially managed conservatively, but as the disease progresses and hemodynamic insufficiency develops, every measure to improve the patient's position on the Frank-Starling curve (Fig 18–8) must be at-

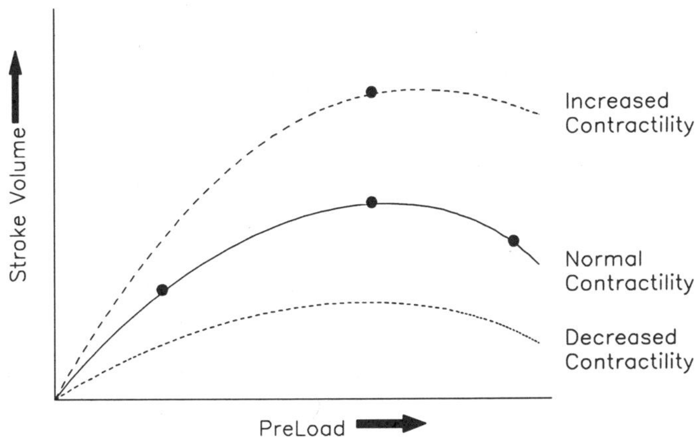

FIG 18–8.
Frank-Starling curve. Volume expansion at any given level of contractility will result in an increase in stroke volume. Once a certain limit of myocardial fiber length is reached, further increases in preload would reduce stroke volume.

tempted. Volume expansion, inotropic support, or afterload reduction, in addition to adequate ventilation and oxygenation, are the mainstays of treatment. These measures must be instituted in a careful and methodic fashion with the guidance of continuous invasive monitoring.

STEROIDS

Even though the use of steroids in septic shock remains controversial, and the original studies of Schumer[97, 98] have not been consistently reproduced,[10] we continue to advocate their use in the pediatric burn patient in whom gram-negative septicemia develops. Originally we were concerned, as others were,[10] with the potential complications and detrimental effects of steroid therapy (Table 18–4). Throughout the years, however, these complications have proved to be more theoretical than factual, or perhaps only of significance with repeated administration of the drug.[99] While we agree wth Blaisdell[10] that most patients who die from infection do so from multiple organ failure or diffuse overwhelming sepsis and not from septic shock, we believe that when given during the early stages of sepsis, steroids can interrupt the progressive downhill course, which was so characteristic of burn septicemia prior to Schumer's studies (Fig 18–9). The mechanisms by which steroids in high doses exert their beneficial effects are probably multiple and for the most part remain to be elucidated.[99] Stabilization of lysosomal membranes[97] is potentially the most important therapeutic effect of steroids in burned patients, but such stabilization requires that the drug be administered prior to the development of frank "septic or endotoxic shock." Thus in the septic patient we advocate the use of steroids (maximum of two doses) at the first sign of hypoxemia (Pa_{O_2} <80 mm Hg while breathing room air). We routinely used methylprednisolone (Solu-Medrol) in a dose of 30 mg/kg of body weight by rapid IV infusion, diluted with 5% dextrose in water over a period of 30 to 45 minutes. Push infusions of the undiluted drug have been associated with sudden deaths and should be avoided. In our experience a clinical improvement usually manifested by a reduction in the respiratory rate and improved oxygenation usually follows a single dose of steroids, but occasionally two consecutive doses given at 6-hour intervals are necessary.

It would be naive to assume that steroid therapy by itself has been solely responsible for the improved survival in the pediatric burn victim.[16, 31] The management of septicemia, endotoxemia, and septic shock is complex and is still highly empirical. Each therapeutic intervention carries with it significant risks, and survival is to a large extent dependent on continuous monitoring of the patient and carefully weighing at each step of the advantages and disadvantages of the various interventions. Despite an early diagnosis, prompt institution of therapy, continuous monitoring, and early use of steroids, a significant number of pediatric burn victims continue to die. We have not reached the 90% survival reported by Schumer,[97] but mortality

TABLE 18–4.
Anti-Inflammatory and Immunosuppressive Effects of Steroids*

Neutrophilic leukocytosis
Impaired granulocyte random movement and chemotaxis
Impaired bactericidal activity of granulocytes and macrophages
Suppression of lymphocyte response to PHA
Delayed hypersensitivity to mumps, *Candida*, and tuberculosis
Lymphopenia (all subpopulations)
Eosinopenia
Anticomplementemic effects
Impaired prostaglandin response
Depression of serum immunoglobulins

*Data from Hirschberg T, Randazzo B, Hirschberg H: Effects of methylprednisolone on the in vitro induction and function of suppressor cells in man. *Scand J Immunol* 1980; 12:33–39; Majewski JA, Alexander JW: The steroid effect on the in vitro human neutrophil chemotactic response. *J Surg Res* 1976; 21:265–268; O'Flaherty JT, Craddock PR, Jacobs HS: Mechanism of anticomplementary activity of corticosteroids in vivo. *Proc Soc Exp Biol Med* 1977; 154:206–209; Rinehart JJ, Balcerzak SP, Sagone AL, et al: Effects of corticosteroids on human monocyte function. *J Clin Invest* 1974; 54:1337–1343.

GROUP	CONTROL	EXPERIMENTAL
Treatment	Saline	Dexamethasone – 3mg/kg or Prednisolone – 30mg/kg
N	85	86
Mortality	32 (38%)	9 (10.5%)
Complications	3 (4%)	4 (5%)

FIG 18–9.
Steroids in the treatment of gram-negative septicemia, a prospective study. (Adapted from Schumer W: Steroids in the treatment of clinical septic shock. *Ann Surg* 1976; 184:333–341.)

continues to decrease and currently approaches 15%. Considering that patients studied by Schumer were not burned, a 15% mortality rate represents a significant accomplishment.

SODIUM BICARBONATE

While prompt correction of imbalances in acid-base metabolism, and in particular metabolic acidosis, seems a reasonable therapeutic objective for the septic patient, the most important intervention should be elimination of the source of excess hydrogen ions, rather than administration of alkaline solutions.[36] In the patient with septic shock, this can be translated into prompt correction of hypovolemia, restoration of cardiac hemodynamics, and maintenance of adequate oxygenation. These patients are usually dehydrated, hypoxic, and severely acidotic, and their supply of oxygen to the tissues is compromised. Peripheral vasoconstriction, decreased myocardial contractility, and low levels of 2,3-diphosphoglycerate are responsible for tissue hypoxia. In order to compensate for this, the increase in hydrogen ion concentration brings about a "rightward shift" of the oxyhemoglobin dissociation curve, and the release of oxygen from hemoglobin is enhanced. Thus, despite a reduction in available oxygen, the excess of hydrogen ions exerts a protective effect upon tissue oxygenation.[45] This compensatory mechanism is lost whenever overcorrection or rapid correction of the acidotic state is induced. Thus the need for caution exists when attempting to correct the pH by administration of sodium bicarbonate.

Another problem associated with rapid correction of acidosis is the consequent rise in Pa_{CO_2}, which invariably occurs as the pH increases. Carbon dioxide diffuses readily across cell membranes and across the blood-brain barrier, while bicarbonate lags behind. The net effect of this phenomenon is worsening of intracellular and cerebrospinal fluid (CSF) acidosis and impairment of organ function and the level of mentation. Also, the drive for ventilation is decreased, and a vicious cycle may develop.[81] The effects of bicarbonate on serum electrolytes and osmolality can be significant as well. Bicarbonate administration lowers levels of serum potassium and calcium and increases the sodium level and the osmolality. Repeated doses of bicarbonate frequently result in hypernatremia and hyperosmolality,[30,56] and, indirectly, intracellular dehydration and acidosis.[74]

Thus in the septic patient sodium bicarbonate is only indicated in the presence of severe metabolic acidosis with a blood pH below 7.2. Assuming normal pulmonary function and maximal respiratory compensation, a pH below 7.2 would be associated with a serum bicarbonate level below 10 mEq/L. The goal of therapy is to increase the bicarbonate level to just above 10 mEq/L (i.e., 12 mEq/L) to partially correct the degree of ionic imbalance.

The conventional formula, and one that we continue to advocate to estimate the dose of sodium bicarbonate, is as follows:

$$\text{Dose (in mEq)} = (12 - [HCO_3^-]) \times (0.5 \times \text{weight [kg]})$$

EXAMPLE.—A 20-kg child presents with arterial blood gases in the following range: pH, 7.17; Pa_{CO_2}; 17; and bicarbonate concentration, 6 mEq/L. The dose necessary to raise the serum bicarbonate level to 12 mEq/L will be as follows: dose (mEq) = (12 − 6) × (0.5 × 20); dose = 60 mEq.

In most cases, we recommend that half of the calculated dose be administered by slow push and that the other half be given by rapid drip over 1 hour. All subsequent doses of bicarbonate are calculated and administered in the same manner. For as long as the pH is greater than 7.2 and the serum bicarbonate level is greater than 10 mEq/L, no further doses of sodium bicarbonate are given. We must emphasize that in the patient with septic shock, bicarbonate therapy is a temporizing measure and that the treatment priority should be to improve circulation and tissue oxygenation.

PHOSPHATE SALTS

Hypophosphatemia is a common complication of chronic illnesses and particularly burn injuries. The consequences of this metabolic disorder are manifold (see Table 7–3, Chapter 7, "Resuscitation of the Burned Child"). Of particular importance to the septic patient are the effects of hypophosphatemia not only on the function of granulocytes and monocytes (decreased chemotaxis, phagocytosis, and killing power), but also on red cell function and the oxyhemoglobin dissociation curve (shift to the left), which effectively impairs the release of oxygen to the tissues. To prevent hypophosphatemia, we routinely administer, throughout the patient's entire hospitalization, intravenous potassium supplements in the form of the phosphate salts. As soon as the patient tolerates fluids given by mouth, the milk program is promptly reinstituted (milk is rich in phosphate). Serum phosphate levels are monitored frequently in our patients, and any deficits that are detected are corrected promptly.

Surgical Intervention Geared at Removal of the Source of Infection

In the burned patient, the burn wound is the most common site for bacterial colonization and the obvious port of entry of organisms to the bloodstream. Thus in most cases, gram-negative septicemia is preceded by the development of burn wound sepsis. The latter has been defined by Teplitz et al.[106] as "the presence of actively proliferating microorganisms exceeding 10^5/gm of burn wound tissue and actively invading subjacent unburned tissue." In most cases this is associated with discolored, purulent, and foul-smelling wounds, but in some cases, infection is not readily apparent to the naked eye. As defined above, burn wound sepsis is associated with a poor prognosis,[47, 84] and in its management the physician is often confronted with a therapeutic dilemma. On one hand, systemic antibiotics are unlikely to yield adequate concentrations in burned, devitalized tissues, and bacterial replication is likely to continue uninterrupted. On the other hand, the surgical risk associated with excisions of large sections of the burn wound is felt to be too high to undertake routinely. The studies of Parks et al.[76] have provided evidence that surgical excision of infected devitalized burn tissues in most cases down to fascia can be accomplished safely in patients with burn wound sepsis and even in the presence of septicemia. By removing the source of infection and the continuous showering of organisms, morbidity and mortality was decreased, and marked improvement in the overall condition of the patient was attained within hours of the operative procedure. In these series, which included 22 children with histologically confirmed burn wound sepsis (burns ranged from 33% to 91% of the total BSA), no intraoperative deaths occurred, and the overall mortality was 14% (3 children died at 2, 5, and 56 days postoperatively). Since initiation of surgical intervention as an adjunct to accepted medical management of sepsis, the overall mortality has remained low,[16] and the procedure is now performed on a routine basis.

CONCLUSIONS

Gram-negative septicemia is a common and often fatal complication of burn injuries. The port of entry of the organism to the bloodstream is primarily the burn wound. Although colonization of open wounds with bacteria is invariably present, septicemia is rare in patients with burns affecting less than 35% of the BSA. Prevention efforts should be directed to patients with large burns and particularly those who are immunocompromised, malnourished, or have other associated pathologic findings. Early detection requires continuous monitoring of the patient. An algorithm for use in burned children is proposed.

Once the diagnosis has been established, a conservative, methodical, and physiologically oriented approach to the management of the patient is recommended. Patients with septic shock require invasive monitoring and cardiopulmonary support, which is best provided in an intensive care setting. Some of the therapeutic principles and modalities, which in our hands have reduced morbidity and mortality, are discussed.

REFERENCES

1. Adams T, Traber DL: The effects of a prostaglandin synthetase inhibitor, Ibuprofen, on the cardiopulmonary response to endotoxin in sheep. *Circ Shock* 1982; 9:481–489.
2. Ablad B: A study of the mechanism of the hemodynamic effects of Hydralazine in man. *Acta Pharmacol Toxicol (Copenh)* 1963; 20 (suppl 1):1–53.
3. Alexander JW: The body's response to infection in *Burns, A Team Approach*. Artz CP, Moncrief JA, Pruitt B (eds): Philadelphia, WB Saunders, 1979, pp 107–119.
4. Alexander JW, MacMillan BG, Stinnett JD, et al.: Beneficial effects of aggressive protein feeding in severely burned children. *Ann Surg* 1980; 192:505–517.
5. Alexander JW, Stinnett JD, Ogle CK, et al: A comparison of immunologic profiles and their influences on bacteremia in surgical patients with a high risk of infection. *Surgery* 1979; 86:94.
6. Askoseljavaara S, Alho A, Sundell B, et al: Endotoxin effect on host defense in burns. *Eur Surg Res* 1979; 11:62.
7. Bachofen M, Weibel ER: Alterations of the gas exchange apparatus in adult respiratory insufficiency associated with septicemia. *Am Rev Respir Dis* 1977; 116:589.
8. Baker CC, Miller CL, Trunkey DD: Predicting fatal sepsis in burn patients. *J Trauma* 1979; 19:641–647.
9. Bhatia SK, and Frolich ED: Hemodynamic comparison of agents useful in hypertensive emergencies. *Am Heart J* 1973; 55:365–373.
10. Blaisdell FW: Controversy in shock research: Con: The role of steroids in sepsis shock. *Circ Shock* 1981; 8:673–682.
11. Bohs CT, Miller TH, Traber DL: Pulmonary vascular response to endotoxin in normal and lymphocyte depleted sheep. *Circ Shock* 1979; 6:13–21.
12. Bostman JL, Wertheimer AI, Zaske D, et al: Individualizing gentamycin dosage regimens in burn patients with gram-negative septicemia: A cost benefit analysis. *J Pharm Sci* 1979; 68:267–272.
13. Brodin B, Von Schenk H, Schildt B, et al: Low plasma fibronectin indicates septicemia in major burns. *Acta Chir Scand* 1984; 150:5–11.
14. Bryant RE, Hood AF, Hood CE, et al: Factors affecting mortality of gram-negative rod bacteremia. *Arch Intern Med* 1971; 127:120.
15. Carvajal HF, Feinstein R, Traber DL, et al: An objective method for eary diagnosis of gram-negative septicemia in burned children. *J Trauma* 1981; 21:221–227.
16. Carvajal HF, Parks DH: Survival statistics in burned children. *J Burn Care Rehabil* 1982; 3:81–84.
17. Cason JS, Lowbury EJL: Prophylactic chemotherapy for burns: Studies on the local and systemic use of combined chemotherapy. *Lancet* 1960; 11:501.
18. Chartrand SA, McCracken G: Staphylococcal pneumonia in infants and children. *Pediatr Infect Dis* 1982; 1:19–23.
19. Chatterjee K, Swan JHC, et al: Effects of vasodilator therapy for severe pump failure in acute myocardial infarction on short-term and late prognosis. *Circulation* 1976; 53:797.
20. Collignon PJ, Sorrell TC, Uther JB: Prevention of sepsis associated with the insertion of

intravenous cannulae. *Med J Aust* 1985; 142:346–348.
21. Cowan DH, Fratianne RB, Ahmed F: Platelet aggregation as a sign of septicemia in thermal injury. *JAMA* 1976; 235:1230–1234.
22. Cuevas P, Ishiyama M, Koizumi S, et al: Role of endotoxemia of intestinal original in early death from large burns. *Surg Gynecol Obstet* 1974; 138:725–730.
23. Curreri PW, Luterman A, Brown DW, et al: Analysis of survival and hospitalization time for 937 patients. *Ann Surg* 1980; 192:471.
24. Davidson I, Gelin LE, Haglind E: Plasma volume, intravascular protein content, hemodynamic and oxygen transport changes during intestinal shock in dogs. *Crit Care Med* 1980; 8:73–80.
25. Dopamine for treatment of septic shock. *The Medical Letter* 1975; 17:13–14.
26. Driscoll DJ, Gillette PC, Duff DF, et al: Hemodynamic effects of dobutamine in children. *Am J Cardiol* 1979; 43:581–584.
27. Driscoll DJ, Gillette PC, McNamara DG: The use of dopamine in children. *J Pediatr* 1978; 92:309–314.
28. Driscoll DJ, Pinsky WW, Entman ML: How to use inotropic drugs in children. *Drug Ther* 1979; 39:124–135.
29. Drueck C, Welch GW, Pruitt BA: Hemodynamic analysis of septic shock in thermal injury: Treatment with dopamine. *Am Surg* 1978; 44:424–427.
30. Edelman IS, Leibman J, O'Meare MP, et al: Interrelationships between serum concentration, serum osmolality, total exchangeable potassium, and total body water. *J Clin Invest* 1958; 37:1236–1256.
31. Feller I: Improvements in burn care since 1965. *NBIE Newsletter* 1980; 1(1):1–4.
32. Glew RH, Moellening RC, Burke JF: Gentamycin dosage in children with extensive burns. *J Trauma* 1976; 16:819–823.
33. Goldberg LI: Cardiovascular and renal actions of dopamine: Potential clinical applications. *Pharmacol Rev* 1972; 24:1–29.
34. Goldberg LI, Hsieh YY, Resnekou L: Newer catecholamines for treatment of heart failure and shock: An update on dopamine and a first look at dobutamine. *Prog Cardiovasc Dis* 1977; 19:327–340.
35. Hartford CE, Bodensteiner JA, Boyd WC, et al: The use of multiple systemic antibiotics in the treatment of patients with burns. *Surg Gynecol Obstet* 1974; 138:837–840.
36. Hazard PB, Griffin JP: Sodium bicarbonate in the management of systemic acidosis. *South Med J* 1980; 73:1339.
37. Heggers JP, Robson MC, Doran ET: Quantitative assessment of bacterial contamination of open wounds by a slide technique. *Trans Soc Trop Med Hyg* 1969; 63:532–534.
38. Hinshaw LB: Myocardial function in endotoxin shock. *Circ Shock* 1979; 1(suppl):43–51.
39. Helwig JT, Council KA (eds): *Sas User's Guide*. Gary, Ind, SAS Institute, 1979.
40. Hocking RR: The analysis and selection of variables in linear regression. *Biometrics* 1976; 32:1–50.
41. Holbrook PR, Taylor G, Pollack MM, et al: Adult respiratory distress syndrome in children. *Pediatr Clin North Am* 1980; 27:677–685.
42. Holder I, Schwab M, Jackson L: Eighteen months of routine topical antimicrobial susceptibility testing of isolates from burn patients: Results and conclusions. *J Antimicrob Chemother* 1979; 5:455–463.
43. Kahn AM, McGrady VL, Rosen VJ: Burn wound biopsy: Multiple uses in patient management. *Scand J Plast Reconstr Surg* 1979; 13:53.
44. Kaplan SL, Vargo TA: Entoform shock in children, in Dickerman JD, Lucey JF (eds): *The Critically Ill Child.* Philadelphia, WB Saunders Co, 1985, pp 45–64.
45. Kaye R: Diabetic ketoacidosis. The bicarbonate controversy. *J Pediatr* 1975; 87:156–159.
46. Kayser FH: Methicillin resistant staphylococci. *Lancet* 1975; 2:650.
47. Kim SH, Mason AD, Lindberg RB, et al: An evaluation of burn wound biopsy. Washington, DC, American Burn Assoc 1981, p 24.
48. Kreger BE, Craven DE, McCabe WR: Gram-negative bacteremia: Reevaluation of clinical features and treatment in 612 patients. *Am J Med* 1980; 68:344–355.
49. Lawrence JC, Lilly HA: A quantitative method for investigating the bacteriology of skin: Its application to burns. *Br J Exp Pathol* 1972; 53:550.
50. Levin D, Perkin RM: Septic shock, in Nelson JD (ed.): *Current Therapy in Pediatric Infectious Diseases*. Philadelphia, BC Decker, Inc, 1986, pp 208–218.
51. Liedberg N, Reiss E, Artz C: Infection in burns: III. Septicemia a common cause of death. *Surg Gynecol Obstet* 1954; 99:151.
52. Lilly HA, Lowbury EJL, Wilkins MD, Cason JS: Staphylococcal sepsis in a burns unit. *J Hyg* (Lond) 1979; 83:429–435.
53. Linares HA: A report of 115 consecutive autopsies in burned children (1966–1980). *Burns* 1982; 8:263–270.
54. Lindahl S: Influence of an end inspiratory

pause on pulmonary ventilation, gas distribution, and lung perfusion during artificial ventilation. *Crit Care Med* 1979; 7:540.
55. Loeb HS, Winslow E, et al: Acute hemodynamic effects of dopamine in patients with shock. *Circulation* 1977; 44:163.
56. Loeb JN: The hyperosmolar state. *N Engl J Med* 1974; 290:1184–1187.
57. Loebl EC, Marvin JM, Heck EL, et al: The use of quantitative biopsy cultures in bacteriologic monitoring of burn patients. *J Surg Res* 1974; 16:1–5.
58. Luderer J, Hayes AH, Dubynsky O, et al: Long-term administration of sodium nitroprusside in childhood. *J Pediatr* 1977; 91:490–491.
59. MacMillan B, Law E, Holder I: Experience with *Candida* infections in the burn patient. *Arch Surg* 1972; 104:509.
60. Marvin JA, Heck EL, Loebl EC, et al: Usefulness of blood cultures in confirming septic complications in burn patients: Evaluation of a new culture method. *J Trauma* 1975; 15:657–662.
61. McAlhany JC, Czaja AJ, Pruitt BA: Antacid control of complications from acute gastroduodenal disease after burns. *J Trauma* 1976; 16:645.
62. McCabe WR: Gram-negative bacteremia. *Adv Intern Med* 1975; 19:135.
63. McManus WF, et al: Burn wound infection. *J Trauma* 1981; 21:753–756.
64. Majeski JA, Alexander JW: The steroid effect on the in vitro human neutrophil chemotactic response. *J Surg Res* 1976; 21:265–268.
65. Miller RR, Vismara LA, Zelis R, et al: Clinical use of sodium nitroprusside in chronic ischemic heart disease: Effects on peripheral vascular resistance and venous tone and on ventricular volume, pump, and mechanical performance. *Circulation* 1975; 51:328.
66. Moncada S, Flower RJ, Vane JR: Prostaglandins, prostacyclin, and thromboxane A_2, in Goodman A, Goodman LS, Gilman A (eds): *The Pharmacological Basis of Therapeutics* (6th ed). New York, MacMillan Publishing Co, 1980, pp 668–681.
67. Moody BJ, Shakespeare PG, Batstone GF: The effects of septic complications upon the serum protein changes associated with thermal injury. *Ann Clin Biochem* 1985; 22:391–396.
68. Morrison DF: *Multivariate Statistical Methods* (2nd ed). New York, McGraw-Hill Book Co, 1976, pp 230–248.
69. Nathan P, et al: A laboratory method for the selection of topical agents to treat infected burn wounds. *Burns* 1978; 4:177–187.
70. Nathan P, Holder I, MacMillan B: Burn wounds: Microbiology, local host defenses, and current therapy. *Crit Rev Clin Lab Sci* 1973; 4:61–100.
71. Neal GD, et al: Burn wound histological cultures. A new technique for predicting burn wound sepsis. *J Burn Care Rehabil* 1981; 2:35–39.
72. Neu HC: The role of *Pseudomonas aeruginosa* in infections. *J Antimicrob Chemother* 1983; 11(suppl B):1–13.
73. O'Flaherty JT, Craddock PR, Jacob HS: Mechanism of anticomplementary activity of corticosteroids in vivo. *Proc Soc Exp Biol Med* 1977; 154:206–209.
74. Ostrea EM, Odell GB: The influence of bicarbonate administration on blood pH in a "closed system": Clinical implications. *J Pediatr* 1972; 80:671–680.
75. Parks DH, Carvajal HF, Larson DL: Management of burns. *Surg Clin North Am* 1977; 57:875–894.
76. Parks DH, Linares HA, Thompson PD: The surgical management of burn wound sepsis. *Surg Gynecol Obstet* 1981; 153:374–376.
77. Perkin RM, Levin DL: Shock in the pediatric patient: I. *J Pediatr* 1982; 101:163–169.
78. Perkin RM, Levin DL, Webb R, et al: Dobutamine: A hemodynamic evaluation in children with shock. *J Pediatr* 1982; 101:977–983.
79. Petersen SR, Umphred E, Warden GD: The incidence of bacteremia following burn wound excision. *J Trauma* 1982; 22:274–279.
80. Pfenninger J, Gerber A, Tschappeler H, et al: Adult respiratory syndrome in children. *J Pediatr* 1982; 101:352–357.
81. Pierce NF, Fedson DS, Brigham KL, et al: The ventilatory response of acute base deficit in humans, time course during development, and correction of metabolic acidosis. *Ann Intern Med* 1970; 72:633–640.
82. Polischuk SA: Tables aiding differential diagnosis of burn sepsis. *Proceedings of the Symposium for Treatment of Burns.* Prague, September 13–15, 1973, pp 158–161.
83. Pollack MM, Reed TD, Holbrook PR: Bedside pulmonary artery catheterization in pediatrics. *J Pediatr* 1980; 96:274–277.
84. Pruitt BA, Foley FD: The use of biopsy in burn patient care. *Surgery* 1973; 73:887–893.
85. Pruitt BA, Goodwin CW: Stress ulcer disease in the burned patient. *World J Surg* 1981; 5:209–222.
86. Pruitt BA, Lindberg RB, McManus WF, et

al: Current approach to prevention and treatment of *Pseudomonas aeruginosa* infections in burned patients. *Rev Infect Dis* 5:(5), 889–897, 1983.

87. Pruitt BA, McManus WF, Kim SH, et al: Diagnosis of treatment of cannula-related intravenous sepsis in burn patients. *Ann Surg* 1980; 191:546–554.
88. Rackow EC, Fein IA, Leppo J: Colloid osmotic pressure as a prognostic indicator of pulmonary edema and mortality in the critically ill. *Chest* 1977; 72:709–713.
89. Rinaldo JE, Rogers RM: Adult respiratory distress syndrome. *N Engl J Med* 1982; 306:900–909.
90. Rinehart JJ, Balcerzak SP, Sagone AL, et al: Effects of corticosteroids on human monocyte function. *J Clin Invest* 1974; 54:1337–1343.
91. Robson MC, Heggers JP: Bacterial quantification of open wounds. *Milit Med* 1969; 134:19.
92. Rosenberg JC: Suppression of the immune response by steroids: Comparative patency of hydrocortisone, methylprednisolone, and dexamethasone. *Transplantation* 1980; 29: 425–428.
93. Rubio T, Riley HD: Serious systemic infection associated with use of in-dwelling intravenous catheters. *South Med J* 1973; 66:633–637.
94. Sasaki TM, Welch GW, Herndon DN, et al: Burn wound manipulation: Induced bacteremia. *J Trauma* 1979; 19:46–48.
95. Sayeed MM: Pulmonary cellular dysfunction in endotoxic shock. Metabolic and transport derangements. *Circ Shock* 1982; 9:335–355.
96. Schlaes DM, Levy J, Wolinsky E: Enterococcal bacteremia without endocarditis. *Arch Intern Med* 1981; 141:578–581.
97. Schumer W: Steroids in the treatment of clinical septic shock. *Ann Surg* 1976; 184:333–341.
98. Schumer W: Septic shock. *JAMA* 1979; 242:1906–1907.
99. Schumer W: Controversy in shock research: Pro: The role of steroids in septic shock. *Circ Shock* 1981; 8:667–671.
100. Shoemaker WC, Czer LSC: Evaluation of the biologic importance of various hemodynamics and oxygen transport variables. *Crit Care Med* 1979; 7:424–431.
101. Shoemaker WC, Schluchter M, Hopkins JA, et al: Fluid therapy in emergency resuscitation. Clinical evaluation of colloid and crystalloid regimens. *Crit Care Med* 1981; 9(5):367–368.
102. Sibbald WJ, Anderson RR, Drieger H, et al: Alveolocapillary permeability in human septic ARDS. *Chest* 1981; 79:133.
103. Skillmann JJ: The role of albumin and oncotically active fluids in shock. *Crit Care Med* 1976; 4:55.
104. Smith R, Linares HA, Jorgensen JH: Bacteremia and postmortem microbiology in burned children. *Am J Clin Pathol* 1975; 63:502–508.
105. Tahlan RN, Keswani RK, Saini S, et al: Correlation of quantitation burn wound biopsy culture and surface swab culture to burn wound sepsis. *Burns* 1984; 10:217–224.
106. Teplitz C: *Pathology of Burns,* in Artz CP, Moncrief JA (eds): *The Treatment of Burns.* Philadelphia, WB Saunders Co, 1969, pp 22–28.
107. Timmons MJ: Are systemic prophylactic antibiotics necessary for burns? *Ann R Coll Surg Engl* 1983; 65:80.
108. Traber DL, Adair TH, Adams T: Hemodynamic consequences of endotoxemia in sheep. *Circ Shock* 1981; 8:551–561.
109. Traber DL, Adams T, Henriksen N, et al: Reproducibility of cardiopulmonary effects of different endotoxins in the same sheep. *J Appl Physiol* 1983; 54:1167.
110. Traber DL, Thomson PD, Blalock JE, et al: Action of an opiate receptor blocker on ovine cardiopulmonary responses to endotoxins. *Am J Physiol* 1983; 245:H189–H193.

110a. Trunkey DD: Inhalation injury. *Surg Clin North Am* 1978; 58(6):1133–1140.

111. Virgilio RW, Smith DE, Zarins CK: Balanced electrolyte solutions: Experimental and clinical studies. *Crit Care Med* 1979; 7:98.
112. Volenec FJ, Clark GM, Mani MM, et al: Burn wound biopsy bacterial quantitation: A statistical analysis. *Am J Surg* 1979; 138:695.
113. Waisbren BA, Mellender JW, Collentine GE: Burn mortality with treatment by parenteral and local antibiotics and total exposure, in Mattes P, Barclay TL, Konickova Z (eds): Research in burns: Transactions of the Third International Congress on Research in Burns. Bern, Hans Huber Publishers, 1971, pp 201–205.
114. Weil MH, Morisette M, Michaels S, et al: Routine plasma colloid osmotic pressure measurements. *Crit Care Med* 1974; 3:229–234.
115. Weil MH, Nishijima H: Cardiac output in bacterial shock. *Am J Med* 1978; 64:920.
116. Weiner N: Norepinephrine, epinephrine, and the sympathomimetic amines, in Goodman A, Goodman LS, Gilman A (eds): *The Pharmacological Basis of Therapeutics* (6th ed). New York, MacMillan Publishing Co, 1980, pp 138–175.

117. Yoran C, Glassman E: The paradoxic effects of tolazoline hydrochloride on pulmonary hypertension of mitral stenosis. *Chest* 1973; 63:843–846.
118. Zapol WM, Kobayashi K, Snider MT, et al: Vascular obstruction causes pulmonary hypertension in severe acute respiratory failure. *Chest* 1977; 71:306.
119. Zapol WM, Snider MT: Pulmonary hypertension in acute respiratory failure. *N Engl J Med* 1977; 296:476.
120. Zawacki BC, Azen SP, Imbus SH, et al: Multifactorial probit analysis of mortality in burned patients. *Ann Surg* 1979; 189:1–5.

SECTION VI

ORGAN FAILURE

19 / Heat and Smoke Injuries Of the Airway

JOEL H. HOROVITZ, M.D., F.R.C.S.(C.)

Pulmonary complications are a major cause of morbidity and mortality in the burn patient. Some 20% to 25% of patients hospitalized for burn treatment develop pulmonary complications. Within that subgroup of burned patients, 40% to 50% will die from these pulmonary complications. Overall, approximately one in three burn deaths is a direct result of involvement of the respiratory tract. Exposure to heat and smoke, especially in an enclosed space, is the cause of the high morbidity and mortality. This morbidity and mortality was first studied systematically after the Coconut Grove fire in 1940.[32] This chapter will review our current state of knowledge in the field of heat and smoke airway injuries.

Three characteristic types of pulmonary dysfunction seen in the burn population are (1) carbon monoxide poisoning, (2) upper airway obstructive disease, and (3) parenchymal (small-airway) dysfunction.[23] The type and severity of the lesion depend on both the quantity and composition of the inhaled substance. The composition of smoke (a suspension of solid or liquid particle in a mixture of gases) is varied and therefore results in a wide spectrum of pulmonary dysfunction. Early studies in the composition and effects of various noxious agents in smoke showed that kerosene smoke had little deleterious effect.[59] Zikria analyzed wood smoke and found high concentrations of aldehydes, including acrolein, which caused pulmonary edema and death in experimental animals. The process of pyrolysis (superheating without combustion) also produces these same substances. Other constituents of smoke, such as the oxides of sulfur or nitrogen, hydrochlorides, and chlorine gas, are all known irritants to the respiratory tract.

CARBON MONOXIDE POISONING

Acute exposure to carbon monoxide (CO), which is the most common constituent of smoke, is responsible for almost all deaths at the scene of a fire. Carbon monoxide is an odorless, colorless gas that has a great affinity for binding with hemoglobin, thus displacing oxygen (O_2) and leading to asphyxia. The combination of CO and hemoglobin produces carboxyhemoglobin (COHb), which does not carry O_2. Since the affinity of CO for hemoglobin is 250 times greater than that of O_2, the O_2-carrying capacity of the blood is greatly reduced, and the oxygen-hemoglobin dissociation curve is shifted markedly to the left. Carbon monoxide poisoning therefore leads to severe cerebral hypoxemia as well as myocardial ischemia. The extent of CO involvement in early morbidity was only appreciated when routine blood gas analysis became widespread. Chronic lung disease and exposure to cigarette smoke commonly result in blood CO concentrations of 8% to 18%. The effects of CO are proportional to blood CO concentration—COHb concentrations greater than 30% are highly symptomatic of CO poisoning while COHb levels of 60% result in convulsions, coma, and a high mortality.

Since the clinical effects of CO exposure are nonspecific, a high index of suspicion is necessary to make a diagnosis. Carboxyhemoglobin levels should always be measured in any burn or smoke-inhalation patient. Since most patients will have been given O_2 to inhale at the scene or during transport, the initial level of CO measured in the hospital will not accurately reflect the depth of exposure. A nomogram[59] or equation[43] can be used to calculate the original CO level.

Since the binding of CO and hemoglobin is reversible, the mainstay of treatment of CO poisoning is oxygen. Administration of pure O_2 at atmospheric pressure is the initial treatment of choice. If the CO level is greater than 45%, then the airway should be controlled, and volume-cycled ventilation with 100% O_2 should be used rather than O_2 by mask. Many of the patients with CO poisoning will be severely acidotic—a harbinger of a high mortality. However, even in these high-risk patients, successful treatment has been reported without resorting to hyperbaric oxygenation.[49] Some concern exists about using hyperbaric O_2 because even short-term hyperoxia may produce significant pulmonary structural changes.[9]

Other effects of CO poisoning have been noted. Hyperamylasemia has been reported in up to 40% of smoke-inhalation patients with CO poisoning.[50] The amylase value was highest on admission and declined over 2 to 3 days. Isoenzyme analysis has shown that the salivary gland is the organ of origin of the amylase. That diabetes insipidus has been reported in severe CO poisoning,[17] reflects the profound cerebral hypoxia that may occur. The great majority of patients with pure CO poisoning is adequately treated with pure O_2. Only rarely will serious sequelae develop in patients who are resuscitated early.

UPPER AIRWAY OBSTRUCTION

The most common pulmonary abnormality in smoke inhalation is upper airway edema leading to airway obstruction.[35] Toxic products from incomplete combustion are highly irritating to the respiratory mucosa. Heat injury per se is very rare because of the efficient temperature-reducing properties of upper airways. This was shown experimentally in animals given large amounts of dry heat; virtually all heat was dissipated well above the level of the carina.[34] The exception to this is the inhalation of moist heat, which produces severe denudation of the tracheobronchial lining. Steam inhalation from ruptured pipes produces a rapid, severe tracheobronchitis, but this is fortunately a rare event.

Upper airway obstruction is clearly due to the inhalation of smoke alone because it frequently occurs in the absence of cutaneous burns.[59] There are several well-described experimental animal models of pure smoke inhalation using wood or cotton combustion.[22] Many investigators have produced pulmonary edema in these types of preparation because the upper airways are bypassed with an endotracheal tube or tracheostomy. A more complete discussion of pulmonary edema is presented in the next section.

Obstructive disease is clinically suspected in patients with the following characteristics: (1) exposure to smoke in an enclosed space, (2) facial or oral burns, (3) singed nasal hairs, (4) wheezing, and (5) a cough producing soot-laden sputum. In addition, a significant number of these patients will have a history of excessive alcohol or drug ingestion prior to the inhalational episode. While this constellation of history and physical findings is highly suggestive of an inhalation injury, enough variability exists to render these factors nonspecific. In patients with severe smoke exposure, conjunctivitis and copious carbonaceous sputum usually imply a prolonged exposure to the noxious products of smoke.

The definitive diagnosis of upper airway obstructive disease is made with the early, and sometimes repeated, use of fiberoptic bronchoscopy.[25] As soon as the patient is hemodynamically stable, bronchoscopy should be done using topical local anesthesia. If marked edema is present in the upper airway, it is probably unsafe to pass the bronchoscope through the vocal cords. A lubricated endotracheal tube placed over the bronchoscope will allow immediate control of the airway if indicated. If the initial examination shows a totally patent airway, then full bronchoscopy can be safely performed. The bronchoscopic examination may be repeated every 12 hours to document the progression of any obstructive disease. There are a significant number of seriously burned patients (burns from explosions, etc.) who require very early endotracheal intubation, and in these patients the diagnosis of airway edema is easily made.

Other modalities have been suggested for the early diagnosis of inhalation injury. The use of xenon 133 lung scan[35] is an accurate technique, but requires equipment that is not readily available in many hospitals. Arterial blood gas analysis is usually normal in patients with obstructive airway problems until very late in the course, at which time it may be too late to intubate, and emergency tracheostomy will be required. When airway control is necessary, it is preferable to avoid early tracheostomy, which is associated with a higher incidence of complications than endotracheal intubation.[31] Chest x-rays are generally not helpful early in the course of an inhalational injury.

In addition to control of the airway, humidified air-oxygen mixtures are a standard treatment adjunct. Some patients may have severe bronchospasm so that a bronchodilator such as aminophylline may have to be administered.

A controversial treatment modality, based primarily on animal data, is the use of corticosteroids for the treatment of inhalation injury. Treatment with corticosteroids has been studied in a controlled trial in 60 patients.[28] Half the group was treated with dexamethasone; their course was no different from the control group. In a similar controlled study, Moylan also concluded that steroids were of no benefit in smoke inhalation. A more recent but uncontrolled study of the use of steroids in pure inhalation injury in large-hotel fire victims failed to show any benefit from the early use of steroids.[45]

Prophylactic intubation with continuous positive-airway pressure (CPAP) has been advocated in the early management of inhalation injury.[54] An animal study showed that a CPAP of 8 cm H_2O maintained oxygenation and reduced pulmonary shunt in experimental smoke inhalation.[8] There are no published trials in humans to the value of prophylactic intubation with CPAP.

The majority of patients presenting with upper airway obstruction can be easily managed with careful attention to bronchopulmonary toilet. If significant airway edema exists, then short-term endotracheal intubation is usually successful. Chronic permanent sequelae of upper airway obstruction are unusual, although bronchiectasis has been reported.

PARENCHYMAL DYSFUNCTION

The least common but most lethal form of pulmonary involvement in burns is parenchymal (small-airway) dysfunction. This is commonly referred to as the adult respiratory distress syndrome (ARDS). The causes of ARDS are listed in Table 19–1. By far the most common antecedent cause is systemic sepsis.[24] In smoke inhalation, numerous additional factors can also be implicated. Some of the factors that have been investigated recently are listed in Table 19–2. A good summary of the relative role of these substances in ARDS has recently been published.[38]

Adult respiratory distress syndrome is presumed to be a direct result of pulmonary endothelial damage (vascular and/or airway), which results in interstitial pulmonary edema and progressive filling and collapse of alveoli. Interstitial blood vessels, particularly pulmonary arterial vessels, can be compressed as well. The result of this fluid accumulation is a spectrum of ventilation/perfusion (V/Q) abnormalities. Lung units with a low V/Q will cause hypoxemia (decreased arterial oxygen pressure [Pa_{O_2}]). Alveoli with absent ventilation

TABLE 19–1.
Known Causes of Adult Respiratory Distress Syndrome

PRIMARY	SECONDARY
Sepsis (systemic or pulmonary)	Ischemic pulmonary injury
Aspiration (blood, acid)	Fluid overload (colloid, electrolyte)
Oxygen toxicity	Microatelectasis
Pulmonary injury	
Microembolization	
Smoke inhalation	

but persistent blood flow are defined as producing a pulmonary shunt (QS/QT). Alveoli with normal ventilation and decreased perfusion cause an increase in dead space. Increased dead space ventilation generally causes hypercapnia (increased partial pressure of CO_2 in arterial blood [Pa_{CO_2}]). Alterations in V/Q in smoke inhalation have been investigated by utilizing the multiple inert gas technique. These authors found that an increase in the occurrence of high V/Q abnormalities and an increase in dead space ventilation occurred early in the course of the inhalation injury. Later in the evolution of the injury, low V/Q abnormalities were more frequent; true shunting did not seem to be a significant factor. This study lends support to the importance of various humoral factors proposed as causative agents in ARDS seen in smoke inhalation patients. In contrast, the nonsmoke inhalation patient with ARDS characteristically has increased QS/QT, which is primarily responsible for the development of early hypoxemia.[7]

Although the hallmark of ARDS is hypoxemia, other physiologic derangements occur: (1) decreased functional residual capacity (FRC), (2) decreased effective compliance of the lungs (C_{eff}), and (3) increased dead-space ventilation (V_D/V_T). The interplay of these factors is shown in Figure 19–1. Central to these abnormalities is an increased extravascular lung water content (EVLW). Tranbaugh et al.[52] measured EVLW in burned patients resuscitated with Ringer's lactate solution. Immediate postburn EVLW was normal in all patients, but patients who later became septic had a marked increase in lung water. Even severe inhalation injury failed to produce high EVLW in this study.[52] The same authors later focused on another group of patients with se-

TABLE 19–2.
Summary of Recently Investigated Etiologic Factors Implicated in ARDS

FACTOR	REFERENCE(S)
Serotonin	Huval, et al., 1984[27]
Fibronectin	Saba, et al., 1983[46]; Fourrier, et al., 1985[14]; Cohler, et al., 1985[6]
Leukocytes	Hammerschmidt, 1983[19]; Hallgren, et al., 1984[18]
Prostaglandins	Brigham, et al., 1983[2]; Gee, et al., 1985[15]
Complement activation	Heideman, 1979[21]; Gelfand, et al., 1983[16]; Solomkin, et al., 1985[48]
Oxygen free radicals	Till et al., 1983[51]; Bulkley, 1983[4]
Chemotaxis	Hechtman, et al., 1984[20]

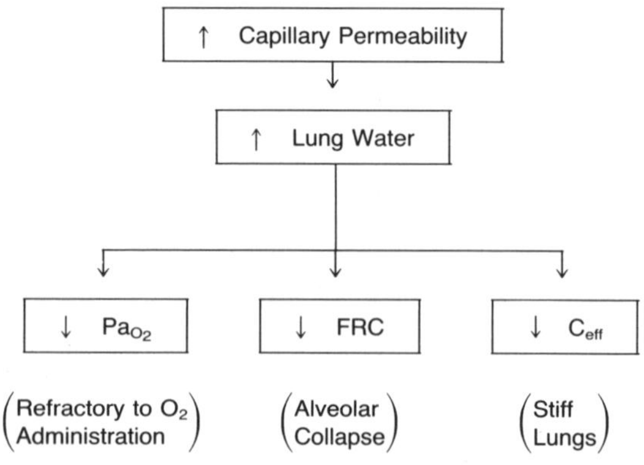

FIG 19–1.
Summary of physiologic derangements in ARDS.

vere inhalation injuries.[53] They found that early increases in EVLW were quite rare (1 of 14 patients), but late increases correlated well with the onset of sepsis. Despite the normal EVLW levels, patients of Tranbaugh all had severe pulmonary dysfunction with hypoxemia. Other authors[41] have studied similar but more severely burned patients and shown that even though the EVLW increases did not correlate well with the severity of inhalation injury, elevated admission EVLW seemed to identify patients with parenchymal inhalation injury.

Treatment of ARDS

Identification of patients at risk for ARDS is the earliest form of treatment.[24] Routine arterial blood gas analysis will identify hypoxemia. Tests of ventilation (Pa_{CO_2}, minute ventilation) and lung mechanics (C_{eff}, respiratory rate) are easily done and when followed serially allow for the early institution of ventilatory support. The most common indication for treatment is a decreased Pa_{O_2}; this is temporarily treated by increasing the inspired O_2 concentration (FI_{O_2}). The ratio of Pa_{O_2} FI_{O_2} is an easy means of tracking ARDS—a decreasing number signifying worsening oxygenation. The airway should be controlled early with a low-pressure, high-volume cuffed endotracheal or nasal tracheal tube. In order to increase FRC and recruitment of collapsed or hypoventilated alveoli, a volume-cycled ventilator is utilized with an initial tidal volume of 10 to 15 ml/kg of body weight. The effects of such treatment can be judged by constructing a compliance curve (expired tidal volume/inspiratory hold pressure) as tidal volume is increased progressively. If adequate oxygenation cannot be achieved with high tidal-volume ventilation, then other methods of increasing FRC must be instituted. Continuous positive-airway pressure or positive end-expiratory pressure (PEEP) are begun when an adequate Pa_{O_2} (>65 torr) cannot be maintained without using a dangerously high FI_{O_2} (>0.5). Positive end-expiratory pressure therapy may be associated with serious side effects and complications.[5, 30, 47] Therefore, PEEP should be increased in small amounts in a stepwise fashion and its effects on O_2 transport monitored at each step until an adequate Pa_{O_2} is achieved.

A more complete discussion of the details of ventilatory therapy is beyond the scope of this review. However, other newer, nonconventional therapies (Table 19–3) advocated will be reviewed.

Of the alternative mechanical therapies, extracorporeal membrane oxygenation (ECMO) has been universally abandoned as ineffective. High-frequency or jet ventilation has been used for treatment of bronchopleural fistula and ARDS,[26, 39] but has not been any more effective than standard PEEP therapy. Even though jet ventilation has been proposed to limit barotrauma, this complication may still be seen with it.[12] At the present time, jet ventilation should still be considered an experimental technique.

Prophylactic CPAP has been mentioned previously. Reports of its use in nonburn patients indicate that early PEEP for mild hypoxemia does not affect the subsequent development of ARDS in high-risk patients.[42] These observations have led to a heightened interest in the pharmacologic treatment of ARDS.

The most controversial adjunctive treatment in respiratory failure has been the use of steroids. Up to 1984, a review of the human and animal data did not provide a clear answer to this question, but the weight of evidence seemed to suggest no benefit from the use of steroids.[13] The most recent randomized

TABLE 19–3.
Alternative Treatment Adjuncts in ARDS

MECHANICAL	PHARMACOLOGIC
Extracorporeal membrane oxygenation (EMCO)	Corticosteroids
	Hypertonic mannitol
Prophylactic CPAP or PEEP	Fibronectin
Jet ventilation	Dipyridamole
	Ibuprofen

study[57] in ARDS patients compared large doses of methylprednisolone with a placebo of mannitol. The results showed that steroids failed to improve pulmonary function and were associated with an increased infection rate. A small group of patients exists with a form of ARDS characterized by idiopathic pulmonary fibrosis.[1] Anti-inflammatory doses of methylprednisolone (125 mg intravenously every 6 hours) were associated with an 85% recovery rate in this high-risk group. The authors attributed their excellent results to the use of steroids. It should be stressed, however, that this type of patient is uncommonly seen and should not provide a basis for the routine use of steroids in ARDS.

The other pharmacologic agents listed in Table 19–3 are all being studied in ARDS models. The published results do not support the use of any of them in patients.[3, 10, 38, 55]

SUMMARY

Pulmonary complications—CO poisoning, upper airway obstruction and acute pulmonary insufficiency—occur frequently in the burn patient. The morbidity and mortality from these complications are high. Early diagnosis and the institution of known effective therapies can limit the deleterious effects of smoke inhalation.

REFERENCES

1. Ashbaugh DG, Maier RV: Idiopathic pulmonary fibrosis in adult respiratory distress syndrome. *Arch Surg* 1985; 120:530–534.
2. Brigham KL, et al: Prostaglandins and lung injury. *Chest* 1983; 83:705–725.
3. Buchman SR, et al: Failure of methylprednisolone, ibuprofen, or prostacyclin to reduce HCl-induced pulmonary albumin leak in dogs. *Surgery* 1984; 96:163–169.
4. Bulkley GB: The role of oxygen free radicals in human disease processes. *Surgery* 1983; 94:407–438.
5. Cane RD, Shapiro BA: Mechanical ventilatory support. *JAMA* 1985; 254:87–92.
6. Cohler LD, Saba TM, Lewis EP: Lung vascular injury with protease infusion: Relationship to plasma fibronectin. *Ann Surg* 1985; 202:240–248.
7. Dantzker DR, et al: Ventilation perfusion distributions in the adult respiratory distress syndrome. *Am Rev Respir Dis* 1979; 120:1039–1048.
8. Davies LK, Poulton TJ, Modell JH: Continuous positive airway pressure is beneficial in treatment of smoke inhalation. *Crit Care Med* 1983; 11:726–729.
9. Davis BW, et al: Pulmonary oxygen toxicity: Early reversible changes in human alveolar structures induced by hyperoxia. *N Engl J Med* 1983; 309:878–882.
10. Dehring DJ, et al: Indomethacin improvement of septic acute respiratory failure in a porcine model. *J Trauma* 1983; 23:725–729.
11. Demling RH, et al: Early lung dysfunction after major burns: Role of edema and vasoactive mediators. *J Trauma* 1985; 25:959–966.
12. Egol A, Culpepper JA, Snyder JV: Barotrauma and hypotension resulting from jet ventilation in critically ill patients. *Chest* 1985; 88:98–102.
13. Flick MR, Murray JF: High-dose corticosteroid therapy in the adult respiratory distress syndrome. *JAMA* 1984; 251:1054–1056.
14. Fourrier F, et al: Compared evolution of plasma fibronectin and angiotensin-converting enzyme levels in septic ARDS. *Chest* 1985; 87:191–195.
15. Gee MH, et al: Arachidonate cyclo-oxygenase metabolites as mediators of complement-initiated lung injury. *Fed Proc* 1985; 44:46–52.
16. Gelfand JA, Donelan M, Burke JF: Preferential activation and depletion of the alternative complement pathway by burn injury. *Ann Surg* 1983; 198:58–62.
17. Halebian P, et al: Diabetes insipidus after carbon monoxide poisoning and smoke inhalation. *J Trauma* 1985; 25:662–663.
18. Hallgren R, et al: Signs of neutrophil and eosinophil activation in adult respiratory distress syndrome. *Crit Care Med* 1984; 12:14–18.
19. Hammerschmidt DE: Leukocytes in lung injury. *Chest* 1983; 83:165–205.
20. Hechtman HB, Valeri CR, Shepro D: Role of humoral mediators in adult respiratory distress syndrome. *Chest* 1984; 86:623–627.
21. Heideman M: The effect of thermal injury on hemodynamic, respiratory and hematologic variables in relation to complement activation. *J Trauma* 1979; 19:239–243.
22. Herndon DN, et al: The pathophysiology of smoke inhalation injury in a sheep model. *J Trauma* 1984; 24:1044–1051.
23. Horovitz JH: Pulmonary complications in the burn patient. *Cutis* 1978; 22:489–494.
24. Horovitz JH: Practical ventilatory management in Najarian JS, Delaney JP (eds): *Emergency*

Surgery. Chicago, Year Book Medical Publishers, 1982, pp 131–141.
25. Hunt JL, et al: Fiberoptic bronchoscopy in acute inhalational injury. *J Trauma* 1975; 15:641–649.
26. Hurst JM, DeHaven CB: Adult respiratory distress syndrome: Improved oxygenation during high-frequency jet ventilation/continuous positive airway pressure. *Surgery* 1984; 96:764–769.
27. Huval WV, et al: Role of serotonin in patients with acute respiratory failure. *Ann Surg* 1984; 200:166–172.
28. Levine BA, et al: Prospective trials of dexamethasone and aerosolized gentamicin in the treatment of inhalation injury in the burned patient. *J Trauma* 1978; 18:188–193.
29. Loke J, Virgulto JA, Smith GJW: Rabbit lung after acute smoke inhalation. *Arch Surg* 1984; 119:956–959.
30. Luce JM: The cardiovascular effects of mechanical ventilation and positive end-expiratory pressure. *JAMA* 1984; 252:807–811.
31. Lund TL, et al: Upper airway sequelae in burn patients requiring endotracheal intubation or tracheostomy. *Ann Surg* 1985; 201:374–382.
32. Mallory TB, Brickley WJ: Management of the Coconut Grove burns at the Massachusetts General Hospital: With special reference to the pulmonary lesions. *Ann Surg* 1943; 117:865–884.
33. Mohsenifar Z, et al: Relationship between O_2 delivery and O_2 consumption in the adult respiratory distress syndrome. *Chest* 1983; 84:267–274.
34. Moritz AR, Henriques FC, McLean R: The effects of inhaled heat on the air passages and lungs: An experimental investigation. *Am J Pathol* 1945; 21:311–331.
35. Moylan JA, et al: Early diagnosis of inhalation injury using ^{133}Xenon lung scan. *Ann Surg* 1972; 176:477–484.
36. Murray IP, et al: Titration of PEEP by the arterial minus end-tidal carbon dioxide gradient. *Chest* 1984; 85:100–104.
37. Nerlich M, Flynn J, Demling RF: Effect of thermal injury on endotoxin-induced lung injury. *Surgery* 1983; 93:289–296.
38. Norwood SH, Civetta JM: The adult respiratory distress syndrome. *Surg Gynecol Obstet* 1985; 161:497–508.
39. O'Rourke PP, Crone RK: High-frequency ventilation: A new approach to respiratory support. *JAMA* 250:2845–2847.
40. Parving HH, et al: Effect of carbon monoxide exposure on capillary permeability to albumin and α_2-macroglobulin. *Scand J Clin Lab Invest* 1972; 29:381.
41. Peitzman AB, Shires T III, Corben WA, et al: Measurement of lung water in inhalation injury. *Surgery* 1981; 90:305–312.
42. Pepe PE, Hudson LD, Carrico CJ: Early application of positive end-expiratory pressure in patients at risk for the adult respiratory distress syndrome. *N Engl J Med* 1984; 311:281–286.
43. Peterson JE, Stewart RD: Predicting the carboxyhemoglobin levels resulting from carbon monoxide exposures. *J Appl Physiol* 1975; 39:633–638.
44. Robinson NB, et al: Ventilation and perfusion alterations after smoke inhalation. *Surgery* 1981; 90:352–363.
45. Robinson NB, et al: Steroid therapy following isolated smoke inhalation injury. *J Trauma* 1982; 22:876–879.
46. Saba TM, et al: Lung vascular permeability after reversal of fibronectin deficiency in septic sheep: Correlation with patient studies. *Ann Surg* 1983; 198:654–662.
47. Shapiro BA, Cane RD, Harrison RA: Positive end-expiratory pressure therapy in adults with special reference to acute lung injury: A review of the literature and suggested clinical correlations. *Crit Care Med* 1984; 12:127–141.
48. Solomkin JS, et al: Complement activation and clearance in acute illness and injury: Evidence for C5a as a cell-directed mediator of the adult respiratory distress syndrome in man. *Surgery* 1985; 97:668–678.
49. Strohl KP, et al: Carbon monoxide poisoning in fire victims: A reappraisal of prognosis. *J Trauma* 1980; 20:78–80.
50. Takahashi M, et al: Hyperamylasemia in acute carbon monoxide poisoning. *J Trauma* 1982; 22:311–314.
51. Till GO, et al: Oxygen radical dependent lung damage following thermal injury of rat skin. *J Trauma* 1983; 23:269–277.
52. Tranbaugh RF, et al: Lung water changes after thermal injury: The effects of crystalloid resuscitation and sepsis. *Ann Surg* 1980; 192:479–490.
53. Tranbaugh RF, et al: Effect of inhalation injury on lung water accumulation. *J Trauma* 1983; 23:597–605.
54. Venus B, et al: Prophylactic intubation and continuous positive airway pressure in the management of inhalation injury in burn victims. *Crit Care Med* 1981; 9:519–523.
55. Vincent JL, et al: Prevention of the adult respiratory distress syndrome with dipyridamole. *Crit Care Med* 1985; 13:783–785.

56. Weigelt JA, Snyder WH, Mitchell RA: Early identification of patients prone to develop adult respiratory distress syndrome. *Arch Surg* 1981; 142:687–691.
57. Weigelt JA, et al: Early steroid therapy for respiratory failure. *Arch Surg* 1985; 120:536–540.
58. Zarem HA, Rattenborg CC, Harmel MH: Carbon monoxide toxicity in human fire victims. *Arch Surg* 1973; 107:851–853.
59. Zikria BA, et al: What is clinical smoke poisoning? *Ann Surg* 1975; 181:151–156.

20 / Cardiovascular Effects of Burns in Children

AMBROSE M. VALLONE, M.D.

The major function of the cardiovascular or circulatory system is to provide tissues with nutrients and oxygen sufficient to meet metabolic needs. Under normal, unstressed, resting conditions, the amount of oxygen delivered to the body is three to four times in excess of oxygen needs. Burns have a major effect both on the level of oxygen delivery and on the level of oxygen needs and can result in tissue hypoxia by producing an imbalance between tissue oxygen needs and delivery. This chapter reviews the components of the oxygen delivery system and the effects that burns have on oxygen delivery and use. In addition, a general approach to the assessment, monitoring, and management of burns in the pediatric patient will be reviewed.

OXYGEN DELIVERY SYSTEM

Systemic oxygen delivery (SOD) is the amount of oxygen delivered to the body in cubic centimeters of oxygen/minute/sq m (Table 20–1). It is equal to cardiac index multiplied by the arterial oxygen content. Arterial oxygen content is the amount of oxygen contained in 100 cc of arterial blood and includes the amount of oxygen dissolved in the plasma plus the amount of oxygen bound to the hemoglobin molecule. The total amount of oxygen consumed by the body (see Table 20–1) is equal to the amount of oxygen delivered to the body (SOD) minus the amount of oxygen returned from the body to the heart, i.e., cardiac index multiplied by mixed venous oxygen content. Mixed venous oxygen content is the oxygen contained in 100 cc of mixed venous blood, which is best obtained from the main pulmonary artery in the absence of intracardiac shunts. Oxygen consumption is normally dependent on total metabolic needs and is independent of SOD. In the normal state, oxygen consumption equals oxygen needs (see Table 20–1). Circulatory failure exists when tissue oxygen needs exceed oxygen consumption (Table 20–2). This may occur with decreases in oxygen delivery, decreases in oxygen extraction, or increases in oxygen

TABLE 20–1.
Oxygen Delivery Relationships

1. Systemic oxygen delivery (SOD) = cardiac index (Q) × arterial oxygen content (Ca)
   SOD(cc/min/sq m) = Q (cc/min/sq m) × Ca*(cc O_2/100 cc)
2. Oxygen consumption (VO_2) = oxygen delivered to body − oxygen returned from body to right ventricle
   VO_2(cc/min/sq m) = Q(cc/min/sq m) × Ca(cc O_2/ 100 cc) − Q(cc/min/sq m) × mixed venous oxygen content ($C\bar{v}$†)(cc O_2/100 cc)
3. Oxygen needs $= VO_2 = QCa - QC\bar{v}$
   $= Q \times (Ca - C\bar{v})$
   $= QCa \times \dfrac{Ca - C\bar{v}}{Ca}$
   = SOD × oxygen extraction

*Ca = arterial oxygen tension (PaO_2, mm Hg) × 0.003 (cc O_2/mm Hg/100 cc) + (hemoglobin [gm/dl] × 1.36 × % hemoglobin arterial oxygen saturation)
†$C\bar{v}$ = partial pressure of O_2 in mixed venous blood ($P\bar{v}O_2$, mm Hg) × 0.003(cc O_2/mm Hg/100 cc) + (hemoglobin [gm/dl] × 1.36 × % mixed venous pulmonary artery oxygen saturation)

TABLE 20–2.
Causes of Circulatory Failure: Oxygen Consumption Less Than Oxygen Needs*

Decreased Q
Decreased heart rate
Decreased stroke volume
Decreased preload
Increased afterload
Decreased contractility
Decreased Ca
Decreased hemoglobin
Decreased arterial saturation
Decreased PaO_2
Increased carbon monoxide
Decreased extraction
Altered hemoglobin oxygen affinity
Maldistribution of flow
Increased oxygen needs
Fever
Pain
Increased work at breathing

*$VO_2 = QCa \times (Ca - C\bar{v})/Ca < O_2$ needs.

needs. The SOD may be decreased by decreasing cardiac output or by decreasing arterial oxygen content. Arterial oxygen content may be decreased by decreasing hemoglobin and by decreasing arterial oxygen tension and saturation. As SOD falls, oxygen consumption is initially maintained, and total metabolic oxygen needs are satisfied by an increase in oxygen extraction.[1, 12] With a further fall in SOD the increase in oxygen extraction cannot compensate for the decrease in delivery, and oxygen consumption falls. At this point unless metabolic needs can be decreased, tissue hypoxia will occur. Despite evidence of tissue hypoxia, vital organ function may still be maintained. Multiple studies using hemorrhage, tamponade, and hypoxia, as well as burns, to lower SOD have shown a preferential redistribution of flow from nonvital organs to vital organs such as the heart and brain.[16, 17, 35] With a further fall in oxygen delivery, the compensatory mechanisms that maintain vital organ oxygen use are no longer adequate, and dysfunction of vital organs may occur, leading to death.

EFFECT OF BURNS ON OXYGEN DELIVERY AND USE

An acute burn can have a significant effect on metabolic needs as well as on all components of the oxygen delivery system, i.e., cardiac output, arterial oxygen content, and oxygen extraction. Multiple animal studies have documented an immediate postburn decrease in cardiac output.[5, 6, 7, 14, 18, 19, 29, 31] Cardiac output falls immediately by 40% to 60%. This fall is followed by a further gradual reduction with a nadir at 12 to 18 hours. If the animal survives untreated, cardiac output gradually returns to preburn values by 36 to 48 hours. Moncrief[31] demonstrated that the decrease in cardiac output is accompanied by a fall in oxygen consumption and evidence of tissue hypoxia, i.e., acidosis and an increase in lactate. Presumably SOD was decreased below the point at which an increase in extraction could maintain body oxygen consumption. Wolfe[46] demonstrated in an animal model that nonsurvivors could be distinguished by a lower cardiac output and oxygen consumption and higher lactate levels. These findings indicate that mortality from burn shock is related to a level of tissue oxygen delivery inadequate to meet tissue needs. Multiple studies in adults have documented a fall in cardiac output if the surface area injury exceeds 20% to 25%.[2, 4, 21, 39, 43] Although data on the measured cardiac outputs in burned children are inadequate, infants and young children, who have a greater surface area/body weight ratio, may indeed be more likely to sustain a fall in cardiac output for a given percent surface area burn.

A significant amount of research has been done to determine the cause of the fall in cardiac output in burns. Cardiac output is equal to the stroke volume (volume ejected with each beat) multiplied by heart rate. Studies have demonstrated a fall in stroke volume in burn patients.[2, 4] Stroke volume is determined by the preload, contractility, and afterload of the heart.[11] Preload refers to the length of the cardiac muscle prior to contraction. In the intact heart it is equivalent to the end-diastolic volume of the heart. A fall in the end-diastolic volume will lead to a fall in stroke volume, the well-known Frank-Starling relationship. Blalock[8] proposed in 1931 that the fall in output was due to fluid loss. It is well known that burns lead to an increase in capillary permeability and a loss of volume from the intravascular space.[22] This capillary leak is most prominent during the first 6 to 12 hours after a burn and may be present throughout the body with burns greater than 30% of the surface area. In addition, the burn results in a breakdown in the skin's protective functions and an increase in external loss of fluid through evaporation. The decrease in intravascular volume is proportional to the depth and extent of the burn. As intravascular volume falls, cardiac output will be maintained initially by an increase in contractility and tachycardia. In general, cardiac output will be maintained until intravascular volume is reduced by more than 15%. With a further reduction of intravascular volume, cardiac output will fall.

Although the reduction in preload or intravascular volume is the major cause of the fall in cardiac output, animal studies have also demonstrated that the fall in cardiac output may occur within minutes of the burn before there is any measurable decrease in intravascular volume or right atrial pressure. In addition, studies in adult burn patients have documented a low stroke volume or stroke work with a normal or increased pulmonary wedge pressure presumably indicating a normal or increased end-diastolic volume.[2, 4] These results may be explained by decreases in contractility or by increases in afterload. Acute metabolic disturbances such as hypoxia, acidosis, or hypocalcemia may result in a decrease in contractility. Some investigators, however, have postulated the presence of "myocardial depressant factors" that may interfere with myocardial contractile function. Although a plasma factor that may decrease contractility has been demonstrated in burn shock in multiple animal experiments[6, 40] and in adult burn patients,[13, 41] its significance remains a question. No studies document the development of "myocardial depressant factors" in children. Clinical reports in adults have documented that the low stroke volume at the normal or elevated filling pressures can be increased by inotropic agents. No reported invasive or noninvasive assessments of contractility in the pediatric burn patient exist. Pediatric clinical experience is minimal with respect to the need for or use of inotropic agents for acute resuscitation in cases uncomplicated by a prior period of prolonged hypotension or hypoxia leading to secondary myocardial damage or dysfunction. Later in the course of treatment severe pulmonary disease requiring elevated levels of positive end-expiratory pressure and sepsis may also produce secondary changes in myocardial function requiring inotropic support. It is unlikely, however, that a primary decrease in contractility contributes significantly to the fall in cardiac output in the acutely burned pediatric patient.

The measurable drop in cardiac output, which may occur before a fall in intravascular volume or right atrial pressure, may in part be related to an increase in afterload.[14, 19] Afterload is the tension developed by cardiac muscle during contraction.[11] Blood pressure and vascular resistance are used as clinical estimates of afterload. Studies have documented an acute increase in systemic and pulmonary vascular resistance in burns.[4, 5, 31] As cardiac output falls, increased activity of the sympathetic nervous system results in an increase in vascular resistance. The increase in resistance can sustain blood pressure or perfusion pressure to vital organs. In addition, vascular resistance changes in different vascular beds vary, which allow a redistribution of flow to vital organs.[17] In most cases, these changes in resistance are beneficial to the organism. Volume resuscitation will increase cardiac output, and systemic and pulmonary vascular resistance will return to normal. Intense sympathetic discharge, however, may acutely increase afterload and contribute to the fall in stroke volume. A sustained increase in systemic resistance despite volume resuscitation may contribute to a low cardiac output.

Experimental animal studies have documented that vasodilators can increase cardiac output when added to volume resuscitation.[24, 25, 30] Vasodilators have also been used in the adult burn patient to increase cardiac output.[39] There is no reported clinical experience with the use of vasodilators to increase cardiac output in the acutely burned pediatric patient, although vasodilators are used to treat hypertension associated with burns in the later stages of injury. The use of vasodilators in the early burn period when patients may be intravascularly volume-depleted may be dangerous. Invasive monitoring would be indicated to document an adequate intravascular volume and an elevated resistance before their use.

Burns acutely decrease SOD by decreasing cardiac output. Burns can also decrease SOD by decreasing arterial oxygen content. Although burns are associated with acute hemolysis and a decreased red cell life span, the loss of intravascular volume results in an early increase in hematocrit. With volume resuscitation the hematocrit may slowly fall. In acutely burned patients, however, arterial hypoxia and carbon monoxide poisoning may decrease arterial oxygen saturation and arterial oxygen content. Burns may also adversely affect oxygen extraction. Carbon monoxide will shift the oxyhemoglobin curve to the left and interfere with oxygen extraction. Acute burns not associated with an elevated level of carbon monoxide in the blood may also result in a shift to the left of the oxygen dissociation curve and possibly limit extraction.[20]

In summary, burns have multiple effects on the oxygen delivery system. The decrease in cardiac output is secondary to a decrease in preload, although changes in contractility and afterload may also play a limited role. Arterial content may be decreased, and changes in the oxygen dissociation curve may affect extraction. In addition, the acute stress with the increased sympathetic output may increase oxygen needs. Under these circumstances oxygen delivery and oxygen consumption may fall below oxygen needs, and tissue hypoxia may occur.

ASSESSMENT, MONITORING, AND MANAGEMENT OF BURNS IN PEDIATRIC PATIENTS

The goal of management is to assure that all tissues receive adequate oxygen to meet their needs. Circulatory failure is the physiologic condition in which oxygen delivery and consumption are below oxygen needs, and therapy must be aimed at increasing oxygen delivery and decreasing oxygen needs (see Table 20–2). The major focus of therapy is to increase oxygen delivery by increasing cardiac output and assuring a normal oxygen content. In most pediatric burn patients adequate cardiac output and perfusion can be attained in the acute phase with volume resuscitation alone. Bradycardia or tachyarrythmias that interfere with output are rare but must be treated if present. Hypoxia, hypocalcemia, hypoglycemia, and significant acidosis (pH less than 7.20) may interfere with cardiac function and require specific treatment. In the later stages, significant respiratory disease requiring mechanical ventilation with elevated levels of positive end-expiratory pressure or sepsis may lead to changes in cardiac function and necessitate inotropic support.[26,45] Oxygen delivery can also be increased by increasing arterial oxygen content to normal. In the acute phase of treatment, this entails maintaining a normal arterial oxygen tension and saturation. Inhalation injury leading to parenchymal and airway damage may lower arterial oxygen tension. Carbon monoxide exposure can lower arterial saturation and shift the oxyhemoglobin dissociation curve, limiting extraction. Elevation of inspired oxygen concentration and intubation for respiratory failure may be needed. Overzealous ventilation or bicarbonate administration may lead to a significant alkalosis and interfere with tissue oxygen extraction and should be avoided.[23] An effort must be made to decrease oxygen demands. Elevated temperatures and pain must be treated. Patients who remain in circulatory shock should be intubated and ventilated not only to ensure adequate arterial oxygen levels and ventilation, but also to decrease the oxygen demand of breathing. The control of ambient temperatures may also affect oxygen or metabolic demands.[32]

Although the goal of management is to assure that all tissues receive adequate oxygen to meet their needs, we cannot measure individual organ oxygen delivery or use and must rely on certain physiologic parameters measured noninvasively and invasively together with our knowledge of normal physiologic responses to guide therapy. Table 20–3 lists parameters commonly used in the clinical setting to assess a patient's circulatory status. As intravascular volume falls, increased sympathetic outflow results in an increase in contractility and *heart rate* to maintain stroke volume. The infant and young child are more dependent on changes in heart rate to maintain flow and can sustain higher rates than adults. With adequate fluid resuscitation one should see a gradual decline in the heart rate. Elevated heart rates may result from fever and pain. The quality of the pulse may be used to assess cardiac output. The *pulse volume* decreases as the stroke volume falls, and peripheral pulses may be more difficult to palpate. A decreased *blood pressure* most likely indicates a low cardiac output in the acutely burned patient. A normal pressure, however, is not an adequate indicator of a normal cardiac output. As output falls, the blood pressure is maintained by an increase in vascular resistance. Initially, diastolic pressure may even increase with a fall in pulse pressure. As cardiac output decreases further, systolic and diastolic pressures fall. The decreased pulse pressure accounts for the de-

TABLE 20–3.

Clinical Parameters Used to Assess Circulatory Status in Burn Patients

Noninvasive Parameters
- Heart rate
- Pulse quality: peripheral pulses
- Respiratory rate
- Blood pressure: pulse pressure
- Skin perfusion: capillary refill time
- Level of consciousness
- Urine output
- Laboratory
  - Urine sodium
  - Urine osmolality
  - Metabolic acidosis
  - Disseminated intravascular coagulation profile
  - Liver function studies
  - Electrocardiogram

Invasive Monitoring
- Intra-arterial pressure monitoring
- Central venous pressure (CVP): normal 2–6 mm Hg; in patients with compromised perfusion, fluids should be administered to increase CVP to 10 mm Hg with assessment of clinical status
- Swan-Ganz catheterization
  - Pulmonary capillary wedge (PCWP) normal 5–12 mm Hg
    - Reflection of filling volume of the left ventricle
  - Pulmonary artery pressure
    - Systolic 15–25 mm Hg
    - Diastolic 8–15 mm Hg
    - Mean: MPAP 10–20 mm Hg
  - Systemic vascular resistance = $\frac{79.9\ (BP - CVP)}{Q} =$ 800–1,600 dyne·sec/cm^5/sq m
  - Pulmonary vascular resistance = $\frac{79.9\ (MPAP - PCWP)}{Q} =$ 80–240 dyne·sec/cm^5/sq m
  - Stroke volume index: 30–60 cc/sq m
  - Arterial mixed venous oxygen content difference: Ca − C$\bar{v}$: normal 3–5.5 vol%
  - Oxygen extraction: $\frac{Ca - C\bar{v}}{Ca}$: normal 26% ± 2%
  - Oxygen consumption: normal 120–200 cc/min
  - Shunt fraction: $= \frac{Cc' - Ca}{Cc' - C\bar{v}}$: normal = <7%
  - Cc′ = pulmonary end capillary oxygen content = Pc′O_2(mm Hg) × 0.003(cc O_2/mm Hg/100cc) + (hemoglobin [gm/dl] × 1.36 × end capillary oxygen saturation)

creased peripheral pulses. Evidence suggests that the infant may be less able to raise vascular resistance and maintain blood pressure in response to a volume loss.[48] Little is known about the timing of the development of normal responses in man, but this may be one factor contributing to the uniformly higher reported mortality in infants with moderate burns.[9, 15]

As systemic blood flow initially falls, a redistribution of flow occurs from "nonvital" to vital organs.[17] Blood flow to the skin, kidneys, muscle, and gastrointestinal system decreases, and blood flow to the heart, brain, and adrenal gland tends to be maintained. With a further drop in cardiac output, flow to the vital organs becomes compromised. A careful clinical evaluation could therefore provide a qualitative assessment of flow. Examination of the unburned *skin* can provide indirect evidence of a fall in cardiac output. When flow is decreased, the skin will be *cool and clammy. Mottling* of the skin may also indicate a decrease in flow, although infants may show mottling secondary to vasospasm related to the ambient temperature without an associated decrease in cardiac output. The *capillary refill time,* obtained by expressing the blood out from an area of skin and determining how long it takes for the area to refill with blood, may also be prolonged, i.e., for a period greater than 5 seconds. An adequate *urine output* in the presence of a normally functioning kidney implies an adequate glomerular filtration rate and renal plasma flow, and presumably a normal output. A decreased urine flow rate with an elevated urine osmolality and low urine sodium concentration may indicate a low cardiac output. Absent or decreased bowel sounds may be associated with decreases in gastrointestinal flow.

Central nervous system blood flow is maintained despite moderate reductions in cardiac output, so a patient may present with tachycardia, a normal blood pressure, low urine output, cool skin, and decreased capillary refill, but be awake and alert. With a greater fall in flow, central nervous system flow is reduced, and the patient may exhibit a change in the *level of consciousness,* lethargy, or irritability. Coronary flow is also maintained until cardiac output is severely reduced. With reductions in coronary flow, myocardial ischemia may occur. The increased sympathetic output will increase myocardial oxygen needs; the increased heart rate may limit time for coronary flow; and the decreased diastolic pressure may limit the driving pressure for coronary flow. The patient may then exhibit arrhythmias, or evidence of myocardial dysfunction. A patient with a severe decrease in cardiac output may be tachycardic or may exhibit various dysrhythmias, be hypotensive, have alteration in consciousness, have cold, clammy skin, and be anuric. The shock state, if prolonged, can lead to disseminated intravascular coagulation and laboratory evidence of liver damage.

A *metabolic acidosis* or an increase in lactic acid may be evidence that tissue oxygen needs are not being met. Arterial blood gas measurements may document a metabolic acidosis with a compensatory respiratory alkalosis, and clinically the patient may exhibit an increase in *respiratory rate* and increased depth of breathing. It is common for patients with large burns to present with a metabolic acidosis, which gradually resolves with successful resuscitation. A persistent or worsening acidosis may be evidence of persistent hypoxia and an inadequate oxygen delivery. The above clinical parameters and their change with volume resuscitation can provide a useful guide to therapy.

Most pediatric burn patients are managed using a specific regimen of fluid resuscitation calculated on the basis of the extent of injury. Fluid resuscitation is then adjusted based on the above clinical parameters.[44] Invasive arterial, central venous pressure, and Swan-Ganz monitoring are available in most pediatric intensive-care settings and can be helpful in the management of specific patients. *Intra-arterial pressure monitoring* provides a more accurate measurement of blood pressure than the cuff sphygmomanometer or doppler instruments in situations where flow may be significantly reduced and resistance increased.[36] Pediatric patients with major burns (greater than 40%) should be managed with arterial lines. A 20-gauge angiographic catheter is used in older children, and a 22-gauge is adequate for infants and younger children. Pressure measurements may be inaccurate with smaller-gauge catheters. The catheters are most often placed in the radial, dorsalis pedis, or posterior tibial arteries, but the femoral and axillary sites may also be used and may provide a better measurement of central blood pressure when blood flow is significantly reduced. The temporal artery should not be used because of the reported incidence of temporal-lobe infarctions. The catheters may be placed using the percutaneous catheter over-the-wire technique or by direct cutdown. The complications include infection and thrombosis, both of which may be more common when the catheters are left in place for longer than 3 days. Proper attention to aseptic technique, gentle flushing and withdrawing of blood, daily changing of a heparin flush solution, and frequent monitoring of perfusion distal to the site will minimize complications.

Central venous pressure (CVP) monitoring can provide a quantitative assessment of a patient's intravascular volume status. In addition, in a patient without cardiopulmonary disease, the CVP will also provide a measure of the left ventricular filling volume of the heart.[36] Multiple factors, however, may affect CVP independently of the intravascular volume. These include (1) right heart function, (2) vasoconstriction, (3) pulmonary artery pressure, and (4) pericardial and intrathoracic pressures.[43] A low CVP most likely represents a low intravascular volume, but may also be seen with conditions resulting in a large negative intrapleural pressure, i.e., inspiratory airway obstruction. In addition, at low CVPs the curve relating CVP to intravascular or right-heart volume is relatively flat, and large changes in volume may occur with little change in CVP. A high CVP may represent a high vascular volume, but may be seen with heart failure, tricuspid valve disease, pulmonary disease, or an elevated intrapericardial or intrathoracic pressure, i.e., from pneumothorax, PEEP, etc. Despite these problems, careful use of the CVP and, particularly, measurement of the change in CVP with volume administration along with observations of the cardiovascular effects, can help the management of patients undergoing rapid vascular volume changes. Several authors recommend the use of CVP monitoring to manage significant burns in infants and small children—a population that has a greater mortality for comparably sized burns.[10, 34] We feel that CVP monitoring may be helpful in infants and small children with extensive burns and is indicated in children who do not respond clinically to the anticipated volume needs. If the patient continues to show poor perfusion, a decreased urine output, a persistent or worsening acidosis, or CNS changes suggesting a low cardiac output, in the face of what seems to be adequate volume resuscitation, then central monitoring is indicated. If the patient has a low central venous pressure, further volume administration is indicated. If the central venous pressure is normal or only minimally elevated, a volume bolus may be given with careful attention to the change in CVP and clinical status. An improved clinical status with no change or a small transient rise in the CVP indicates that the volume was needed. A large increase in CVP (greater than 3 mm Hg) with little change in clinical status probably indicates that inotropic support is needed. In this situation further monitoring with a Swan-Ganz catheter is indicated.[37]

The clinical use of the Swan-Ganz catheter is well established in adults and children.[28, 38, 47] Table 20–3 lists the information provided by its use. The pulmonary capillary wedge pressure is used as an indirect measure of left atrial pressure. In the absence of mitral valve disease, arrhythmias, or severe left ventricular dysfunction, the mean left atrial pressure is a measure of the left ventricular end diastolic measure. The left ventricular diastolic pressure reflects left ventricular end-diastolic volume or preload of the heart. The PCWP may be a better reflection than the CVP of preload of the left ventricle in patients with cardiac dysfunction or pulmonary disease, and in patients with shock from various etiologies. More importantly, cardiac output can be determined by the thermodilution technique.[33] Systemic oxygen delivery can then be calculated by measuring arterial oxygen tension, saturation, and hemoglobin. Systemic and pulmonary vascular resistances can be calculated to provide an indirect measurement of the afterload of each ventricle. The measurement of the stroke volume index, PCWP, systemic resistance, and their changes with interventions can provide a measure of the contractility of the heart. The catheter also provides access to pulmonary arterial–mixed venous blood. The measurement of a mixed-venous oxygen tension less than 27 torr may be predictive of tissue hypoxia.[27] The arterial–mixed venous oxygen content difference can provide an indirect assessment of cardiac output if oxygen consumption is normal. In the presence of an unchanging oxygen consumption, a widening arterial–mixed venous oxygen content difference is a sign of a falling cardiac output. Oxygen extraction can be calculated and is a measure of the relationship of oxygen delivery to oxygen consumption. An increased extraction may be seen with a decreased oxygen delivery or an increased oxygen need. Calculation of the intrapulmonary shunt fraction (portion of the cardiac output not oxygenated after one passage through the lungs) provides an indirect assessment of the extent of pulmonary involvement. In the presence of a significant right to left intrapulmonary shunt, changes in the arterial oxygen tension may be secondary to changes in cardiac output and oxygen consumption, as well as the extent of pulmonary dysfunction or shunt. These changes can be best interpreted with the aid of the hemodynamic variables provided by the Swan-Ganz catheter. Finally, the effect of therapeutic interventions can be noted not only on cardiac output and oxygen delivery, but on oxygen needs by the calculation of oxygen consumption. Katz et al. and Pollack et al. provide information on the technique of catheter insertion and use. Catheters can be placed in children of all ages at the bedside with few complications and can provide accurate data. The Swan-Ganz catheter is routinely used by some clinicians to help guide fluid resuscitation in adults with extensive burns.[3] More frequently, such monitoring is used in adults with cardiovascular disease or significant pulmonary disease. Most clinicians do not believe that the Swan-Ganz catheter is needed in the routine fluid resuscitation of the pediatric burn patient, but it may be useful in the following situations: (1) patients who fail to respond to volume resuscitation and have normal or elevated CVP; (2) septic shock; (3) patients with evidence of cardiac dysfunction, cardiomegaly, clinical evidence of failure with pulmonary edema, and poor perfusion; (4) patients with pulmonary disease requiring elevated levels of positive end expiratory pressure; and (5) patients in whom afterload reducing agents are used.

In summary, the goal of therapy is to assure that oxygen delivery is adequate to meet oxygen needs. The control of ambient temperature, treatment of pain, and the use of mechanical ventilation when the work of breathing is significantly increased can decrease oxygen needs. Most of our therapy is aimed at increasing oxygen delivery by increasing cardiac output and maintaining a normal oxygen content. Volume resuscitation alone results in an adequate cardiac output in most patients. Noninvasive clinical parameters are sufficient to guide therapy in most patients, but invasive monitoring may be useful in selected patients.

REFERENCES

1. Adams RP, Dieleman LA, Cain SM: A critical value for O_2 transport in the rat. *J Appl Physiol* 1982; 53:660–664.
2. Agarwal N, Petro J, Salisbury RE: Physiologic profile monitoring in burned patients. *J Trauma* 1983; 23:577–583.
3. Aikawa N, Ishibiki K, Naito C, et al: Individ-

ualized fluid resuscitation based on haemodynamic monitoring in the management of extensive burns. *Burns* 1982; 8:249–255.

4. Aikawa N, Jeevendra-Martyr JA, Burke JF: Pulmonary artery catheterization and thermodilution cardiac output determination in the management of critically burned patients. *Am J Surg* 1978; 135:811–817.
5. Asch MJ, Feldman RJ, Walker HL, et al: Systemic and pulmonary hemodynamic changes accompanying thermal injury. *Ann Surg* 1973; 178:218–221.
6. Baxter CR, Cook WA, Shires GT: Serum myocardial depressant factor of burn shock. *Surg Forum* 1966; 17:1–2.
7. Baxter CR, Shires GT: Physiological response to crystalloid resuscitation of severe burns. *Ann NY Acad Sci* 1968; 150:874–894.
8. Blalock A: Experimental shock: VII. The importance of local loss of fluid in the production of low blood pressure after burns. *Arch Surg* 1931; 22:610–616.
9. Bocanegra MD, Bazan AA, Jelarde NZ, et al: Clinical evaluation of the administration of large volumes of plasma in the treatment of severely burned children. *Surgery* 1978; 83:558–564.
10. Boswick JA, Thompson JD, Kershner CJ: Critical care of the burned patient. *Anesthesiology* 1977; 47:164–170.
11. Braunwald E, Ross J: Control of cardiac performance, in Berne RM, Sperelakis N, Geiger SR (eds): *Handbook of Physiology,* section 2: *The Cardiovascular System.* American Physiologic Society, 1979, pp 533–580.
12. Cain SM: Oxygen delivery and uptake in dogs during anemic and hypoxic hypoxia. *J Appl Physiol* 1977; 42:228–234.
13. DeSantis D, Phillips P, Spath MA, et al: Delayed appearance of a circulating myocardial depressant factor in burn patients. *Ann Emerg Med* 1981; 10:22–24.
14. Dobson EL, Warner GF: Factors concerned in the early stages of thermal shock. *Circ Res* 1957; 5:69–74.
15. Durtschi MB, Kohler TR, Finley A, et al: Burn injury in infants and young children. *Surg Gynecol Obstet* 1980; 150:651–656.
16. Fell C: Changes in distribution of blood flow in irreversible hemorrhagic shock. *Am J Physiol* 1966; 210:860–868.
17. Ferguson JL, Merrill GF, Miller HI, et al: Regional blood flow redistribution during early burn shock in the guinea pig. *Circ Shock* 1977; 4:317–326.
18. Fozzard HA: Myocardial injury in burn shock. *Ann Surg* 1961; 154:113–119.
19. Gilmore JP, Handford SW: Hemodynamic response of the dog to thermal radiation. *J Appl Physiol* 1956; 8:393–398.
20. Greenburg AG, Frank H, Perkin RM: The left shifted oxyhemoglobin curve in the burn patient. *J Trauma* 1976; 16:573–578.
21. Hardy JD, Neely WA, Wilson FC, et al: Thermal burns in man: V. Cardiac output during early therapy. *Surg Gynecol Obstet* 1955; 101:94–98.
22. Hayashi H, Yoshinager M, Koono M, et al: Endogenous permeability factors and their inhibitors affecting vascular permeability in cutaneous arthus reactions and thermal injury. *Br J Exp Pathol* 1964; 45(4):419.
23. Hazard PB, Griffin JP: Sodium bicarbonate in the management of systemic acidosis. *South Med J* 1980; 73:1339–1342.
24. Hilton JG: Effects of sodium nitroprusside on thermal trauma depressed cardiac output in the anesthetized dog. *Burns* 1984; 10:318–322.
25. Hilton JG: Effects of verapamil on thermal trauma depressed cardiac output in the anesthetized dog. *Burns* 1984; 10:313–317.
26. Jardin F, Farcot JC, Boisante C: Influence of positive end-expiratory pressure on left ventricular performance. *N Engl J Med* 1981; 304:387–392.
27. Kasnitz P, Druger GL, Yorra F, et al: Mixed venous oxygen tension and hyperlactemia. *JAMA* 1976; 236:570–574.
28. Katz RW, Pollack MM, Weibley RE: Pulmonary artery catheterization in pediatric intensive care. *Adv Pediatr* 1983; 30:169–191.
29. Michie DD, Goldsmith RS, Mason AD, et al: Hemodynamics of the immediate postburn period: I. Hemodynamic alteration produced by thermal burns. *J Trauma* 1963; 3:111–119.
30. Michie DD, Goldsmith RS, Mason AD: Effects of hydralazine and high molecular weight dextran upon the circulatory responses to severe thermal burns. *Circ Res* 1966; 13:468–473.
31. Moncrief JA: Effect of various fluid regimens and pharmacologic agents on the circulatory hemodynamics of the immediate postburn period. *Ann Surg* 1966; 164:723–749.
32. Moncrief JA: Burns. *N Engl J Med* 1970; 288:444–454.
33. Moodie DS: Measurement of cardiac output by thermodilution in pediatric patients. *Pediatr Clin North Am* 1980; 27:513–523.
34. Munster AM: The early management of thermal burns. *Surg* 1980; 87:29–40.
35. Neutze JM, Wyler F, Rudolph AM: Changes in distribution of cardiac output after hemorrhage in rabbits. *Am J Physiol* 1968; 215:857–864.
36. Notterman DA: Invasive hemodynamic moni-

toring, in Zimmerman SS, Gilden JH (eds): *Crit Care Pediatr.* WB Saunders Co, 1985, pp 43–54.

37. Perkin RM, Levin DL: Shock in the pediatric patient: II. *Therapy* 1982; 101:319–332.
38. Pollack MM, Reed TP, Holbrook PR, et al: Bedside pulmonary artery catheterization in pediatrics. *J Pediatr* 1980; 96:274–276.
39. Pruitt BA, Mason AD, Moncrief JA: Haemodynamic changes in the early postburn patient: The influence of fluid administration and of a vasodilator (hydralazine). *J Trauma* 1971; 11:36–48.
40. Raffa J, Trunkey DD: Myocardial depression in acute thermal injury. *J Trauma* 1978; 18:90–93.
41. Rosenthal SR, Hawley PL, Hakim AA: Purified burn toxic factor and its competition. *Surgery* 1972; 71:527–536.
42. Shoemaker WC: Monitoring of the critically ill patient, in Shoemaker WC, Thompson WL, Holbrook PR (eds): *Society of Critical Care Medicine Textbook of Critical Care.* Philadelphia, WB Saunders Co, 1983, pp 369–400.
43. Shoemaker WC, Vladeck BC, Bassin R, et al: Burn pathophysiology in man. I. Sequential hemodynamic alterations. *J Surg Rev* 1973; 14:64–73.
44. Vure FE, Joseph M, Beer S, et al: A practical approach to the treatment of burn shock in childhood. *Burns* 1981; 8:245–248.
45. Weisel RD, Vito L, Dennis RC, et al: Myocardial depression during sepsis. *Ann J Surg* 1977; 133:512–520.
46. Wolfe RR, Miller HI: Cardiovascular and metabolic responses during burn shock in the guinea pig. *Am J Physiol* 1976; 231:892–897.
47. Wyse SD, Pfitzner J, Rees A, et al: Measurement of cardiac output by thermodilution in infants and children. *Thorax* 1975; 30:262–265.
48. Young M, Cotton D: Arterial and venous blood pressure responses during a reduction in blood volume and hypoxia and hypercapnia in infants during the first two days of life. *Pediatr* 1966; 37:733–742.

21 / Gastrointestinal Complications in Burned Children

GEORGE J. FUCHS III, M.D.
WALLACE A. GLEASON, JR., M.D.

Burns are an important child health problem in the United States and are the leading cause of nonvehicular accidental death with a peak incidence occurring among children 1 to 5 years of age.[10] Many life-threatening complications may accompany burn injury, one of the most notable of which involves the gastrointestinal (GI) tract. GI complications were first described by Swan in 1823 in a young boy dying of a burn injury in which gastric erosions were observed. Twenty years later in 1842 Curling recognized acute duodenal ulceration as a life-threatening complication of burns, and the association was established.[17] Although Curling's ulcer has since become defined as either a gastric or duodenal ulcer in a patient with thermal injury, it is clear that clinically significant mucosal abnormalities are not confined to ulcers alone but also include more superficial erosions of the stomach and duodenum.

GASTRODUODENAL DISEASE IN BURN PATIENTS

The true incidence of Curling's ulcers is difficult to evaluate as most cases in children have been diagnosed at autopsy. Autopsy data would suggest, however, that the incidence of Curling's ulcer, in addition to more superficial mucosal changes in the stomach and duodenum is 2 to 3 times higher in children than in adults.[13, 23]

With the development and widespread use of fiberoptic endoscopy, the natural history of the upper gastrointestinal response to thermal injury has been further elucidated. Although these studies have been in adults, and occasionally in adolescents, it is likely that these findings can be extrapolated to events as they occur in children. Serial endoscopic examination has revealed that gastritis may develop as early as 5 hours after the burn injury. By 72 hours, approximately 75% of patients with large burns involving more than 30% of their body surface demonstrate superficial gastric disease.[5] Detection of gastric ulcers is very unusual before 4 days after injury, but when present, gastric ulcers develop within areas of severe superficial gastritis.[6] As shown in Table 21–1, 16% to 26% of patients with large burns ultimately develop gastric ulcers, one third of whom will have multiple gastric ulcers.

In the duodenum, this temporal sequence is much the same. Superficial mucosal erosions may be evident by 12 hours after injury, and by 72 hours can be demonstrated in 67% of patients. Ulcers, however, are rare prior to 72 hours but are usually seen by the second or third week after the burn. Duodenal ulcers will eventually develop in almost one third of patients and, as with gastric ulceration, always occur against the background of diffuse superficial mucosal disease.

It is of interest that isolated gastric and duodenal disease rarely occur as isolated events. Greater than 80% of patients will

TABLE 21–1.
The Incidence of Gastroduodenal Disease in Adult Burn Patients

REFERENCE	BURN SIZE, % TOTAL BODY SURFACE AREA	GASTRIC EROSIONS, %	GASTRIC ULCERS, %	DUODENAL EROSIONS, %	DUODENAL ULCERS, %
Czaja et al., 1974[6]	≥23	78	22	28	82
Czaja et al., 1975[7]	≥23	49	16	41	32
Czaja et al., 1976[8]	≥20	83	26		

have simultaneous superficial or ulcerative gastric and duodenal disease. Overall, 25% of all patients with Curling's ulcers will have ulcers in both the stomach and duodenum.[6, 7]

Pathogenesis

The precise pathogenesis of gastroduodenal erosion remains undefined, yet certain factors are known to initiate and aggravate mucosal damage. Of note is the increasing incidence of Curling's ulcer with increasing burn size.[4, 19] The temporal sequence of the morphology and histopathology of the lesions, as well as direct measurements of mucosal blood flow, implicate as the basic etiology mucosal ischemia due to altered submucosal blood flow in the immediate postburn period.[6, 12] The histological characteristics are consistent with infarction necrosis with microvascular congestion, edema, mucosal hemorrhage, and epithelial cell necrosis. In many cases the superficial lesions appear to represent early mucosal sloughs and nascent ulceration. The immediate postburn period is characterized by a normal or even an initial suppression of gastric acid secretion, perhaps due to increased catecholamine production. Hyperacidity, therefore, is not considered to be a contributing factor in the early genesis of mucosal disease. Using timed gastric collections, however, patients with both gastric and duodenal disease secrete significantly more acid after the first 48 to 72 hours than burn patients with normal or only mildly inflamed mucosa.[5, 8] This eventual hyperacidity against the background of an increasingly susceptible ischemic gastric mucosa correlates temporally with the development of ulcerations. In addition to back diffusion of gastric acid across the damaged mucosa, autolysis by pepsin further contributes to the evolution of the ulcer. Progression of the initial gastroduodenal lesions as well as the development of new lesions is associated with further episodes of mucosal ischemia elicited by submucosal shunting of blood flow due to septic episodes or hypoxia of respiratory insufficiency. Focal areas of infarction due to septic emboli or hemoconcentration have also been implicated as less frequent causes of gastroduodenal lesions.

Clinical Manifestation

The clinical picture of postburn gastroduodenal disease is variable. Gastrointestinal complaints may be masked by the superimposed symptoms related to the burn itself or by those of other associated complications such as sepsis. And, as with all illness in children, the limited expressive capabilities of younger children may lead to a delay in diagnosis.

Table 21–2 lists presenting signs and symptoms. Most patients with mucosal lesions of the stomach and duodenum are asymptomatic and have an uncomplicated course. Evolution of mucosal injuries to an increasing number of superficial lesions or to frank ulcer formation may be occurring silently while other more emergent complications of burn injuries such as sepsis, hypotension, and respiratory insufficiency develop. In patients who have symptoms of gastrointestinal complications, bleeding is the first indication in half of patients, the majority of whom present with hematemesis and the remainder with melena.[4, 19] Duodenal ulcers hemorrhage more commonly than gastric ulcers, and duodenal lesions located posteriorly bleed more commonly than those located anteriorly.

Surprisingly, short of hemorrhage there is a paucity of other signs or symptoms, such as nausea and vomiting, to suggest gastrointestinal disease.[1] This is particularly true in children. In one series, up to 49% of children with Curling's ulcers who ultimately died were never symptomatic.[4] In prospective studies of postburn duodenal disease in adults, the majority of patients were asymptomatic and would have remained undiagnosed without routine endoscopic examination.[5, 7] Even patients who perforate may remain asymptomatic. Perforation occurs in less than 15% of patients and when present is usually painless, only to be discovered at the time of surgery or autopsy. The clinical picture, therefore, emphasizes the need for vigilant monitoring of burn patients in an anticipation of gastrointestinal involvement.

Diagnosis

Early diagnosis of gastroduodenal mucosal disease in children with thermal injury solely on a clinical basis is difficult. However, given its high frequency, the physician managing the burn patient must have a high index of suspicion for its presence.

Routine testing of stool for occult blood may herald the onset of disease. Ileus is almost always present in the immediate postburn period and requires a nasogastric tube for decompression and the prevention of aspiration. One must therefore distinguish occult bleeding due to irritation of the gastric lining attributable to the nasogastric tube from bleeding of more malignant causes. Contrast x-ray examination of the upper GI tract is insensitive and does not reliably demonstrate the extent of mucosal disease, particularly that of a more superficial nature. In view of the frequent coexisting ileus and the occasional perforation in the asymptomatic patient, contrast studies in patients with thermal injuries must be used with caution.

Endoscopy is the procedure of choice as prompt diagnosis allows early therapy. In instances of severe bleeding, endoscopy may accurately locate the site and consequently be of assistance to the surgeon in the event that surgical intervention is required. Hematemesis or melena are the most common presenting signs, but generally indicate an already advanced lesion. Since endoscopic changes are seen as early as 5 hours after injury, early endoscopy is recommended. Early lesions appear as punctate hemorrhages and superficial

TABLE 21–2.
Clinical Characteristics of Burned Children With Curling's Ulcer

	ABRAMSON, 1965*	BRUCK, 1972†
No. of children	90	63
Mean age, yr (range)	4.7 (11 wk–12 yr)	4.3 (5 wk–13 yr)
Hemorrhage, no. (%)	44 (49)	32 (51)
Hematemesis, no. (%)	—	23 (37)
Melena, no. (%)	—	20 (32)
Perforation, no. (%)	12 (13)	4 (6)
Epigastric pain, no. (%)	—	1 (2)
Asymptomatic, no. (%)	—	31 (49)

*Data from Abramson DJ: Curling's ulcer in childhood: Review of the literature and report of five cases. *Surgery* 1964; 55:321–336. (Literature review of autopsy cases between 1823 and 1963.)

†Data from Bruck HM, Pruitt BA: Curling's ulcer in children: A 12-year review of 63 cases. *J Trauma* 1972; 12:490–496. (Retrospective review of autopsy, surgical, and "clinical" cases.)

erosions interspersed with more normal appearing mucosa. In adult patients, development of frank ulceration is most frequently in the fundus, but antral lesions are not uncommon. In children, many reports suggest that ulcers are most frequently found in the duodenum, although more recent studies indicate a gastric predominance as in the adult burn patient.[4, 21] Acute duodenitis is characterized by erythema, edema, and friability as well as mucosal punctate erosions. Ulcerations of the gastric mucosa are generally multiple, while duodenal ulcers are more frequently solitary and characteristically shallow. The sharp margins of the ulcers reveal minimal gross inflammatory changes or edema. Biopsy specimens frequently demonstrate microvascular congestion and hemorrhage as well as inflammatory changes. In those patients with active bleeding in whom endoscopy is nondiagnostic, radionuclide scanning with 99^{m} technetium pertechnetate–labeled red blood cells may be considered. One of the potentially limiting factors of this technique is the requirement of a bleeding rate of greater than 0.5 ml/minute.

Treatment

Therapy for upper gastrointestinal mucosal disease in patients with thermal injury adheres to the same principles as applied to gastroduodenal disease of similar nature such as peptic disease, mucosal disease following head injury, and stress ulcers. Of major importance is the correction of concomitant predisposing conditions; intravascular repletion with blood products should be established in the patient with hypovolemic shock; coexistant sepsis should be treated with appropriate antibiotics after a complete evaluation of possible sources; and adequate respiratory function should be assured with artificial ventilation, if necessary.

Subsequent therapy is usually directed at control of upper gastrointestinal hemorrhage, as this is the predominant presenting feature and one of the most life-threatening complications. A large-bore nasogastric tube should be inserted that permits gastric decompression, minimizes the risk of vomiting and aspiration, and may provide information about the rate of bleeding. Saline lavage may control the bleeding in many patients. Instillation of antacids through the nasogastric tube should then be undertaken in order to maintain a neutral gastric pH as shown in Table 21–3. A mixture or alternation of aluminum hydroxide and magnesium hydroxide is preferred to avoid the complication of constipation with the former and diarrhea with the latter if either agent is used alone. Should constipation or diarrhea occur, the proportion of aluminum and magnesium may be altered to increase tolerance.

The additional use of a histamine H_2-antagonist is probably a useful adjunct to antacid therapy in the presence of severe bleeding. Although not yet approved for use in children less than 16 years of age, there has been widespread and sufficient experience in children with the use of cimetidine, and to a lesser extent with ranitidine, that clearly suggests these agents should not be withheld in life-threatening gastroduodenal mucosal disease. These agents are potent inhibitors of gastric acid production and have proven to be important additions to the therapy for ulcer disease. It must be remembered that antacids impair the absorption of orally administered cimetidine and ranitidine if given simultaneously. A staggered dosing regimen or use of the parenteral preparations obviates this problem. Of particular importance in the burn patient is the observation of an increased cimetidine clearance correlating with the size of the burn.[15] The gastric pH should therefore be monitored since a higher or more frequent dose may be required for effective alkalinization. Potential side effects of cimetidine are few, but include gynecomastia or neutropenia in selected patients. Ranitidine is more potent, longer acting, and probably has fewer significant toxic side effects than cimetidine although there is comparatively less experience with this drug.

The most recent agent introduced for use

TABLE 21–3.
Drug Therapy for Gastroduodenal Mucosal Disease in the Pediatric Burn Patient

AGENT	RECOMMENDED DOSE	COMMENTS
Antacids		
Magnesium/aluminum hydroxide	Active bleeding: 60–80 ml/1.73 sq m/hr by continuous nasogastric infusion* or 15–30 ml every 2 hr Prophylaxis: 15–30 ml every 3–6 hr	Drug of choice; must maintain gastric pH ≥4; may inhibit absorption of histamine H_2-antagonist if given simultaneously; contraindicated with ileus or perforation
Histamine H_2-antagonist†		
Cimetidine	5–10 mg/kg every 4–6 hr, orally or intravenously	Need to modify dose to maintain gastric pH ≥4; modify dosage in patients with renal or hepatic disease
Ranitidine	Children: 1.25–1.90 mg/kg every 12 hr orally‡ Adults: 100 mg orally two times daily or 50 mg three to four times daily intravenously	As with cimetidine; parenteral dose in children not well established
Cytoprotection†		
Sucralfate	250–500 mg orally four times daily	Efficacy in children not established

*Data from Silverman A, Roy CC (eds): *Pediatric Clinical Gastroenterology*. St. Louis, CV Mosby Co, 1983, pp 162–189.
†Not approved by FDA for children under 16 years of age.
‡Data from Blumer JL et al.: Pharmacokinetic determination of ranitidine pharmacodynamics in pediatric ulcer disease. *J Pediatr* 1985; 107:301–306.

in gastroduodenal mucosal disease is sucralfate, a complex polyaluminum hydroxide salt of sucrose sulfate. In an acid environment sucralfate binds to the ulcer tissue and provides a mechanical protective barrier. It also stimulates prostaglandin synthesis, and in this manner actively enhances cellular repair. Sucralfate is minimally absorbed so that toxic side effects are rare. Constipation, which occurs in approximately 2% of adult patients, is its only appreciable side effect. However, until further randomized control studies are performed, its role in children with thermal injury and acute gastroduodenal mucosal disease remains to be established.

Indications for surgical intervention include massive bleeding, intractable bleeding, or perforation. When the volume of blood replaced exceeds 60% of the total blood volume of the pediatric burn patient, an operative procedure should be considered.[4, 25] In general, the consensus favors early rather than late surgical intervention. The frequent coexistence of sepsis as well as the heavy bacterial density of the burn wound in a patient who is already nutritionally debilitated due to the initial burn injury makes a surgical procedure particularly unattractive.

Many types of surgical procedures have been employed ranging from highly selective vagotomy and pyloroplasty to total gastrectomy, although no single approach has emerged as the procedure of choice. Because they are considered the most simple, rapid, and atraumatic, some have stated a preference for vagotomy and pyloroplasty. A gastrotomy and thorough inspection of the mucosa is recommended as part of any surgical procedure because of the high frequency of multiple ulcers and their occurrence in both the duodenum and stomach.

Prophylaxis

The initiation of gastrointestinal pathology occurs within the first hours after a burn and results from ischemia. Adequate intravenous fluids should therefore be administered in the immediate postburn period to minimize vascular compromise of the upper gastrointestinal tract. After the development of the initial lesion, there is further damage from the backflow of gastric acid and from autolysis by pepsin that is derived from pepsinogen in an acid environment. For this reason, medical prophylaxis is directed at alkalinization of the luminal contents. The efficacy of antacids in the prevention of gastrointestinal bleeding in adult patients with burns has been clearly established. Patients who receive antacids each hour as needed to maintain a gastric pH of 7 or greater demonstrate significantly less hemorrhage.[16] There are no studies of the prophylactic benefit of histamine H_2-antagonists in burn patients; however, trials of cimetidine versus antacids in the prophylaxis of stress ulcers in critically ill patients have demonstrated comparable but not superior efficacy of cimetidine.[11, 18] Of the two agents, antacids have been the more consistently effective prophylactic agent. A combination of antacids with a histamine H_2-antagonist is used in many centers, even though there have been no randomized controlled studies in burn patients showing its superiority over the use of antacids alone.

Preliminary studies demonstrate efficacy with the prophylactic use of sucralfate in preventing hemorrhage from stress ulcers in critically ill adults.[3] Its extremely low toxic potential and ease of administration makes it a potentially attractive drug in the pediatric population. However, until the appropriate studies of the use of the drug in children are conducted, its use as the sole prophylactic agent cannot be recommended.

ESOPHAGUS

In a postmortem review of 54 children with thermal injury, 7.4% were reported to have ulceration of the esophagus.[13] Other reports indicate that lesions in the esophagus are unusual, but when present they are almost always the result of a nasogastric tube.[20] The incidence and severity of mucosal lesions increases as the duration of nasogastric intubation increases. Conservative management of the esophageal ulcer is usually sufficient, and emphasis is placed on the use of Silastic rather than hard plastic feeding tubes, as well as their early removal.

ILEUS

Impaired intestinal motility is a common early complication in patients with burns of greater than 25% of their total body surface.[20] Motility is usually restored soon after correction of the hypovolemia that occurs in the early shock phase. Recurrence of an ileus later in the hospital course suggests sepsis; an evaluation of the patient for a possible source is required as are considerations for antibiotic therapy. Intravenous alimentation may be necessary until resolution of the ileus enables the resumption of enteral feedings.

OTHER

Pancreatitis occurs rarely and may simply be due to contiguity with duodenal inflammation or the result of generalized sepsis.[7, 20] Other uncommon gastrointestinal complications of burn injury include superior mesenteric artery syndrome and hepatic dysfunction due to hepatocellular damage most likely as a result of hypotension.[9, 22]

Other abnormalities encountered in the gastrointestinal tract of burn patients include isolated cases of focal and multifocal ischemic necrosis and ulceration of the distal small bowel and colon, perhaps due to large doses of vasopressors. Septic infarct of the small and large bowel as a consequence of bacteremia has also been reported.[13]

Bacterial infection and sepsis remain serious problems and are implicated in the majority of patients who ultimately die due to thermal injury. Loss of the skin barrier and the multifaceted impairment of specific and nonspecific immune mechanisms have largely been held responsible.[10] An impaired intestinal mucosal barrier as a site of entry for enteric organisms, and ultimately as a source of sepsis in burn patients, has been proposed. This concept is supported by the high incidence of sepsis due to enteric organisms, and by investigations in animal models that demonstrate translocation of enteric organisms from the intestinal tract to mesenteric lymph nodes and other visceral organs.[14]

REFERENCES

1. Abramson DJ: Curling's ulcer in childhood: Review of the literature and report of five cases. *Surgery* 1964; 55:321–336.
2. Blumer JL, et al: Pharmacokinetic determination of ranitidine pharmacodynamics in pediatric ulcer disease. *J Pediatr* 1985; 107:301–306.
3. Borrero E, et al: Comparison of antacid and sucralfate in the prevention of gastrointestinal bleeding in patients who are critically ill. *Am J Med* 1985; 79 (suppl 2C):62–64.
4. Bruck HM, Pruitt BA: Curling's ulcer in children: A 12-year review of 63 cases. *J Trauma* 1972; 12:490–496.
5. Czaja AJ, McAlhany JC, Andes WA, et al: Acute gastric disease after cutaneous thermal injury. *Arch Surg* 1975; 110:600–606.
6. Czaja AJ, McAlhany JC, Pruitt BA Jr: Acute gastroduodenal disease after thermal injury: An endoscopic evaluation of incidence and natural history. *N Engl J Med* 1974; 291:925–929.
7. Czaja AJ, McAlhany JC, Pruitt BA Jr: Acute duodenitis and duodenal ulceration after burns: Clinical and pathological characteristics. *JAMA* 1975a; 232:621–624.
8. Czaja AJ, McAlhany JC, Pruitt BA Jr: Gastric acid secretion and acute gastroduodenal disease after burns. *Arch Surg* 1976; 111:243–245.
9. Czaja AJ, Rizzo TA, Smith WR Jr, et al: Acute liver disease after cutaneous thermal injury. *J Trauma* 1975; 15:887–894.
10. Demling RH: Burns. *N Engl J Med* 1985; 313:1389–1398.
11. Haloran LG, et al: Prevention of acute gastrointestinal complications after severe head injury: A controlled trial of cimetidine prophylaxis. *Am J Surg* 1980; 139:44–48.
12. Kamada T, et al: Gastric mucosal hemodynamics after thermal or head injury. *Gastroenterology* 1982; 83:535–540.
13. Law EJ, Day SB, MacMillan BG: Autopsy findings in the upper gastrointestinal tracts of 81 burn patients. *Arch Surg* 1971; 102:412–416.
14. Maejima K, Deitch EA, Berg RD: Bacterial translocation from the gastrointestinal tracts of rats receiving thermal injury. *Infect Immun* 1984; 43:6–10.
15. Martyn JA, Greenblatt DJ, Abernathy DR: Increased cimetidine clearance in burn patients. *JAMA* 1985; 253:1288–1291.
16. McAlhany JR, Czaja AJ, Pruitt BA: Antacid control of complications from acute gastroduodenal disease after burns. *J Trauma* 1976; 16:645–649.
17. Nordstrom H, Nettelblad H: Curling's ulcer—a serious complication of the burned patient. *Scand J Gastroenterol* 1984; 105(suppl):14–18.
18. Priebe HJ, et al: Antacid versus cimetidine in preventing acute gastrointestinal bleeding: A randomized trial in 75 critically ill patients. *N Engl J Med* 1980; 302:426–430.
19. Pruitt BA, Foley FD, Moncrief JA: Curling's ulcer: A clinical-pathology study of 323 cases. *Ann Surg* 1970; 172:523–539.
20. Pruitt BA: The burn patient: II. Later care and complications of thermal injury. *Curr Probl Surg* 1979; 16:1–95.
21. Pruitt BA, Goodwin CW: Stress ulcer disease in the burned patient. *World J Surg* 1981; 5:209–222.
22. Reckler JA, et al: Superior mesenteric artery syndrome as a consequence of burn injury. *J Trauma* 1972; 12:979–985.
23. Sevitt S: Duodenal and gastric ulceration after burning. *Br J Surg* 1967; 54:32–41.
24. Silverman A, Roy CC, (eds): *Pediatric Clinical Gastroenterology*. St. Louis, CV Mosby Co, 1983, pp 162–189.
25. Williams JW, Pannell WP, Sherman RT: Curling's ulcer in children. *J Trauma* 1976; 16:639–644.

22 / Neurologic Complications of Burns in Childhood

EDWARD M. KAYE, M.D.
IAN J. BUTLER, M.D., F.R.A.C.P.

The first documented study of neurological complications of burns in childhood occurred in 1832, when Dupuytren described "intensive cerebral congestion" in the autopsies of burned children.[18] The causes of neurologic manifestations in burns were initially attributed to cerebral edema,[21] a burn "toxin"[11, 25] or demyelination.[17] Multifactorial causes for burn-related encephalopathy were subsequently postulated by Allgower and Siegrist[1] and included asphyxia, carbon monoxide poisoning, and acute circulatory insufficiency as pathophysiologic mechanisms. The incidence of neurological problems associated with burns has varied from 1% to 85%,[30] but based on more contemporary literature, the incidence appears to be declining.[3] Children in general appear to have neurologic complications more commonly than adults.[32]

Central nervous system dysfunction occurring with thermal burns is defined as burn-related encephalopathy. This chapter outlines the multiple etiologies of this encephalopathy that may occur in the burn-injured child. Although the effect of burns on the spinal cord and autonomic nervous system is virtually unknown, peripheral nervous system mechanisms of pain in burns is discussed.

BURN-RELATED ENCEPHALOPATHY

Clinical Features

Incidence

The incidence of burn-related encephalopathy in more recent series of childhood burns has varied from 5% to 14% (Table 22–1). The onset of symptoms following the burn may range from a few hours to several weeks with the mean duration between 12 and 16 days (see Table 22–1). In a review of 83 patients with seizures following burns, peak latency was determined to be between 18 and 24 hours with the incidence decreasing linearly until the fifth day following the burn.[16] The severity of the burn does not necessarily correlate with the frequency or degree of neurological symptoms[10, 42] although in many instances severe burns were more frequently associated with encephalopathy or seizures.[16]

Neuropsychiatric Manifestations

The typical neurologic features of the pediatric burn victim may include coma; lethargy; irritability; agitation; disorientation; delirium, including hallucinations; vomiting; respiratory arrest; muscular twitching; cognitive or be-

TABLE 22–1.
Summary of Clinical Features in Burn-Related Encephalopathy

DATA	AUTHORS		
	ANTOON ET AL. (1972)	MCMANUS ET AL. (1974)	MOHNOT ET AL. (1982)
No. of patients in series	20	36	13
Incidence of encephalopathy (%)	14	6.6	5
Mean surface area of burns (%)	42	51	30
Mean age (yr)	4.8	4.96	3.0
Mean time from burn to symptoms (days)	16.25	12.8	16.6
Incidence of seizures	11/20	36/36	9/13
Mortality	10/20	12/36	1/13

havioral changes; and seizures.[3, 16, 27, 30, 41, 42] There is no specific clinical pattern to these neurologic symptoms, primarily because the etiologies are so diverse.[3] Psychiatric problems that may mimic symptoms seen in other encephalopathies occur frequently in children with burns.[5] One study demonstrated a 40% incidence of behavioral problems, a 26% occurrence of cognitive problems, and a 34% incidence of both following burns in children.[16] Neuropsychiatric problems were also recorded in 14 of 39 adult victims following the famous Coconut Grove fire.[9]

CONVULSIONS

Convulsions are one of the most common manifestations of a burn-related encephalopathy. The incidence of convulsions in burn patients has been reported to be approximately 2%.[34] It is difficult to estimate the incidence of seizures in burn encephalopathy because most reports include seizures as an important or sole criterion for diagnosing the encephalopathy.[3, 16, 27, 30] Most of the seizures have been described as generalized, but focal seizures also occur.[3, 16, 27, 30, 34] In one report,[16] right-sided seizures were seen slightly more often, but this predominance has not been observed in other series.[3, 27, 30] The latent period from the burn to the seizure onset may vary from a few hours to weeks.[27] The latent interval most likely varies according to the etiology of the seizure, with metabolic causes being associated with earlier onset of seizures in some cases.[16, 27] Etiologies for the convulsions are not always determined, but appear to be similar to those for burn-related encephalopathy. Causes have included hyponatremia, fever, hypertension, hypoxia, cerebral edema, previous seizures, medications, and topical drug applications.[16, 27, 34, 43]

ELECTROENCEPHALOGRAPHY

The electroencephalogram (EEG) has been used as a clinical test in burn victims to document encephalopathy and to follow patients with seizures. In 1965, Petersen et al.[32] described nonspecific changes in the EEGs of 21 of 58 consecutive burn patients of all ages. In 18 of these 58 patients, diffuse slow waves with some focal changes were noted that seemed to correlate positively to the degree of burn. Later, diffuse slow waves were demonstrated in 10 patients with burn-related coma.[14] In describing two cases, Hall[12] noted high-amplitude waves (1 to 4 cycles/second), especially posteriorly, which improved with the clinical course. Electroencephalographic changes in a series of 40 patients with burns consisted of excessive slow activity in 88%, especially over the occipital area, and epileptiform discharges in another 10%.[15] All chronic cases in this study and 88% of acute cases demonstrated EEG abnormalities. The EEG abnormalities in the same report were observed 3 to 11 days after the burn and were unrelated to the onset of seizures, which usually occurred in the first 48 hours. The EEG of burn victims has been consistently abnormal as shown by one study in which 9 of 10 adult burn victims manifested low-voltage activity in the θ and δ ranges.[2] Mohnot et al.[30] described excessive slow waves in 4 of 6 patients and Prekop et al.[33] recorded EEG slowing in all patients studied.

PAIN MECHANISMS

Burns are associated with hyperalgesia or increased sensibility of the skin to stimuli. This hyperalgesia is expressed as spontaneous pain and a decreased pain threshold. There are two forms of hyperalgesia: primary hyperalgesia, which occurs directly within the burn area, and secondary hyperalgesia, which occurs outside of the injured region.[35] The area of primary hyperalgesia shows increased sensitivity to both heat and mechanical stimuli, while in secondary hyperalgesia only mechanical stimuli produce the altered sensation.[13, 35] This sensory dissociation suggests that there may be different mechanisms for primary and secondary hyperalgesia, and possibly different mechanisms for mechanically and thermally induced hyperalgesia.[35]

Different types of pain afferents mediate the heat-induced hyperalgesia following thermal injury. Depending on the type of skin, both C-fiber and A-fiber nociceptive afferents may be involved in the heat-induced hyperalgesia.[29] The cause of the mechanically induced hyperalgesia in primary and secondary hyperalgesia is not known, but it has been postulated to occur on the basis of enhanced sensitivity of central neurons.[45]

PATHOLOGY

The first neuropathologic description of the brain from a burn victim was recorded by Dupuytren in 1832.[18] The description was that of intensive cerebral and meningeal congestion. Several authors, such as Riehl,[36] believed that cerebral edema was inevitably associated with burns. In many of the early reports cerebral edema was the only pathologic finding. In one report, 2 of 7 children died with autopsy evidence of cerebral edema.[31] Six autopsied cases were reported in which cerebral edema demonstrated by widening of gyri, narrowing of sulci, uncal and tonsillar herniation, and microscopic interstitial edema were present.[41] A detailed neuropathologic study carried out in two patients demonstrated dilated surface blood vessels, gyral swelling, sulcal obliteration, uncal notching of temporal lobes, but no evidence of cerebellar herniation.[25] In a series of 39 autopsy studies, 17 showed macroscopic evidence of cerebral and meningeal edema.[18] Cerebral edema was noted in six children who died from burns, many of whom appeared to have relatively minor burns.[10] Hughes et al.[16] found cerebral edema in 26% of patients with burns, but this was not necessarily the cause of seizures or death. More recent studies have not demonstrated this high incidence of cerebral edema. Edema was suspected in 5 of 72 cases from one series, but confirmed in only one autopsied patient. In a neuropathologic study of seven children who died from burns, cerebral edema was documented in only one patient.[3]

Other neuropathologic changes have been noted in burn patients. Mallory and Brickley[26] noted cortical ganglion cell degeneration in one case. Later, ganglion cell degeneration was demonstrated in the cortex, hypothalamus, and basal ganglia with lesser involvement of the brain stem.[41] In one report, ganglion cells from the cortex, hypothalamus, caudate nuclei, lentiform nuclei, and thalamic nuclei were affected in two patients, while only one case demonstrated cerebellar Purkinje cell loss.[25] In this last study, hemorrhages were seen within the white matter in both cases, along with ventricular dilation and white matter loss in one case. Diffuse degenerative changes in white matter, with large areas of perivascular demyelination, were reported in one postmortem study.[11] An area of partial demyelination within the cerebrum and degenerative changes within the cerebellar cortex were observed in one autopsied patient and were thought to be due to cerebral edema and anoxia.[42] Hydrocephalus, cortical atrophy, and gliosis were discovered in a neuropathologic study of a child who died three years after a burn injury.[40]

In a neuropathologic study reviewing the findings of seven children who died of burn-related complications, Antoon et al.[3] delineated various factors that might have caused the encephalopathy. In three of these children, no pathologic lesion could be found. One had evidence of *Pseudomonas* meningitis, while another demonstrated pseudolaminar necrosis of the cerebral and cerebellar cortices. Two children had an increase in brain weight, one due to microabscesses and one from cerebral edema.

ETIOLOGIES

The association between neurologic symptoms and burns evolved gradually during the early part of the century. As mentioned previously, Dupuytren (1832) noted cerebral edema in children who died from burns. In 1928, Kruse[21] described a 14-month-old child who manifested blindness, progressive hydrocephalus, and mental deterioration associated with second-degree burns. Kruse[21] suggested that the neurological findings were caused by cerebral edema. Riehl[36] believed that all patients dying from burns developed cerebral edema. Cerebral edema in burn patients has been recognized both clinically,[16, 33] and by numerous neuropathologic observations.[10, 18, 25, 31]

Causes for the cerebral edema are not completely understood, but a number of hypotheses have been suggested. In 1936, Globus and Bender[11] reported neuropathologic findings in a burn-injured child consisting of diffuse degeneration of white matter and larger perivascular areas of demyelination. They considered these changes to be similar to multiple sclerosis and thought that the causal agent could be a burn-related toxin. Several authors have championed a "burn toxin" as the etiology for the neuropathologic changes and edema,[25, 41] but no specific toxin has ever been discovered.

It has become apparent in the last several years that there is more than one etiology for burn-related encephalopathy (Table 22–2). Sevitt,[39] in 1957, suggested shock, anoxia, uremia, infection, and direct exposure of the skull to heat as causes for burn encephalopathy. The recognition of hypoxemia as a cause for some of the initial neurologic symptoms was made by Allgower and Siegrist in 1957.[1] They postulated that asphyxia, carbon monoxide poisoning, and acute circulatory insufficiency with cerebral vascular congestion, were causes for the encephalopathy. Further studies noted anoxia as a contributory factor in neurologic complications of burns.[3, 19] The importance of hypoxemia and overhydration with water intoxication and hyponatremia was noted in several series.[18, 19, 31, 37] Late-onset coma has been reported to occur with gram-negative sepsis, which improved after application and growth of skin homografts.[14]

Several recent series describing encephalopathies in burn victims have been able to determine an etiology for most of the neurological complications observed. Antoon and coworkers[3] determined that of 20 cases of encephalopathy, 9 were due to hypoxia (usually in the first 48 hours) and the others were due to hyponatremia, sepsis, shock, and cortical venous thrombosis, with only 1 case in which the etiology was unknown. Fever has been noted as an etiology,[42] as has hyperten-

TABLE 22–2.
Etiologies for Burn-Related Encephalopathies

Hypoxia (including carbon monoxide poisoning)
Hypovolemia-ischemia
Metabolic disturbance
Hyponatremia
Acidosis
Hypocalcemia
Hyperglycemia
Infection
Meningitis
Microabscesses
Sepsis
Fever
Cortical venous thrombosis
Hypertension
Complications of therapy

sion.[24, 42] In a recent series of cases, multiple metabolic derangements due to hyponatremia, hypoxemia, acidosis, and sepsis were determined as causes for neurologic symptoms in burned children.[30]

NEUROLOGIC COMPLICATIONS OF BURN THERAPY

Some of the causes of burn encephalopathy have been recognized as a complication of specific burn therapy. Tannic acid, which was a mode of external therapy beginning in 1925, was noted to cause hepatic pathologic lesions and a secondary encephalopathy.[28] Silver nitrate, which was used topically on the burn wounds, caused a loss of sodium and chloride ions due to a chemical action on burn surfaces.[6] Another topical agent, hexachlorophene, has been associated with an encephalopathy in burn patients. Symptoms such as seizures, diplopia, nausea, vomiting, irritability, and weakness have been attributed to hexachlorophene.[8, 22] A similar encephalopathy has been noticed in neonates receiving hexachlorophene.[20] Experimentally, burns have been shown to increase hexachlorophene absorption by 2½ times.[7]

Many of the antibiotics used routinely in burn victims may cause neurologic sequelae. Hearing loss, hypocalcemia, hypomagnesemia, and hypokalemia have been reported in burn patients with the use of topical neomycin, bacitracin, polymyxin B, and colistin.[4] Colistin was also thought to cause two cases of late-onset burn-related encephalopathy.[23]

Seizures and respiratory arrest have been noted to occur following the use of topical lidocaine, tetracaine, and cocaine.[43]

PROGNOSIS

In the first reports concerning burn-related encephalopathy, it appeared that the prognosis was quite poor. Kruse[21] noted blindness, progressive hydrocephalus, and mental deterioration in one child with burn encephalopathy. A case first reported by Roth[38] and later by Bender[5] was noted to have hydrocephalus, cortical atrophy, mental impairment, aphasia, and athetosis. In a series of six burned patients, one developed a spastic hemiplegia with mental retardation.[10] Neuropsychiatric sequelae of burn encephalopathy were reported by Bender[5] and, later, Woodward[44] noted that 81% of burned children developed emotional disturbances compared to 14% of a random control group. Beginning in the last decade, however, the frequency of long-term neurological complications from childhood burns has decreased greatly.[3, 30]

The mortality of patients with burn encephalopathy was initially thought to be quite high. In one series, 2 of 6 encephalopathic children died,[42] and in another case series, 5 of 6 children died from neurological complications following relatively minor burns.[10] Even in reports with a low frequency of the neurologic sequelae in survivors, mortality rates of 33% to 50% have been noted in neurologically affected burn patients.[3, 27] In a more recent report of burn-related encephalopathy in children, only 1 of 13 patients died and 11 patients were neurologically normal.[30] The gradual improvement in the morbidity and mortality of children with burn-related encephalopathy is no doubt a consequence of improved management of burns, especially in regard to fluid and electrolyte replacement.

SUMMARY

The causes of burn-related encephalopathy in children are considered to be multifactorial. Initially, anoxia, acidosis, shock, and carbon monoxide poisoning may be significant factors. Later, during resuscitative efforts, overhydration, hyponatremia, and other electrolyte imbalances may cause seizures or cerebral edema. Factors such as temperature elevation, sepsis, and bacterial meningitis are frequent causes of delayed-onset encephalopathy. The therapy of burns, which may include administration of topical preparations, antibiotics, or anesthetics, can also produce neurologic problems. The EEG is an invaluable tool to document the presence and improvement of neurologic symptoms. Close laboratory monitoring of electrolytes, fluid balance, and infections may prevent a significant portion of neurologic problems in the burned child.

REFERENCES

1. Allgower M, Siegrist J: *Verbrennungen: Pathophysiologie, Pathologie, Klinik, Therapie.* Berlin, Springer-Verlag, 1957.
2. Andreasen NJC, et al: EEG changes associated with burn delirium. *Dis Nerv Syst* 1977; 38:27–31.
3. Antoon AY, Volpe JJ, Crawford JD: Burn encephalopathy in children. *Pediatrics* 1972; 50:609–616.
4. Bamford MFM, Jones LF: Deafness and biochemical imbalance after burns treatment with topical antibiotics in young children. *Arch Dis Child* 1978; 53:326–329.
5. Bender L: Burn encephalopathies in children. *Arch Pediatr* 1943; 60:70–87.
6. Burke JF, Bondoc CC, Morris PJ: Metabolic effects of topical silver nitrate therapy in burns covering more than 15% of the body surface. *Ann NY Acad Sci* 1968; 150:674–681.
7. Carroll FE, et al: Absorption of antimicrobial agents across experimental wounds. *Surg Gynecol Obstet* 1967; 125:974–982.
8. Chilcote R, et al: Hexachlorophene storage in a burn patient associated with encephalopathy. *Pediatrics* 1977; 59:457–459.
9. Cobb S, Lindemann E: Neuropsychiatric observations. *Ann Surg* 1943; 117:814–824.
10. Emery JL, Reid DAC: Cerebral edema and spastic hemiplegia following minor burns in young children. *Br J Surg* 1962; 50:53–56.
11. Globus JH, Bender MB: Disseminated toxic degenerative encephalopathy (disseminated sclerosing demyelination) secondary to extensive and severe burns. *J Nerv Ment Dis* 1936; 83:518–529.
12. Hall KV: Encephalopathy complicating burn injuries in children. *Scand J Plast Reconstr Surg* 1968; 2:59–63.
13. Hardy JD, Wolff HG, Goodell H: Experimental evidence on the nature of cutaneous hyperalgesia. *J Clin Invest* 1950; 29:115–140.
14. Haynes BW, Bright R: Burn coma: A syndrome associated with severe burn wound infection. *J Trauma* 1967; 7:464–475.
15. Hughes JR, Cayaffa JJ, Boswick JA: Seizures following burns of the skin: III. Electroencephalographic recordings. *Dis Nerv Syst* 1975; 36:443–447.
16. Hughes JR, et al: Seizures following burns of the skin: II. Conditions associated with these seizures. *Dis Nerv Syst* 1973; 35:347–353.
17. Hughes L: Burns with cerebral complications. *Med J Aust* 1947; 2:122.
18. Jaworska M, Hanc I: Cerebral tissue reaction to burn trauma in children. *Acta Chir Plast* 1965; 7:52–57.
19. Jeffs JV, Edwards GE, Hoyle JR: Induced hypothermia in the management of burns encephalopathy. *Br J Plast Surg* 1966; 19:361–363.
20. Kimbrough RD: Review of recent evidence of toxic effects of hexachlorophene. *Pediatrics* 1973; 51:391–394.
21. Kruse F: Enzephalitis und amauruse nach verbrennung. *Dtsch Med Wochenschr* 1928; 54:1039–1041.
22. Larson DL: Studies show hexachlorophene causes burn syndrome. *Hospitals* 1968; 42:63–64.
23. Lindsay WK, Murphy EG, Birdsell DC: Thermal burn encephalopathy. *Can J Surg* 1965; 8:165–171.
24. Lowrey GH: Hypertension in children with burns. *J Trauma* 1967; 7:140–144.
25. Madow L, Alpers BJ: Brain changes in patients with extensive body burns. *Arch Neurol Psychiatry* 1954; 72:440–451.
26. Mallory TB, Brickley WJ: Pathology: With special reference to the pulmonary lesions. *Ann Surg* 1943; 117:865–884.
27. McManus WF, Hunt JL, Pruitt BA: Postburn convulsive disorders in children. *J Trauma* 1974; 14:396–401.
28. Mettler FA: Burn encephalopathy as a diagnosis. *J Med Soc NJ* 1974; 71:817–823.
29. Meyer RA, Campbell JN: Myelinated nociceptive afferents account for hyperalgesia that follows a burn to the hand. *Science* 1981; 213:1527–1529.
30. Mohnot D, Snead OC, Benton JW: Burn encephalopathy in children. *Ann Neurol* 1982; 12:42–47.
31. Morrison B: A study of burns and scalds in children. *Arch Dis Child* 1947; 22:129–151.
32. Petersen I, et al: An electroencephalographic and psychiatric study of burn cases. *Acta Chir Scand* 1965; 129:359–366.
33. Prekop R, et al: Brain edema in burned children. *Acta Chir Plast* 1984; 26:184–192.
34. Raine PAM, Azmy A: A review of thermal injuries in young children. *J Pediatr Surg* 1983; 18:21–26.
35. Raja SN, Campbell JN, Meyer RA: Evidence for different mechanisms of primary and secondary hyperalgesia following heat injury to

the glabrous skin. *Brain* 1984; 107:1179–1188.
36. Riehl G: Zur verbrennungsfrage. *Arch Dermatol Syph* 1931; 169:409–415.
37. Rosenbloom C, Kravath R: Neurological disturbances following minor burns. *Lancet* 1969; 2:1423.
38. Roth N: Encephalopathy due to burns. *Arch Neurol Psychiatry* 1941; 45:980–983.
39. Sevitt S: *Burns: Pathology and Therapeutic Applications*. London, Butterworth, 1957.
40. Ule G, Doose H: On the pathological anatomy of prolonged brain damage after burns (post combustion encephalopathy). *Arch Kinderheilk* 1960; 161:155–161.
41. Walker J, Shenkin H: Studies on the toxemia syndrome after burns: II. Central nervous system changes as a cause of death. *Ann Surg* 1945; 121:301–313.
42. Warlow CP, Hinton P: Early neurological disturbances following relatively minor burns in children. *Lancet* 1969; 2:978–982.
43. Wehner D, Hamilton GC: Seizures following topical application of local anesthetics to burn patients. *Ann Emerg Med* 1984; 13:456–458.
44. Woodward J: Emotional disturbances of burned children. *Br Med J* 1959; 1:1009–1013.
45. Woolf CJ: Evidence for a central component of post injury pain hypersensitivity. *Nature* 1983; 306:686–688.

23 / Autopsy Findings in Burned Children

HUGO A. LINARES, M.D.

Burns are not a simple injury, but a very complicated disease, of which the numerous and various degrees constitute so many affections, which present marked characters, variable results, particular complications. . . .[29]

Indeed, the anatomical observations on severe burns during the past two centuries, specially after the report on five burn autopsies performed by Cumin in 1823 and the works by Dupuytren, have confirmed that a vast ensemble of morphological multisystem lesions evolves from the severe physiopathological derangement occurred in the severe burn patient.[11, 17]

The contribution of autopsy material to the better understanding of the perplexities of the burn illness cannot be underestimated. A careful morphological evaluation of the anatomohistological lesions and their clinical correlation can provide an invaluable critical analysis and give relevant information about important complications, unsuspected lesions, therapeutic effects, or previous diseases.

The burn autopsy can provide not only an appropriate morphological analysis but a dynamic interpretation of sequential pathogenesis. The autopsy should be oriented to an adequate investigation and retrospective evaluation of the entire clinical course of the burned patient. The history and magnitude of the injury and the clinical course and complications of therapy should be reconstituted to achieve a dynamic sequence of events. Thus, a properly conducted autopsy has as much practical value, as it represents a learning experience. The pathological information presented herein encompasses an 18-year period beginning in 1966, in which a complete postmortem examination was performed in 146 burned children. In 131 cases (89.7%) the burn occurred from exposure to flame, whereas only 15 cases (10.2%) were due to scalds.

CAUSES OF DEATH

In most of the cases, assessment of the actual mechanism of death is a very difficult task. Thus, it is pertinent to remember Cohennheim, who stated that people do not die because they develop pulmonary edema, but that they develop pulmonary edema because they are about to die.[33]

Frequently, the establishment of the cause of death is closer to the subjective judgment of the observer than to any other objective evidence and, in most cases, selecting a single cause of death for each burned patient is neither easy nor always possible.[3, 14, 37] The only pathognomonic burn lesions are those occurring in tissues that are directly exposed to the thermal source (skin and/or orificial mucosa). If the patient survives long enough, the autopsy findings will be related to the complications rather than to the burn itself. In these cases, representing the vast majority, death can be attributed to multiple causes that often are very difficult to interpret (multiple-organ failure). Furthermore, studies during life and at autopsy do not always result in an adequate and satisfactory explanation of the events[37] and the pathophysiologic disturbances leading to death may leave no anatomical traces.[49]

Table 23–1 lists as the cause of death the lesion that was felt to represent the major contributing factor as well as its concurrent association with documented sepsis (positive blood cultures and invasion of viable tissue by microorganisms). Autopsy findings resulting from complications that may have also contributed to the final event are described later.

Table 23–1 shows the lung as the most affected organ. Thus, the causes of death could be classified as lung related and not lung related. Of the total of 146 cases, 115 (79%) had significant pulmonary pathologic findings, which were considered a major contributory cause of death. Sepsis was documented in 90 of these (78%). In the remaining 31 cases (21%) death was attributed to other factors. Twenty four cases of this group (77%) were also associated with documented sepsis.

The larger group of pulmonary complications (43%) is listed under the title of "pulmonary distress." The lung has a limited reactional pattern and different types of injuries usually elicit a similar anatomopathological response; thus, "pulmonary distress" describes the lesions reported elsewhere as shock lung, posttraumatic pulmonary insufficiency, progressive pulmonary consolidation, congestive atelectasis, traumatic wet lung, respirator lung, Da Nang lung, and many others.[5, 19]

The classical lesions of pneumonia or bronchopneumonia (hematogenous or airborne) were considered to be a major contributory cause of death in 36.5% of the lung-related cases.

Cause of Death According to Survival Time

Death within 48 hours

Ten children (7%) died within 48 hours after burn, five from fluid imbalance or "shock lung," three from inhalation injury, one from aspiration pneumonia, and one from pulmonary embolism. There was only one case of documented sepsis in this group, a child with a severe inhalation injury.

Death during days 3 to 7 after burn

Thirty-one patients (22%) died during this period, most of them with "pulmonary distress" (17 cases). There were four cases of inhalation injury, two of disseminated intravascular coagulation, two of bronchopneumonia, two of fluid and electrolyte imbalance and one each of aspiration, pulmonary embolism, acute renal failure, and massive atelectasis

TABLE 23–1.
Major Causes of Death (146 Autopsies), 1966–1984

LUNG RELATED*		OTHERS†	
"Pulmonary distress"	50	Fluid imbalance	7
Pneumonia/bronchopneumonia	42	Disseminated intravascular coagulation	6
Inhalation injury	11		
Aspiration pneumonia	7	Postoperative shock	4
Pulmonary embolism	2	Gastrointestinal bleeding	4
Pulmonary edema	2	Candidiasis	2
Massive atelectasis	1	Acute heart failure	2
		Acute renal failure	1
		Pancarditis	1
		Septic encephalitis	1
		Mucormycosis	1
		Intestinal infarction	1
		Metabolic encephalopathy	1

*Total no. of cases, 115 (79%); associated with sepsis, 90 (78%).
†Total no. of cases, 31 (21%); associated with sepsis, 24 (77%).

due to displacement of endotracheal tube. Fifty-eight percent of these patients had concurrent sepsis.

DEATH DURING THE SECOND WEEK

Twenty-two patients (16%) died during the second week. Of these, nine had lesions compatible with "pulmonary distress," five had bronchopneumonia, two had inhalation injury, two had gastrointestinal bleeding, and one each had aspiration pneumonia, postoperative shock, acute heart failure, and pancarditis. Fifty-nine percent of these patients had concurrent sepsis.

DEATH AFTER THE THIRD WEEK

Eighty-three patients (57%) died between 14 and 21 days postinjury. There were 35 cases of bronchopneumonia and 23 cases of "pulmonary distress." The rest of the patients died as a result of other complications listed in Table 23–1. In this group, concurrent sepsis confirmed at autopsy was present in 93% of the cases.

Causes of Death According to Age

For the 35 children under 2 years of age, the main cause of death was "pulmonary distress" (ten cases). Of the remaining, eight had bacterial pneumonia, five had fluid and electrolyte imbalance, three had inhalation injury, three had aspiration pneumonia, two had postoperative shock, and there was one case each of disseminated intravascular coagulation, gastrointestinal bleeding, acute heart failure, and septic encephalitis. In this group, sepsis was confirmed in 56% of the cases.

In the 2- to 4-year-old group (47 patients), bacterial pneumonia and pulmonary distress were present in 33 of the cases and inhalation injury in 2 cases. Sepsis occurred in 77% of the cases.

Pulmonary complications were also the most frequent contributory cause of death for children 5 to 16 years of age (47 of 63 cases). One of the patients was an 18-year-old girl who died of severe acute pulmonary edema and sepsis. In the group of patients over 5 years of age, sepsis was present in 90% of the cases.

Cause of Death According to Mortality Risk

The mortality risk of the patients was calculated according to age, percentage of body area burned, and percentage of third-degree burn.[50] As expected, pulmonary complications represented the most important factor contributing to death in all groups. Bronchopneumonia/pneumonia (40% of the cases) was the major contributing factor in the 45 patients with a mortality risk of less than 30%. This was followed by "pulmonary distress" (20% of the cases). In the 34 patients with a mortality risk between 31% and 69%, "pulmonary distress" was present in 36% of the cases, followed by bronchopneumonia/pneumonia in 24% of the cases. In 67 patients with more than 70% risk of mortality, "pulmonary distress" was the most significant factor in 43% of the cases followed by bronchopneumonia/pneumonia in 24% of the cases. Sepsis was present in 66% of patients with less than 30% mortality risk; in 82% of patients with 31% to 69% mortality risk, and in 80% of patients with more than 70% mortality risk.

GENERAL FINDINGS AND COMMENTS

Sepsis

Sepsis remains one of the most dangerous complications of burn injury. In our series, documented sepsis (positive blood cultures and invasion of viable tissues) was present in 114 cases (78%). The most frequent source of infection was the burn wound (67%) followed by intravenous catheters (10%) and airborne sepsis (8%). The source of sepsis was undetermined in 13% of the cases. The predominant infecting microorganisms, were in order of importance, *Pseudomonas aeruginosa* (52%), *Escherichia coli* (34%), *Klebsiella pneumoniae* (32%), *Candida* sp. (30%), and *Staphylococ-*

cus aureus (25%). Secondary viral infection (herpes virus, cytomegalovirus or papilloma virus) was present in 8% of the cases.

The problem of sepsis in the burned patient is of such magnitude that we currently advocate continuous monitoring. The burn wound should be inspected daily for the presence of hemorrhagic, vesicular, or necrotic areas; gray, dark brown, or black spots; or other unusual changes (Fig 23–1). The suspected areas should be biopsied and the sample subjected to microbiological cultures and histopathological studies. The specimens for both laboratories should be taken from the same area (one biopsy sample divided in half usually suffices). The only requisite is that the specimen for studies must include surrounding viable tissue. In our laboratory the biopsy sample is processed in Paraplast and stained for bacteria and fungi within 2 to 4 hours.[28]

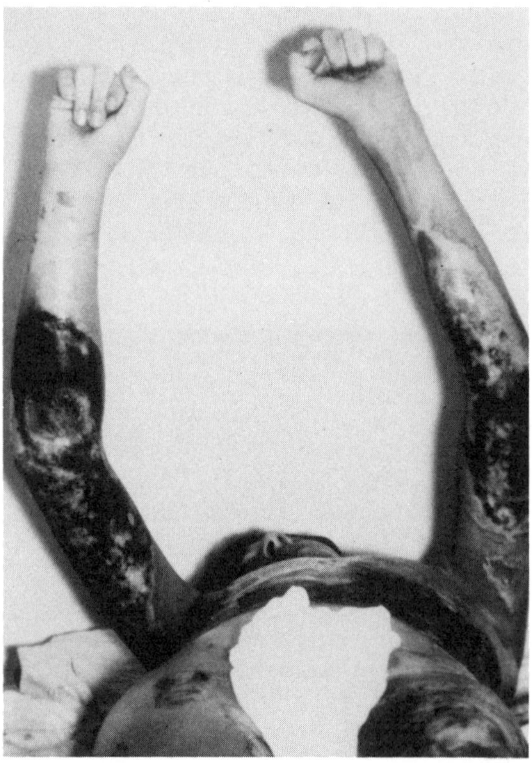

FIG 23–1.
Patient with mucormycosis infection (black discoloration).

Burn wound sepsis is suspected when the burn wound is the site of proliferating microorganisms exceeding 10^5/gm of tissue, and there is active invasion of subjacent unburned tissue.[44] We define septicemia as a systemic disease (or syndrome) caused by the persistent presence of pathogenetic microorganisms and/or their toxic products in the blood and/or in body tissues, resulting in physiologic derangement.[27] The presence of bacteria on or within the necrotic eschar cannot be considered sufficient evidence of burn wound sepsis, but as a site of primary colonization it has potential capability for bacterial overgrowth and invasion of surrounding viable tissue. The likelihood of infection and invasion increases with wound depth.

The morphological sequence includes the presence of microorganisms over the surface of the burn wound (contamination), within the burn eschar (colonization), within the surrounding viable tissue (invasion), and within vessels with or without tissue metastasis (septicemia) (Figs 23–2 to 23–5).

Skin cultures should always be accompanied by histologic examination of the same tissue. The latter will help to differentiate between tissue invasion and surface contamination and will prevent unnecessary therapy. Although a bacterial count of 10^5/gm of tissue or more is likely to indicate bacterial invasion, this is not invariably true. Only the histological sections can indicate the level of infection. We have observed invasion of viable tissue with bacterial counts less than 10^5/gm of tissue, and have found only superficial colonization in many cases where the bacterial count exceeded 10^5/gm of tissue. Both studies are usually complementary; the cultures define the type and quantity of microorganisms and the histological sections help define the level of infection.

The histological diagnosis of burn wound sepsis requires differentiation between tissue necrosis due to thermal injury and that due to invading microorganisms; thus, an experienced pathologist should be consulted. The presence of polymorphonuclear leukocytes in

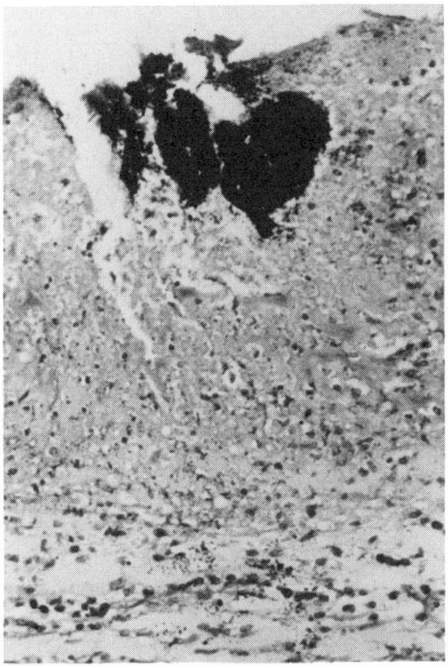

FIG 23–2.
Skin. Full-thickness skin burn with superficial gram-positive cocci colonization (dark clumps) (Gram stain, original magnification ×56.2).

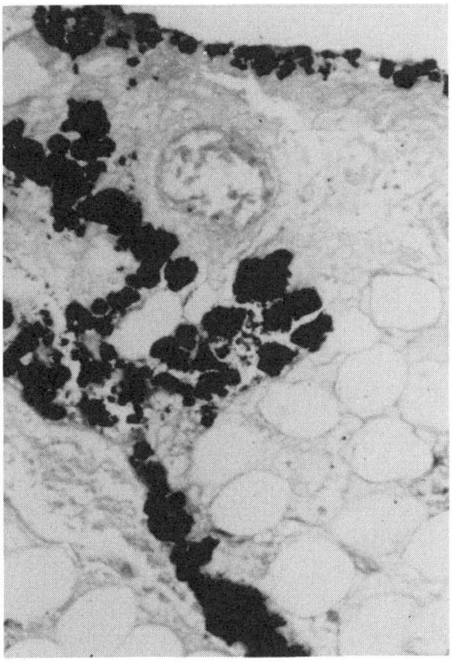

FIG 23–3.
Skin. full-thickness skin burn with gram-positive cocci showing invasion (dark clumps) (Gram stain, original magnification ×156.25).

the burn wound is not always indicative of infection as they may accumulate and persist in the aseptic wound.[45] Conversely, some gram-negative bacteria, mainly *Pseudomonas* sp., may elicit only a minimal cellular response.

The evaluation of sepsis should include microbiological and histopathological findings along with the clinical assessment of the patient. Blood cultures may be negative or the cultured organisms may be altered due to antibiotic therapy. The burn wound biopsy,[35, 45] is a valuable procedure as it can also detect other local or systemic complications and uncover the presence of fungal or viral infec-

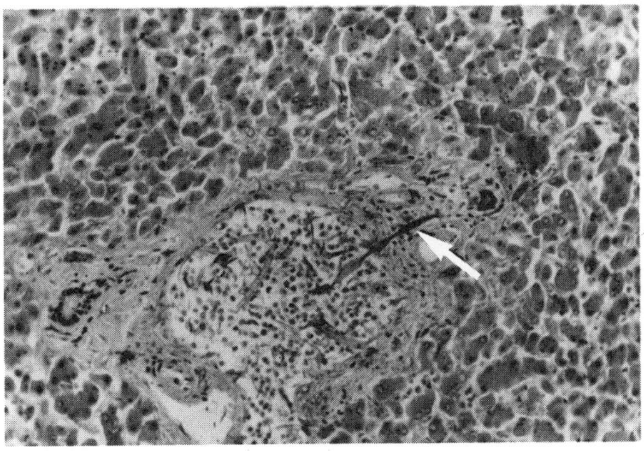

FIG 23–4.
Liver mycosis. Several fungal elements invading hepatic tissue (arrow) (PAS stain, original magnification ×156.25).

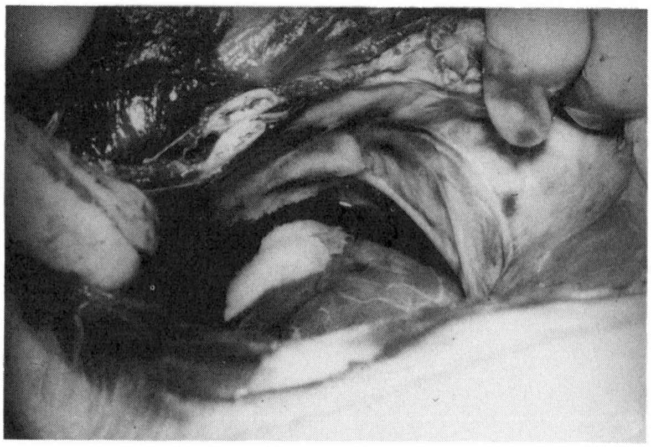

FIG 23–5.
Lung mycosis. Cotton-like fungal elements growing over pleural surface.

tions. These infections have a low yield of culture isolation, require specific techniques for detection, and are frequent laboratory contaminants; thus, without the benefit of wound biopsy these are difficult to recognize early.[25]

At autopsy it is necessary to take an adequate number of sections from the burned and unburned skin as well as sections from venous cutdown areas. Multiple, deep, parallel incisions of the burn wound should be made, looking for discoloration of subcutaneous tissue, hemorrhages, or other suspicious zones (Fig 23–6). If no suspicious areas are seen, random sections should be taken for histological studies and bacterial and fungal cultures. Cardiac blood cultures, if properly obtained, can also be very valuable in assessing sepsis.[40] Cultures from different organs (especially from lung tissue), may be taken as well.

Respiratory System

Pulmonary complications are frequent in patients with severe thermal injuries, and along with sepsis constitute the most important factors influencing morbidity and mortality in burn patients. Lung damage may also result as a nonspecific pulmonary response to body tissue injury or sepsis.[9]

Of our 146 cases of burn fatalities in children, pulmonary damage was a major contributory cause of death in 115 cases (79%) and, as expected, the association with sepsis was remarkably high (78%).

Upper respiratory tract

Most of the lesions of the upper respiratory tract appeared to have been caused by endotracheal tubes or tracheostomy tubes. A few

FIG 23–6.
Burn wound sepsis. Transversal section of skin with multiple sites of bacterial invasion (dark spots) (hematoxylin-eosin transparency, original magnification ×1).

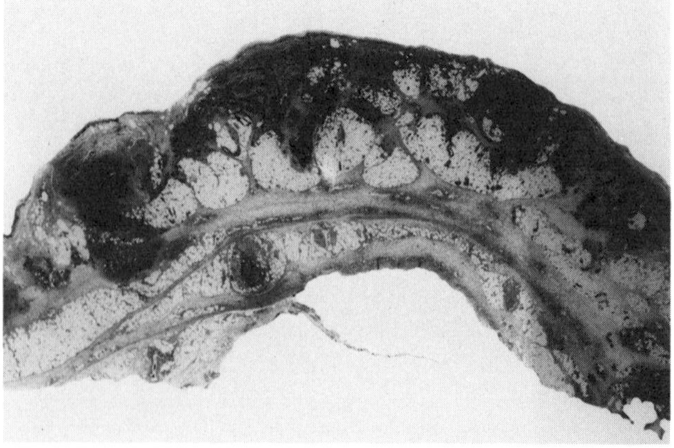

lesions were due to inhalation injury (coagulation necrosis). Forty-five cases in our series (31%) revealed severe necrotizing lesions in the upper airways; of these, 15 had undergone tracheostomy. Damage to the upper respiratory tract is commonly seen following tracheostomy, and the potential for severe complications involving the entire respiratory system is always present; thus, tracheostomies must be performed only when specifically indicated.[36] The tracheostomy site must be carefully monitored for possible complications, such as infection with opportunistic organisms, which can invade through the damaged mucosa and lead to the development of severe necrotizing tracheitis, pneumonia, and intrapulmonary bleeding.

The upper respiratory tract along with pharynx and esophagus were also the site for opportunistic viral infection in 8% of our cases.

INHALATION INJURY

Although the incidence of inhalation injury was only 8% in our series, the reader must understand that the diagnosis of inhalation injury at autopsy is not always possible. The classical coagulation necrosis of the tissues and the deposition of carbonaceous material may no longer be present if the patient had a prolonged survival or if there are laryngotracheal lesions secondary to intubation. However, in many occasions, carbonaceous material may be detected in the pulmonary parenchyma.

Direct thermal injury to the lower airways is extremely rare except in those patients subjected to the effect of hot gases or high-pressure steam from sudden explosions or similar accidents. The extension of the damage usually depends on the time of exposure, intensity and type of inhalant. Hot, dry air almost never reaches the lower respiratory tract with a damaging temperature. This is because of rapid dissipation of heat through the air passages. In contrast, steam can produce serious damage even to the pulmonary parenchyma because of its high thermal conductivity.[6, 31] The most common occurrence of inhalation injury takes place when the fire occurs in a closed area, thus exposing the patient to the inhalation of smoke. Smoke contains a variety of toxic products of combustion, which may cause a severe inflammatory reaction in the entire tracheobronchial tree including lung parenchyma. The resulting respiratory injury is associated with a high mortality rate. The predominant morphological features of inhalation injury include acute tracheobronchitis which varies in severity from marked congestion, edema and leukocytosis, to a severe necrotizing process accompanied by sloughing of the mucosa. The progressive separation of the necrotic epithelium with the formation of pseudomembranous casts may cause a complete or partial obstruction of the airways and result in atelectasis and pneumonia.[20] The pseudomembranous exudate is mainly composed of cellular debris, mucus, fibrin and polymorphonuclear leukocytes. Usually there is no pseudomembranes in bronchioles but changes progressing to a peribronchial pneumonia. The pulmonary parenchyma shows lesions similar to that described in "pulmonary distress" such as congestion, interstitial and alveolar edema, neutrophilic infiltration, occasional hyaline membranes and microthrombi, septal edema, atelectasis, hyperplasia of pneumonocytes (type II), macrophage activity, and edema of subpleural septa and peribronchiovascular spaces.

PROGRESSIVE RESPIRATORY INSUFFICIENCY

A progressive deterioration of pulmonary function has been recognized as a frequent, and often fatal, complication in patients who have suffered severe burns. The respiratory insufficiency is manifested by an increased respiratory effort followed by a progressive decrease in compliance, increased resistance, decreased arterial oxygen tension, and pulmonary arteriovenous shunting.[5]

This clinical syndrome and its variants has been described under the variety of terms (see above). The more common morphological features are interstitial and intra-alveolar edema and hemorrhages, intra-alveolar proteinaceous and cellular debris, hyaline membranes, and fibrin microthrombi (Fig 23–7). Although numerous factors have been implicated in the genesis of this type of pulmonary insufficiency, its pathogenetic mechanisms remain unclear. Increased awareness, early diagnosis, and prompt institution of therapy are essential to a reduction in morbidity and prevention of irreversible lung damage. It is of particular importance to note the possibility of concurrent iatrogenic oxygen toxicity.[38]

OTHER FINDINGS

Congestion and edema are probably the most common lung lesions that in varying degrees of severity are found in practically every single burn autopsy.

Other findings include bronchopneumonia/pneumonia, atelectasis, hemorrhages, abscesses, emphysema, macrophages activation, septal megakaryocytosis, and other minor alterations (Fig 23–8).

Cardiovascular System

The cardiovascular system disclosed anatomic lesions in 47 of our cases (32%). There were six cases of nonspecific myocarditis, all coinciding with gram-negative septicemia; two cases of gram-negative bacterial endocarditis; two cases of pancarditis due to gram-positive microorganisms; one case of endocarditis-myocarditis due to *Candida* sp.; and one case of nonbacterial thrombotic endocarditis. Subendocardial hemorrhages were seen in 13 cases, most of which were septic. Subendocardial ischemic lesions involving single fibers or group of fibers were present in 28.7% of the cases, including acute infarction of the papillary muscles of the left ventricle in 8% of

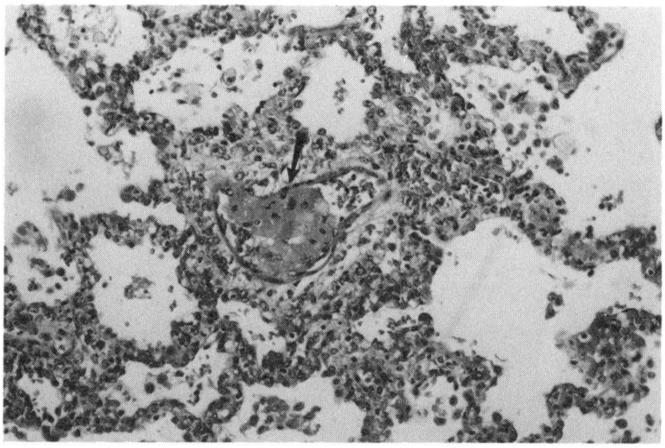

FIG 23–7.
Lung. Fibrin microthrombi *(arrow)* (hematoxylin-eosin, original magnification ×156.25).

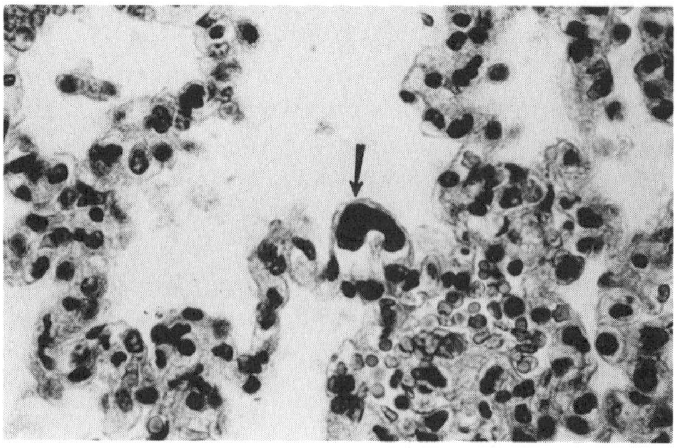

FIG 23–8.
Lung. Septal megakaryocyte *(arrow)* (hematoxylin-eosin, original magnification ×312.5).

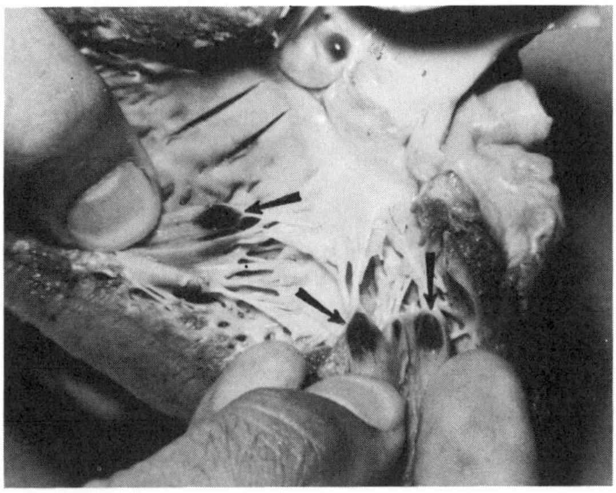

FIG 23–9.
Heart. Papillary muscle hemorrhage *(arrows).*

cases. Ventricular subendocardial hemorrhages and focal myocardial lesions are often described in association with shock, but their significance is still uncertain[39] (Fig 23–9).

In two cases there was severe arterial thrombosis due to invasive phycomycosis *(Mucor),* which prompted amputation of the left arm in both cases. Pulmonary artery embolism as a cause of death occurred in two cases; severe deep vein thrombosis was present in two cases (superior vena cava and iliac veins, respectively). There was one case of focal necrosis of the endocardium of the right ventricle due to an intravenous catheter lodged in the area. An unusual source of sepsis was the presence in one case of a subendothelial *Pseudomonas* abscess, 2 cm in diameter, which was ulcerated and located 3 cm below the initiation of the descending thoracic aorta (Fig 23–10).

Digestive System

ESOPHAGUS

Thermal burns of the esophagus are rare. Due to immediate reflex ejection elicited by ingestion of hot liquids, injuries to the esophagus are usually self-limited and superficial due to the immediate reflex ejection elicited by the heat. In contrast, chemical burns constitute a significant problem, not only because of the difficulties in the immediate management, but also because of the frequent complications and unavoidable sequelae that frequently develops.

The severity of the lesion is related to the nature, amount, contact time, and concentration of the agent ingested.[13] The severity of the injury varies from one area to another depending on the consistency of the corrosive agent, esophageal peristalsis and/or spasm.[46] As a result, the irregular topography of the ulceration will also lead to irregular scarring and stenosis.[32] In most cases the damage is progressive because of the sequential chemical reactions produced within cells or tissues that persist even after the death of the patient.

The rapid transit time of concentrated acids (usually thin liquids) and the resistance of the esophageal squamous epithelium lead to major corrosive effects in the stomach rather than in the esophagus. The latter is only

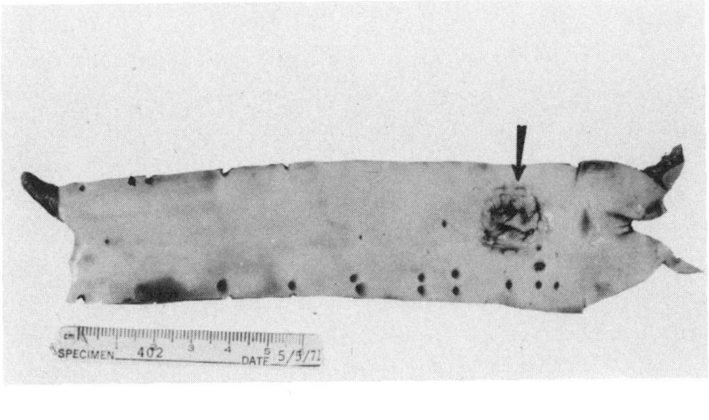

FIG 23–10.
Aorta. *Pseudomonas aeruginosa* abscess *(arrow).*

rarely affected.[1, 22, 41] However, injury to the esophagus can also occur after vomiting of the corrosive substance. This can also produce further injury to the lips, skin around the mouth, and even the larynx. In addition, strong acids cause almost immediate coagulative necrosis of the tissue, probably due to protein precipitation. This will impede further penetration, and therefore will produce more superficial lesions than the alkalis.

Strong alkalis are at least partially neutralized by the acid gastric environment but produce maximum effects in the esophagus where the transit time is decreased due to the usual thickness of the liquids involved. In this case the cardial spasm is most likely to succeed making the passage of the substance to the stomach more difficult. Alkalis remove water from cells and tissues and have a saponifying effect on lipids and precipitate proteins forming alkali-albuminate linkages. The precipitates redissolve in an excess of water and produce the so-called colliquation necrosis, as opposed to the coagulation necrosis caused by acids. Thus, the lesions produced by alkalis are highly destructive, leading in some cases to the perforation of the organ.[8] The corroded areas are soft, gelatinous, and friable, showing a brownish discoloration.

In a broad sense, the healing process of esophageal lesions follows the characteristics of burns elsewhere in the body. The necrotic tissue is sloughed and replaced by a granulating bed. The elicited inflammatory process, fibroblastic activity, contraction, and scar formation will eventually result in fibrosis and stricture formation. The severity of the lesion and the length of healing time will depend on the depth of necrosis and extent of injury.

The esophagus, like other organs, can occasionally be affected by the systemic effects of burn sepsis. Hyperemia, edema, petechiae, and superficial ulcerations or erosions may be present. In addition, bacteria, fungi, or virus can seed the organ via the bloodstream or from the oral cavity. However, these types of lesions are not very common, seldom cause severe problems per se in the course of the disease, and at most constitute a final event in a critically burned patient.

In our series, 37 children (25%) disclosed acute, superficial erosive esophagitis at time of autopsy, and 34 of them had concurrent septicemia. True ulcerations were observed in only four cases; all of these were located in the lower portion of the organ.

Stomach and Duodenum

Acute digestive tract bleeding constitutes a common gastrointestinal complication of severe burn injury. The initial postburn congestion and hyperemia of the mucosa frequently evolves into a diffuse bleeding, which can also originate not only in a nonspecific, superficial, and inflammatory process, but also in erosions and/or ulcerations, with subsequent possibility of hemorrhage and perforation, a life-threatening complication. These lesions compatible with the so-called "stress ulcer syndrome" have been associated not only with burns, but also with several other conditions, such as trauma, major surgery, sepsis, central nervous system lesions, respiratory disturbances, acute myocardial infarction, hepatic cirrhosis, and anti-inflammatory drugs.[21]

Erosions and ulcers can be seen through the entire gastrointestinal tract from esophagus to rectum, but the stomach and the duodenum have been the sites of greatest predilection for these types of lesions. This may be due to the fact that gastroduodenal mucosa (especially stomach) is a labile tissue likely to be affected by any stressing stimulus. The first large collection of published cases is attributed to the English surgeon, Thomas B. Curling, who in 1842, published an article on acute ulceration of the duodenum in cases of burn. He reported 12 cases and mentioned 7 more, totaling 19. However, not all the cases were based on his own observations nor were all of them ulcerations. Twelve of the 19 cases were duodenal ulcers, 5 were duodenitis, and 2 were reported as normal duodenum. Eleven of the 12 ulcers were from postburn patients and the remaining 1 was a case of duodenal ulceration posthyperemesis gravidarum previously reported by Hodgkin.

From that time on, the gastroduodenal ulcerations postburn were better known under the name *Curling's ulcer*, despite the fact that similar lesions were described years earlier.[10, 16, 29, 43] Through the years, confusion has arisen concerning the definition of the lesions according to the depth of penetration. Thus, ulcerations that do not penetrate the muscularis mucosa have been reported by some authors as erosions, while others call ulcers any lesion ranging from superficial loss of the mucosa to transmural penetration.

We prefer to use the descriptive term *acute gastrointestinal focal necrosis*, proposed by Stremple et al.,[42] ranging from the superificial epithelial necrotic lesion to complete necrosis of the wall, comprising single or multiple lesions and located in any segment of the gastrointestinal tract. The muscularis mucosa is the boundary used to differentiate superficial lesions (erosions) from deep lesions (ulcerations) (Fig 23–11).

Within the first hours after a severe burn, gastroduodenal congestion and edema are likely to occur, and by the end of the first day a focal or diffuse hemorrhagic gastroduodenitis may be established. In this case, confluent pinpoint mucosal hemorrhages, sometimes alternating with focal areas of ischemia, can be seen mainly over the fundus and great curvature of the stomach and in the first pars of the duodenum.

The mucosa appears pink-red in color. It is soft and friable and bleeds easily. Also, it shows scattered dark-red or black blood clots which, when wiped off, reveal minute, shallow, round to oval erosive lesions. These lesions lie between the rugal crests and involve only the mucosa. The rugal pattern of the stomach does not show significant alterations. At any given time, a varying age and severity of the lesions may be present. These vary from simple focal hyperemia or small yellowish edematous areas with hyperemic margins to petechial hemorrhages and mucosal erosions. The bleeding is usually diffuse originating from the multiple erosive areas.

By the end of the first week, the superficial erosive lesions have a tendency to heal, but in a certain number of cases, the loss of substance can involve the muscularis mucosae and penetrate deeply, constituting a frank ulceration. The superficial or deep lesions are generally unique or double in the duodenum where they are mainly located over the posterior wall of the first pars, and usually are multiple in the stomach (predominantly in the fundus and the anterior wall of great curvature). The lesions show minimal to moderate inflammatory edema and induration of the margins (especially in the duodenum) and have a circumscribed, punched-out appearance.

The sizes vary from 1 to 2 mm in diameter to 3 to 4 cm in diameter, the larger lesions being predominantly located in the duodenum. The shape also has a wide geometrical variety from an irregular, dentate, stellate, or serpentine appearance to a linear, oval, or circular configuration.

The ulcer base is generally clear and gray-yellow; occasionally a bleeding vessel can be seen. However, a dark-brown staining of the floor of the lesion may be seen as the result of the acid digestion of blood originated from the exposed tiny vessels of the floor. Hemorrhages (hematemesis, "coffee-ground" vomitus, melena) and, sometimes, perforation are the most frightening complications. Acute ulcers have a tendency to heal in a relatively short time and no scars will form if the process has not reached the muscular coat of the organ.

Occasionally, the focal necrosis has a linear appearance that may be due to the mechanical action of the nasogastric tube, although in these cases no severe complications are likely to occur.

The incidence of acute focal gastroduodenal necrosis in burns is very difficult to determine due to the multiple variables involved. In many cases, the gastrointestinal complaints are minimal and are not even reported. Also,

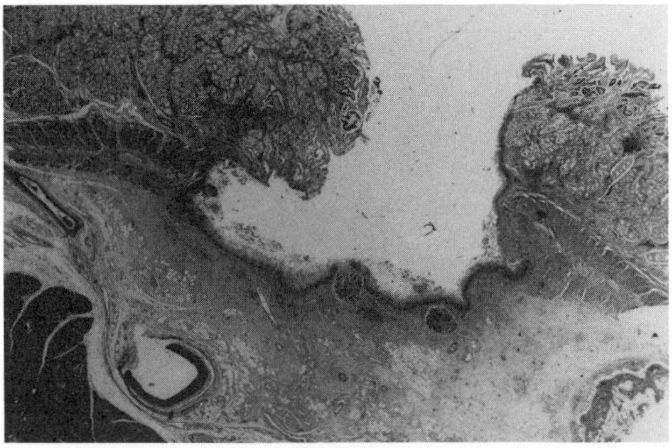

FIG 23–11.
Duodenum. Curling's ulcer. Note the depth of penetration involving most of the wall of the organ (hematoxylin-eosin transparency, original magnification ×1).

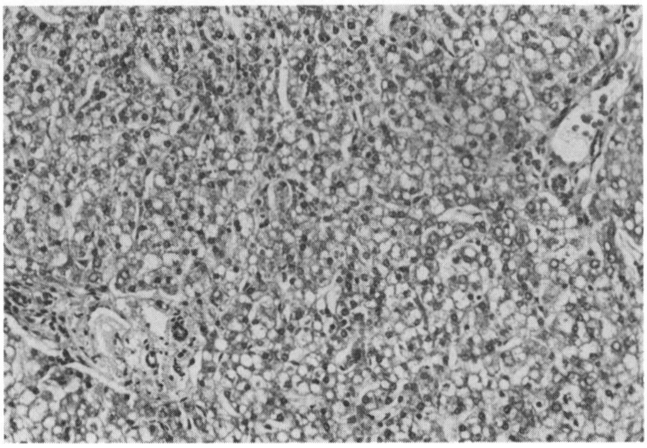

FIG 23–12.
Liver. Diffuse fatty metamorphosis (empty droplets) (hematoxylin-eosin, original magnification ×56.25).

the results of the studies based on clinical cases or autopsy reports will differ considerably. Often the gastroduodenal lesions of burned patients who have died are not detected because the autopsy is partially realized or is not performed at all. Significant variations can be observed if the pathologist differentiates between erosions and ulcerations or reports only lesions invading the muscularis mucosae. Some of the patients die in the first days after burn, before an erosion or ulceration can develop; on the other hand, there are also a number of ulcerations following burn injury that go on to healing without significant clinical symptoms.

In our series, 31 patients showed stomach and/or duodenal ulcerations at autopsy with concurrent sepsis in 23 cases (74%). The majority of the ulcers (65%) occurred after the third week postburn. Of the 31 cases, 16 patients had ulcers in the duodenum, 12 in the stomach, and 3 in both the duodenum and the stomach. Of the 31 cases with ulcers at the time of the autopsy, 29 (94%) had more than 50% total surface burned. In four cases, the ulcers were the major contributing factor to the fatal outcome due to severe gastrointestinal bleeding in three of the cases, and peritonitis after perforation in one case.

Liver

A variable degree of hepatic dysfunction is always present in the burned patient. This is usually related to the severity of the injury.

In our series, hepatomegaly was the most common finding. Liver fatty metamorphosis was present in 75 (57%) of the cases (Fig 23–12). Fifty-four of these had sepsis. In 27 cases the fat had a predominant centrilobular distribution, while in 12 cases the distribution was periportal; in the remaining 36 cases the pattern was diffuse. Fatty changes per se are reversible and their significance depends on the cause and severity of accumulation.

Central necrosis was present in 8 cases and intrahepatic cholestasis was seen in 21 of the cases, all concurrent with sepsis. Most of the cases of intrahepatic cholestasis were observed in patients receiving also total parenteral nutrition.[7] A marked deposition of a dark brown granular pigment occurring within the Kupffer cells of some patients receiving intravenous infusions of a lipid emulsion was also observed.[47] No metastatic septic lesions were seen except in four cases (two abscessed due to *Candida* sp., one mucormycosis invasion, and one case of herpes virus infection). Proliferation of Kupffer cells were also a common finding in cases of severe burns mostly associated with sepsis.

Kidneys

Advances in fluid resuscitation therapy have greatly diminished or altogether prevented renal complications following a severe burn injury.

The kidneys are able to function properly even with only 20% of their normal capacity; however, this enormous reserve can be jeopardized because of the severe hemodynamic changes that occur during the shock phase. The cardiovascular disturbances, the neuroendocrine response, the electrolytes alterations, the tissue damage, the massive demands for exogenous fluid administration, and the subsequent reabsorption of burn edema form part of the complex mechanisms directly affecting the function of the kidneys. Thus, a state of kidney dysfunction is frequently present in extensive burns during the immediate postburn period and in sepsis and shock from other causes.

The morphological lesions observed in the kidney do not always coincide with the degree of the functional impairment, but an association between acute renal failure and the so-called "acute tubular necrosis" can be usually demonstrated. Martineau and Hartman[30] review the renal pathologic changes reported in extensive burns since 1923. The most frequent lesions observed in the early and late postburn period were congestion; interstitial and submucosal hemorrhages; hyaline thrombi in the glomerular loops and granular thrombi in the large vessels; hemorrhagic and anemic infarctions; glomerular endothelial hyperplasia; interstitial edema; hyaline, granular, and hemoglobin casts; and a variety of degenerative changes in the tubules (albuminous and vacuolar degeneration, degenerative fatty infiltration, and tubular necrosis, particularly involving the proximal convoluted tubule and Henle's loop). Tubular hemoglobin casts and bilateral necrosis were found only in the first 72 hours, while acute interstitial nephritis and metastatic abscesses were late findings (after 72 hours). In their own study of 84 experimentally burned dogs and 20 human cases, Martineau and Hartman[30] found degenerative tubular changes, capillary congestion, tubular casts from the products of intravascular hemolysis, and lesions due to infection.

The most common lesion in our series of autopsies was acute tubular necrosis (43%). All cases of acute tubular necrosis was associated with clinical renal failure; however, in 12 other cases of clinical renal failure no morphological changes were seen at autopsy. Acute tubular necrosis and renal failure developing later in the course of the illness was always associated with pulmonary lesions and/or septicemia. In addition, there were 15 cases (10%) of pyelonephritis and 7 cases (5%) of interstitial nephritis.

Urinary Bladder

The most frequent lesion was mucosal hemorrhage due to indwelling urinary catheters (73%). There were ten cases of nonspecific cystitis and three of *Candida* sp. cystitis.

Adrenal

True adrenal insufficiency is rare in burned patients.[39] The lesions found in adrenals in our series were mostly associated with shock or septic complications and were not directly related to the final event. There were 38 cases of hemorrhages, of which 34 were bilateral. Thirty-three of these cases were associated with documented sepsis.

Lymphoid Tissue

Considerable interest has focused on the immune system and the immunological defects in patients with severe thermal injury.[18, 24] In this series of autopsies, lymphocyte depletion was the common denominator in all the lymphoid tissues examined (nodes, spleen, thymus, gastrointestinal tract). A marked depletion of lymphocytes from the thymic-dependent areas was a common finding early in the postburn period and for as long as 114 days postburn (the longest survival time in our 146 autopsies). This change was associated with a progressive increase of pyroninophilic cells resembling plasmablasts and plasma cells in the bursal-dependent areas of the nodes.[26]

The spleen showed ischemic type infarcts in 10 of the cases and, in 16 cases, acute splenitis associated with sepsis was seen.

Brain

Cerebral symptoms in burn patients are being increasingly reported in recent years, and although usually not fatal, burn encephalopathy may be a relatively common process.[2, 39] More than 90% of the cases showed generalized edema and a focal or diffuse loss of neurons as well as perivascular transudates, diapedesis hemorrhages, and other lesions associated with toxic-hypoxic alterations.[48] There was one case of acute metabolic encephalopathy with central pontine myelinolysis related to severe hyponatremia/hypo-osmolarity.[15, 23]

Disseminated Intravascular Coagulation

Disseminated intravascular coagulation (DIC) is not uncommon following severe thermal injuries. Most severely burned patients will undergo transient episodes of DIC as a consequence of the large postburn tissue destruction and/or sepsis. However, in some cases this syndrome will evolve into a fatal complication. Lesions compatible with DIC were found in 23 cases, but only in severe cases were the lesions generalized and severe enough to be considered a contributory cause of death. Sepsis was present in 18 of the cases including the cases in which disseminated intravascular coagulation was listed as the primary cause of death.

Other Lesions

A number of lesions were encountered in different organs such as focal hemorrhagic necrosis of the intestine (eight cases), pneumatosis intestinalis (two cases), peripancreatic fat necrosis (two cases) and many others; all of these were felt to have resulted from secondary complications. There were also several cases of pancreatic acinar ectasia with dilatation of the pancreatic ducts and inspissation of pancreatic secretion.[4] An increased risk for complications was noted with the insertion of a peritoneal dialysis catheter, especially when it was inserted throughout burned tissue. In five of the six cases in which this procedure was performed, the patients developed catheter-related sepsis.

The association with low-flow states frequently evolves in ischemic lesions throughout the entire gastrointestinal tract. The most common changes are those of intestinal mucosal necrobiosis and muscular banding.

REFERENCES

1. Alford BR, Harris HH: Chemical burns of the mouth, pharynx and esophagus. *Ann Otol* 1959; 68:122–128.
2. Andreasen NJC, Hartford CE, Knott JR: Cerebral deficits after burn encephalopathy. *N Engl J Med* 1974; 290:1487–1491.
3. Argamaso RV: Pathology, mortality and prognosis of burns. *Can Med Assoc J* 1967; 97: 445–449.
4. Baggenstoss AH: The pancreas in uremia: A histopathologic study. *Am J Pathol* 1948; 24:1003–1017.

5. Blaisdell FW: Respiratory insufficiency syndrome: Clinical and pathological definition. *J Trauma* 1973; 13:195–199.
6. Brinkmann B, Puschel K: Heat injuries to the respiratory system. *Virchows Arch Anat Pathol Anat Hist* 1978; 379:299–311.
7. Cano N, Gerolami A: Intrahepatic cholestasis during total parenteral nutrition. *Lancet* 1983; 1:985.
8. Citron BP, et al: Chemical trauma of the esophagus and stomach. *Surg Clin North Am* 1968; 48:1303–1311.
9. Clowes GHA, et al: The nonspecific pulmonary inflammatory reactions leading to respiratory failure after shock, gangrene and sepsis. *J Trauma* 1968; 8:899–914.
10. Cooper S: Pathology of burn and scalds. *London Med Gazette* 1839; 23:837–838.
11. Cumin W: Cases of severe burn with dissections, and remarks. *Edinburgh Med Surg J* 1823; 19:337–344.
12. Curling TB: On acute ulceration of duodenum in cases of burn. *Trans R Med Chir Soc Lond* 1842; 25:260–281.
13. Daly JF, Cardona JC: Acute corrosive esophagitis. *Arch Otolaryngol* 1961; 74:629–634.
14. Delarue J, et al: Les lesions viscerales des grands brules. *Ann Anat Pathol* 1962; 7:53–85.
15. Dreyfus PM: Nutritional disorders of the nervous system, in Wyngaarden JB, Smith LH (eds): *Cecil Textbook of Medicine*. Philadelphia, WB Saunders, 1982, vol 3, p 2048.
16. Dupuytren G: *Lecons Orales de Clinique Chirurgicale*. New York, Collins and Hannay, 1833.
17. Dupuytren G: *Lecons Orales de Clinique Chirurgicale: XII. Des brulures*. Paris, G. Bailliere, vol 4, 1839.
18. Farrell MF: Study of lymphocyte depletion and serum complement perturbations following acute burn trauma. *Surgery* 1973; 73: 697–701.
19. Fishman AP: Shock lung: A distinctive nonentity. *Circulation* 1973; 47:921–929.
20. Herndon DN, et al: The pathophysiology of smoke inhalation injury in a sheep model. *J Trauma* 1984; 24:1044–1051.
21. Hinchey EJ, et al: The stress ulcer syndrome. *Adv Surg* 1970; 4:325–392.
22. Hodgsen JH: Corrosive stricture of the stomach. *Br J Surg* 1959; 46:358–361.
23. Kleinschmidt-DeMasters BK, Norenberg MD: Rapid correction of hyponatremia causes demyelination: Relation to central pontine myelinolysis. *Science* 1981; 211:1068–1070.
24. Leguit P: Immunological studies in burn patients: I. Lymphocyte transformation in vitro. *Int Arch Allergy Appl Immunol* 1983; 44: 101–105.
25. Linares HA, Larson DL: Opportunistic phycomycosis in burn patients: A report of two cases requiring amputation of the left arm. *Burns* 1977; 4:129–132.
26. Linares HA, Beathard GA, Larson DL: Morphological changes of lymph nodes of children following acute thermal burns. *Burns* 1978; 4:165–170.
27. Linares HA: A report of 115 consecutive autopsies in burned children: 1966–1980. *Burns* 1982; 8:263–270.
28. Linares HA: Technical notes on the use of biopsy in the diagnosis and treatment of septic burns. *Rev Arg de Quern* 1983; 1:8–10.
29. Long J: Post-mortem appearances found after burns. *London Med Gazette* 1840; 25:743–750.
30. Martineau PP, Hartman FW: The renal lesions in extensive cutaneous burns. *JAMA* 1947; 134:429–436.
31. Moritz AR, Henriques FC, McLean R: The effects of inhaled heat on the air passages and lungs: An experimental investigation. *Am J Pathol* 1945; 21:311–338.
32. Nosny P: Esophageal burns caused by absorption of caustic liquids. *Presse Med* 1964; 72:1429–1433.
33. Orth J: What is the cause of death? *Berlin Klin Wochenschr* 1908; 45:485–490.
34. Parks DH, Linares HA, Thomson PD: The surgical management of burn wound sepsis. *Surg Gynecol Obstet* 1981; 153:374–376.
35. Pruitt BA, Foley FD: The use of biopsies in burn patient care. *Surgery* 1973; 73:887–893.
36. Pruitt BA: Other complications of burn injury, in Artz CP, Moncrief JA, Pruitt BA (eds): *Burns; A Team Approach*. Philadelphia, WB Saunders, 1979, p 523.
37. Sevitt S: Reflections on mortality and causes of death after injury and burns. *Injury* 1972; 4:151–156.
38. Sevitt S: *Reactions to Injury and Burns*. London, Heinemann, 1974.
39. Sevitt S: A review of the complications of burns, their origin and importance for illness and death. *J Trauma* 1979; 19:358–369.
40. Smith RF, Linares HA, Jorgensen JH: Bacteremia and postmortem bacteriology in burned children. *Am J Clin Pathol* 1975; 63:502–508.
41. Steigmann F, Dolehide RA: Corrosive (acid) gastritis. *N Engl J Med* 1956; 254:981–989.
42. Stremple JF, et al: The stress ulcer syndrome. *Curr Probl Surg* 1973; April, pp 1–64.
43. Swan J: Case of severe burn. *Edinburgh Med Surg J* 1823; 19:344–345.
44. Teplitz C, et al: *Pseudomonas* burn wound

sepsis: I. Pathogenesis of experimental *Pseudomonas* burn wound sepsis. *J Surg Res* 1964; 4:200–221.

45. Teplitz C: The pathology of burns and the fundamentals of burn wound sepsis, in Artz CP, Moncrief JA, Pruitt BA (eds): *Burns: A Team Approach*. Philadelphia, WB Saunders, 1979, p 45.
46. Terracol J, Sweet RH: Disease of the esophagus. Philadelphia, WB Saunders, 1958.
47. Thompson SW: The pathology of parenteral nutrition with lipids. Springfield, Ill, Charles C Thomas, 1974.
48. Unterharnscheidt FJ, Linares HA: Morphological findings in the CNS after thermal burn: A preliminary report. Proceedings of the Sixth American Burn Association Meeting, Cincinnatti, Ohio, 1974, p 52.
49. Wartman WB: Mechanisms of death in severe burn injury: The need for planned autopsies, in Artz CP (ed): *Research in Burns*. Philadelphia, FA Davis, 1962, p 6.
50. Zawacki B, et al: Multifactorial probit analysis of mortality in burned patients. *Ann Surg* 1979; 189:1–5.

SECTION VII

REHABILITATION

24 / Hypertrophic Healing: Controversies and Etiopathogenic Review

HUGO A. LINARES, M.D.

Skin, the largest organ of the body, is not only an easy target for many external sources of injury, but is also the most accessible to direct observation. Despite the frequent description of skin diseases that can be found in the ancient literature, descriptions of deforming scars and contractures did not begin to appear in the medical literature until the 16th century. This lack of early information on scars might be a consequence of short or inadequate descriptions, or the terminology used by the fathers of medicine may not be comprehended in terms of contemporary discussions of these entities.[11]

The following is an excerpt from the Edwin Smith papyrus, a medical text from 1600 B.C., in which the word "wound" appears 142 times: "The existence of swelling on his breast, large, spreading, and hard. Touching them is like touching a ball of wrappings. . . . " This may have been written in reference to a case of hypertrophic healing.[21] Also, in the Bible, Leviticus 13, mostly dedicated to leprosy, could refer to hypertrophic healing: "If a man had a boil on his skin which later healed, should now in the place of the boil have a white scab or a pink blotch. . . . "

In African tribes, the practice of deliberately producing hypertrophic scars or keloids as facial or body markings has been in use for centuries and is still used today. Literature from the Yoruba people, around the 10th century and beyond, indicates that the Yorubas not only knew about keloids but understood some of the specifics of their character and presentation.[121]

Ambroise Paré, in the 16th century, described hypertrophic scars and contractures and advised on treatment: "If the scar is too big, or high, it shall be plained by making convenient ligation, and straight binding to the part, a plate of lead rubbed over with quicksilver . . . more so one must be careful if burns affect the palpebrae or the lips, or the fingers or the throat or the axillae or the joint of the knee or of the arm, for these parts should not stick together. . . . "[74]

The first full description, however, was probably the reference by Retz,[133] in his book *Treatise on Skin Diseases and Things of the Mind*, to a "fatty hernia," and in which he describes the case of a woman with hypertrophic scars and a thick contracture band on her left arm.

Alibert,[3] who named the lesion first "cancroides" and later "keloids," introduced the differentiation between keloids arising spontaneously (true keloids) and those arising after trauma (false keloids). This differentiation led to the controversy about keloids and hypertrophic scars that still continues, almost 200 years later.

THE DISTINCTIONS BETWEEN KELOIDS AND HYPERTROPHIC SCARS

"The first observers have wisely given to the diverse diseases which they have the opportunity to discover, analogue names to the things which they represent. I will imitate their example naming under the title of Cancroides, the peculiar tumors which I am going to discuss"[3] (Fig 24–1). The name reflected the small, bifurcated prolongations extending out from the borders of the lesion that he sometimes saw, which resembled the claws of a crab. A few years later, and because of the analogy between the words "cancroide" and "cancer," he renamed it "keloid."[4] Soon afterward, and without explanation, he used the word "cheloid."[5] In these works, he described

MALADIES DE LA PEAU.

LES CANCROIDES.

QUELQUES CONSIDÉRATIONS SUR LES CANCROÏDES.

CCCLXX. Les premiers observateurs ont judicieusement donné aux diverses maladies qu'ils ont eu occasion de découvrir, des noms analogues aux choses qu'elles représentent. J'imiterai leur exemple, en désignant sous le titre de *Cancroïdes*, les tumeurs singulières que je vais décrire. En attendant que des faits plus nombreux m'éclairent davantage sur leur nature, je vais exposer leurs principaux phénomènes.

CCCLXXI. Par un double rapport, les Cancroïdes semblent se lier aux affections dartreuses et aux affections cancéreuses. Formeroient-elles un genre intermédiaire? Ce qu'il y a de positif, c'est qu'il s'opère quelquefois à leur surface une desquammation furfuracée qui a la plus grande ressemblance avec les écailles herpétiques. Souvent ces écailles ne s'apperçoivent point. D'une autre part, il est des circonstances où le développement de ces tumeurs est accompagné de douleurs vives, pungitives et lancinantes, comme dans le cancer.

CCCLXXII. J'estime que l'étude des Cancroïdes est d'une très-grande importance en pathologie. En

Tome I. 27

FIG 24–1.
Copy of the title page on "Cancroides" from Alibert's *Precis sur les Maladies de la Peau,* ed 2. Paris, 1822, p 417. (Used by permission.)

several cases as "cancroides," "keloids," or "cheloid" without further distinction. Some of them seem to have been spontaneous tumors, whereas others clearly had their origin in previous excoriations of the skin.

During the second and third decades of the 19th century, he initiated the controversy that still divides the scientific community. In his book *Traite Complet des Maladies de la Peau,*[6] Alibert stated that it is essential to distinguish between true keloids (keloides genuina) and false keloids (keloides spuria). True keloids have a lancinating, pungent, burning pruritus, especially strong in bad weather and electrical storms, with a painful sensation similar to that of a cancerous lesion. The false keloid, on the other hand, results only from inflammation of a scar after burns or after any ulceration produced by the "morbus limphatic," such as scrofula or syphilis.[6]

Although this division was generally accepted in the beginning, the so-called "false keloid" (always originating from a previous lesion) started to be designated as cicatrix, warty tumors of the cicatrix,[61] cicatricial keloid,[155] or vegetations of the cicatrix.[50] Rayer is probably the first to describe a keloid developing from a burn scar.[132]

The first review of published cases seems to be that of Dieberg,[41] who divided the lesions into three categories: spontaneous keloid, cicatricial keloid, and verrucous tumor of the cicatrix. Then, Virchow[157] proposed that the term keloids be used only for lesions of spontaneous origin, but a few years later stated that these spontaneous lesions seemed to be a class of sarcoma.[157]

Later in the 19th century, the division between keloids and scars began to be seriously challenged, and "hypertrophic" became a differentiating term. According to Hutchinson,[67] keloid was essentially a disease of the scar tissue and probably never originated from normal skin. Langhans[93] believed that a true keloid was a heterologous, independent tumor, whereas the keloid originating from a scar could be better termed "hypertrophic scar." However, Curling[37] never accepted this differentiation and asserted that the keloid of Alibert was not a disease of the skin, but one of scar tissue.

In describing a case of spontaneous keloids in the fingers, Volkmann[158] complained that the French had been very "generous" with the word keloid, which they had used many times to designate small fibromas or even hard sarcomas of the skin. It is in Kaposi's chapter on keloids, however, that the disputed histological differentiation of these lesions was first made.[62] He described the true keloid as having skin with "rete ridges" and "dermal papillae," which according to him, means that the keloid had developed in previously healthy dermis. In hypertrophic scars, rete ridges and dermal papillae are absent because the development of the scar requires a loss of substance. This loss is replaced by scar tissue, but this scar never spreads superficially beyond the limits of the initial injury, whereas keloid invades the adjacent healthy corium, transgressing those limits.

Finally, he described a third lesion, the cicatricial keloid, which have rete ridges and dermal papillae in the borders of the lesion but not in the center, because it is really a hypertrophic scar surrounded by a keloid, and thus a combination of cicatrix and keloid. Kaposi affirmed that the keloid differs from hypertrophic scar only histologically. The closer the structure of the skin (papillae and skin anexae) resembles the normal state, the closer the lesion is to being a true keloid.

This description added another dimension, that of structural appearance, which gave rise to new controversies.

Several articles then appeared that claimed that there was no sense in establishing a division in the group of keloids because they were intermediate forms between the cicatrical keloid and the idiopathic one. Histologic examination could not always differentiate among lesions, and the pressure of the so-called spontaneous keloid on the epidermis could also produce atrophy of the rete ridges and papillae.[9] Piffard[129] stated that it was difficult to exclude trauma from the etiology of the true keloid, which could develop from the most trivial wound. Thus, the term "spontaneous keloid," used when a previous injury cannot be confirmed, was used only for clinical convenience and not to express a histological differentiation; true and false keloids must be considered anatomically identical.[34, 145] Duhring[45] stated further that spontaneous keloids arise spontaneously, whereas the cicatricial keloids result from burns, cuts, and wounds of all kinds. Microscopically they are identical in structure.

Keloid has also been regarded as an autoinfected fibroid hypertrophy of scar tissue, a concept that assumes that all keloids are true and all are cicatricial.[68] Warren,[160] however, thought that it was advisable to retain the classification of true and false keloid, although he believed that the so-called true keloid probably developed from a minute scar or blister. He also divided the scars into three categories: (1) hypertrophic scars due to an excessive formation of cicatricial tissue; (2) contracted scars, due to an attempt at absorption of larger cicatricial surfaces; and (3) normal scars, which represent the more or less imperceptible tissue that forms the line of union of the well-adjusted edges of the wound.

Schutz[137] indicated that keloids should be classified as a hyperplasia of scar tissue and Unna[153] differentiated between a permanent and a transitory variety. According to him, hypertrophic scars are a special form of keloid that develops on the base of granulation tissue and disappears with it—a transitory keloid. On the other hand, keloids could be distinguished from hypertrophic scars and other transitory keloids by their independent extension, their long persistence, and their tendency for recurrence—a fibroma limited to the cutis. The suggestion by Kaposi that hypertrophic scars do not exceed the limits of the initial injury was supported by Thorn, who described a tendency for keloids to grow peripherally, and for hypertrophic scars to maintain a strict permanence within the limits of the initial injury.[149] Not everyone, however, agreed.[164]

Thus, at the turn of the century, only two theories were generally accepted: (1) that keloids always begin in scar tissue, and (2) that all forms of keloid have a tendency to resolve and disappear. The distinction between hypertrophic scar and aggressive keloid were thought to be one of degree only.[69]

At the beginning of this century, the controversy was limited to differentiation between two entities: keloid and hypertrophic scar. But a new structural element of discrepancy was introduced by Goldman in 1901[57]: the behavior of the elastic tissue. He analyzed the common and the differential characteristics of the two processes. He concluded that hypertrophic scars and keloids have in common a previous injury to the skin, a hyperplasia of the connective tissue that always originates in the dermis and is limited to it, and the absence of elastic fibers. The adipose subcutaneous tissue never participates, even if it is damaged by the injury. In hypertrophic scars, the destruction of the elastic fibers is localized mainly to the papillary layer of the dermis, which explains the defective regeneration of the papillae that results from the lack of the "subepithelial elastic skeleton." This "skeletal" deficiency makes it vulnerable to the permanent deformation caused by external forces (tension, pressure, etc.). In keloids, the destruction of the elastic tissue predominates in the reticularis layer of the dermis. Also, in hypertrophic scars, the newly formed connective bundles are more delicate because they resemble more the connective tissue of the dermal papillae—a clear difference from the appearance in keloids.

These conclusions stimulated serious controversies again. Ravogli[131] was a strong supporter of the differences described by Goldman, but opposite views were shared by others. Among them, Gottheil insisted that the so-called true and false keloids were the same disease, and attributed the confusion to the inability to demonstrate the preexisting injury. In a critical review published in 1909, Heidengsfeld[64] concluded that a difference between true and false keloids was not possible, either clinically or histologically, and that keloids and hypertrophic scars could not be differentiated on histological grounds. He found no dermal papillae in spontaneous keloids, although they were preserved in false keloids and regenerated in cicatricial tissues.

Following an observation of Kaposi that keloids exceed the limits of the initial injury and invade normal tissue, Stelwagon[146] wrote that this invasive nature was the main characteristic that separated them from hypertrophic scars. This concept has been expanded on and supported by other workers since that time.[8, 22, 48, 54, 80, 91, 107, 147] In 1935, Geschickter[55] proposed that keloids should be classified as tumors of the dermis occurring at the site of a previous injury.

Despite all the controversies, a differentiation between the two entities was subsequently felt to be pointless—the pathologic changes in both cases were essentially the same, their treatment was similar,[51] and they differed only in the degree of proliferative tendency.[19, 56, 88, 100, 106, 128, 163] Furthermore, during the last 30 years modern methods of analysis have failed to add new information, and controversy lingers.

According to Lagrot et al.,[91] hypertrophic scars and keloids are two different aspects of the same pathologic state (the disease of the cicatrix), but while hypertrophic scars cure spontaneously, keloids are a chronic definite state. Differences have also been justified on the basis of tissue cultures[30]; x-ray diffraction analysis[65]; histoenzymologic activity[90]; amino acid pattern[33]; presence of HLA antigens[94]; or presence of antinuclear antibodies.[73]

Based on anatomical studies, Asboe-Hansen[8] still maintained that keloids differ from hypertrophic scars in a number of respects; they are shiny and rounded, grow beyond the traumatized area, and have ample mucinous substance, higher water content, numerous mast cells, and dense collagen fibril structures. Also, their growth is deep and subepidermal loose tissue is not present, nor are epidermal appendages. Pruritus does not occur, and spontaneous regression is rare. An interesting concept was proposed by Mancini and Quaife[106] at the conclusion of a detailed and elegant experimental work in which they regarded the hypertrophic scar as just one of several stages that the healing of a keloid might fix upon, and proposed the term "hypertrophic healing" to encompass all lesions known as keloids and hypertrophic scars.

A few years later, however, Blackburn and Cosman[17] insisted that histological differences can be demonstrated—that keloids have conspicuous thick, glassy, faintly retractile, pale-staining collagen bundles in an abundant mucinous ground substance, with relatively few fibroblasts and, usually, with no foreign-body reaction. Recently, the entities were again differentiated by clinical appearance, although the authors separated out an intermediate category—scars with an appearance somewhere between the two that have characteristics of both.[22] In fact, the inclusion of an intermediate category is probably recognition of the concept of continuity in the evolution of the process.

Since agreement exists that both keloids and hypertrophic scars originate from a previous lesion of the skin, we support the concept that hypertrophic scars are morbid variants of keloids and that they constitute similar abnormalities within the spectrum of human wound healing and scar maturation. In our opinion the differences are only quantitative, with keloids representing the most severe degree of hypertrophic scarring. Figure 24–2, obtained from a histological section of a burn scar, clearly depicts the diagnostic dilemma. If that section is divided in two and the two sections are examined by different pathologists, it is likely that they will yield different diagnoses. The time has come for the controversy to be put to rest and efforts should be directed toward identifying appropriate therapeutic modalities. The concept of "hypertrophic healing" proposed by Mancini and Quaife[106] lends itself to a unifying practical approach, and we support it.

MORPHOLOGIC APPEARANCE

Hypertrophic scars or keloids are fully epithelialized dermal lesions, raised above the level of the skin, which vary widely in shape, size, color, and consistency. These variations are usually related to the extension of the injury, site of the lesion, time of evolution, and individual susceptibility. Early (so-called immature) hypertrophic scars in certain areas (such as the lobules of the ears or shoulders) tend to be prominent, nodular, pedunculated or semipedunculated (reflecting herniations of the skin), round or oval, smooth and shiny, hard, somewhat elastic, red or pink, and in continuity with the surrounding normal skin. If the scar involves large areas of the skin, it usually has an irregular surface and is firm, somewhat elastic, red or pink, and is rarely elevated more than 10 to 15 mm above the level of the surrounding skin. The edges are usually more prominent than the rest of the scar and end abruptly, sometimes with finger-like or claw-like prolongations. In some scars, minute pinkish, bluish, or purplish superficial blood vessels, arranged in a delicate net-like fashion, can be distinguished. Occasionally, the scar may have isolated, scattered, fine hair-like appendages. The lesions appear to exceed the limits of the previous injury and do not adhere to the subcutaneous tissue.

After a certain period of time, usually months and sometimes years, they became broader and more irregularly outlined, and they flatten, soften, and blanch during a long process called maturation of the scar.

As sections are cut, the scar tissue presents a particular resistance to the knife, the surface appears whitish or grayish and dense, with fascicular or nodular structures, which are sometimes translucent and always limited to the dermis.

Light Microscopy

The microscopic appearance of hypertrophic scars depends on the stage in their evolution, which may be why some investigators

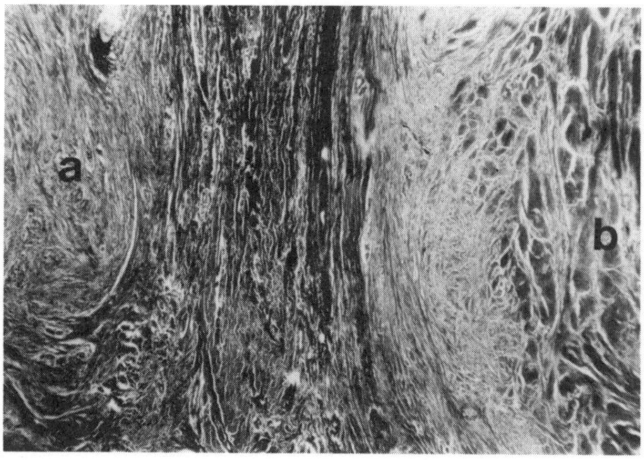

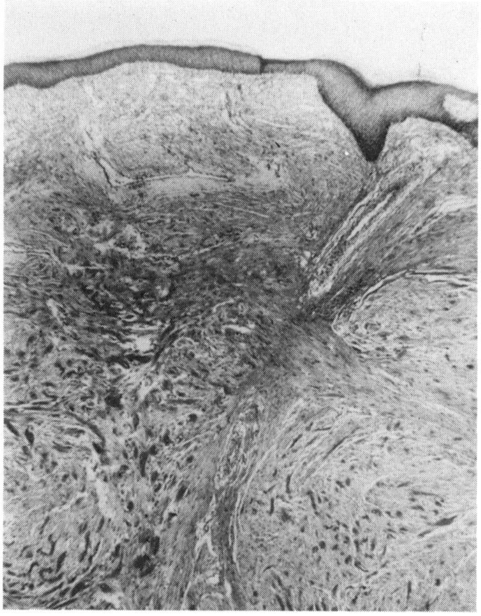

FIG 24–2 (above).
Hypertrophic healing showing two different collagen patterns in the same section. According to Blackburn and Cosman (see text), area *a* should be diagnosed as hypertrophic scar, and area *b* should be diagnosed as keloid (hematoxylin-eosin, original magnification ×156.25).

FIG 24–3 (right).
Hypertrophic healing. Absence of rete ridges. The collagen fibers of the dermis run in a predominant whorl-like arrangement with areas of nodular pattern (hematoxylin-eosin, original magnification ×43.75).

still try to differentiate between hypertrophic scars and keloids. The appearance varies greatly, ranging from an early, active, immature hypertrophic scar to a late, inactive, mature stage. Changes are also related to the site of the scar and to gross anatomy. Pedunculated or semipedunculated round or oval hypertrophic scars that are located mainly in areas such as the lobules of the ear or shoulders, have a tendency to have very broad, thick collagen fibers in a haphazard array. Under the microscope, it is also possible to see that "invasion" of surrounding normal tissues does not occur, but that the overgrown scar pushes apart the surrounding normal tissue without invading it. In scars that have formed pedunculated or semipedunculated structures, the collagen fibers can be seen to be growing in an exophytic tumoral fashion, pushing the epithelium upward like herniations of the tegument, which suggests that the tumoral appearance and excessive growth are limited by the particular characters of the opposing superficial layers of the skin in the affected area and on its resistance to deformation.

Microscopic changes in the epidermis are notably diverse. It may appear acanthotic, with prolongations of the rete ridges and hyperpigmentation, or it may be thin and smooth, with the rete ridges absent. The abnormalities of the interface between epidermis and dermis are usually related to the extent of the injury and the pressure from the nodular formations lying too close to the epidermis. Only one morphologic abnormality is ever observed in the papillary layer of the dermis (which is composed of loosely arranged, nonoriented collagen fibers grouped in fine bundles)—a physical compression of the fibers from the underlying dermal scar. In this circumstance, the collagen fibers tend to reorganize into a compressed pattern, with an orientation parallel to the surface of the skin.

The reticularis layer of the dermis, which is the layer in which the lesion develops, is composed of young connective tissue, particularly rich in ground substance, collagen fibers, cells, and blood vessels. In early stages, hypertrophic scars contain a greatly increased number of cells—most of which are fibroblasts and myofibroblasts—and numerous blood vessels. The collagen fibers adopt an irregular, curvilinear, whorl-like arrangement, which in most cases progresses to distinct nodular forms. The fiber bundles increase in thickness and the nodular areas become highly compacted; whorls and nodules can often be seen in the same section. Also, the nodules often become more clearly delimited and appear to be surrounded by thicker collagen fibers, which form a septal-like capsule[98, 103] (Figs 24–3 to 24–6).

These structures never involve the subcutaneous tissue, from which they are often separated by somewhat compact parallel bands of connective tissue with nearly normal characteristics. The increased cellular population is composed of young, active fibroblasts and myofibroblasts. Mast cells appear increased over the number observed in normal skin. Plasma cells and lymphocytes are usually present at the beginning of the formation of the scar and form a perivascular cuff, which may persist for a long time as scattered foci or chronic inflammation. The vascular structure is prominent and the capillary network appears to follow the arrangement of the collagen fibers. The skin appendages are atrophic, destroyed, or displaced by the scar. At times they do not slough, but do elicit a foreign-body reaction. Usually, no elastic tissue can be found except in the papillary areas of the dermis and in the normal dermal areas surrounding the scar. The interstitium shows a significant amount of ground substance (glycosaminoglycans), which has been shown to contain an elevated amount of chondroitin-4-sulfate.[140]

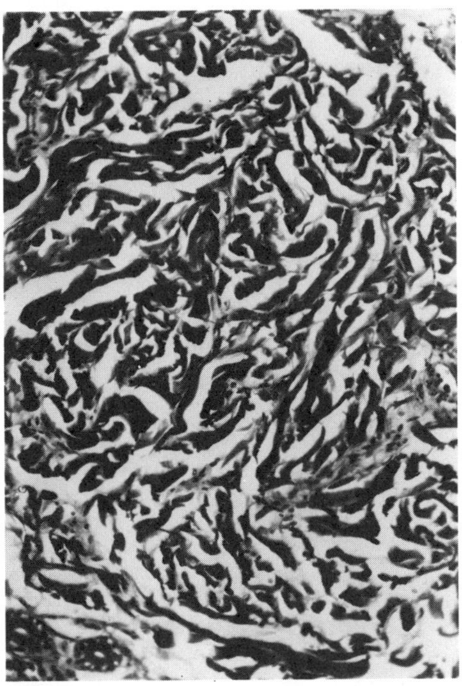

FIG 24–4.
Normal skin. Collagen bundles of the dermis are arranged in a three-dimensional, loose network. Compare with Figures 24–5 and 24–6 (hematoxylin-eosin, original magnification ×156.25).

With time, the thickened hyaline fibers of nodules and whorls become elongated and the elastic fibers reappear. This is indicative of a regression pattern, which proceeds toward "mature" scar. The reorientation of the collagen fibers in a parallel arrangement, as found with nonhypertrophic healing, is accompanied by a progressively reduced number of fibroblasts and myofibroblasts, and a pronounced decrease in vascularization, which corresponds to the flattening, blanching, and softening of the matured scar described above, although the tissue structure never recovers its original appearance.

Scanning Electron Microscopy

Under the scanning electron microscope (SEM) the nodules appear as fused masses of tissue in stark contrast to the adjacent collagen filaments and fibers.[103] The individual collagen filaments present in normal skin are rarely seen. The dermal matrix appears as an adhesive mass of material, as though the filaments were "glued" together.[81] Fiber diameter is about one half to three quarters that in

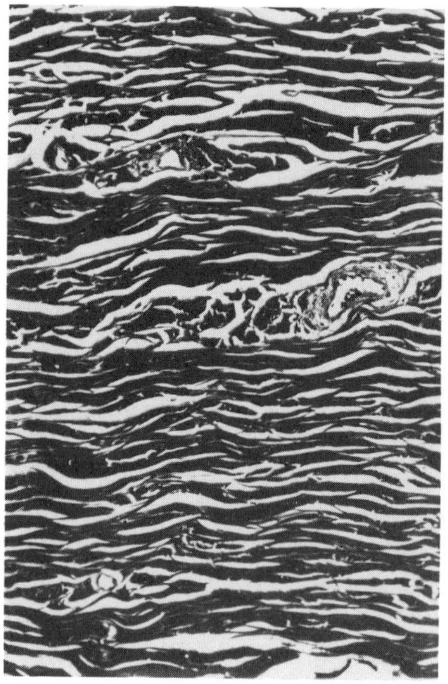

FIG 24–5.
Nonhypertrophic scar. Collagen bundles of the dermis are arranged in a predominant parallel pattern. Compare with Figures 24–4 and 24–6 (hematoxylin-eosin, original magnification ×156.25).

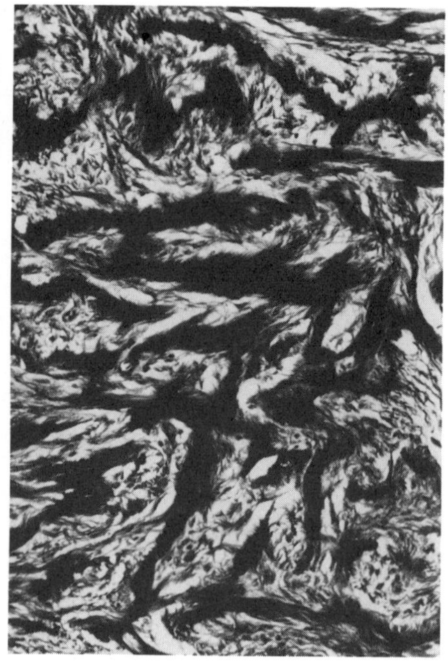

FIG 24–6.
Hypertrophic scar. The thick collagen bundles of the dermis are arranged in a predominant whorl-like pattern. Compare with Figures 24–4 and 24–5 (hematoxylin-eosin, original magnification ×156.25).

normal skin, and cross-stranding is frequent.[77] The large bands of collagen appear also to be oriented in every direction except directly across the wound.[66]

Transmission Electron Microscopy

The nodules of hypertrophic scars consist of tightly packed collagen with a reduced amount of total interstitial space. The collagen filaments have a predominant diameter of 600 Armstrong. The lumen of the vessels is often partially or completely occluded, and the basal lamina in most of the vessels is greatly thickened.[98]

In early stages, the number of fibroblasts and myofibroblasts is significant. Fibroblasts have an active appearance, with vast arrays of rough endoplasmic reticulum and Golgi membranes.[82] Myofibroblasts appear with folded or grooved nuclei containing fine contractile filaments, and with a variable number of free ribosomes, mitochondria, glycogen, vacuoles, and pinocytotic vesicles.[72]

The structural appearance of hypertrophic scars under electron microscopy parallels that under light microscopy at any stage of hypertrophic healing.

ETIOPATHOGENESIS

Why some individuals develop a hypertrophic scar and others subjected to the same injurious stimulus do not remains an enigma. The only general agreement about mechanisms concerns the precondition of injury to the skin, which may be as small as the bite of an insect or as large as that resulting from surgery, lacerations, or burns.

A scar develops along a predictable course;

to heal in a hypertrophic manner, the lesion must have reached the deeper layers of the dermis reticularis. Although abnormal healing can develop after even a minimal puncture wound, it is most frequent when the process of repair requires the formation of granulation tissue. This tissue is essentially an inflammatory tissue, but with certain special characteristics which imply that repair is, at least, initiated in a manner that should support systematic and orderly restitution of the damaged or destroyed site.[99] This is demonstrated by the granulation tissue, the aim of which is to "clean" the site of the injury by an efficient phagocytic activity, to "fill" the gap produced by the loss of tissue (through the activity of new fibroblasts, which infiltrate the area and begin synthesizing the necessary products for new connective tissue), and to "feed" the new tissue through the proliferation of newly formed blood vessels. These small vessels grow in a perpendicular orientation to the surface, and can be seen on inspection of the wound bed as slightly protruding small red granules, which characterize the appearance of "granulation tissue."

The organization of vessels, new cells, and extracellular materials, and their maturation within the granulation tissue, are extremely important in determining the future course of the healing.[99] In normal healing, development of young connective tissue in the granulation tissue (consisting primarily of fibroblasts and collagen fibers) follows a typical pattern. At the surface of the granulation, these structures are parallel to the vertical proliferating capillaries. In the lower layers, however, the collagen fibers have a transverse orientation with respect to the vessels and are parallel with respect to the surface of the skin. By the time the wound is covered with new epithelium (or by the time that a graft is fixed), all the collagen fibers of the dermis will have acquired a predominant parallel orientation with respect to the surface that is characteristic of normal mature scars. By the fourth week after the injury, following development of granulation tissue and its contraction and after epithelial covering has taken place, the wound will have begun to evolve along a normal or hypertrophic healing process.

What triggers the young scar to initiate the process of hypertrophy is still unknown. The latter follows a specific sequence of events. The collagen fibers of the dermis adopt a characteristic whorl-like arrangement or a nodular pattern.[99] The fibroblasts become dominant and active again, and the vascular proliferation responsible for the classical erythema of the scar makes its appearance. The collagen fibers increase in thickness, forming whorls or nodules that are progressively more compact, and in a time that varies from a few weeks to a few months, an abnormal, disfiguring mass of tissue—reddened, elevated, and hard—develops over the healed area.

Hypertrophic healing occurs in burns because the tissue that is destroyed is unavailable to form a good scar, which forces the granulation tissue to make only retractile tissues.[60] In addition to individual characteristics such as sex, race, and age, a number of variables seem to influence the development of hypertrophic healing: constitutional predisposition, familial predilection, local causes, character of the blood vessels and connective tissue fibers, the nature of a ground substance, endocrine factors, autoimmunity, infection and inflammation, and several other possibilities.

Constitutional Predisposition (Diathesis)

Alibert[3] observed that most of his patients with keloids were women, and concluded that a radical weakness of the lymphatic system was responsible for keloids. Dieberg[41] maintained that the disease had a tendency to reccur because it is a cacochymia. According to Curling,[37] the tendency of the scar to grow is constitutional, although the local peculiarities of the scar are important to the production of the keloid. Justus also believed in a predispositional factor, linking the hyperthyroid state to a tendency to form keloids.[76] Although the exact etiologic factors in the production of keloids are not known, the wide variations in the disease might suggest some sort of fibroblastic diathesis, which varies in intensity among races and individuals.[118]

Familial Predilection

Many examples have been reported of hypertrophic healing occurring in families. Alibert[6] described a case of a father and his son who had similar lesions on the chest. In another report, in a black family, a 14-year-old boy, four of his siblings, his father, and two paternal uncles had similar if not identical lesions situated mostly on the back and at the same cervical level.[23] Hebra described a case involving a mother and three daughters, and Hutchinson cites another affecting father and daughter.[62]

A process similar to what Darwin called sexual selection was supported by Bohrod,[20] who described the tendency for keloid formation as a hereditary physicochemical difference: a fibroblastic diathesis. Bloom[19] reviewed 31 familial cases of keloid in the literature and added the pedigree of an Italian family with 14 affected members in five generations. The pedigree indicated that the predisposition to keloids was inherited through a regular, dominant, autosomal mechanism. However, Omo-Dare,[122] in Africa, studied the families of 68 persons and concluded that the predisposition to keloid formation is inherited as an autosomal recessive character.

On the basis of studies of normal skin and keloid cultures from a single patient, Russell et al.[135] suggested that expression of the keloid phenotype is restricted to cells isolated from the keloid nodule as a direct result of an inherited or somatic "keloid mutation." Keloids have also been associated with some genetic diseases such as the Rubenstein-Taybi syndrome[138] or Goeminne syndrome.[165]

Local Causes

The individual peculiarity of a scar, or the circumstances surrounding its development, have been suggested to be important.[37] In some instances, the nature or the intensity of an irritant may be the important factor, as in the case described by Welander,[162] in which keloids developed in the same tattooed design, but only where it was tattooed with red pigment and not with blue. An interesting theory was published by Pautrier,[124] who said that keloids never undergo a true recurrence; the new keloid is produced by the new local surgical trauma. Another implied factor is the manner in which local skin tension is applied. Keloids rarely occur in areas where there are frequent changes in the tension of the skin, such as in the skin creases.[118] The vascular response produced by exogenous foreign bodies (such as dressings) and endogenous foreign bodies (such as keratin or injured hairs) may also cause a hypertrophic healing.[115] The interplay between the local and systemic factors in dealing with particles acting as foreign bodies, exogenous or endogenous, is ultimately responsible for the peculiar type of foreign-body granuloma that forms the basis of scar hypertrophy and keloids.[56]

Local susceptibility may also be a factor. Most susceptible are the presternal region and upper back. Less susceptible are the lower back, abdomen, lower limb, postaxial upper limb, central face, and genitalia.[36] Other authors have been unable to demonstrate the local nature of the keloid process.[32] It was also suggested that hypertrophic healing has also been represented as an overactive local healing process due to an increase in energy production that takes place by means of cell respiration.[79]

Blood Vessels

Warren[159] was probably the first to call attention to the pathology of blood vessels in keloids, but numerous investigators continue to study the phenomenon today. The vessels, especially in the center of the tumor, become obliterated by the pressure of the surrounding connective tissue and provide the starting point of the new growth. They are affected pathologically far beyond the tumor and are the avenue through which keloid relapse occurs.[35] Crocker saw the tumor surrounded by numerous dilated and cellular vessels, and advised the surgeon to cut very widely during the removal to get beyond the diseased vessels and avoid relapse. In another publication, Warren[160] wrote that the development of a keloid probably begins with a growth of cells in the adventitia of the arterioles, which later become fusiform cells, and finally fibers. His hypothesis is that as bundles of the fibers form around the arteries, the tissue of the dermis is gradually compressed and that different bundles, thus uniting, form the keloid growth. The tendency for recurrence is evidently due to the involvement of the walls of blood vessels, at some distance beyond the borders of the tumor.

Schutz[137] also supported the idea that keloids develop from a growth of the adventitial cells of the vessels, and Unna[153] added that while there is an individual histological predisposition of the cutaneous vessels, the growth is due to the interstitial thickness of the collagen tissue. However, Thorn[149] refuted these theories on the basis that keloids contain no smooth muscle.

The activity of the blood vessels has been regarded as an important factor in the origin of keloids for the past 20 years. The genesis and maintenance of keloids may be a consequence of local intracapillary hemagglutination, produced by partially depolymerized ground substance in an area subject to trauma.[13] The blood vessels of hypertrophic scars differ from those of mature scars and normal skin, not only in quantity but in quality.[43] Hypoxia seems to be an integral factor in the generation of hypertrophic healing.[144] The morphological evidence is the observation of microvascular occlusion, partial or total, encountered in most microvessels, apparently due to an excess of endothelial cells[86] and to the leakage and deposition of blood products into the wound and lesion.[84]

Connective Tissue Fibers

Goldmann[57] noted that the lack of regeneration of elastic tissue in scars could be the cause of regression of the keloid. He stated that whichever of the proposed theories of causation was applied, the result would always be the same because of the damage to the same structural element, the elastic fiber. Keloid is to the skin as an aneurysm is to the artery. The destruction, or degeneration, of the elastic fibers could be the predisposing factor in the production of the keloid.[131] This notion was disputed by Heidingsfeld who believed the absence of the elastic fibers was the result of pressure atrophy and had no etiologic significance. In atrophic lesions of skin, such as stria atrophica and similar conditions, elastic fibers are completely absent.[131] It is possible that the elastic tissue, temporarily absent in scars, could have a contributory role in the genesis of hypertrophic healing. Fragments of altered elastin, remaining for a long time as foreign bodies, could be contributing to the persistence of a chronic inflammatory response, or the immunological response elicited by the injured elastic fibers could be interfering with the normal pathway of biosynthesis of elastin.[101]

While abnormalities in collagen have also been implied,[151] studies using x-ray diffractional analysis and electron microscopy have shown no abnormalities in the collagen fibers.[10] Most of the studies in this area have been directed to the analysis of the balance between collagen synthesis and degradation.[34, 128] The rate of collagen production was found to be elevated significantly in hypertrophic healing, which partly explains an abnormal deposition of collagen.[29] Keloid fibroblasts may lack the ability to respond appropriately to orientational stress and may not be able to lay down collagen along the lines of force to counteract the stress. Collagen is synthesized, but since it is "wrongly" aligned, the cohesive forces are only those of fibril-fibril interaction; therefore, the cells still have some stress placed on them when the normal amount of scar tissue has been laid down. This collagen synthesis continues until the strength of the keloid tissue is equal to that of normal surrounding tissue, at which time the process begins to lay down the mass of scar tissue.[66] Collagen synthesis is greater than degradation and is caused by the increased synthesis of each fibroblast, rather than increased fibroplasia. Keloid collagenase activity is similar to that of normal skin.[28] The increased collagen synthesis, moreover, is not related to altered collagen types.[27] The increased amount of serum α-globulins in abnormal scars may inhibit collagenase activity, which produces the excessive accumulation of collagen.[42]

A different intramolecular and intermolecular cross-linking of collagen was also reported to be present in an appreciable amount in hypertrophic scars, while it was virtually absent in normal skin.[113] The Cohen group found also that the serum from patients with keloids does not contain a factor or factors that significantly modifies the in vitro growth kinetics or collagen synthesis of keloid-derived or normal dermal fibroblasts. The altered collagen synthesis by keloid fibroblasts is neither related to abnormal cell growth nor decreased collagen degradation, although in vitro some collagen synthesis may be associated with an increase in trypsin-activated collagenase.[110-112] The production of collagenase was found to be controlled to some extent by the epidermis.[47]

Cells

The possible role of the adventitial cells of the blood vessels was described by Schutz (see above) who also described the presence of plasma cells, round cells, and numerous mast cells, especially in the periphery near the vessels, where the keloid grows and develops.[137] The amount of mast cells present in the abnormal scarring was also noted by other investigators.[8, 83, 98, 126]

Ground Substance

Much has been published during the past 30 years regarding the ground substance. Changes in interstitial material related to collagen or elastin have been said to be significant in the etiology of hypertrophic healing.[49] Although the collagen content seems to be similar, keloids have a higher content of mucopolysaccharides (glycosaminoglycans) than normal scars or normal skin.[44, 141, 143] The amount of glycosaminoglycans and sialoglycoproteins that are excessively soluble, such as those found in immature granulation tissues, is increased. The greatest amount, in addition to B isomer, corresponds to chondroitin-4-sulfate and chondroitin-6-sulfate.[14]

The increased amount of glycoproteins and glycosaminoglycans reflects the higher metabolic activity in hypertrophic scars[139, 141] and the increase suggests that proteoglycans may form an environment of collagen synthetic products, and may perform an important role in the process of change from postburn (granulation) to hypertrophic healing.[148] The whorl (or "nodular regions") characteristic of hypertrophic scars are the actively proliferating areas, and the presence of chondroitin-4-sulfate is related to this proliferation.[102, 140] The increases of chondroitin-4-sulfate may be due to abnormalities in the activity of hyaluronidase.[2]

A significantly increased collagen-proteoglycan interaction has also been suggested to be a factor in human hypertrophic scars, as compared with nonhypertrophic scars.[97]

Endocrine Causes

According to Garb and Stone, hormonal stimulation is the main or the important contributing cause of keloid formation.[54] Thirty-four percent of their cases occurred during the second decade of life, when the hormonal stimulation is very high. They also observed that in some cases after menopause, the lesions disappeared or spontaneous involution occurred. Others have reported hypercalcemia with increased calcium in keloid tissues,[126, 127] and attributed the formation of keloids to physiochemical disturbances of the connective tissue and humors of the body. The keloids arise because of delayed elimination of necrotic tissue and delayed epithelialization. The calcium metabolism disturbances were thus attributed to parathyroid malfunction. Observation of a series of 38 patients with keloids and hyperthyroidism (including the experimental production of the disease) led Justus[76] to believe that keloids and thyroid function had some particular relationship.

Geschickter and Lewis[55] found increased estrogen content in a keloid from the ear and theorized that the disease resulted from a localized endocrine disturbance. Several authors described the tendency of keloids to grow during pregnancy.[31, 71] Trusler and Bauer[152] found that plethoric persons have a greater tendency toward hypertrophic healing than anemic ones. The observation that keloids are more common in dark-skinned people led to the belief that keloids are linked to an aberration of melanocytic stimulating hormone (MHS).[89]

Autoimmunity (Hypersensitivity)

The underlying cause of keloid formation could be the hypersensitivity of fibroblasts, and of the vascular endothelial cells, to any agent that acts on the protein of these cells and has the power to induce them to proliferate.[48] Chytilova and co-workers[26] were able to produce keloids on rabbits in the course of autoimmune disease produced by the repeated injection of lyophilized autologous skin. The presence of IgG in keloids suggests that an intradermal agent may be responsible for this type of lesion.[27a, 120] Differences in immunoglobulin content were also found by other researchers.[18, 85]

Persons who carry HLA-B14 or HLA-Bw16 antigens have been shown to have a greater risk of developing keloids.[94] Osman et al. developed a sebum-autoimmune theory based on the assumption that sebaceous glands may secrete sebum intradermally after injury. The sebum would thus act as an antigen, initiating an autoimmune granulomatous response that may progress to formation of keloid.[123] Differences also in immunoglobulin content were found by other researchers.[18, 84]

Infection, Inflammation

Several investigators supported the belief that keloids were infections of tuberculous character[39, 59, 117, 136,] or secondary to syphilis.[58] Cases have also been reported after varicella,[108, 150] herpes zoster,[71] and erysipelas.[160] One theory proposed that parasites were involved.[40]

The sclerosis observed in keloids may be inflammatory in origin, analogous to the process in discoid lupus erythematosus and scleroderma. This theory stems from the observation of a perivascular lymphocytic inflammatory infiltrate that is a consistent finding, especially in early lesions and in the periphery of the older ones.[92]

Other Theories

Keloids are local benign dermatomas. The recurrence has been said to be due, probably, to a local nerve damage.[12] Alternatively, the disease was considered to be a connective tissue growth of an inflammatory character, probably caused by a variety of agents (chemical, bacterial, etc.), acting on the dermis, in special local, regional, or general conditions.[7] Local factors such as infections, foreign bodies, and ischemia have been considered,[156] as well as differences in concentrations of potassium, magnesium, iron, and copper,[130] and differences in enzymatic activity.[70, 79]

Robinson et al.[134] described a specific stimulator of growth in the serum of patients with keloids. According to Marshall and Rosenthal,[107] the "trigger" mechanism in keloid formation appears to be the extravasation of lymph (localized edema). They stated that in the case of burns, the formation of excess fibrous growth may be due, in part, to the great amount of serous exudate that seeps from the wound area and remains stagnant in the burned tissue for some time: a fibroblastic response to extravasated serum.

As factors of pathogenetic significance, Asboe-Hansen[8] listed predisposition, youth, growth, central nervous system disturbances, individual dysfunction, endocrine dysfunction, postinjury edema, and inflammation or local tension. Others found also that the anabolic phase was disproportionately accelerated.[80] The relative increase in type III collagen, concomitant increased levels of glycosaminoglycans, and high cell density are all related to cyclic adenosine monophosphate (AMP), which may modulate the differentiated state of fibroblasts in an abnormal way for reasons not yet known.[142]

Current Views

Despite the many questions still unanswered, significant advances have occurred during the past 15 years in the understanding of cicatrization in general and hypertrophic healing in particular. The core of the problem seems to be loss of balance between synthesis and degradation of collagen—an alteration of that equilibrated turnover that makes all the elements of the skin work in a coordinated manner to accomplish its complex biological function. Contraction of the wound may be the most important mechanism in the interplay of forces in fibers and cells that are set into action to close the gap in a manner as close as possible to the previous healthy state.[25, 160] In the past, it had been attributed to changes in the granulation tissue, such as fibrillar shortening of collagen[16]; secondary dehydration[38]; centripetal expansion of the surrounding tissue[46, 154]; sphincter-type activity[24, 63]; or the presence of a specialized area in the borders of the wound.[161]

This concept was developed further with the suggestion that the contraction of a wound could be due to the contractile activity of the fibroblast.[1]

Thus, the most significant advance during recent years was the identification of cells in granulation tissues, of a specific, contractile nature, which share common characteristics with fibroblasts and myoblasts. These cells were properly called myofibroblasts.[53, 105]

More recently, the restoration and tissue strength following injury has been suggested to result from the formation of a myofibroblast-reticulum network.[52] The appearance of myofibroblasts following the deposition of the early collagen fibers within granulation tissues suggests that a certain number of fibroblasts acquire contractile activity to manipulate the spatial orientation of the newly synthesized collagen fibers. The presence of increased numbers of myofibroblasts in hypertrophic healing could be the direct result of the apparent excess of collagen, which would impair the activity of the myofibroblasts and render them unable to control a proper fibrillar arrangement toward normal repair.[96] As important as the cellular contractility are the forces interacting between the collagen fibers, which in turn appear to depend on collagen fibril size, density, and architecture "en masse."[52] Interactions of fibronectin with native collagen during collagen fibril formation and its possible role in the regulation of the size of collagen fibers,[87] as well as the biophysical implications,[114] are of interest relative to this interaction.

The physical properties of the collagen fibers are closely related to their biological development, as is the environmental matrix—mainly glycosaminoglycans, occurring as proteoglycans. The relationship that glycosaminoglycans bear to the fibrous proteins, and to the water and microions of the intercellular matrix, presumably accounts for the general physical architecture and properties of the connective tissue.

Recent progress in molecular biology has shown that many cell functions are brought about by an interaction among macromolecules.[15] The binding between macromolecules therefore has far-reaching physiological implications.[75, 104]

The study of proteoglycans in hypertrophic scars can be of great interest because the organization of collagen fibrils in tissues may be related to amounts and kinds of proteoglycans,[119] and because the binding of proteoglycans to collagen can influence fibril formation.[95] Further, the presence of great amounts of chondroitin-4-sulfate in hypertrophic scars has been suggested as a contributing factor in sulfate in the overabundance of collagen deposition by serving as an obstacle to the collagenase attack on the collagen molecule.[102] Preliminary results suggest that link-stabilized aggregates of proteoglycans are inhibitory to mammalian collagenase.[116]

The areas of future research should include the study of the factors that influence the structure, migration, function, and modulation of the cells that control the synthesis and degradation of the intercellular matrix. The immunologic and genetic interference should be thoroughly explored. Biochemical analysis and structural events could be important in determining the role of the sulfated glycosaminoglycans in the development and aggregation of collagen fibers.

Several possible mechanisms might be involved in producing the excessive amount of collagen deposition that is characteristic of these scars: an actual increase in the rate of collagen synthesis; the presence of inhibitors for the enzymatic breakdown of collagen and/or glycosaminoglycans; the absence or defective production of the specific enzymes; the presence of physical barriers opposing a proper enzymatic attack; growth activity promoted by sulfated proteoglycans; or other causes, yet unknown. Determining whether these phenomena occur concomitantly, identifying the predominant mechanism of hypertrophic scar formation so common in burned children, and pinpointing the triggering mechanism for this abnormal healing process are all tasks that remain.

Acknowledgment

Marilyn A. Thompson, Director of Editorial Services, The University of Texas Medical Branch at Galveston, was technical editor of the manuscript for this chapter.

REFERENCES

1. Abercrombie M, Flint MH, James DW: Wound contraction in relation to collagen formation in scorbutic guinea-pigs. *J Embryol Exp Morphol* 1956; 4:167–175.
2. Alexander SA, Donoff RB: The histochemistry of glycosaminoglycans within hypertrophic scars. *J Surg Res* 1980; 28:171–181.
3. Alibert JLM: *Description des Maladies de la Peau Observees a l'Hospital Saint-Louis et Exposition des Meilleurs Methodes Suives pour leur Traitement.* Paris, Barrois l'Aine et Fils, 1806, p 113.
4. Alibert JLM: Note sur la keloide. *J Univ Sci Med* 1816; 2:207–216.
5. Alibert JLM: *Quelques Recherches sur la Cheloide en Memories de la Societe Medicale d'Emulation.* Paris, Migneret, Crochard, and Gabon, 1817, pp 744–752.
6. Alibert JLM: *Traite Complet des Maladies de la Peau.* Paris, Cormon et Blanc, 1833.
7. Arcangeli M, Torchiana L: Contributo allo studio della istologia ed istogenesi del cheloide. *Arch Ital Chir Biol* 1925; 12:210–235.
8. Asboe-Hansen G: Hypertrophic scars and keloids: Etiology, pathogenesis and dermatologic therapy. *Dermatologica* 1960; 120:178–184.
9. Babesiu V: Ein Beitrag zur Histologie des Keloids. *Arch Derm Syphilol* 1880; 12:238–245.
10. Bairati A, De Petris S: Ricerche sulla natura ed ultrastruttura dei cheloidi: II. Indaginin diffrattografiche e di microscopia elettronica. *Boll Soc Ital Biol Sper* 1963; 39:1222–1224.
11. Banerjee BN, Dutta AK: Cross section of dermatology through the evolution of history. *Indian J Dermatol* 1968; 13:73–81.
12. Barduzzi D: Sulla patogenesi e sulla terapia del cheloide. *Boll Sez Cult Sci Med R Accad Fisiocr Siena* 1887; 5:72–74.
13. Barnard RD, Garnes AL, Oppenheim A: Hemagglutinative vasoocclusion in the pathodynamics of keloids. *Am J Surg* 1961; 101:192–197.
14. Bazin S, et al: Degre de maturation du collagene dans des cicatrices normalies et cheloidiennes. *CR Acad Sci Paris* 1970; 270:1638–1640.
15. Berkaloff AJ, et al: *Biologie et Physiologie Cellulaires.* Paris, Hermann, 1981.
16. Billingham RE, Russell PS: Studies on wound healing, with special reference to the phenomenon of contracture in experimental wounds in rabbits' skin. *Ann Surg* 1956; 144:961–981.
17. Blackburn WR, Cosman B: Histologic basis of keloid and hypertrophic scar differentiation. *Arch Pathol* 1966; 82:65–71.
18. Bloch EF, et al: General immune reactivity in keloid patients. *Plast Reconstr Surg* 1984; 73:448–451.

19. Bloom D: Heredity of keloids: Review of the literature and report of a family with multiple keloids in five generations. *NY State J Med* 1956; 56:511–519.
20. Bohrod MG: Keloids and sexual selection: A study in the racial distribution of disease. *Arch Dermatol Syphilol* 1937; 35:19–25.
21. Breasted JH: *The Edwin Smith Surgical Papyrus*. Chicago, The University of Chicago Press, 1930.
22. Brody GS, Peng STJ, Landel RF: The etiology of hypertrophic scar contracture: Another view. *Plast Reconstr Surg* 1981; 67:673–684.
23. Burnett WJ: A case of cheloidea, with some remarks on cheloid growths. *Am J Med Sci* 1853; 26:369–374.
24. Burrows MT: Studies on wound healing. *J Med Res* 1924; 44:615–643.
25. Carrell A, Hartmann A: Cicatrization of wounds: I. The relation between the size of a wound and the rate of its cicatrization. *J Exp Med* 1916; 24:429–450.
26. Chytilova M, Kulhankek V, Horn V: Experimental production of keloids after immunization with autologous skin. *Acta Chir Plast* 1959; 1:72–79.
27. Clore JN, Cohen IK, Diegelmann RF: Quantitative assay of types I and III collagen synthesized by keloid biopsies and fibroblasts. *Biochem Biophys Acta* 1979; 586:384–390.
27a. Cohen I, et al: Immunoglobulin, complement, and histocompatibility antigen studies in Keloid patients. *Plast Reconstr Surg* 1979,63:689–695.
28. Cohen IK, Diegelmann RF, McCoy B: Elevated collagen synthesis in cultured keloid fibroblasts. *Surg Forum* 1977; 28:526–527.
29. Cohen IK, Keiser HR, Sjoerdsma A: Collagen synthesis in human keloid and hypertrophic scar. *Surg Forum* 1971; 22:488–489.
30. Conway H, et al: Differential diagnosis of keloids and hypertrophic scars by tissue culture technique with notes on therapy of keloids by surgical excision and decadron. *Plast Reconstr Surg* 1960; 25:177–182.
31. Cosman B, et al: The surgical treatment of keloids. *Plast Reconstr Surg* 1961; 27:335–358.
32. Cosman B, Wolff M: Correlation of keloid recurrence with completeness of local excision: A negative report. *Plast Reconstr Surg* 1972; 50:163–166.
33. Craig RDP: The chromatography of burns and allied scars, in Matter P, Barclay TL, Konickova A (eds): *Research in Burns: Transactions of the Third International Congress on Research in Burns*, Prague, Sept 20–25. 1970. Bern, Hans Huber Publ, 1971, pp 417–423.
34. Craig RDP, Schofield JD, Jackson SS: Collagen biosynthesis in normal human skin, normal and H.S. and K. *Eur J Clin Invest* 1975; 5:69–74.
35. Crocker HR: The anatomy of keloid in an early stage. *Br Med J* 1886; 2:544.
36. Crockett DJ: Regional keloid susceptibility. *Br J Plast Surg* 1964; 17:245–253.
37. Curling H: Case of multiple keloids of scars (Alibert's keloid) in which the indurations are white instead of red. *Br Med J* 1870; 1:284.
38. Cuthbertson AM: Contraction of full-thickness skin wounds in the rat. *Surg Gynecol Obstet* 1959; 108:421–432.
39. Darier J: *A Textbook of Dermatology*. Philadelphia, Lea & Febiger, 1920.
40. Deneriaz J: *Etude sur la cheloide*, these de doctorat. Berne, 1887.
41. Dieberg C: Ueber die mit dem Namen "Keloid" bezeichneten Gwschwulst-forman. *Dtsch Klin* 1852; 33:369–373, 35:387–391, 37:403–405.
42. Diegelmann RF, Bryant CP, Cohen IK: Tissue alpha-globulins in keloid formation. *Plast Reconstr Surg* 1977; 59:418–423.
43. Donoff RB, Burke JF: Abnormality of hypertrophic scar blood vessels. *J Surg Res* 1978; 25:251–255.
44. Donoff RB, Swann DA, Schweidt SH: Glycosaminoglycans of normal and hypertrophic human scar. *Exp Mol Pathol* 1984; 40:13–20.
45. Duhring LA: *A Practical Treatise on Diseases of the Skin*, ed 3. Philadelphia, JB Lippincott Co, 1888.
46. Edwards LC, Dunphy JE: Wound healing: I. Injury and normal repair. *N Engl J Med* 1958; 256:224–233.
47. Erlich HP, Buttle DJ: Epidermis promotion of collagenase in hypertrophic scars organ cultures. *Exp Mol Pathol* 1984; 40:223–234.
48. Filips L: Practical observations on the treatment of keloids and potential keloids. *Med Records* 1939; 150:379–383.
49. Findlay GH, Stoughton RB: Spontaneous keloid with unusual histological features. *Arch Dermatol* 1955; 71:599–601.
50. Follin E: Etude sur les vegetations des cicatrices. *Gaz Hop* 1849; 75:299–306.
51. Fomon S: *The Surgery of Injury and Plastic Repair*. Baltimore, Williams & Wilkins, 1939.
52. Forrest L: Current concepts in soft connective tissue wound healing. *Br J Surg* 1983; 70:133–140.
53. Gabbiani G, Ryan GB, Majno G: Presence of modified fibroblasts in granulation tissue and

their possible role in wound contraction. *Experientia* 1971; 27:549.
54. Garb J, Stone MJ: Keloids: Review of the literature and a report of 80 cases. *Am J Surg* 1942; 58:315–335.
55. Geschickter CF, Lewis D: Tumors of connective tissue. *Am J Cancer* 1935; 25:630–655.
56. Glucksmann A: Local factors in the histogenesis of hypertrophic scars. *Br J Plast Surg* 1951; 4:88–103.
57. Goldmann E: Zur Pathogenese und Therapie des Keloids. *Beitr Klin Chir* 1901; 31:581–615.
58. Gougerot H: A propos d'une syphilide sur cheloide. *Ann Mal* 1914; 9:363.
59. Gougerot H, Lamy P: Cheloides et tuberculose: Observation de cheloide sur les cicatrices operatoires d'adenites tuberculeuses. *Gazette des Hôpitaux* 1908; 99:1179.
60. Guerin A: Physiologie pathologique de la cicatrisation des brulures. *Compte Xendus Association Française pour l'Avance des Sciences* 1894; 23:789–793.
61. Hawkins C: On warty tumors in cicatrices. *London Med Gazettte* 1833; 13:481–482.
62. Hebra F, Kaposi M: *On Diseases of the Skin Including the Exanthemata.* London, The New Sydenham Society, 1874, vol 3, p 272.
63. Hegemann G: Experimentelle Studie uber die Bedeutung und die Ursachen der Wundkontraktion bei der Wundheilung. *Beitr Klin Chir* 1950; 180:229–242.
64. Heidingsfeld ML: Keloid: A comparative histologic study. *JAMA* 1909; 53:1276–1281.
65. Holmstrand K, Longacre JJ, de Stefano GA: The ultrastructure of collagen in skin, scars and keloids. *Plast Reconstr Surg* 1961; 27:597–607.
66. Hunter JAA, Finlay JB: Scanning electron microscopy of normal human scar tissues and keloids. *Br J Surg* 1976; 63:826–830.
67. Hutchinson J: London hospital reports. 1864, vol 1, p 92.
68. Hutchinson J: On keloid. *Arch Surg (London)* 1892; 4:228–240.
69. Hutchinson J: On the nature of keloid of scars. *Edinburgh Med J* 1897; 1:5–9.
70. Im MJC, Hoopes JE: Alpha-naphthyl acid phosphatase activity in normal human skin and keloids. *J Invest Dermatol* 1971; 57:184–189.
71. Jacobsson F: The treatment of keloids at Radiumhemmet, 1921–1941. *Acta Radiol* 1948; 29:251–267.
72. James WD, Besanceney CD, Odom RB: The ultrastructure of a keloid. *J Am Acad Dermatol* 1980; 3:50–57.
73. Janssen de Limpens AMP, Cormane RH: Studies on the immunologic aspects of keloids and hypertrophic scars. *Arch Dermatol Res* 1982; 274:259–266.
74. Johnson T: *The Works of That Famous Chirurgeon Ambrose Parey.* London, M Clark 1678, p 519.
75. Junqueira LCU, Montes GS: Biology of collagen-proteoglycan interaction. *Arch Histol Jpn* 1983; 46:589–629.
76. Justus J: Beobachtungen und Experimente zue Aetiologie des Keloides. *Arch Dermatol Syphilol* 1919; 127:274–326.
77. Kemble JVH: Scanning electron microscopy of hypertrophic and keloid scar. *Postgrad Med J* 1976; 52:219–221.
78. Kemble JVH, Brown RFR: Histochemistry of hypertrophic scars and keloids. *Proc R Soc Med* 1974; 67:257–258.
79. Kemble JVH, Brown RFR: Enzyme activity in human scars, hypertrophic scars and keloids. *Br J Dermatol* 1976; 94:301–305.
80. Ketchum LD, Cohen IK, Masters FW: Hypertrophic scars and keloids. *Plast Reconstr Surg* 1974; 53:140–154.
81. Kischer CW: Collagen and dermal patterns in the hypertrophic scar. *Anat Rec* 1973; 179:137–146.
82. Kischer CW: Comparative ultrastructure of hypertrophic scars and keloids. *Scan Electron Microsc* 1984; 1:423–431.
83. Kischer CW, Bailey JF: The mast cell in hypertrophic scars. *Texas Rep Biol Med* 1972; 30:327–338.
84. Kischer CW, Shetlar MR, Chvapil M: Hypertrophic scars and keloids: A review and new concept concerning their origin. *Scan Electron Microsc* 1982; 4:1699–1713.
85. Kischer CW, et al: Immunoglobulins in hypertrophic scars and keloids. *Plast Reconstr Surg* 1983; 71:821–825.
86. Kischer CW, Thies AC, Chvapil M: Perivascular myofibroblasts and microvascular occlusion in hypertrophic scars and keloids. *Hum Pathol* 1982; 13:819–824.
87. Kleinman HK, Wilkes CM, Martin GR: Interaction of fibronectin with collagen fibrils. *Biochemistry* 1981; 20:2325–2330.
88. Knapp TR, Daniels JR, Kaplan EN: Pathologic scar formation. *Am J Pathol* 1977; 86:47–63.
89. Koonin AJ: The aetiology of keloids: A review of the literature and a new hypothesis. *S Afr Med J* 1964; 38:913–916.
90. Kurnatovski A, Pruszczynski M: The histoenzymological pattern of the keloids and hyper-

trophic scars. *Acta Chir Plast* 1968; 10:232–236.

91. Lagrot F, et al: Essai de traitement des cheloides. *Ann Chir Plast* 1956; 1:33–34.
92. Lambert WC, Elam WD, Anderson WA: Are keloids an inflammatory disease? *Arch Dermatol* 1984; 120:1607.
93. Langhans T: Ein Fall von Keloid. *Arch Pathol Anat Physiol* 1867; 20:330–341.
94. Laurentaci G, Dioguardi D: HLA antigens in keloids and H.S. *Arch Dermatol* 1977; 113:1726.
95. Lilja S, Barrach HJ: An electron microscopical study of the influence of different glycosaminoglycans on the fibrillogenesis of collagen type I and II in vitro. *Virchows Arch A* 1981; 390:325–328.
96. Linares HA: Myofibroblasts in hypertrophic scars: Cause or consequence? *Cirugiá Plastica Iberolatinoamericana* 1979; 5:207–213.
97. Linares HA: Measurement of collagen-proteoglycans interaction in hypertrophic scars. *Plast Reconstr Surg* 1983; 71:818–819.
98. Linares HA, et al: The histiotypic organization of the hypertrophic scar in humans. *J Invest Dermatol* 1972; 59:323–331.
99. Linares HA, et al: On the origin of the hypertrophic scar. *J Trauma* 1973; 13:70–75.
100. Linares HA, Larson DL: Early differential diagnosis between hypertrophic and nonhypertrophic healing. *J Invest Dermatol* 1974; 62:514–516.
101. Linares HA, Larson DL: Elastic tissue and hypertrophic scars. *Burns* 1976; 3:4–7.
102. Linares HA, Larson DL: Proteoglycans and collagenase in hypertrophic scar formation. *J Plast Reconstr Surg* 1978; 62:589–593.
103. Linares HA, Larson DL, Bauer PS: Influence of mechanical forces on burn scar contracture and hypertrophy, in Krisek TJ, Hoopes JE (eds): *Symposium on Basic Science in Plastic Surgery.* St Louis, CV Mosby Co, 1976, vol 15, pp 101–128.
104. Lindal V, Hook M: Glycosaminoglycans and their binding to biological macromolecules. *Ann Rev Biochem* 1978; 4:385–417.
105. Majno G, et al: Contraction of granulation tissue in vitro: Similarity to smooth muscle. *Science* 1971; 173:584.
106. Mancini RE, Quaife JV: Histogenesis of experimentally produced keloids. *J Invest Dermatol* 1962; 38:143–181.
107. Marshall W, Rosenthal S: Pathogenesis and experimental therapy of keloids and similar neoplasms in relation to tissue fluid disturbances. *Am J Surg* 1943; 62:348–357.
108. Matheis H: Exanthematische Keloide nach Varizellen. *Dermatologica* 1943; 143:319–327.
109. Maximow AA, Bloom W: *A Textbook of Histology.* Philadelphia, WB Saunders Co, 1930.
110. McCoy BJ, Cohen IK: Effects of various sera on growth kinetics and collagen synthesis by keloid and normal dermal fibroblasts. *Plast Reconstr Surg* 1981; 67:505–509.
111. McCoy BJ, Cohen IK: Collagenase in keloid biopsies and fibroblasts. *Connect Tissue Res* 1982; 9:181–185.
112. McCoy BJ, Galdun J, Cohen IK: Effects of density and cellular aging on collagen synthesis and growth kinetics in keloid and normal skin fibroblasts. *In Vitro* 1982; 18:79–86.
113. Moriguchi T, Fujimoto D: Crosslink of collagen in hypertrophic scars. *J Invest Dermatol* 1979; 72:143–145.
114. Motegi K: Consideration of the formation and biological significance of hypertrophic scar. *J Maxillofacial Surg* 1984; 12:123–127.
115. Mowlem R: Hypertrophic scars. *Br J Plast Surg* 1951; 4:113–120.
116. Muir H: Proteoglycans: State of art. *Semin Arthritis Rheum* 1981; 11:7.
117. Naegeli J: Recherches experimentales sur des animaux. *Bull Soc Fr Dermatol Syphilol* 1931; 38:949–950.
118. Nason KH: Keloids and their treatment. *N Engl J Med* 1942; 226:883–885.
119. Oegema TR, et al: The effect of proteoglycan on the formation of fibrils from collagen solutions. *Arch Biochem Biophys* 1975; 170:698–709.
120. Oluwasanmi JO, Ajayi OO: Immunofluorescent study of keloids. *Ghana Med J* 1974; 13:177–180.
121. Omo-Dare P: Yoruban contributions to the literature on keloids. *J Natl Med Assoc* 1973; 65:367–406.
122. Omo-Dare P: Genetic studies on keloid. *J Natl Med Assoc* 1975; 67:428–432.
123. Osman AAA, Gumma KA, Satir AA: Highlights on the etiology of keloid. *Int Surg* 1978; 63:33–37.
124. Pautrier LM: Comment se pose le probleme des cheloides. *Bull Soc Fr Dermatol Syphilol* 1931; 38:895–903.
125. Pautrier LM, Woringer F: Anatomie pathologique des cheloides. *Bull Soc Fr Dermatol Syphilol* 1931; 38:932–939.
126. Pautrier LM, Woringer F: Recherches histochimiques du calcium dans les cheloides. *Bull Soc Fr Dermatol Syphilol* 1931; 38:961–965.
127. Pautrier LM, Zorn M: Calcemie: Teneur en calcium de la peau dans les cheloides et les acnes cheloidiennes. *Bull Soc Fr Dermatol Syphilol* 1931; 38:953–961.

128. Peacock EE Jr, Madden JW, Trier WC: Biologic basis for the treatment of keloids and hypertrophic scars. *South Med J* 1970; 63:755–760.
129. Piffard HF: *A Treatise on the Materia Medica and Therapeutics of the Skin*. New York, W. Wood, Co, 1881, p 197.
130. Psillakis JM, et al: Water and electrolyte content of normal skin, scars, and keloid. *Plast Reconstr Surg* 1971; 47:272–274.
131. Ravogli A: A false or cicatricial keloid. *JAMA* 1904; 43:279–302.
132. Rayer P: *Traite des Maladies de la Peau*, p1, XV. Paris, Atlas, 1835.
133. Retz N: *Des Maladies de la Peau et de Celles de l'Esprit*, ed 3. Paris, Mequignon, 1790, pp 155–158.
134. Robinson DW, Corbett E, Hamilton TR: Some observations on connective tissue growth and tissue culture in relation to keloid formation: A preliminary report. *Surg Forum* 1952; 2:505–510.
135. Russell JD, Russell SB, Trupin KM: Differential effects of hydrocortisone on both growth and collagen metabolism of human fibroblasts from normal and keloid tissue. *J Cell Physiol* 1978; 97:221–230.
136. Sabourad R: *Elementary Manual of Regional Topographical Dermatology*. New York, Rebman Co, 1906, p 25.
137. Schutz J: Ein Fall von sogenanntem wahren keloid combiniert mit narben-keloid. *Arch Dermatol Syphilol* 1894; 29:25–38.
138. Selmanowitz VJ, Stiller MJ: Rubinstein-Tabi syndrome. Cutaneous manifestations and colossal keloids. *Arch Dermatol* 1981; 117:504–506.
139. Shetlar MR, et al: The hypertrophic scar, glycoprotein and collagen components of burn scars. *Proc Soc Exp Biol Med* 1971; 138:298–300.
140. Shetlar MR, Shetlar CL, Linares HA: The hypertrophic scar: Location of glycosaminoglycans within scars. *Burns* 1977; 4:14–19.
141. Shetlar MR, et al: The hypertrophic scar: Hexosamine containing components of burn scars. *Proc Soc Exp Biol Med* 1972; 139:544–547.
142. Shoshan S: Wound healing. *Int Rev Connect Tissue Res* 1981; 9:1–26.
143. Sibeleva KF, Zenkevich GD, Laufer AL: Mucopolysaccharides and collagen in human keloids. *Vopr Med Khim* 1961; 11:55–60.
144. Sloan DF, et al: Tissue gases in human hypertrophic burn scars. *Plast Reconstr Surg* 1978; 61:431–436.
145. Starr L, Pepper W (eds): *A System of Practical Medicine*. Philadelphia, Lea Bros Co, 1886, vol 4, p 685.
146. Stelwagon HW: *Treatise on Diseases of the Skin*. Philadelphia; WB Saunders Co, 1907, p 603.
147. Sturim HS: Keloids versus hypertrophic scars. *RI Med J* 1968; 51:103–105.
148. Takama H: Correlative changes of collagen and proteoglycans in the hypertrophic post burn scar. *Dermatology* 1976; 86:375–377.
149. Thorn J: Ueber spontanes keloid. *Arch Klin Chir* 1895; 51:618–636.
150. Traub EF: Keloids as sequel to varicella. *Arch Dermatol Syphilol* 1944; 49:278–279.
151. Trawinski H: Zur Kenntnis des disseminierten Spontankeloids. *Arch Dermatol Syphilol* 1909; 96:303–338.
152. Trusler HM, Baur TB: Keloids and hypertrophic scars. *Arch Surg* 1948; 57:539–552.
153. Unna PG: *The Histopathology of the Diseases of the Skin*. New York, McMillan Co, 1896, p 839.
154. Van Den Brenk HAS: Studies in restorative growth processes in mammalian wound healing. *Br J Surg* 1956; 43:525–550.
155. Velpeau J: Leçon sur la nature et le traitement de la keloide. *Gaz Hop* 1845; 18:229–236.
156. Verrier E: Estudio sobre la patogenia de las cicatrices operatorias fibrosas hipertroficas o queloideas. *Med Ibera* 1930; 24:273–276.
157. Virchow R: *Vorelesungen Uber Pathologie*. Berlin, A Hirschwald, 1864.
158. Volkmann R: Ein Fall von aechtem (spontanem) keloid der finger und der zehen. *Arch Klin Chir* 1872; 13:374–379.
159. Warren JC: *Uber Keloid*. Vienna, Sitzungsberichte der K.K. Academie der Wissenschaften zu Wien, vol 47, 1868.
160. Warren JC: Hypertrophies and degenerations of cicatrices and cicatricial tissue. *Trans Am Surg Assoc* 1893; 11:41–79.
161. Watts GT, Grillo HC, Gross J: Studies in wound healing: II. The role of granulation tissue in contraction. *Ann Surg* 1958; 148:153–160.
162. Welander L: *Nordiskt Med Arkiv* no. 3, 1896.
163. Whitehill JL: Prophylaxis of surgical keloids. *Arizona Med* 1954; 11:399–402.
164. Wilms M: Zur pathogenese des keloids. *Beitr Klin Chir* 1899; 23:149–166.
165. Zuffardi O, Fraccaro M: Gene mapping and serendipity: The locus for torticollis, keloids, cryptorchidism and renal dysplasia (31430, McMusick) is at Xq28, distal to the G6PD locus. *Hum Genet* 1982; 62:280–281.

25 / Preserving Function and Minimizing Deformity: The Role of the Occupational Therapist

PATRICIA FADER, O.T.R.

The overall goals of burn care are to preserve life, minimize disability, and provide emotional support to the burned child. Rehabilitation services are primarily directed at preserving the child's physical function and supporting the child emotionally through the use of activity.

During the acute phase of the burn, the therapist strives to minimize edema and avoid the deleterious effects of bedrest. Since the pain of the burn injury may cause the child to voluntarily immobilize areas of the body, the therapist must encourage active range of motion from the first day of injury. As the burn wound heals, spontaneously or via postburn grafting, prevention of deformity by minimizing the effects of burn scar contracture and hypertrophic scar formation take priority. Since both functional and cosmetic deformity occur during the active phase of hypertrophic scar formation, burn patients must be followed up on an outpatient basis until the burn scar matures. Mature burn scar also lacks the elasticity of normal skin, so children may need to be followed up by the burn team throughout the growing years to prevent functional limitations.

The traditional role of the occupational therapist in the case of burn patients has been to provide splinting, pressure treatments, adaptations to activities of daily living, adaptive equipment, and exercise through the use of activity. The occupational therapist also assesses the developmental needs of the pediatric burn patient to determine if there is a need for therapeutic intervention. The therapist works closely with physical therapy and child life therapy personnel, and although the delineation of roles may differ in various hospital settings, the objectives of rehabilitation and techniques are similar.

An effective rehabilitation program requires the support of physicians and nurses. The therapist communicates the rehabilitation needs of the burn patient to the burn team and coordinates all therapeutic interventions with the medical treatment. Communication must take place at daily medical rounds or at scheduled patient care conferences. In addition, time must be spent educating the nursing staff to the purpose and value of the rehabilitation process, as well as teaching the necessary skills to follow through with the rehabilitation program.

WORKING WITH THE PEDIATRIC PATIENT

Participation of the child (patient) is essential to the successful attainment of the rehabilitation goals. Several approaches may be necessary to obtain cooperation. Children respond well to consistency and established routines.[36] One way of achieving consistency is with scheduling so that medical, rehabilitation, and relaxation times occur at regular intervals. Many children respond to rewards for cooperation, such as stickers or extra play time. Children with behavioral problems may respond to contractual agreements between the child and burn staff that outline the desired behaviors as well as the consequences for cooperative or uncooperative behaviors. Some children may respond to socialization and will try to imitate the behavior they may observe in another child.

To obtain cooperation, the therapist must establish good rapport with the child. Several suggestions for developing rapport have been advanced.[20] If trust is to be developed, the therapist must be honest. If a treatment is painful, the child must be apprised of it, and its advantages and disadvantages must be discussed. Only promises that can be kept should be made. The rehabilitation procedures should be explained thoroughly and in simple language, allowing the child to ask questions before beginning. Major changes in the treatment program should be explained in detail and in advance. Children should be allowed to cry during painful treatments without scolding. However, the older child should be encouraged to verbally express feelings, fears, or questions in an understandable manner. If the child does well, he should be praised and criticism and irrelevant behavior should be ignored. All commands must be repeated as often as necessary and all actions explained. If possible, choices should be provided. Bedside visits at times when no treatments are required can be an effective means of establishing rapport.

EVALUATION

The initial evaluation of the pediatric burn patient is similar to that of the adult and includes information that can be obtained from the medical record as well as by inspection. The therapist must be aware of previous medical history, social history, and other injuries that may have impact on the rehabilitation program. To anticipate problems and specific needs during the rehabilitation phase, such as joint contracture, hypertrophic scarring, long-term bed rest, traction, or immobilization of a body part, the therapist must evaluate the type, depth, extent, and location of the injury. A superficial burn injury that heals conservatively in less than 2 weeks does not usually lead to hypertrophic scarring or burn scar contractures. Deep partial-thickness burns, on the other hand, are often associated with hypertrophic scarring and contractures. In general, the longer the wound remains open, the more likely the patient will be to develop a hypertrophic scar. Deep partial- and full-thickness burns that have been autografted can form hypertrophic scars, particularly at the graft edges and in areas where the graft did not adhere. The location of a deep burn over joint areas will alert the therapist to the possibility of burn scar contractures.[7, 13, 27, 38] Active range of motion is indicated, but may be limited initially by edema and pain. Elevation of the extremity usually decreases edema formation.

The therapist's initial evaluation is used to plan a rehabilitation program that minimizes disability and deformity and coordinates efforts with other members of the burn team. Burned children must be reevaluated frequently and checked for range of motion, ability to perform activities of daily living, strength, and endurance. Complications related to pressure or scarring can usually be anticipated and prevented. Sensory loss as well as hypersensitivity should be noted. All treatment modalities are reviewed, and the rehabilitation program is revised as often as necessary to attain optimal functional and cosmetic results.

POSITIONING

Positioning is a technique that is used to preserve a functional state and to prevent burn scar contractures. It is most commonly used for patients restricted to bed rest, but it can be used with the upright sitting or standing postures, as well. The goal is to attain a position that opposes the forces of contracture, provides safe joint alignment, and main-

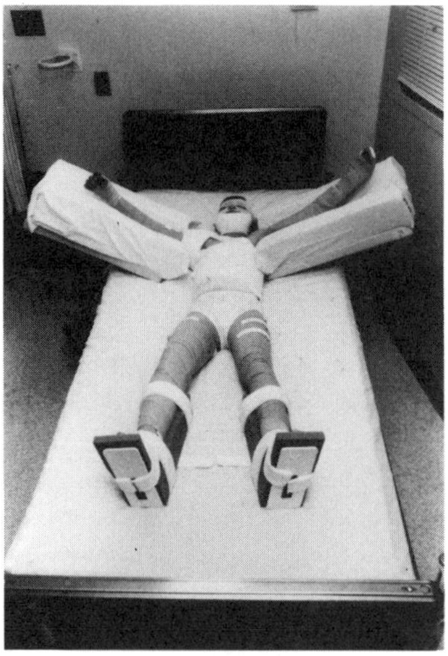

FIG 25–1.
Burn patient in supine position.

tains tendon balance without causing stretch or pressure injuries to the peripheral nerves or skin. In general, only the affected joints require positioning. However, critically ill patients who are likely to remain supine for long periods or those with extensive injuries may benefit from total body positioning. Common factors that may affect positioning are edema, donor sites, grafted areas, and respiratory function. It is difficult to manage a total positioning program with patients on the air-fluidized bed, but partial positioning can usually be accomplished. Effective positioning should be encouraged from day 1 and the results monitored. The supine position is preferred for the severely burned patient (Fig 25–1).

Burns of the ear require special attention to prevent pressure necrosis and folding of the helix. Pressure can impair circulation to the ear's cartilage and contributes to the development of chondritis. This is a common sequela of ear burns.[17] A pillow under the head may result in pressure to the ears and should not be used. A foam "doughnut" with the hole over the ear may be used to protect the ear.

Burns of the anterior neck must be carefully positioned to minimize a neck flexion contracture. Pillows should be avoided; instead, a small foam or cloth roll placed under the neck, or a foam roll placed lengthwise along the spinal column, can maintain slight neck extension. The latter will also permit retraction of the scapula.[25] Other alternatives include a neck extension pillow, which can also be used to hyperextend the neck and position the head,[12] or a short mattress, which can be used with medically stable patients to hyperextend the neck.

Burns of the axilla may severely limit arm rotation at the level of the shoulder. To minimize axillary contracture, the shoulder must be positioned at 90° of abduction and 15° to 20° of horizontal adduction. In older children, positioning of the shoulder can be accomplished using commercially available abduction trays, which are secured with an aluminum frame that slides under the mattress. Arm slings fastened to overhead traction bars or pillows placed on bedside tables are other methods used to abduct the older child's shoulders. Small children can be positioned using foam wedges that fit snugly inside the bed or crib rails. The arm can be secured to the foam with Velcro. Another successful way of positioning small children is with the "papoose device," which is a foam bed fitted to the child with axillary wedges glued into place.[22] The child is secured into position with Velfoam straps. The forearm is positioned in supination, with the wrist supported in slight extension. The burned hand is elevated and, if splints are unavailable, placed in a functional position with the hand open and positioned around a cloth roll.

The trunk of the body is positioned in a straight posture. This is especially important if there are unilateral trunk burns, to avoid contractures in a scoliosis-like position.[26] The hips are positioned in 0° of extension with no internal or external rotation and abducted 10°

to 15°. The position of comfort is with the hips externally rotated, with the knees flexed, and the lateral aspects of the legs resting against the bedrail. If sustained over long periods, this position may lead to pressure damage of the peroneal nerve just below the knee.[16] Dislocation of the hip in debilitated burn children has been attributed to a combination of factors, including poor positioning and contractile forces from the burn scar.[9] The knee must be supported at 0° of extension, and the feet must be maintained at 0° of dorsiflexion to preserve the length of the Achilles tendon. A small roll placed under the ankle helps to prevent decubitus ulcers in this area. A foot board used to position the feet must be covered with thick foam to prevent pressure necrosis to the volar surface. In small children, the papoose board can also be used to position the legs and feet. An abduction wedge and foam foot rest are glued onto the foam bed, and the child's legs are secured using Velfoam straps.[22] Figure-of-eight wrapped elastic bandages help to maintain the ankle position, but the ankle must be held in dorsiflexion while the wrap is applied.

Positioning in the prone position may be required in children when the back is grafted or used as a donor. A prone mattress is cut short at the ankle to allow the feet to rest in dorsiflexion. The mattress should also be cut so that the shoulders are positioned at 15° to 20° of horizontal adduction and 90° of abduction. The head can be supported by the mattress and turned side to side, or the mattress can be cut at the base of the neck and the head supported with a small foam pillow under the forehead, thus aligning the head with the airway (Figure 25–2).

Although not ideal, side-lying positioning may be needed for postural drainage, to relieve pressure from long-term bed rest, or to comply with grafting procedures. Under these circumstances, the extremities are extended, the shoulders are flexed to 90°, and the body is aligned straight.

When the patient sits up, the shoulders can be positioned to 90° on a foam-covered bedside table (Figure 25–3). Skyhooks may also be used to position the shoulder. If burned, the lower extremities can be elevated on a second chair with the feet in dorsiflexion against a foam-covered foot board. The burned lower extremity should not be allowed to dangle during the acute phase of the injury, as the blood may pool in the lower leg, causing bleeding and possible graft loss. Pooling of blood, edema, bleeding, and graft loss are common complications. Proper posture must be emphasized to the ambulatory patient, as well. Children with flexion hip contractures should not be allowed to sit for long periods and may require a high desk that can be used while standing upright at school.

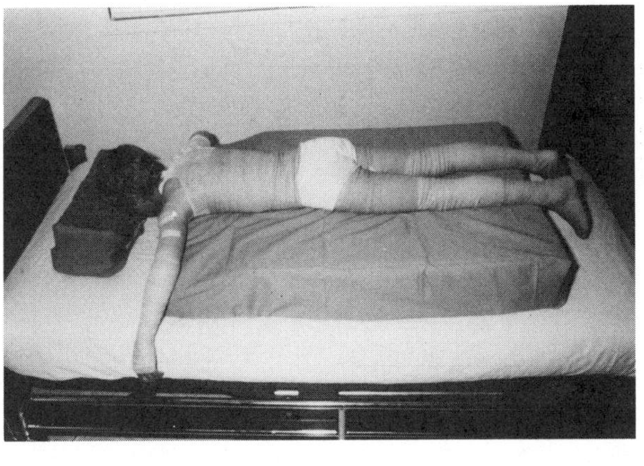

FIG 25–2.
Burn patient in prone position.

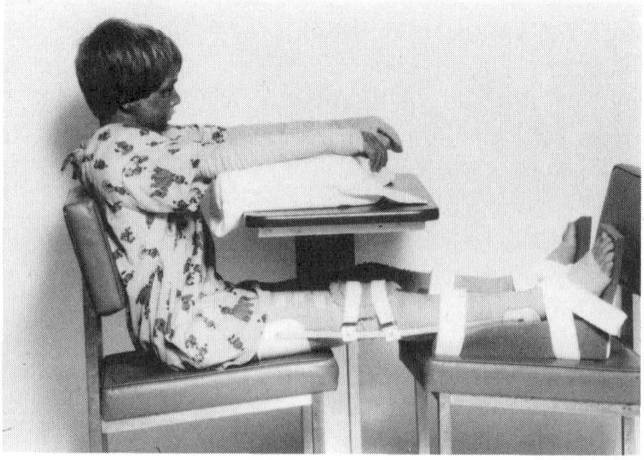

FIG 25–3.
Burn patient in sitting position with shoulders at 90 degree angle.

An overhead walker is used by some burn centers to position axilla burns while the patient is ambulatory.[32]

SPLINTING

Splinting is a form of positioning and can be used to obtain the same goals. Splinting may be needed to immobilize a body part, such as following a grafting procedure, in cases of exposed tendons, etc. Many types of materials can be used for splinting in the burn patient. Low *thermoplastic* materials are the most popular, as they are easy to modify and to clean. High-heat plastics, silicone (Silastic Esomere), plaster, and various foams have also been used for splinting. Foams are frequently used in conjunction with low *thermoplastic* materials. Closed-cell foam is preferred because it can be cleaned. Open-cell foam can be used, but must be changed frequently to prevent infection, since it cannot be cleaned.

Deep dermal burns of the hands should be splinted within 24 hours of the injury. Other splinting can be delayed until problems with positioning, range of motion, or patient cooperation are noted. Small children may require early splinting, as they have difficulty understanding positioning. Splints required to immobilize a body part after a surgical procedure can be fabricated in the operating room or in the recovery room. Surgical splints can be fitted over a thin gauze layer or over bulky dressings. The grafted area is immobilized until approximately the fifth postoperative day. At that time, active range of motion, play, and activities of daily living are initiated, and the splint-wearing schedule is decreased. Once bulky dressings are removed, the surgical splints will need to be modified to fit the patient; thereafter, frequent checks will minimize pressure problems. It is recommended that splints be removed at least every 4 hours for thorough cleaning, and that fitting checks be done daily. Examination of the skin for pressure marks, wound maceration, loss of sensation, or hypersensitivity must be practiced frequently. Small children are particularly difficult to fit with splints and should be monitored closely. They are less likely than older children or adults to complain of pain. Splints are contoured to the patients and must fit closely to the body part to prevent shifting, which can occur if the splint is too large. The shifting of a splint may cause poor positioning of the body part, as well as pressure or friction leading to skin breakdown. Thus, it is recommended that splints be secured with gauze wrap or elastic wraps, which are better for this purpose than are straps. However, elastic wraps, if applied incorrectly, can cause edema and restrict circulation, so they must be used with caution. All personnel need to be taught the skill of applying the splints. Other alternatives include us-

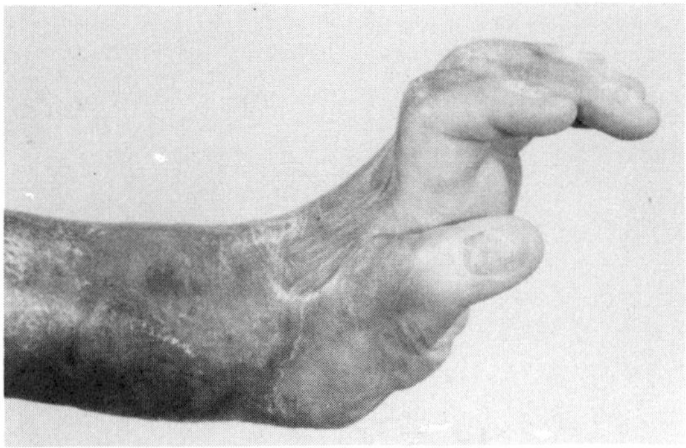

FIG 25–4.
Example of burn contracture of the hand.

ing tubular elastic cotton gauze or wide Velfoam straps for application.

Deep dermal burns of the dorsum of the hand require splinting to maintain a good position. The anticipated deformities from burn scar contraction are metacarpophalangeal joint (MCP) hyperextension, interphalangeal (IP) flexion, radial deviation, thumb adduction with extension, and flattening of the palmar arches. This is referred to as the "intrinsic minus" position (Fig 25–4). The hand is splinted in an antideformity position with the hand supported in MCP flexion, IP extension, slight ulnar deviation, and palmar abduction of the thumb. The MCP joints are flexed 40° to 70° to maintain the length of the collateral ligaments and stretch the burn scar. It is easier to position the thumb in palmar abduction if the MCP joints are not fully flexed. The IP joints are positioned in full extension. The wrist is positioned in 0° to 30° of extension to maintain tendon balance while preventing both extension and flexion burn scar contracture of the wrist (Fig 25–5). Initially, the burned hand is removed from splints for passive and active exercise and voluntary movement. Less MCP flexion may be needed to maintain the IP joints in extension and the thumb in palmar abduction when splinting is done in young children. In some cases, splinting material can be thinned by heating and rolling the material with a rolling pin, or the material can be purchased in ¹⁄₁₆-in. sheets. This grade is particularly useful for splinting in babies.

The extensor hood mechanism of the fingers is especially vulnerable to injury from deep dermal burns. Actively exercising or passively moving the proximal interphalangeal (PIP) joint into full flexion can cause further damage to the tendon sheath. If the central slip is ruptured, exercise of the PIP joint will cause the lateral bands to move in a volar direction, shifting anterior to the axis of joint rotation.[9, 21, 37] In this position, the lateral bands of the extensor hood mechanism will flex instead of extending the finger at the PIP joint. Initially, only the lack of full finger extension will be noted, but if untreated, the finger will eventually assume the position of a boutonnière deformity. Therefore, precautions should be taken with the hand that has sustained deep dermal burns over the PIP joint. Since it is difficult to assess the depth of burn injury accurately, hands suspected of extensor hood mechanism damage should be splinted within 24 hours of admission and with the IPs in full extension. Passive range of motion to the PIP joint is not used with

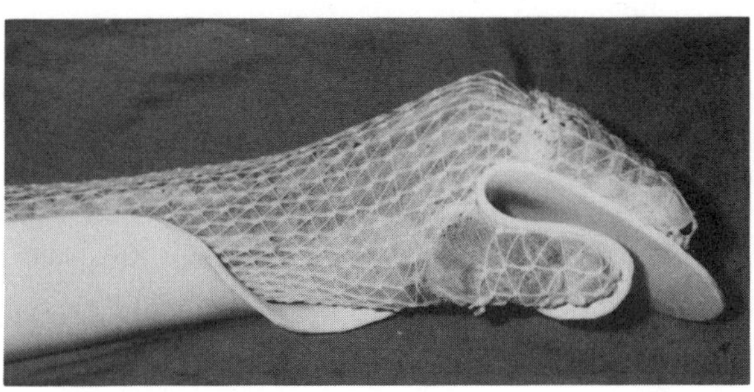

FIG 25–5.
Burned hand positioned in splints to prevent burn scar contracture. Note full interphalangeal extensions, metacarpophalangeal flexion, thumb abduction, and slight extension of the wrist.

these patients. The therapist evaluates the hand by gently beginning active range of motion and observing the depth of the wound. If the patient is unable to fully extend a finger, injury to the extensor hood mechanism is suspected. The PIP joint is then immobilized in extension for 4 to 6 weeks to allow healing of the extensor hood mechanism with the lateral bands in a functional position. Exercise to the MCP and distal interphalangeal (DIP) joint must be continued during this period. Flexion exercise of the DIP joint helps to reduce deformity by pulling the extensor mechanism distally, thereby reducing the volar shift of the lateral bands and retraction of the medial extensor tendon.[18] Finger extension splints may be helpful in maintaining extension during the patient's bath, exercise, or other periods when the hand splints are removed. After 4 to 6 weeks of immobilization, supervised gentle active range of motion is initiated. If no extensor lag is noted, the active range of motion is progressively increased.

The extensor to the DIP joint can also be injured from deep dermal burn injuries that, if untreated, may result in a mallet finger deformity. To treat this injury, the DIP joint is splinted in extension for 4 to 6 weeks to allow healing. Swan-neck deformities have been observed in burn injuries to the hand. If a swan-neck deformity is noted, the PIP joint should be splinted in slight flexion.

Deep palmar burns may also require splinting as a positioning technique to prevent burn scar contracture. During the acute phase, palmar burns are splinted on the dorsal surface of the hand to prevent maceration of the wound (Fig 25–6). It is possible to use a volar splint to position the palmar burn if the splint is removed frequently to prevent wound maceration. The anticipated scar deformity is flexion of the fingers, flexion and adduction of the thumb, and shortening of the palm. These hands are splinted with the fingers in extension, the thumb in radial abduction with slight flexion at the MCP, and the wrist extended 0° to 30°. The splint can be fabricated to abduct the fingers.

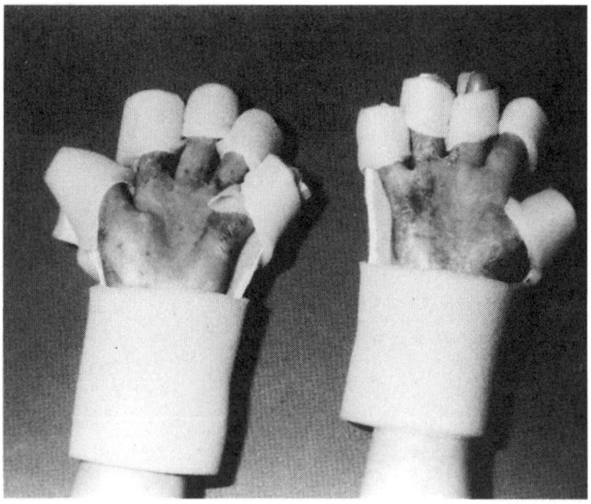

FIG 25–6.
Palmar hand burns positioned with the metacarpophalangeal joints of the fingers in extension with dorsal splints.

Circumferential burns to the hand are initially positioned with neutral extension of the IP joints, 30° to 45° of MCP flexion, 0° to 30° of wrist extension, and the thumb midway between palmar and radial abduction. As with all hand burns, the hand must be monitored closely and revisions in the splint or splinting program made as needed.

Preservation of the palmar arches is essential for proper rehabilitation of the severely burned hand. Flattening of the palmar arch will affect the patient's ability to obtain full flexion of the MCP joints. The splint can be fabricated to support the contour of the arch; however, this may be difficult to accomplish in small children. To provide support to the palmar arch, a round piece of contoured adhesive foam can be secured to the splint, or palmar pads can be fabricated out of silicone fitted directly on the palm of the patient's hand.

Silicone (Silastic Esomere) splints can also be used to position a young child's hand. A bivalve silicone mitt is advantageous in that the splint provides total contact, and the hand cannot slip out of position. Mallick and Carr[23] have reported the use of silicone mitts following grafting in acute burns. Flesch also reported the use of plaster casting for splinting hands in small or uncooperative children.[11]

Traction devices used to position the burn hand include the hayrake, the halo, and the traction hand splint. Traction splinting is used to correct hand deformities (i.e., boutonnière),[27] or to position the hand postgraft without applying pressure over the new graft (Fig 25–7). Traction pulls the digits into extension at the IP joints, and the thumb is palmarly abducted. There are several ways in which rubber-band traction is applied to the fingertips, including dressmaker hooks glued to the fingernails,[19] pulp hooks,[35] Kirschner wires, and suture loops.[23] The traction splint is incorporated into the splint distal to the fingers to provide a base for the rubberband traction. The rubber-band traction is then attached to the splint extension and the fingers. The patient is observed closely to prevent loss or loosening of fingernails, as well as to detect pressure areas that can be caused by traction splinting.

The anticipated burn scar contracture resulting from anterior, lateral, or medial burns of the elbow is a flexion contracture. To prevent contracture, the elbow is splinted in extension. Two styles of splints have been traditionally used: the three-point extension splint[39] and the low thermoplastic conformer.[29] Both styles of splints are fabricated with the length reaching from the insertion of the deltoid to 1 to 1½ in. proximal to the radial or ulnar styloid. Shorter conformers may allow some elbow flexion, thus not controlling the contracture as well. Longer splints may cause pressure over the bony prominences of the wrist or may slip up into the anterior axilla. Both splints are fitted to the anterior arm with the wrist positioned in neutral or full supination. Arm conformers are not recommended for use over the posterior surface of the arm. A posterior conformer can apply pressure over the ulnar nerve, cause skin breakdown to the elbow, or slip proximally into the axilla, causing pressure to the radial nerve. Usually the arm splint is fitted over the hand splint (if both splints are required) since the hand splint is more difficult to fit.

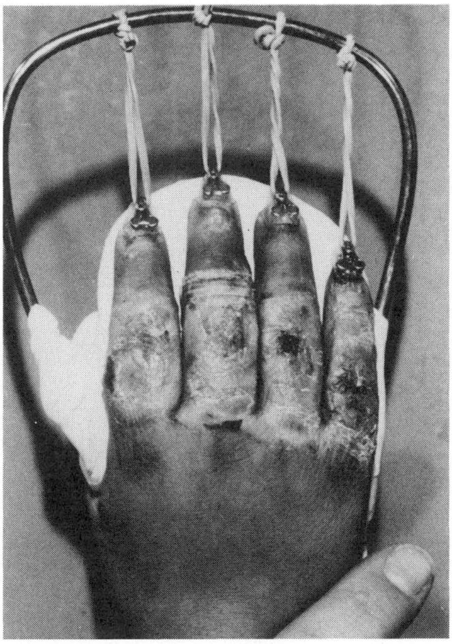

FIG 25–7.
Burned hand positioned in rubber-band traction splint. Dressmaker hooks are glued to the fingernails of the patient.

The anticipated contracture from posterior, medial, or lateral burns of the knee is a flexion contracture. The knee is splinted with posterior leg conformers or three-point splints similar to the elbow conformer (Figs 25–8 and 25–9). The length of the leg conformer is measured from the proximal midthigh to 1½ in. proximal to the lateral malleolus. It is possible to fit a leg conformer to the medial aspect of the leg if the splint is flared around the patella.

If three-point splints are used to position the elbow or knee, caution is required to prevent the joint from being forced into hyperextension. Splints are removed periodically to encourage exercise, to be cleaned, and for proper fitting checks. The elbow and knee pads on the three-point splints can be applied by sewing parallel Velcro straps to the sheepskin. One strap is applied to the arm above the elbow, and the other strap is applied distally to the elbow.

Several other styles of splints have been

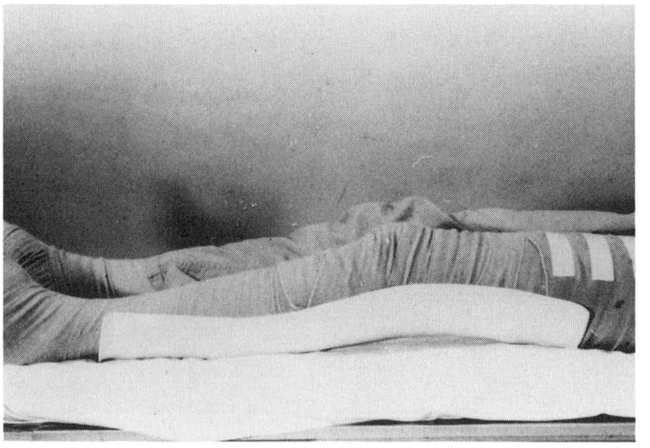

FIG 25–8.
Leg conformer on posterior leg to maintain knee extension. Leg conformer will be applied with an elastic wrap.

used to immobilize the elbow and knee joints in young children. A modified three-point splint fabricated out of low thermoplastic material without aluminum bars is easy to make and controls well the knee joints of young children.[23]

Burns to the lateral or anterior surface of the neck may cause grotesque flexion contractures with loss of range of motion, length, and contour. As the contracture progresses, it will also distort the facial features. The neck is splinted during the acute hospitalization period when positioning fails to maintain the neck length, range of motion, and contour. Although low thermoplastic splinting can be used in the acute hospitalization period to prevent contractures, the application and fit are difficult, due to bulky dressings.

The soft collar works well before the burn is healed. The soft collar is a foam crescent covered with stockinette; it is secured by sewing Velcro to each end of the stockinette so that the collar fits snugly around the neck. A soft collar will minimize neck contracture; however, it may not completely maintain the neck's contour. The child should be able to tolerate a low thermoplastic neck splint 6 to 10 days postgrafting. The low thermoplastic neck conformer is fitted onto the patient's neck while the patient is sitting up. These splints are applied with Velcro attachments[39] and must fit snugly to apply pressure to the neck. It is recommended that a low thermoplastic material that does not shrink while cooling be used. Some therapists fabricate two splints: one for use in the supine position and one in the sitting position. The neck splint or splints are worn day and night, but

FIG 25–9.
Three-point leg splint applied to the leg to maintain knee extension.

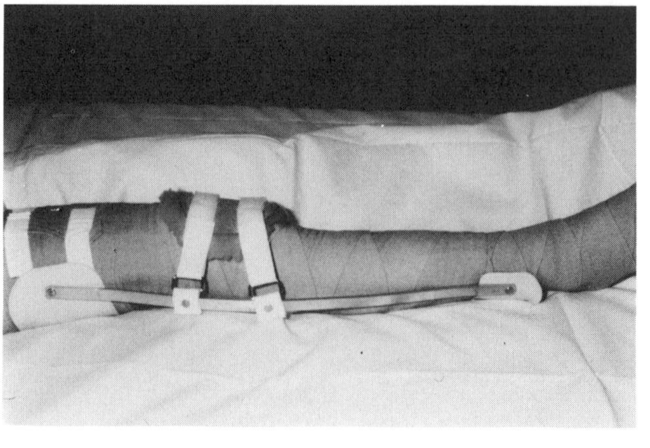

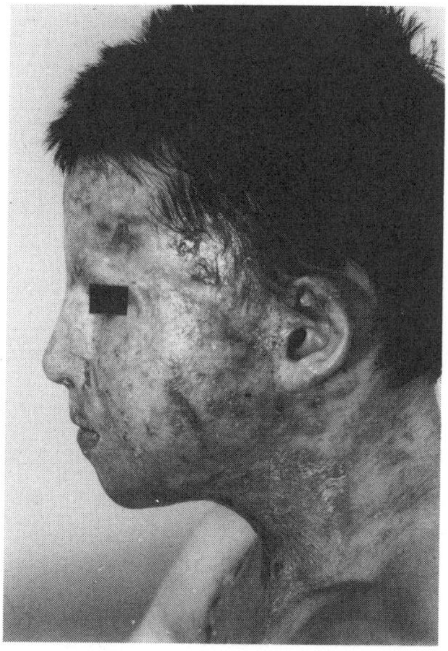

FIG 25–10.
Patient with burn scar contracture of the neck.

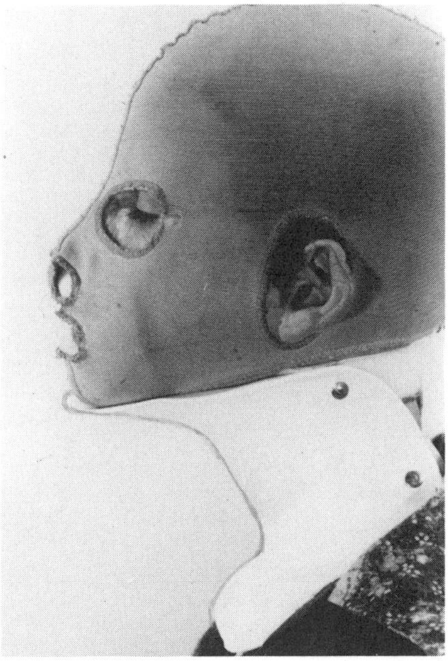

FIG 25–12.
The same patient (see Fig 25–10) in a neck conformer.

are removed for meals, exercise, and to allow airing of open wounds to prevent maceration. The splint is flared away from the child's chin to allow for normal mouth closure and growth of the mandible. Flaring the splint away from the mandible also directs the pressure to the neck and provides a better neck contour[10] (Figs 25–10 to 25–13). Although an uncommon complication of burns, Zuker et al.,[42] reported sleep apnea in three children, which may have been complicated by pressure directed over the mandible. Hard plastic neck conformers can be fabricated from transparent high-heat plastics. However, taking the negative impression, pouring the positive mold, and molding the transparent plastic onto the positive mold must be done quickly, or the neck will contract further and the splint will fit poorly.

Two other commonly used styles of neck splints are the "Watusi" multiring collar[23] and the black ring neck collar. The black ring collar is fabricated out of insulation tubing of various sizes. A low thermoplastic strip is fitted into the contour of the black ringand a Velcro ring attachment is attached to the low thermoplastic strip. The black ring is fitted around the neck snugly to apply pressure (Fig

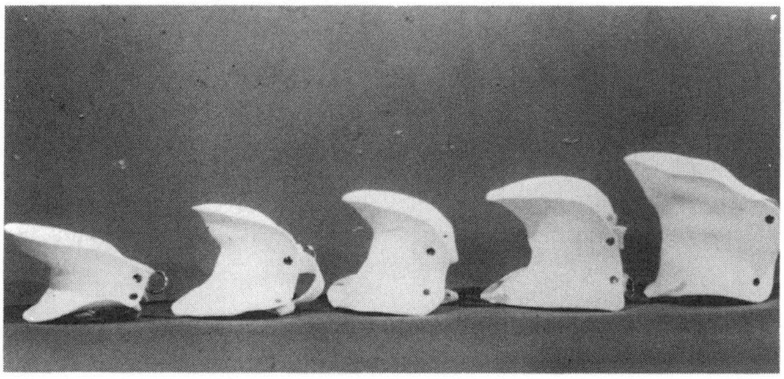

FIG 25–11.
The neck splints used on the same patient (see Fig 25–10) the following 2 weeks. Splints were used serially and changed every 2 to 3 days.

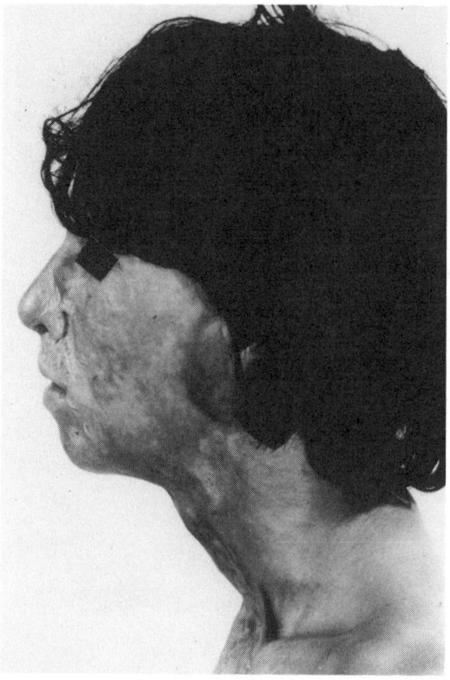

FIG 25–13.
The same patient (see Fig 25–10) 1½ years postburn. The neck conformer was discontinued at this time.

25–14). The ring neck splints are especially helpful with noncompliant wearers of the hard neck conformers or with patients who have already developed a neck contracture. All neck splinting needs to be checked regularly to prevent skin breakdown. Splints need to be revised as the neck length and contour improve.

Microstomia is a common sequela of facial burns around the mouth and of electrical burns of the mouth so common in young children. Mouth splints vary from very simple to those requiring skill with orthodontic materials and techniques. The simplest splint, described by Gorham in 1977, is a low thermoplastic splint that spreads the corners of the mouth and is held between the teeth by the patient. Generally, this splint is useful with cooperative adults, but children do not comply well with its use.[14] Another fairly easy-to-fabricate device described in 1976 consists of two plastic conformers that fit the commissures of the mouth and are applied with an elastic band around the head.[8] A variation of this splint applies the conformers with nonelastic straps. Precaution is necessary with this splint style to prevent skin breakdown of the commissures of the mouth. It has been used with children with some success and should be fabricated to fit with a face mask. Hartford et al.,[15] described a microstomia prevention device that consisted of two steel bars and two plastic conformers fitted to the commissures of the mouth. A screw allows the appliance to be adjusted. Alternative, yet similar, designs are in use as well (Fig 25–15). One commercially available appliance is adjusted dynamically with rubber-band traction. These styles of appliances have been used successfully with cooperative children.

A static acrylic commissural conformer fitted over the child's palate with commissure posts at the corners of the mouth, initially described by Coleleugh and Ryan,[6] is currently the most successful mouth splint used in young children (Fig 25–16). The appliance can be fabricated to be easily removed or may

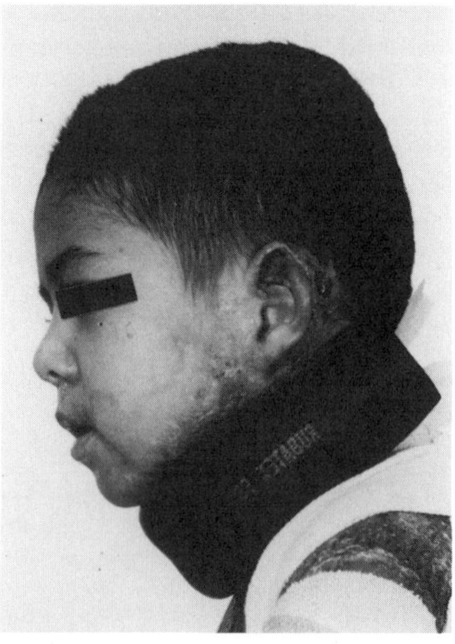

FIG 25–14.
Patient in a black ring conformer.

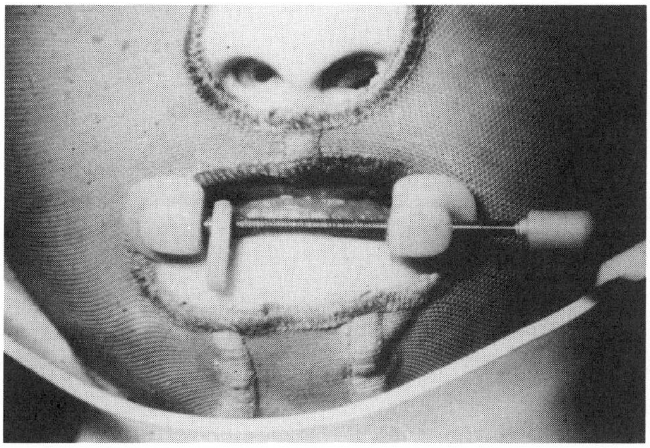

FIG 25–15.
A variation of a microstomia prevention device. This variation was designed by Roland Morales, medical sculptor.

be fixed to the teeth of noncompliant patients.[2] Babies without teeth have been treated by applying mouth-expanding projections onto the clear plastic face mask to maintain the commissures of the mouth.

Nasal and ear openings may gradually be occluded by scar. Small, hollow tubes can be fitted into the opening to prevent this. In small children, a string is attached to the tubes and taped to the face mask to minimize loss of the device.

Scars in the axilla region or on the anterior or posterior trunk in close proximity to the shoulder region can contract, limiting the range of motion of the shoulder. Scar contractures can limit all motions of the shoulder. Diligence with positioning is necessary to prevent an axilla contracture. Axilla splints can be used to position the burn patient while the patient is on bed rest; however, other positioning techniques may be easier and are equally successful. Axilla splints, particularly conformers, may also be used while the patient is upright, although the pull of gravity may make it difficult to fit this splint. The axilla splint is usually not well accepted for use at home unless it is worn only at night, since the splint places the child in a nonfunctional, activity-limiting position. Despite obvious problems, axilla splints can be a valuable adjunct to other therapy techniques. Figure-of-eight wrapped axilla pads can also be used. These thick, semicircular sponges are placed diagonally into the axilla and wrapped in place with an elastic wrap in a figure-of-eight design, intersecting over the cervicodorsal spine. This technique splints the arms slightly away from the body and applies pressure to the axilla region. Full range of motion will only be achieved with a vigorous exercise program.

The anticipated contracture of the ankle is

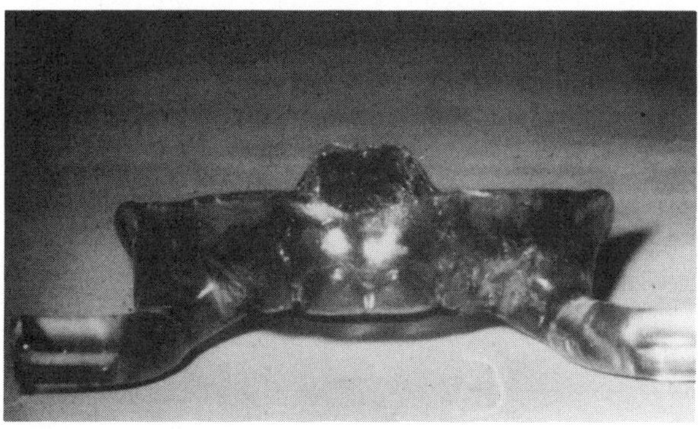

FIG 25–16.
A static acrylic commissural conformer, which is fitted to the child's palate with the commissural posts at the corners of the mouth.

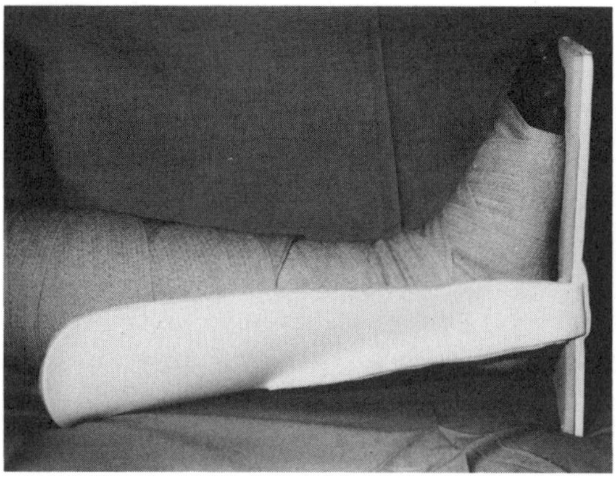

FIG 25–17.
Low thermoplastic splint fabricated to prevent plantar flexion deformity. The area over the heel and Achilles tendon is cut out to prevent pressure to these areas. The splint can be applied with straps or elastic wrap.

in plantar flexion with inversion, and is partly caused by shortening of the Achilles tendon. The ideal position of the ankle is 5° to 10° of dorsiflexion to maintain Achilles tendon length; however, this position is difficult to achieve. The position with the ankle at 0° of dorsiflexion is acceptable, but also difficult to maintain.[40] There are commercial foot splints available that are designed to maintain 0° of dorsiflexion and prevent decubitus ulcers of the heel. Most of these are available in children's sizes. Low thermoplastic splints can also be fabricated to prevent plantar flexion deformity. The area over the heel and Achilles tendon is cut out to prevent pressure necrosis. A platform can be added to the distal end of the splint to lift the heel off the bed, as well as to control rotation of the hip (Fig 25–17). The knee will need to be supported to prevent hyperextension in this style of splint. High-top tennis shoes that are lined with sheepskin can be used to position the ankle or to apply pressure to the dorsal aspect of the foot while the burn scar is fragile. However, these types of shoes are difficult to find in small children's sizes. After the foot is well healed, high-top orthopedic shoes with a padded tongue, double sole, and arch support can be used to maintain neutral dorsiflexion and to control burn scar contracture. Silicone boots molded to the foot have also been used with children to maintain the foot in a functional position.[41] The patient is able to walk in both the shoes and silicone boots. Splints or shoes will need to be removed periodically each day to allow weight bearing and performance of exercises to maintain range of motion and strength of the foot and ankle. Early ambulation is an important factor in maintaining full ankle range of motion.

Hyperextension of the toes is an expected deformity if the foot is burned over the dorsal surface. If the ankle is not splinted, a sole plate can be used to position the toes in a

FIG 25–18.
A sole plate or foot plate is made to conform to the volar surface of the foot and applied with an elastic wrap.

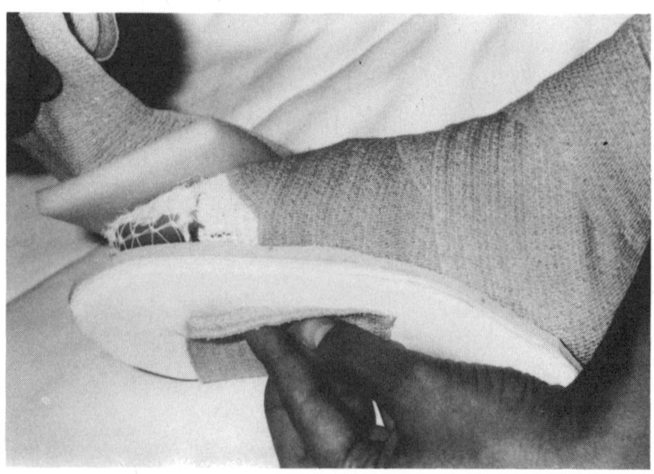

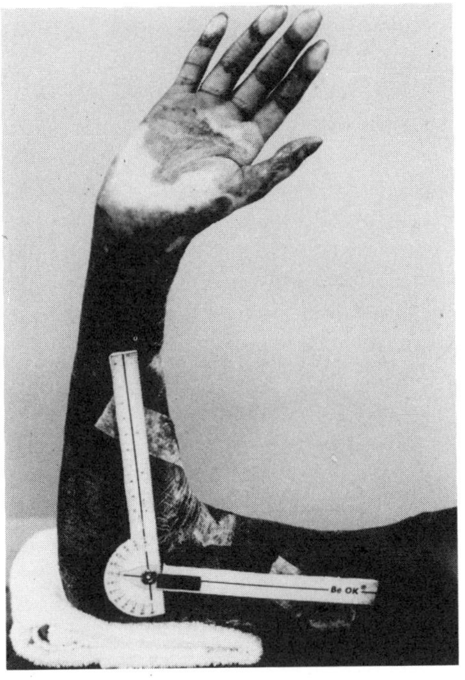

FIG 25–19.
Serial splinting is a technique used with active burn scar to modify joint contracture. This is an arm with a 90° contracture.

neutral position. The sole splint is a piece of low thermoplastic material conformed to the shape and contours of the volar surface of the foot (Fig 25–18). The sole plate is applied with a wide strap or with an elastic wrap over the toes to maintain extension. This splint may require padding to evenly distribute the pressure over the volar surface of the foot. The splint is not designed for use while the patient is ambulatory.

Serial splinting is a valuable technique for the burned child who has developed a burn scar contracture at the joint, and can modify the contracture quickly, provided it is caused by burn scar shortening and not by tendon shortening or soft tissue adhesions. Serial splinting simply refers to splinting with frequent revisions. This technique is most successful if the splint is conformed to the patient and applied with an elastic wrap, since the splint and pressure will work together to soften the burn scar contracture. The technique involves the fabrication of contoured splints that conform to the body part. In the case of an elbow or knee contracted in flexion, the splint is made to conform to the joint at the maximum extension and stretch that the scar will allow. Blanching of the skin is often noted when the skin is at maximum stretch. The child then wears the splint constantly, except for pressure checks and brief periods of exercise. The older child is instructed to try to extend the arm or leg away from the conformer. Generally, improvement will be noted in range of motion by the next day, and the splint is revised to fit the arm or leg with the maximum extension the scar contracture will allow. This process is repeated until the joint is in full extension (Figs 25–19 to 25–

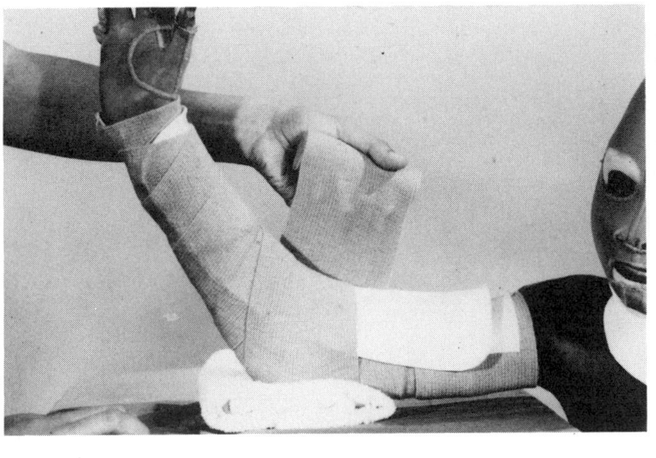

FIG 25–20.
The same area as shown in Figure 25–19 immediately after sustained stretch exercise, being fitted with a conforming splint applied with an elastic wrap.

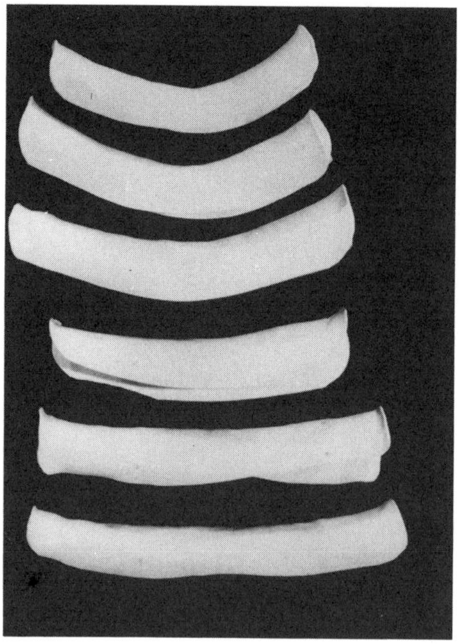

FIG 25–21.
Splints used on the patient shown in Figure 25–19 were revised daily until full extension was achieved.

22). A splinting schedule is then designed to maintain this position and an exercise and activity program initiated to obtain full range of motion. It is also possible to use serial splinting with the neck, wrist, axilla, and hand, with varying degrees of success. The ankle does not usually respond to serial splinting as described above, since the Achilles tendon is shortened. Heel cord shortening may respond to a shoe with a built-up heel that is gradually reduced in height so that the heel is slowly stretched by the weight of the body during ambulation.

Silicone has been used in conjunction with serial splinting to apply more even pressure to the burn scar. The silicone (Silastic) mitt has also been used to serially modify contractures of the child's hand.

Dynamic splinting is beneficial for patients with tendon shortening or soft tissue adhesions; however, it does not apply even pressure over burn scar. It must be used with caution, as it may cause friction or pressure over fragile skin. During the rehabilitation phase, dynamic splinting can be very valuable to provide a slow passive stretch to a body part for short periods of time. Small children may need to be supervised during the periods of splint wear, since the dynamic elements of the splint are easy to remove or position incorrectly.

PRESSURE

Hypertrophic burn scar formation is a common result of deep dermal burns and becomes observable 6 weeks to 3 months after the burn wounds have healed. One predictive factor is the length of time required for the burn wound to heal. Usually, hypertrophic scar does not form over wounds that have healed conservatively in less than 14 days. A high percentage of burn wounds that heal after 21 days will form hypertrophic burn scar.[7] The value of mechanical pressure techniques used to suppress hypertrophic scar formation

FIG 25–22.
Patient shown in Figure 25–19 with full area extension achieved by serial splinting in 14 days.

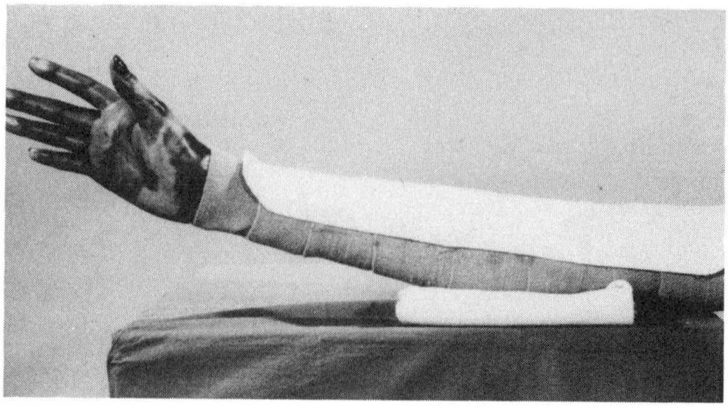

and obtain better cosmetic results are well accepted. Pressure is applied continuously to active burn scar until it matures approximately 12 to 18 months after healing. Pressure is removed from active burn scar for only short periods during the day to maintain cleanliness. However, controversy exists regarding how much pressure is required to suppress the raising of hypertrophic scar. The literature varies, recommending anywhere from 5 to 24 mm Hg of pressure.[1, 33] Tailored burn garments vary the amount of pressure applied to different body parts, ranging from as little as 5 mm Hg of pressure to the head and as high as 25 to 32 mm Hg of pressure to the ankles of the leg supports.[3, 5]

Currently, pressure is applied to burn scars in a variety of ways, including elastic wraps, tubular elastic, premade tubular elastic garments, and tailor-made burn garments. In addition, conforming splints can apply pressure. The advantage of elastic wraps is easy application, causing little friction to the patient's skin. This makes elastic wraps a pressure technique that can be used during the acute hospitalization period. The disadvantage of elastic wraps is that they can be applied too tightly or in an uneven manner, causing edema and impaired circulation. The family and staff must be trained before using this pressure technique. Elastic wraps apply adequate pressure to the extremities and may be used on children who are difficult to fit due to rapid growth or chronic wound problems. Elastic wraps can also benefit the patient without the financial resources to purchase expensive pressure techniques (Fig 25–23).

Tubular elastic bandage pressure can also be used as a temporary dressing during the acute hospitalization or before burn garments can be tolerated by the patient. Like elastic wraps, tubular elastic bandage is valuable in fitting the growing child and is an alternative pressure technique for patients who cannot afford tailor-made burn garments. Some patients tolerate or accept tubular elastic pres-

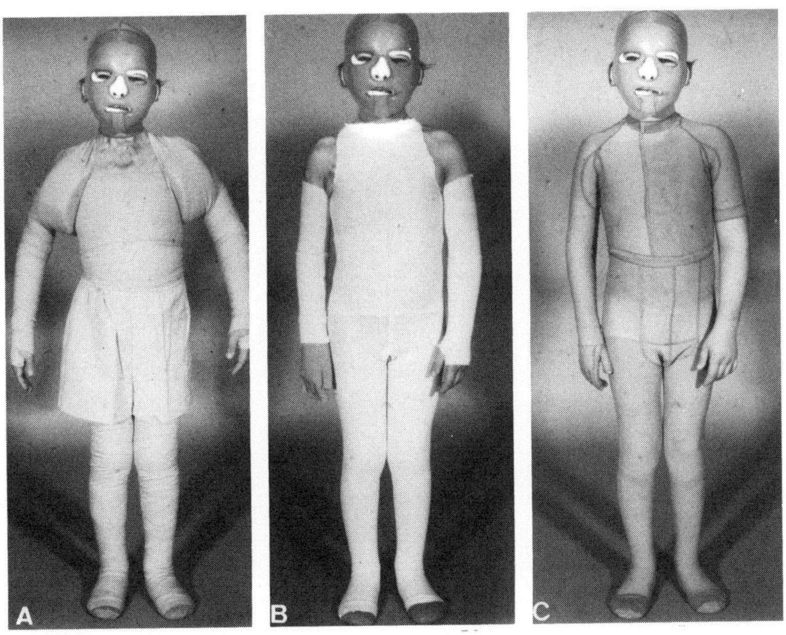

FIG 25–23.
Burn child demonstrating three separate types of pressure wrap techniques. **A,** elastic wrap bandage pressure. **B,** ready-made tubular elastic and tubular elastic garments. **C,** tailor-made garments (i.e., Jobst).

sure better than the tailor-made burn garments. Tubular elastic bandage has the advantage of easy application and cannot be applied too tightly if the patient is properly fitted[34] (see Fig 25–23).

Ready-made garments are commercially available and useful for applying pressure to burn scar. Generally, these garments are used until a tailor-made garment is fitted. Gloves, chin straps, vests, and leotards are available in various sizes. Currently, ready-made gloves are not available for the young child with less than a 6-in. palm circumference. Although ready-made chin straps for young children are not available either, most chin straps can be easily revised to fit the young child. Some therapists construct temporary garments for burn patients.[4]

Tailor-made burn garments (i.e., Jobst) are commercially sold by several companies (see Fig 25–23). These garments are engineered to apply adequate pressure to various body parts without impairing the circulation. Tailor-made garments are recommended for the cooperative patient whose skin is able to tolerate the pressure and application of the garments. Inserts of foam or silicone are applied under the pressure garment to increase or direct pressure to a specific body area. Inserts can be used over joint areas or areas of concavity over which the elastic garment spans. Inserts can be used over raised scars as well.

Pressure to the neck may partially be applied by the head garment or by a turtleneck attachment to the tailor-made vest. However, a neck splint is usually required to apply adequate pressure to the neck. Axilla pressure is difficult to obtain using only the burn garment. Figure-of-eight elastic-wrapped axilla pads are worn over the burn garment to achieve adequate pressure to the axilla region. To direct pressure to the concave area of the chest, pressure inserts are used over the sternum.

Pressure devices can also be used to prevent scar webbing between each of the fingers and the thumb. Burn scar webbing between the fingers is not only cosmetically deforming, but also functionally limits finger flexion. Webbing of the thumb space limits thumb abduction. The pressure glove is fitted down into web space. Slant inserts may improve the fit of the glove into the web spaces of the fingers. The simplest web-space insert is a foam square with two slits, which are drawn over the middle two fingers. As the glove is applied over the foam, the foam fits tightly into the web spaces (Fig 25–24). This style of web spacer can also be used to prevent webbing of the toes. It is possible to place foam into the thumb web space as well. Other materials used to prevent web contractures are worn under the glove and include low thermoplastic, silicone, or Otoform web spacers. It is possible to apply traction to the web spaces with rubber-band traction attached to a wrist strap and thermoplastic conformers inserted in the web space; however, skin breakdown may occur. Pressure applied with an elastic-wrap technique can be used until a glove can be tolerated.[32] Another pressure alternative is the use of a Coband wrap. Coband, a self-adherent elastic tape, is used to apply pressure to the hand, and is useful for decreasing hand edema. Coband is wrapped in a distal-to-proximal fashion, ap-

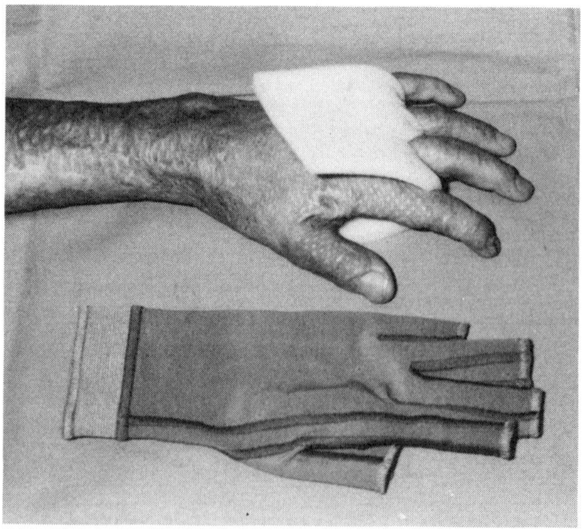

FIG 25–24.
A foam web spacer is effective in minimizing finger web space contracture when worn under a pressure glove.

plied cautiously to assure that it is not wrapped too tightly or is uneven. To prevent skin breakdown over fragile skin areas, a gauze dressing is applied under the Coband.

Pressure devices can be a valuable addition to pressure garments used on the lower extremity. Hip flexion contractures can benefit from a silicone or foam insert over the anterior hip region applied under pressure garments. High-top shoes or silicone boots can apply additional pressure to the ankle and dorsum of the feet.

The face can be grotesquely deformed by hypertrophic burn scar and contractures. Elastic garments span over the concavities of the face so pressure inserts and face masks have been designed especially for the face. The oldest method of applying directed pressure to the face is with a low thermoplastic splint fitted to the facial contours and applied with straps.[28] Two other styles of face mask are now accepted: the silicone face mask ap-

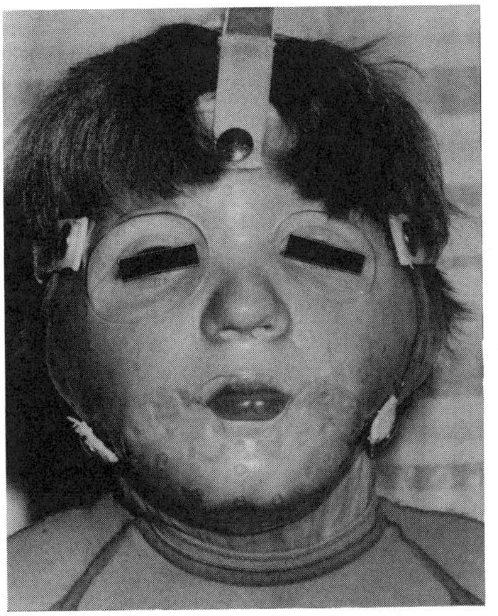

FIG 25–26.
Transparent face mask applied with straps.

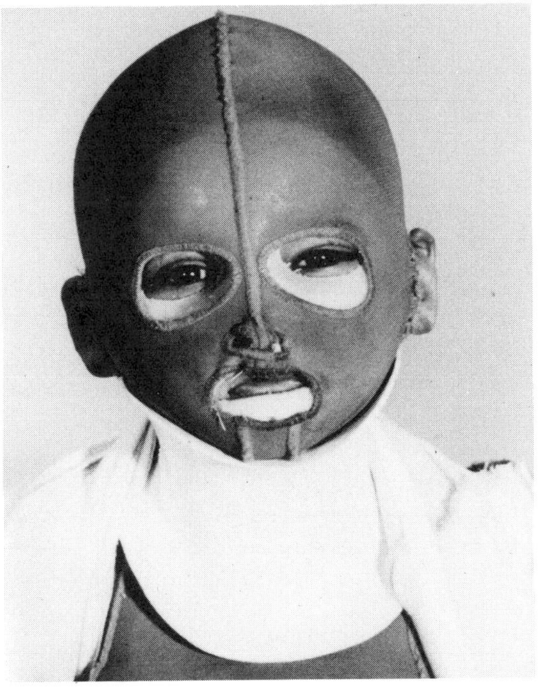

FIG 25–25.
Silicone conformer worn under a face mask pressure garment.

plied under a burn garment (Fig 25–25) and the transparent face mask (Fig 25–26) applied with straps.[27, 31] Both styles of face mask are fabricated using a positive mold of the face, and each style is reported to obtain good clinical results in the control of hypertrophic scar on the face. It has been reported by several authors that the patient's acceptance of the transparent face mask appears to be better than that of the silicone face mask, apparently due to the feeling that the transparent face mask is esthetically more pleasing. Some parents of young children have been noted to prefer the wearing of the softer silicone material. This may be because the silicone face mask applied under a burn garment is more difficult for young children to remove.

Face masks which apply pressure must be used with caution in small children. Head circumference measurements should be obtained at frequent intervals and graphed. Delays in head growth must be detected early. Caution is recommended for children wearing chin straps or face masks regarding the uncommon complication of sleep apnea.[42]

Young children may fear the loss of parental love because their appearance is changed when wearing a face mask. The parents' verbal and nonverbal communication will affect the child's response to the rehabilitation equipment. Verbal expressions of love by the parents are reassuring to the child. Young children may have difficulty understanding the appearance change caused by the face mask. Play activities can be used to prepare the child for this change in appearance. Play may consist of family members putting on and taking off a face mask in the child's presence and explaining to the child that they are the same person with or without a face mask on. Doll and puppet play can also be used to ease the child's apprehension. Older children often fear peer response to the splints, garments, burn scar, and, especially, the face mask. Educating the child to the purpose and importance of rehabilitation equipment can be beneficial. Most children over the age of 6 years will understand long-term results. A program that introduces the child back to their classmates and school can minimize peer rejection. The program should explain the burn, garment, and splints, and answer the children's questions.

Dry skin is a common problem in burn patients and a skin lubricant should be used over healed skin. Lubricating the skin may decrease the itching of the burn scar. Patients are instructed to avoid exposure to the sun during the active phase of scar formation, as their skin will sunburn quickly and this can cause a discoloration of the scar. The patient should wear a sunblock under the pressure garments if expected to be in the sun for long periods of time.

Some children enjoy appliqués, embroidery, or plastic motifs on their burn garments.[24] These can be used as long as they do not interfere with the stretch of the garment or irritate the skin.

RECONSTRUCTIVE SURGERY

During reconstructive surgery the burn patient may require splints postsurgery for positioning and immobilization and to promote graft adherence. Split-thickness skin grafts and, to a lesser extent, full-thickness skin grafts, may contract following reconstructive surgical procedures. Once the graft is healed, splinting is generally used for nightwear only. Patients with neck grafts may require continuous splinting that is removed only for bath, exercise, and meals. Pressure techniques can be used to prevent hypertrophic scar from forming at the graft's edges.

ACTIVITIES OF DAILY LIVING

As the medical status of the child permits, age-appropriate activities of daily living are encouraged by the burn team. The parents are instructed in the importance of their child's independence in activities of daily living, and their support is elicited. Feeding, grooming, and toilet skills are evaluated so that assistance devices and training can be provided according to the patient's needs. Assistance devices are gradually discontinued or revised as the child's functional ability improves. Adaptive clothing may be necessary for independent performance of toilet skills, which are important to the school-aged child. The child's functional ability in performing activities of daily living is followed until the child gains age-appropriate independence.

DEVELOPMENT

A significant number of young children are burned as a result of child abuse or neglect and may have unrecognized developmental delays.

The therapist must evaluate the developmental history provided by the parent and observe the child's behavior during the hospitalization. Since manifested delays can be due to regression from pain, recent physical trauma, or the sudden hospitalization, the patient is only screened for possible delay. If a possible developmental delay is observed, the child is referred for further developmental testing to be done after the hospital discharge.

Play activity is encouraged for all hospitalized children, since not only is play a form of exercise, but also a way many children can express their feelings. Play also provides socialization with other children.

DISCHARGE PLANNING

Although rehabilitation is initiated early in the hospitalization, treatment continues after the child's hospital discharge. The therapist will continue to see the child on an outpatient basis or will refer the family for rehabilitation services that are available locally. However, for optimal results, a large part of the rehabilitation program must take place in the child's home. The family needs to have both the knowledge and skill to effectively use positioning, splinting, pressure, performing activities of daily living, exercise, and developmental play with their burned child.

Educating the family begins during the early hospitalization when the purpose of rehabilitation treatments are explained to the family. The problems of hypertrophic scarring and skin contracture are difficult for most people to conceptualize. It is therefore recommended that the family see a slide program on hypertrophic scar and skin contracture with an explanation of the purpose of positioning, splinting, pressure, and exercise in minimizing the cosmetic and functional deformity. The therapist must develop a home program with the family and child that is effective and realistic for the family to accomplish. The home care program is presented verbally and a written copy given to the family. Since most families are stressed during the child's hospitalization, repetition of information may be necessary. The family must also begin to develop skills, including the application of splint and pressure, as well as encourage exercise and activities of daily living. To develop skill, the family will need to participate actively in the child's care before discharge. The family is given a hospital telephone number for use if they have questions concerning the child's care after discharge.

REFERENCES

1. Baur PS: The healing of burn wounds. *Clin Plast Surg* 1977; 4:389–407.
2. Bennett GK, Carter B: Fixed dental appliances in the treatment of electrical burns to the commissure, abstract 55. 16th annual meeting of the American Burn Association, 1984.
3. Blair KL: *Prevention and Control of Hypertrophic Scarring and Contractures by the Application of the Custom-made Jobskin Pressure Garments.* Toledo, Jobst Institute, 1977.
4. Bruster JM, Pullium G: Gradient pressure. *Am J Occup Ther* 1983; 37:485–488.
5. Cheng JCY, et al: Pressure therapy in the treatment of post-burn hypertrophic scar—a critical look into its usefulness and fallacies by pressure monitoring. *Burns Incl Therm Inj* 1984; 10:154–163.
6. Coleleugh RG, Ryan JE: Splinting electrical burns of the mouth in children. *Plast Reconstr Surg* 1976; 58:239–241.
7. Deitch EA, et al: Hypertrophic burn scars: Analysis of variables. *J Trauma* 1983; 23:895–898.
8. Denton BG, Shaw SE: Mouth conformer for prevention and correction of burn scar contracture. *Phys Ther* 1976; 56:683–688.
9. Evans EB: Preservation and restoration of joint function in patients with severe burns. *JAMA* 1968; 204:91–96.
10. Fader P: A self-instructional package: Neck conformer. *J Burn Care Rehabil* 1985; 6:124–127.
11. Flesch P: Casting the young and the restless, abstract 120. 17th annual meeting of the American Burn Association, 1985.
12. Fowler D: A neck extension pillow for the burn patient. *Occup Ther*, vol 261, August 1981.
13. Garcia-Velasco M, et al: Compression treatment of hypertrophic scars in burn children. *Can J Surg* 1978; 21:450–452.
14. Gorham SA: A mouth splint for burn microstomia. *Am J Occup Ther* 1977; 31:105–106.
15. Hartford CE, et al: An appliance to prevent and treat microstomia from burns. *J Trauma* 1975; 15:356–360.
16. Helm P: Neuromuscular considerations, in Fisher S, Helm P (eds): *Comprehensive Rehabilitation of Burns.* Baltimore, Williams & Wilkins, 1984, pp 235–241.
17. Johnson C, et al: *Burn Management.* New York, Raven Press, 1981.
18. Kilgore ES, Graham WP (eds): *The Hand: Surgical and Nonsurgical Management (Tendons).* Philadelphia, Lea & Febiger, 1977.

19. Kilulu M, Von Prince MP, et al: Application of fingernail hooks in splinting of burned hands. *Am J Occup Ther* 1970; 24:556–559.
20. Klinzing DR, Klinzing DG: *The Hospitalized Child: Communication Techniques for Health Personnel.* Englewood Cliffs, NJ, Prentice-Hall Inc, 1977.
21. Larson DL, et al: Repair of the boutonniere deformity of the burned hand. *J Trauma* 1970; 10:481–487.
22. MacDonald LB, et al: The papoose: Device for positioning the burn child's axilla. *J Burn Care Rehabil* 1985; 6:61–63.
23. Mallick M, Carr J: *Manual on Management of the Burn Patient.* Pittsburg, Hamarville Rehabilitation Center, 1982.
24. McLean NR, Warren EA: A simple device to encourage the unwilling child to wear a pressure garment. *Br J Plast Surg* 1983; 36:529–580.
25. Nicosia JE, Petro J: *Manual of Burn Care.* New York, Raven Press, 1983.
26. Parent L: Burns, in Trombly CA (ed): *Occupational Therapy for Physical Dysfunction,* ed 2. Baltimore, Williams & Wilkins, 1983, pp 399–408.
27. Parks D, et al: Late problems in burns. *Clin Plast Surg* 1977; 4:547–560.
28. Petersen P: A conformer for the reduction of facial contractures: A preliminary report. *Am J Occup Ther* 1977; 31:101–104.
29. Reardon J: Occupational therapy treatment of the patient with thermally injured upper extremity, in Salisbury RE, Pruitt BA (eds): *Burns of the Upper Extremity,* Major Problems in Clinical Surgery Series. Philadelphia, WB Saunders, 1976, vol 19, pp 227–247.
30. Rivers E: A compression hand wrap. *J Burn Care Rehabil* 1984; 5:291–293.
31. Rivers E: The transparent face mask. *Am J Occup Ther* 1979; 33:100–113.
32. Rivers E, et al: Decreasing axillary releases after burn healing: A result of self-directed exercise with an overhead walker, abstract 115. 16th annual meeting of the American Burn Association, 1984.
33. Robertson JC, et al: Pressure therapy for hypertrophic scarring: Preliminary communication. *J Br Soc Med* 1980; 73:348–354.
34. Rose MP, Deitch FA: The effective use of a tubular compression bandage, Tubigrip, for burn scar therapy in the growing child. *J Burn Care Rehabil* 1983; 4:197–201.
35. Sandel E, et al: Finger pulp hooks—a method of positioning, abstract 114. 15th annual meeting of the American Burn Association, 1983.
36. Smith JM, Smith DEP: *Child Management: A Program for Parents and Teachers.* Champaign, Il, Research Press Co, 1976.
37. Tanigawa MC, et al: The burned hand: A physical therapy protocol. *Phys Ther* 1974; 54:953–958.
38. Willis BA, et al: Positioning and splinting the burned patient. *Heart Lung* 1973; 2:696–700.
39. Willis BA: The use of orthoplast isoprene splints in the treatment of the acutely burned child: A preliminary report. *Am J Occup Ther* 1969; 23:57–61.
40. Wright P: Fundamentals of acute burn care and physical therapy management. *Phys Ther* 1984; 64:1217–1231.
41. Zuker RM, Thomson HG: Effective management of deep scald burns to the feet. *J Burn Care Rehabil* 1984; 5:288–290.
42. Zuker RM, et al: Obstructive sleep apnea following burns to the face and neck, abstract 126. 17th annual meeting of the American Burn Association, 1985.

26 / Psychosocial Care of the Severely Burned Child

MARY KNUDSON COOPER, Ph.D., L.P.C.
CYNTHIA M. THOMAS, A.C.S.W., C.S.W.

Hospitalization for a severe burn injury is one of the most traumatic types of hospitalizations a child can experience. A child who is burned has just undergone a terrifying and painful experience. Emergency hospitalization for a burn injury and the subsequent treatment are also terrifying and painful. In addition, the child is suddenly separated from his familiar environment and is placed in a strange, frightening place where his parents are no longer in control and where he is being hurt by strangers. Hospitalization for a burn injury is relatively long, averaging about 30 days, and often extends over several months. During this time the child is necessarily subjected to many painful procedures, such as daily tankings, debridement of dead tissue, dressing changes, blood tests, and numerous surgical procedures. It is also necessary to keep the burn patient moving, when every movement hurts, to maintain respiratory function and joint flexibility. Skin grafting procedures, on the other hand, require that the child be immobilized for up to 10 days, often in uncomfortable positions.

Most of the emphasis in burn treatment traditionally has focused on the physical aspects of care, on survival, and on maintaining optimal physical functioning after the burn injury. Although the physical aspects of a burn injury are critically important, the psychosocial impact of a burn is equally so. Both of these aspects must be taken into account during treatment for the burned child to return to society as a functional human being.

THE PSYCHOSOCIAL CONTEXT

Children who are burned are individuals who are members of families with a particular socioeconomic and cultural background. They must function in the context of these social relationships when they return home. For this reason, it is important to understand the child's psychosocial environment before the burn and during hospitalization, to plan adequately for in-hospital care and follow-up care postdischarge.

A childhood burn injury must be viewed as a crisis for the child and his family. It is a sudden, traumatic change that alters the life of the victim and those closest to him. It is usually an experience that requires new coping skills and leaves both the child and the family emotionally vulnerable.

Research into the effects of hospitalization on children has documented the emotional impact of this experience.[43, 52, 78, 114, 137, 138, 146] Emotional responses such as separation anxiety, regression, anger, fear, and depression are commonly described.

The behaviors seen in burned children are basically similar to those seen with other types of hospitalizations, but tend to be more extreme.[6, 22, 30, 53, 84, 144] Children of all ages who have a relatively large burn (25% of the total body surface or more) commonly manifest extreme anxiety and pain, including body tenseness, shivering, and rhythmic movements.[139] They sometimes grind their teeth or bite their lips or the insides of their mouth raw, especially during bouts of sepsis.

Although " burn psychosis," characterized by a confused sensorium and irrational thought patterns, is more commonly seen in adults than children, it is common in adolescents and is also seen in younger children, especially during septic episodes. Regression is universal among hospitalized children, but is often exteme in burn patients (both children and adult). A weaned child will demand a bottle, and a toilet-trained child will defecate in bed instead of calling the nurse for a bedpan. The regression of young children, although they often become more dependent and demanding, is not nearly as striking as it is in the adolescent. It has been said, in fact, that *all* burn patients regress to a 2-year-old's level, including adults.

Although burn patients are usually conscious and lucid during much of their hospital course, their cognitive processes seem to regress. An adolescent, for instance, may respond to a request with behavior typical of a 2-year-old, even though his mother may say that he was a relatively mature, responsible adolescent before the injury. In talking to burned children after recovery regarding incidents during acute hospitalization, they often do not remember the incident and say that they "couldn't have acted like that."

Several factors can account for the relatively extreme response to burns: (1) the suddenness of the transition from the family to hospital environment, (2) the severity of the physical trauma and required treatment, (3) extreme pain, and (4) the relatively long hospitalization.

One of the most upsetting aspects of hospitalization for a burned child is that the parents, who have been a source of protection and support, are no longer in control. Even with liberal visiting hours, children of all ages fear abandonment. This fear is particularly evident in infants and young children, but can be seen even in adolescents, due to the regression that commonly accompanies hospitalization.[71]

Developmental Differences

Studies of response to hospitalization have recognized that a child's developmental stage is related to differences in response.[155] For infants and toddlers, separation anxiety is particularly acute. They are fearful and withdrawn and can become extremely agitated when their parents leave. In extreme cases, infants in particular can withdraw into a state of emotional shock in which they are unresponsive to pain, which is difficult to distinguish from the behavior of an abused child.[56, 67, 76, 110]

School-aged children (6 to 12 years) who suffer burns are predominantly boys.[17, 73, 86, 87, 104, 134] Although these children manifest some separation anxiety, the main concern in this age group is the restriction of behavior and activity. Often, they become agitated, angry, and manipulative. Although school-aged children have a better understanding of what is happening to them than do younger children, they often have distorted ideas about the accident and why the painful treatment procedures are being done.

Adolescents tend to respond to a burn injury as an adult. The most important issue for this age group is loss of control. The most significant aspects of self-esteem to adolescents (or adults) is their loss of control over their life.[71, 136] In a burn unit, the patient is almost totally out of control. He is often dependent on others to feed him and to help him with personal bodily functions. He is powerless to prevent the staff from carrying out necessary treatment procedures and is reduced to being as dependent as a young child.

This dependency and feeling of powerlessness are probably responsible for the extreme regression often seen in adolescent (and often adult) burn patients. Such patients often become unrealistic and demanding and throw temper tantrums. They are more likely to have sleep disturbances and disorientation, and seem to be more sensitive to pain. They

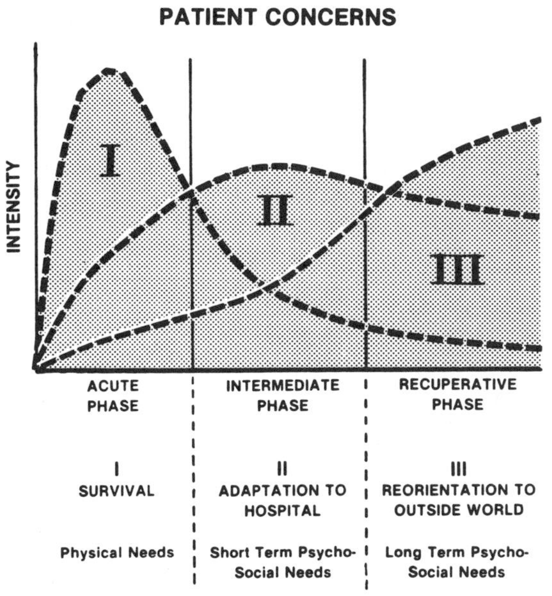

FIG 26–1.
Phases of response and adaptation to acute hospitalization in burned patients.

can become manipulative and, because of their size, be difficult to handle.

In addition, they are also acutely aware of their body image and very concerned about acceptance by peers. They are very likely to become depressed, especially when nearing discharge from acute care, when they must begin to think about returning to the outside world.

PHASES OF ADAPTATION

A number of articles on the psychologic response to burns have recognized phases of response and adaptation to acute hospitalization for burns.[64, 75, 101, 165] Three phases have generally been recognized during acute hospitalization, which can be summarized as (1) the acute phase, (2) the intermediate phase, and (3) the recuperative phase. An additional phase, called the resocialization phase, can be added; this refers to the adjustment process after discharge. The first three phases can be related to patient concerns during hospitalization, as shown in Figure 26–1.

The Acute Phase

The acute phase includes the period immediately following the burn accident and can last several weeks. It is the critical medical phase, during which concern with survival is paramount. Medical complications such as shock, electrolyte imbalances, edema, and infection, which are common in severe burns, can cause changes in the patient's sensorium. Symptoms include confusion, delirium, hyperactivity, and sleep disturbances, which are often associated with organic brain syndrome. The patient is usually less concerned with the long-term implications of the injury than with survival, although adolescents may be acutely aware of the former as well.

The Intermediate Phase

The intermediate phase begins when the patient's initial condition is stabilized, and can last from several weeks to several months, depending on the extent of the injury and subsequent complications. During this phase, the child is fully conscious and aware of what is going on around him. He is adapting to the hospital routine and is acutely aware of short-term psychosocial needs, such as scheduling of treatments and family visiting. Behavioral management often becomes a problem during this phase.

The Recuperative Phase

The recuperative phase includes the latter part of the hospital stay and the early post-hospitalization period. The latter part of acute hospitalization is a period of initial recuperation, which consists largely of physical therapy and preparation for discharge. At this time, the child (excluding infants and young preschool children) usually becomes very concerned about facing the outside world. Because of changes in the body due to disfigurement and disability, there is often a period of considerable anxiety as the child begins the process of resuming life outside the hospital.

The Resocialization Phase

The resocialization phase ideally begins during the last part of acute hospitalization, if opportunities are provided for the child to begin interacting with other persons in and outside the hospital. This phase is most acute during the first year after discharge when the child often must wear pressure garments, splints, and braces to prevent contractures across joints and severe disfigurement.[46, 72, 125] This phase may last for several years, however, and often involves reconstructive plastic surgery to restore optimum function and appearance.

PSYCHOSOCIAL CARE

The Family as the Unit of Treatment

In providing emotional care for a child, it is useful to regard both the child and the family as the object of treatment.[101] The child and the family are experiencing many of the same emotions. Since the child's parents are responsible for the child's general well-being, they also need emotional support.

Parents and other family members are under considerable emotional stress, which makes it difficult for them to provide optimal emotional support to the child. It is common for parents to have difficulties sleeping and eating. Previous physical problems that are stress related, such as hypertension, ulcers, migraine headaches, asthma, and diabetes, are often aggravated by the added stress.

Although the need for emotional support from parents (or other family members) is usually met by having someone visit or stay with the child, this can be a further source of stress for the family. Normal family functioning is disrupted when one or both parents spend a lot of time at the hospital or leave home to be with a child who is being treated at a large burn center distant from the home community. If there are other children in the family, they are often without a mother or are farmed out to other relatives or friends. The siblings frequently are emotionally upset by the accident and the separation, and may have nightmares or behavior problems of their own.

The financial stress of a burn injury is also substantial. The cost of care in a specialized burn facility averages more than $1,000 per day. Even with insurance, this places a heavy drain on the family's financial resources, especially if both parents need to work to provide for the family.

One of the main sources of emotional stress for parents and other family members is guilt. *All* parents feel guilty about the burn accident, whether they were actually involved or not. They feel that somehow they have failed in their role as protector of their child. They are going through a process of imagining what they could have done, or not done, that could have prevented the accident. Having to observe their child in pain and being powerless to stop it, accompanied by the knowledge that their child will be permanently disfigured and possibly disabled, adds to the guilt.

The Role of the Burn Team in Psychosocial Care

The psychosocial care of the burned child is the responsibility of the burn team as a whole, including physicians, nurses, paramedical personnel, and social work and mental health specialists. Most burn facilities have at least part-time support from social worker and psychiatric or psychological support, but most do not have full-time professionals to provide these services. Children's hospitals or specialized burn facilities for children usually have schoolteachers and child life or recreational specialists as well. Hospital chaplains are also available at most hospitals.

Often, mental health and social work personnel are thought of as a luxury and not as necessary personnel. From the authors' experience in a specialized regional burn center for children and a children's intensive care unit (ICU) in a private hospital associated with a university, this type of support is essential in the care of burned children. Most social work and mental health specialists who are assigned part-time to a burn facility are overwhelmed and must necessarily limit their interventions to what many term "Band-Aid" support.[3] The seriousness of the trauma and the long hospitalization, with subsequent follow-up care and reconstructive procedures, require complicated planning and coordination and are very time consuming. Because of the high incidence of suspected abuse and neglect among burned children (ranging from 15% to 20% in children 5 years and under), considerable time must be spent with these families and appropriate referral agencies.[4, 56, 69, 77, 103, 110, 122] Even more competent families require social and emotional support from professionals because of the serious, long-term implications of the injury.

One of the most important functions that social work and mental health professionals can perform is to provide information to the other members of the burn team regarding the psychosocial needs of the burned child and his family. The types of information that are provided include:

1. Information about the child's family and home environment (usually gathered by the social work staff).
2. Information about the psychosocial impact of a traumatic injury on a child and family, with special attention to the child's developmental stage and preburn adjustment.
3. Consultation regarding psychiatric medication and behavioral management of the child and family.
4. Information relevant to coordination of discharge planning.

ACUTE PHASE

If all members of the burn team understand what type of behavior to expect, based on knowledge of the emotional impact of trauma, and have information about the particular characteristics of the child and family, it is much easier to assess their behavior and to recognize when special interventions are necessary. During the acute phase, for example, the main concern of the family as well as the child is survival. Parents are usually very distraught and often do not really hear what they are told, especially regarding permanent disfigurement. Their role at this early stage is important, however, because what the burned child needs most at this time is emotional sustenance and support. This can be provided by the nursing staff and other members of the burn team as well, but the parents' mere presence is probably more reassuring to the child than anything else.

Visiting hours can be a problem with a critically burned patient. Burns in children are sometimes treated in ICUs, which may intensify the child's fear and separation anxiety if parents cannot visit for more than a few minutes at a time. It is also very stressful for parents to be allowed to see their child only for short periods when they are in a strange and technically complex environment and where their child is obviously frightened and in pain.[164]

Many burn units also practice strict isolation procedures to prevent infection, the main cause of death in burns. Parents are sometimes not allowed to hold or even touch their children, which increases their anxiety and guilt. An unpublished study conducted in 1973 at the Shriners Burn Institute in Galveston indicated that there was no significant difference in the rate of infection when strict isolation procedures were followed and when staff and visitors were not required to wear gowns and masks, but thorough hand-washing procedures were observed.[93] Most burn facilities now allow parents to touch their children and to hold babies, which is important in providing emotional sustenance.[118]

In approximately the past 5 years, a number of burn facilities, particularly those located in children's hospitals, have allowed rooming-in and/or unlimited visiting hours. These options, which would not have been considered 10 years ago, have been found to be very successful, especially when the parents have been allowed to assist in the child's treatment.[84] This type of arrangement requires coordinated teamwork within the burn team regarding communication with the child's family. When good communication is maintained, it has been found that the parents and the child are more cooperative, less anxious, and have a better understanding of treatment procedures and the process of recovery. Both nurses and physicians comment that parents can be encouraged to take care of themselves by resting and leaving the burn unit when necessary, and that parents do not become overwhelmed and exhausted, as they often do when they must wait in hallways and waiting rooms.

INTERMEDIATE PHASE

During the intermediate phase, when concern with survival is not as acute, both the patient and the family tend to focus on short-term psychosocial needs. They are adapting to the hospital environment and learning its rules. During this phase, both children and parents are very sensitive to changes in rules and schedules. They may become upset, for instance, if the usual time for tubbing is changed, or if the physician changes his mind about the need for surgery. Even something as simple as ordering chocolate milk and getting white milk on the food tray can precipitate an emotional outburst. Burn patients and their families are emotionally labile at this time, and often express anger, grief, depression, and anxiety over seemingly minor things. Although this can be upsetting to the staff, both the child and the family members sometimes must ventilate their emotions. For children, this usually takes place on the unit and may involve family members as well. Giving them privacy to do this, without jeopardizing the child's physical condition, is important, particularly if the child must be told that a family member or friend has died in the burn accident.

It is helpful to parents if they can also express their emotions away from the burn unit; for this they should have access to a mental health professional. Group meetings with other parents are also very helpful in allowing the parents to support each other by sharing their experiences and feelings while they gain information about burn treatment and the long-term implications of a serious burn injury.[2, 27, 108] If the child is being treated in the locality where he lives, social and emotional support can be provided by outpatient support groups or by a network of recovered burned children and their families. When families must travel from a distance to be with their child, a residential facility is sometimes provided by the hospital or a private source, such as the Ronald McDonald Houses, which allows parents of hospitalized children to provide each other support while staying close to their child.

Although the opportunity to ventilate feelings should be provided, it is very important that the staff, particularly the nursing staff, provide a consistent structure for treatment procedures and scheduling. Not that schedules can't be changed, but both the child and family are less anxious if they know what is being done and why. They both require structure and consistency in their new environment and they are reassured when they find it.

The physician should inform the family regularly about the child's condition. Often, he must repeat the same thing several times because parents may not really hear what is being said the first time. The uncertainties inherent in burn treatment (e.g., the need for and timing of surgical procedures, the length of hospitalization) cause parents continual anxiety. Regular information from the physician and reinforcement from the nursing and paramedical staff helps to ease this anxiety and builds trust in the staff's ability. Since almost all of the treatment procedures for a burn injury are painful, it is especially important for the burned child and family to understand why treatments are being done. Children also need to know what to expect. Even young children can understand if procedures are explained in simple terms. Play therapy with dolls and puppets has been found to be very effective in reducing anxiety in children facing surgery, including burn patients.[97, 119, 157]

It is during the intermediate phase that most of the behavioral problems arise on the burn ward. Young children, including school-aged children, often have distorted ideas about the burn accident and about treatment procedures and may view the treatment as punishment.[15] Since nurses are usually the ones who must administer the painful treatment procedures, they are often seen by both the child and the family as "punishers." A natural resentment can develop between nurses and parents, especially if the nurses are viewed as having taken over the care of the child. The burned child can sense the parents' loss of control and often shows anger and resentment toward both the nurses and parents, intensifying the resentment between them. This can become particularly acute if the parent is suspected of neglecting or abusing the child, and is thus directly responsible for the child's condition.

This tension is best minimized through communication, particularly about the necessity and benefit of treatment procedures and unit policies. Tender loving care (TLC) is also important. When nurses and other medical personnel can understand the parent's anxiety and emotional lability without taking it personally, and show that they care about the child, the family will show more understanding and appreciation in return. Parental involvement in the care of the child also makes the parents understand how difficult the care actually is and will help them to be more understanding of the persons who must administer it.

If serious problems develop between medical personnel and the burned child or the family, a mental health professional or another member of the burn team who is skilled in this type of interaction can act as a mediator to help restore the balance.

Sometimes a mental health professional is required to help set up a behavioral management program in which the entire burn team participates. A number of studies have revealed that behavior modification is helpful during this phase.[147, 149, 163, 168] Since regressive behavior is common during this phase, it is important for staff and parents to understand that regression is normal. Although it is important to reinforce mature behavior that is consistent with the child's developmental stage, it is unrealistic to expect it all of the time. Often the child responds better when his regressive needs are met, for instance, by touching and reassurance that may seem more appropriate for a much younger child.

The management of pain often becomes a problem during the intermediate phase, since burn patients are usually fully conscious and alert at this time and very aware of their pain. In terms of the commonly accepted distinction between acute and chronic pain,[152] the pain from a severe burn injury is acute or "responsive" pain,[51] which is the direct response to tissue damage. With reference to the descriptive classifications of pain,[116, 117, 129] a burn injury causes extremely intense thermal pain. The temporal, spatial, and affective aspects of burn pain vary depending on the type of burn, the duration of treatment required, and the mental state of the patient. The pain is usually most intense when the burn patient is manipulated or moved, and is excruciating when dressings that stick to the wound are removed or when the wound is debrided.

There is probably a difference in the intensity and perhaps the type of pain in second- and third-degree burns. In second-degree burns only the outer epidermal and part of the dermal layers of the skin are destroyed, leaving the nerve endings in the deeper dermal layers intact. Second-degree burns are described by patients as "burning" continuously, not just when the patient is moved or manipulated. One explanation for this continuous burning pain is that bradykinin, a peptide implicated in continuing pain, is released after tissue damage.[70, 98]

A third-degree burn that destroys all layers

of the skin is commonly thought of by medical personnel as not painful, since all the nerve endings in the skin are destroyed. Although it is true that a burn patient does not feel the pain of a pinprick applied to the dead tissue (eschar), third-degree burns do hurt. When the dead tissue covering a third-degree wound is removed and the wound is exposed to air or is manipulated, the pain is excruciating. Even without a physiological explanation such as bradykinin release to account for the pain, the activation of the nerves around the periphery of the burn, which are still intact, is sufficient to cause extreme pain. From the personal experience of one of the authors as a burn patient, and from many years of working with burn patients, it is clear that pain from a burn injury, whether it is a second- or third-degree injury, is often excruciating, overwhelming, and unbearable.

The literature on pain is replete with references to the multidimensional nature of pain. The primary distinction is between "sensory pain," caused by tissue damage, and "suffering," which is a complex process involving the individual's response to pain, including mental anguish.[70, 99, 151, 158]

Pain from a severe burn, like any other pain, has a large component of suffering. There is no question of "psychogenic" vs. "physical" pain. Tissue damage is the primary component of a burn injury. Although there have been no studies in the literature to date on the relationships between the extent of the wound and the perception of pain in burn injuries, the general literature on pain is full of examples of the lack of a consistent relationship between these two aspects of pain[11, 162, 167] as well as cultural, age, and sex differences in the expression of pain.[32, 33, 55, 60, 115, 148, 152, 153] Pain appears to be a very individualistic phenomenon, which makes experimental studies of various types of treatment difficult, unless the patient acts as his own control.

Interestingly enough, medical personnel who work with burns consistently underestimate the severity of burn pain when compared to patients' ratings.[66, 128] It is also commonly accepted by most medical personnel that children, especially babies, do not feel pain in the same way as do adults and adolescents. Burned children do express extreme pain behavior during treatment procedures, but appear to be able to put it out of their minds and recover faster than do adults. Perhaps differences in cognitive development are responsible for the ability of adolescents and adults to anticipate pain and worry more about it. They are also more aware of what has happened to them, both in terms of the reality of the hospitalization and the significance of their injury. No one really knows how babies and young children experience pain; however, and it seems unrealistic to assume that they do not actually *feel* as much pain as adolescents and adults.[45, 159]

Pain control in burns consists of several treatment modalities, including medication, various types of relaxation therapy, and hypnosis. A recent survey of 93 burn facilities in the United States found that there was considerable variation in the types and extent of use of medication for pain.[127] Morphine and morphine derivatives, including methadone, were used by two thirds of the units for painful treatment procedures such as tubbing and debridement,[26, 120] separately and in combination with mood-altering drugs.[9, 10] About half of the units used psychotropic drugs such as diazepam (Valium), hydroxyzine (Vistaril), chlorpromazine (Thorazine), and chlordiazepoxide (Librium) for debridement. Subanesthetic doses of ketamine and self-administered nitrous oxide have also been successfully used to produce an amnesia for painful procedures.[44, 50, 150]

When adults were compared with children, Perry and Heidrich[127] found that children were more likely to receive no pain medication. Seventeen percent of the facilities surveyed said they would not medicate the 3-year-old child described in the hypothetical example used in the questionnaire, which seems to support the contention that children tend to be undermedicated for acute pain.[45, 112]

Relaxation therapy and biofeedback are

specific techniques that have been used successfully to reduce pain and anxiety in burns.[39, 83, 105, 161] Hypnosis has also been found to be helpful for both adults and children.[12, 38, 40, 65, 95, 111, 141, 160]

Some differences in the effectiveness of hypnosis have been noted between adults and children. Schafer,[141] in his study of 20 burn victims, found that children were less successful in achieving hypnotic analgesia and in learning autohypnosis. Wakeman and Kaplan,[160] however, found that children 7 to 18 years old were more successful than adults in the use of hypnosis, and requested significantly less pain medication than adults. Bernstein[12] also found that hypnosis was successful on a pediatric burn unit and stated that it is particularly successful in reaching isolated and depressed children.

It is generally recognized that hypnosis is effective with children.[36, 70, 123] It has been used successfully even with infants and preschool children.[54] Many authors suggest that children are more susceptible to entering a trance state because their stage of cognitive development allows more fantasy than is common among adults, and because they are less fearful of losing control.

The experience of one of the authors with relaxation therapy and hypnosis has indicated that the key to their effectiveness is the establishment of good rapport.[81, 82] Since burn patients are highly motivated to try anything that will help in pain control, it is usually effective if a relationship of trust is established. The most common reason for an adult to refuse hypnosis or to have little success is that he is afraid someone will "take over his mind." The most common reason for lack of success in children is that they are sometimes unwilling to give up types of behavior that they have utilized to cope with pain, such as increased body tension and the use of rhythmic movements or sounds. These may indeed be ways of achieving a trance state by blocking out the painful stimuli, but they do not appear to reduce the expression of anxiety and pain.

Several studies have combined either medication or some type of relaxation therapy with behavioral contracting[149] and "stress inoculation techniques," and found them effective in reducing negative behavior and the expression of anxiety and pain.[47, 163]

It is the authors' contention that more attention should be paid to systematic pain control programs in burn treatment of both adults and children and that effective pain control is a moral as well as a practical responsibility in burn care. Effective techniques that do not compromise the recovery process are available. Simple relaxation techniques can be taught to nursing and paramedical staff and do not require a full-time professional. This, in addition to the selective use of medication for painful procedures such as tanking and debridement, makes medical care more comfortable to give as well as to receive. In addition, a systematic program of pain control gives the patients and their families, as well as the staff, more control over the most stressful aspects of burn care.

RECUPERATIVE PHASE

During the recuperative phase, before the child is discharged from the hospital, the child and family are concerned primarily about returning to the outside world. Both are concerned about the child's appearance and physical functioning. They are also concerned about explaining things to relatives and friends and about returning to school. Anxiety about returning to school and acceptance by peers is especially intense for adolescents, since this is a time when they are acutely aware of their bodies, their relationships with peers, and their developing sexual identity.

Coordinated discharge planning is essential during this phase, and has been shown to be effective in promoting patient and family compliance with follow-up care, especially for large burns.[132] Many burn facilities now have a social worker or nurse burn specialist who is responsible for the coordination of discharge planning, and weekly meetings with the entire burn team are common.[23, 48, 61, 62, 68]

In preparation for discharge, the child's physical care must be taught to a parent or other responsible adult. Referrals for necessary follow-up care, such as physical and occupational therapy and social agencies, must be made at this time. Arrangements for the child to return to school must also be made. Ideally, the child will have been receiving schooling as part of the hospital program. Most teaching hospitals have a school program staffed by special education teachers who can arrange for the child to be withdrawn from his home school and enrolled in the hospital program. They usually arrange to use the child's books from the home school so that continuity can be maintained, and can arrange for information regarding the child's progress to be sent to the home school prior to his return. Sometimes the child will require temporary placement in special education classes because of physical disability, but it has been found that most children can return to their regular class with minor adjustments for the child's special needs.

Experience with burned children indicates that children who go back to school within a few weeks after discharge tend to make a positive adjustment and that children who are taught by a homebound teacher tend to become isolated, depressed, and stuck in the "sick role."[8] A study of children's long-term adjustment to burn injuries found that 90% of children who had access to a schoolteacher in the hospital maintained their appropriate grade level and were able to return to regular school.[109] A number of burn facilities have developed a team that provides a liaison with the child's home school, which can consist of a social worker, nurse, or teacher, as well as a member of the local fire department and, sometimes, interested parents.[28] They usually visit the school and present information on burn prevention and on the special needs of the burned child who is returning to school. This type of program has been effective in helping both school personnel and other children to understand the rehabilitation process and prevents the teasing and fear of the burned child that can occur without this understanding. Children and their parents report that if other children know what happened and why the burned child is required to, for instance, wear pressure garments and splints, they are generally accepting and supportive.

For a realistic preview of what it will be like when the child goes home, parents' discussion groups, particularly those that include parents of recovered or recovering burned children are extremely effective. They can provide information that persons on the burn team only know secondhand. In addition, they can help both the child and the family develop an understanding of what has happened and begin to integrate it into their lives.[28, 29, 96] Play therapy for younger children and "rap groups" for adolescents are also useful before discharge. If possible, it is helpful if the child and family are able to go out on a pass from the hospital before discharge, for a preview of what it will be like to go home. One of the most difficult things for older children, adolescents, and parents to cope with is peoples' stares and questions.[83] If they are able to go out of the hospital before discharge, children have the opportunity to begin to experience what it will be like to rejoin the outside world before they are also overwhelmed with the logistics of the follow-up care and readjustment to home life, for which professional support is available. Some burn facilities have developed a network of recovered burn survivors who can also help both the child and family in their return to normal life. Others have developed group visits to local amusement parks and summer camps that allow the burned children to participate in normal activities in a supportive context.

SOCIAL AND EMOTIONAL ADJUSTMENT TO BURNS

The resocialization process that includes reintegration into the child and family's social world and emotional adjustment to the injury can take many years. The first 1 to 2 years after the injury are described as being the most difficult because of the required follow-up care, the necessity of wearing pressure garments, recurrent skin breakdown, itching, the strain of resuming normal activities and the emotional intensity of the adjustment to the changes that have occurred. Although severe burn injuries can result in permanent disability—usually the loss of digits on hands and feet, and circulation problems in the feet that cause recurrent breakdown—they usually do not result in incapacitating physical disabilities. With the use of splints and pressure garments, disabilities due to scar contractures across joints can be prevented.[46, 72] Although pressure garments also prevent the most serious scar formation, permanent disfigurement always reults from deep second- or third-degree burns.

Literature on children's adjustment to disability due to congenital deformities, chronic illness, and traumatic injury indicates that the adjustment process is complex. Contrary to expectations, the severity of the disability or injury is not the most important variable in adjustment. Instead, family support, especially parental acceptance of the child's condition, is recognized as being crucial for the child's adjustment, whether it is spina bifida, polio, spinal cord injury, cancer, or burns.[5, 42, 79, 91, 130, 140]

Studies of children's adjustment to burns are somewhat contradictory. A number of early studies concluded that approximately 50% of the children in their samples showed signs of emotional disturbance several years after the injury.[6, 7, 13, 20, 22, 113, 126, 165] A number of studies, however, found that burned children, including adolescents with facial burns, were well adjusted 1 to 5 years postburn, as judged by their participation in age-appropriate activities.[16, 80, 143] Wright and Fulwiler,[166] on the other hand, found that mothers of burned children were significantly more depressed than mothers of a group of normal controls. Goldberg[59] also found that burned children had significantly lower self-esteem and were more likely to be behind in school than children with congenital heart defects.

Several recent long-term follow-up studies with large samples of adults and children found that the adjustment of adults and young adults burned in childhood was not influenced by the severity of the injury or sex.[1, 19, 41, 83, 91] In these studies, social support, especially family support, was the best predictor of adjustment. Those with high social support were better adjusted than those with low social support, controlling for the size of the injury, sex, age at time of the burn injury, and time since the burn.

Two studies of burn rehabilitation, one prospective[89, 94] and one retrospective,[19, 49] indicated that there was an initial drop in general functioning at 3 to 6 months after discharge from acute care, with recovery to near preburn functioning at 12 to 18 months after discharge. The latter study, which included both children and adults, found that children and adolescents were the most likely to return to preburn functioning. Persons older than 20 years at the time of the burn were somewhat less likely to regain their preburn levels of functioning, and people older than 50 years when burned were more likely to regain psychosocial functioning but less likely to regain physical functioning. Both studies showed that preburn general functioning was closely related to postburn functioning.

The Adjustment Process

The adjustment process includes three interrelated contexts, (1) the severity of the injury, (2) compliance, and (3) the characteristics of the child and family. These variables can be illustrated in Figure 26–2. Further research is needed to discover how these variables are interrelated, and how interventions at various times affects outcome.[84a]

A retrospective study of 126 young adults who were burned in childhood indicated that this population had generally good social and emotional adjustment and normal self-esteem an average of 8 years postburn.[83, 91] The sample was representative of the original 160 identified subjects, and the respondents did

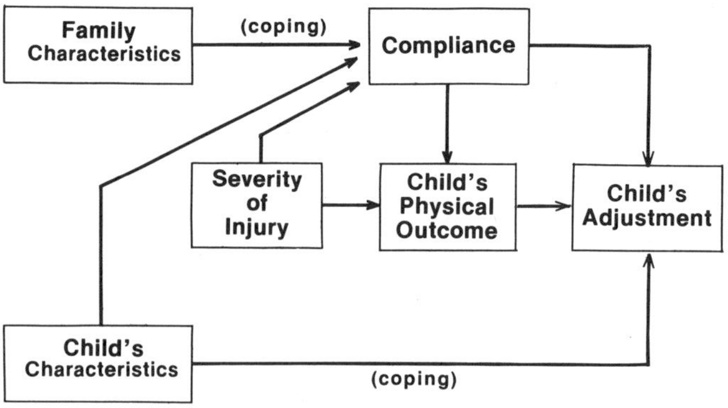

FIG 26–2.
The adjustment process in the burn child and variables that impact on the process.

not differ from those who could not be contacted in terms of age, sex, and extent of burn. Most of the subjects were active participants in society, as evidenced by their involvement in numerous social networks relative to the family, education, occupation, and community and leisure time activities.

Although there was considerably more variation in the subjects' emotional adjustment as measured by their responses to the study's narrative questions, most subjects showed a positive emotional adjustment to their burn injury. However, they indicated that they had encountered many difficulties along the way, including feelings of being left out and difficulties with starting or resuming school activities, peer relationships, and dating and intimate relationships. Ninety percent of the respondents said that adjusting to disfigurement was the most difficult aspect of adjustment.

From these young persons' responses and from clinical experience, it is clear that the process of adjustment is a complex process that involves both internal acceptance and external participation in society. Furthermore, the adjustment takes time and requires both internal strength and emotional support from persons who care. This study clearly showed that social support was the most significant predictor of adjustment. Variables such as "internal strength" or "coping ability" are much more difficult to measure, but appear to be important as well.[25, 63]

The emotional adjustment to burns involves internal changes in the person's "self-concept" (an internal concept of self). The self-concept develops over a lifetime and is formed by a person's experiences, including other persons' reactions to him.[37, 136] A central part of the self-concept is the "body image," which is the way in which a person conceives of himself physically.[107, 142, 145] After a severe burn, the body is changed, and this change must be integrated into a person's body-image and self-concept.[57, 58, 121, 142, 145] To do this, a person must accept the fact that he is a worthwhile person in spite of the changes.

The process by which this kind of acceptance takes place has been called the "grief process" by Kubler-Ross.[92] Although Kubler-Ross worked mainly with dying patients, this process has been related to adjustment to any emotional loss, such as divorce, amputation, etc.[21, 88, 100, 131, 154, 156] Kubler-Ross has identified six stages of grief, which are presented in Figure 26–3. These stages can be identified in both the burned child and the family. At first, there is a stage of emotional numbness, when nothing seems real, followed by denial that the burn injury could be as bad as it is. Then comes anger and guilt, when one asks, "Why me?"; "Why my child?"; "Why now?"; "What did I do wrong?"; "How could I have let this happen?" During this stage, both the child and the family reexperience the burn accident in their minds, trying to figure out why it happened and what they could have done to prevent it.

The first three stages often take place while the child is still in the hospital. It is important

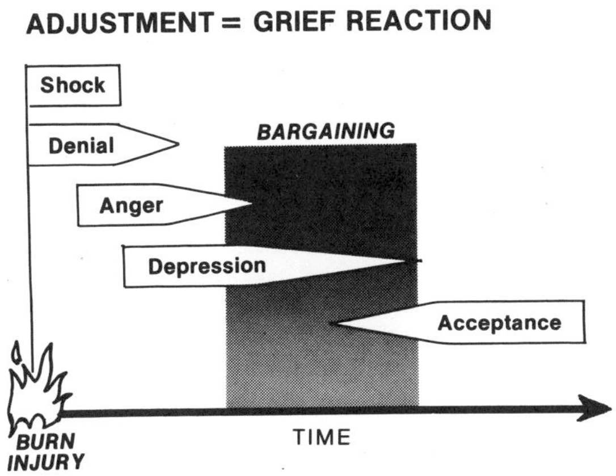

FIG 26–3.
Schematic representation of Kubler-Ross's six stages of grief that constitute adjustment in the burn patient and the relationship of these stages to time of the burn. (Adapted from Kubler-Ross E: *On Death and Dying.* New York, Macmillan Publishing Co, 1969.)

to be aware of this process to understand the child and family's emotional needs. Often, depression also occurs during the acute hospitalization, but just as often depression does not begin until after discharge, when the real impact of the injury sometimes becomes overwhelming.

Although these stages tend to occur one after another, there is a shifting back and forth; just because a person is depressed does not mean he is finished with denial and anger. "Bargaining" involves putting off acceptance with such statements as, "I'll be all right after my nose is reconstructed," etc. Since burn patients, especially growing children, often require extensive reconstructive surgery involving repeated adjustment to a new appearance, the process of adjustment is prolonged over many years.

The child's developmental stage is also an important variable in emotional adjustment. A young child may not be concerned about his appearance, but may reactivate the active grieving process during adolescence and young adulthood. The grief process is an individual process and varies according to the magnitude of adjustment required, the social context, and the characteristics of the individual. Vanderpool[156] found that the expression of emotions during the grief process was significantly affected by the person's age; younger persons, particularly adolescents and young adults, expressed more anger than older persons or younger children.

The outcome of a severe burn injury in childhood is not necessarily negative, as is assumed by many people. The authors have learned through personal and professional experience that acute pain and suffering and the emotional trauma that always follow any significant loss are not necessarily negative. In fact, this experience can have a very positive impact on a person's life. Both the burn survivors themselves and their families are transformed from being caught up in school and work, distracted by the stresses of everyday life, to becoming acutely aware of the significance of life and the importance of caring for others and sharing their experiences. Material possessions, status, and even conventional standards of beauty become meaningless, because burn victims have faced pain and loss and found that they have survived and become aware of something they had all along but could not see. Although most people are intellectually aware that they can get hurt and that they will ultimately die, they have no emotional awareness of either. It is our belief that through the experience of pain and suffering one becomes emotionally and, thus, existentially aware of both.

Improvements in burn care and rehabilitation are taking place at a very rapid rate and survival of very large burns is becoming commonplace, particularly among children.[31] It is encouraging that concern with pain control, behavioral management, and long-term follow-up care have become recognized as essential in burn care. It is this concern with the quality of life that makes the improvements in survival worthwhile.

REFERENCES

1. Ablon J: Reactions of Samoan burn patients and families to severe burns. *Soc Sci Med* 1973; 7:167–178.
2. Abramson M: Group treatment of families of

burn-injured patients. *Social Casework* 1975; :235–241.

3. Addison C: Tolerating stress in social work practice: The example of a burns unit. *Br J Social Work* 1980; 10:341–356.
4. Ajoub C, Pfeifer D: Burns as a manifestation of child abuse and neglect. *Am J Dis Child* 1979; 133:910–914.
5. Anderson FJ, et al: Adjustment of adolescents to chronic disability. *Rehabil Psychol* 1979; 26:177–185.
6. Andreasen NJC, Noyes AS: Factors influencing adjustment of burn patients during hospitalization. *Psychosom Med* 1971; 34:517–525.
7. Andreasen NJ, Noyes R, Hartford CE: Factors influencing adjustment of burn patients during hospitalization. *Psychosom Med* 1972; 34:517–525.
8. Baker G: Personal communication, 1982.
9. Beaver WT: Interaction of narcotics and mood altering drugs: A brief historical review, in Bonica JJ, Albe-Fessard D (eds): *Recent Studies of the Nature and Management of Acute Pain: A Symposium.* New York, HP Publishing Co, 1976, pp 8–41.
10. Beaver WT, Feise G: Comparison of the analgesic effects of morphine, hydroxyzine, and their combination in patients with postoperative pain, in Bonica JJ, Albe-Fessard D (eds): *Advances in Pain Research and Theory.* New York, Raven Press, 1976, pp 553–557.
11. Beecher HK: Relationship of significance of wound to pain experienced. *JAMA* 1956; 161:1609–1613.
12. Bernstein NR: Observations on the use of hypnosis with burned children on a pediatric ward. *Int J Clin Exp Hypn* 1965; 13:1–10.
13. Bernstein NR: *Emotional Care of the Facially Burned and Disfigured Child.* Boston, Little Brown & Co, 1976.
14. Bezzeg EE, et al: The role of the child care worker in the treatment of severely burned children. *Pediatrics* 1972; 50:617–624.
15. Bibace R, Walsh ME: Developmental stages in children's conceptions of illness, in Stone G, Cohen F, Adler N (eds): *Health Psychology.* San Francisco, Josey-Bass, 1979.
16. Blades BC, Jones D, Munster AM: Quality of life after major burns. *J Trauma* 1979; 19:556–558.
17. Borland BL: Prevention of childhood burns: Conclusions drawn from an epidemiologic study. *Clin Pediatr* 1967; 6:603–695.
18. Bowden ML, Feller I: Family reaction to a severe burn. *Am J Nurs* 1973; 73:140–144.
19. Bowden ML, Feller I: *Progress in Burn Rehabilitation: A Report of Three Studies.* Ann Arbor, Mich, National Institute for Burn Medicine, 1982.
20. Bowden ML, Jones C, Feller I: *Psychosocial Aspects of a Severe Burn: A Review of the Literature,* supplement to the International Bibliography on Burns. Ann Arbor, Mich, National Institute for Burn Medicine, 1979.
21. Bowlby J: Grief and mourning in infancy and early childhood, in Eissler RS, et al (eds): *The Psychoanalytic Study of the Child.* New York, International University Press, 1960.
22. Breslin P: The psychological reactions of children to burn traumata: A review. *Ill Med J* 1975; 148:595–602.
23. Bristow O, Stickney C, Thompson S: *Discharge Planning for Continuity of Care.* New York, National League of Nursing, 1976.
24. Brodland GA, Andreasen NJC: Adjustment problems of the family of the burn patient. *Social Casework* 1974; 55:13–18.
25. Bulman RJ, Wortman CB: Attribution of blame and coping in the 'real world': Severe accident victims react to their lot. *J Pers Soc Psychol* 1977; 35:351–363.
26. Butzer S, et al: Methadone: An old analgesic rediscovered. Paper presented at the American Burn Association Meeting, April, 1979, New Orleans.
27. Cahners SS: Group meetings for families of burned children. *Health Soc Work* 1978; 3:165–172.
28. Cahners SS: Group meetings benefit families of burned children. *Scand J Plast Reconstr Surg* 1979; 13:169–171.
29. Cahners SS: A strong hospital-school liaison: A necessity for good rehabilitation planning for disfigured children. *Scand J Plast Reconstr Surg* 1979; 13:167–168.
30. Campbell L: Special behavioral problems of the burned child. *Am J Nurs* 1976; 76:220–224.
31. Carvajal HF, Parks DH: Survival statistics in burned children. *J Burn Care Rehabil* 1982; 3:81–84.
32. Christopherson VA: Sociocultural correlates of the pain response. *Soc Sci* 1971; 46:33–37.
33. Clark WC, Mehl L: Thermal pain: A sensory decision theory analysis of the effect of age and sex on d'. various response criteria and 50% pain threshold. *J Abnorm Psychol* 1971; 78:202–212.
34. Cobb S: Social support as a moderator of life stress. *Psychosom Med* 1976; 38:314.
35. Cook DW: Psychological adjustment to spinal cord injury: Incidence of denial, depression

and anxiety. *Rehabil Psychol* 1979; 26:97–104.
36. Cooper LP: Norms of hypnotic susceptibility in children. *Dev Psychol* 1969; 1:113.
37. Coopersmith S: *The Antecedents of Self-Esteem.* San Francisco, WH Freeman Co, 1967.
38. Crasilneck HB, et al: Use of hypnosis in the management of patients with burns. *JAMA* 1955; 158:103–106.
39. Cromes GF, McDonald M, Robinson C: The effects of relaxation training on anxiety and pain during burn wound debridement. Paper presented at American Burn Association, March 1980, San Antonio.
40. Dahinterova J: Some experiences with the use of hypnosis in the treatment of burns. *Int J Clin Exp Hypn* 1967; 15:49–53.
41. Davidson TN, et al: Social support and post-burn adjustment. *Arch Phys Med Rehabil* 1981; 26:274–278.
42. Davis F: *Passage Through Crisis: Polio Victims and Their Families.* New York, Bobbs Merrill & Co, 1963.
43. Duffy JC: Emotional reactions of children to hospitalization. *Minnesota Med* 1972; 55:1168–1170.
44. Demling RH, Ellerbe S, Jarrett F: Ketamine anesthesia for tangential excision of burn eschar: A burn unit procedure. *J Trauma* 1978; 18:269–270.
45. Eland JM, Anderson JE: The experience of pain in children, in Jacox A (ed): *A Source Book for Nurses and Other Health Professionals.* Boston, Little Brown & Co, 1977, pp 453–473.
46. Evans EB, Larson DL, Yates S: Preservation and restoration of joint function in patients with severe burns. *JAMA* 1968; 204:843–896.
47. Fagerhaugh SU: Pain expression and control on a burn unit. *Nurs Outlook* 1974; 22:645–650.
48. Feller I, et al: The team approach to total rehabilitation of the severely burned patient. *Heart Lung* 1973; 2:701–706.
49. Feller I, et al: A comprehensive rehabilitation program for severe burns, grant #G008003019, final report. 1982.
50. Filkins SA, et al: Self-administered anesthetic: A method of pain control. *J Burn Care Rehabil* 1981; 2:33–34.
51. Fordyce WE: *Behavioral Methods for Chronic Pain and Illness.* St Louis, CV Mosby Co, 1976.
52. Freud A: The role of bodily illness in the mental life of children, in Eissler RS, et al (eds): *The Psychoanalytic Study of the Child.* New York, International University Press, 1952, pp 69–81.
53. Galdston R: The burning and healing of children. *Psychiatry* 1972; 35:57–66.
54. Gardner GG: Hypnosis with infants and preschool children. *Am J Clin Hypn* 1977; 19:158.
55. Gelfand S: The relationship of birth order to pain tolerance. *J Clin Psychol* 1963; 19:406.
56. Gillespie RW: The battered child syndrome: Thermal and caustic manifestations. *J Trauma* 1965; 5:523–533.
57. Goffman I: Studies in adjustment to visible injuries: Evaluation of curiosity by the injured. *J Abnorm Psychol* 1948; 43:13–28.
58. Goffman I: *Stigma: Notes on the Management of Spoiled Identity.* Englewood Cliffs, NJ, Prentice-Hall, 1963.
59. Goldberg RT: A comparative study of the adjustment of children with invisible and visible handicaps: Congenital heart disease and facial burns. *J Counsel Psychol* 1974; 4:428–432.
60. Gonda TA: The relation between complaints of persistent pain and family size. *J Neurol Neurosurg Psychiatry* 1962; 25:277–281.
61. Gordon M: Role of the discharge-planning and outpatient clinic nurses. *J Burn Care Rehabil* 1980; 1:30–32.
62. Granite U: Multidisciplinary discharge and rehabilitation planning for burn patients: Psychosocial implications. *Q Rev Burns* 1979; 5:30–34.
63. Hamburg DA, Adams JE: A perspective on coping behavior: Seeking and utilizing information in major transitions. *Arch Gen Psychiatry* 1967; 17:277–284.
64. Hamburg D, Hamburg B, DeGoza S: Adaptive problems. *Psychiatry* 1953; 16:1–20.
65. Hartley RB: Hypnosis for alleviation of pain in treatment of burns: Case report. *Arch Phys Med Rehabil* 1968; 49:39–41.
66. Heidrich G, Perry S, Armand R: Nursing staff attitudes about burn pain. *J Burn Care Rehabil* 1981; 2:259–261.
67. Helfer RE, Kempe CH (eds): *The Battered Child,* ed 2. Chicago, University of Chicago Press, 1974.
68. Helm PA, et al: Burn rehabilitation: A team approach. *Surg Clin North Am* 1978; 58:1263–1278.
69. Hight DW, Bakalor HR, Lloyd JR: Inflicted burns in children: Recognition and treatment. *JAMA* 1979; 242:517–520.
70. Hilgard ER, Hilgard JR: *Hypnosis in the Relief of Pain.* Los Altos, Calif, William Kaufman Inc, 1975.
71. Hofmann AD, Becker HP, Gabriel R: *The*

Hospitalized Adolescent: A Guide to Managing Ill and Injured Youth. New York, The Free Press, 1976.

72. Huang TT, Blackwell SJ, Lewis SR: Ten years of experience in managing patients with burn contractures of axilla, elbow, wrist, and knee joints. *Plast Reconstr Surg* 1978; 6:70–76.
73. Innes RL, et al: The study of the etiology and epidemiology of burn injuries in children, in Matter P, Barlay TL, Kanckova Z (eds): *Research in Burns.* Bern/Stuttgart, Hans Huber, 1971, pp 437–442.
74. Johnson M: Assessment of clinical pain in Jacox A (ed): *Pain: A Source Book for Nurses and Other Health Professionals.* Boston, Little Brown & Co, 1977, chap 6.
75. Jorgensen JA, Brophy JJ: Psychiatric treatment modalities in burn patients. *Curr Psychiatr Ther* 1975; 15:85–92.
76. Justice B, Justice R: *The Abusing Family.* New York, Human Science Press, 1976.
77. Keen JH, Lendrum J, Wolman B: Inflicted burns in children. *Br Med J* 1975; 5:268–269.
78. Kenny TJ: The hospitalized child. *Pediatr Clin North Am* 1975; 22:583–593.
79. Kessler MS, Milligan WL: Effect of age-of-disability onset on self-esteem and anxiety in wheelchair bound individuals. *Rehabil Psychol* 1979; 26:105–112.
80. Kibbee E: Life after severe burns in children. *J Burn Care Rehabil* 1981; 2:44–47.
81. Knudson MS: Where burn care also eases inner hurt. *Patient Care* 1979; 13:86–103.
82. Knudson-Cooper MS: Biofeedback and relaxation therapy in the treatment of severely burned children. *J Burn Care Rehabil* 1081; 2:102–110.
83. Knudson-Cooper MS: Adjustment to visible stigma: The case of the severely burned. *Soc Sci Med* 1981; 15B:31–44.
84. Knudson-Cooper MS: Emotional care of the hospitalized burned child. *J Burn Care Rehabil* 1982; 3:109–116.
84a. Knudson-Cooper MS: What are the research priorities in the behavioral areas for burn patients? *J Trauma* 1984; 24:1045–1053.
85. Knudson-Cooper MS, Long C, Stephenson E: *The Burned Child Returns to School.* Galveston, Tex, Shriners Burns Institute, 1982.
86. Knudson-Cooper MS, Leuchtag A: The stress of a family move as a precipitating factor in children's burn accidents. *J Human Stress,* June 1982; pp 32–38.
87. Knudson-Cooper MS, Leuchtag A, Bunce H: Psychosocial antecedents of childhood burn injuries. Paper presented at 6th International Congress for Burn Injuries, August 1982, San Francisco.
88. Knudson-Cooper MS, Baker SB: Ontological interpretations of children's burn accidents. Paper presented at the 6th International Congress for Burn Injuries, August 1982, San Francisco.
89. Knudson-Cooper MS: Antecedents and consequences of childhood burn injuries, in Wolraich M, Routh D (eds): *Advances in Developmental and Behavioral Pediatrics.* Greenwich, Conn, JAI Press, vol 3, 1980.
90. Knudson-Cooper MS, et al: Recovery curves for adult victims. *J Burn Care Rehabil,* in press.
91. Knudson-Cooper MS, Bee D: Predictors of psychosocial adjustment and self-esteem in young adults burned in childhood. *Soc Sci Med,* in press.
92. Kubler-Ross E: *On Death and Dying.* New York, Macmillian Publishing Co, 1969.
93. Larson DL: Personal communication, 1975.
94. Larson DL, et al. A comprehensive medical rehabilitation approach for severe burns, Rehabilitation Services Administration grant DHEW 13-P-59298/6, final report, 1982.
95. LeBau WL: Adjunctive trance therapy with severely burned children. *Int J Child Psychother* 2:80–92.
96. Leeder CJ: Families of burn victims receive help through regular group meetings. *Burns* 1978; 5:89–91.
97. Levinson P, Ousterhout MD: Art and play therapy with pediatric burn patients. *J Burn Care Rehabil* 1980; 1:42–46.
98. Lim RKS: Pain. *Ann Rev Physiol* 32:269–288.
99. Livingston WK: *Pain Mechanisms.* New York, MacMillan Press, 1943.
100. Lindemann E: Symptomatology and management of acute grief. *Am J Psychiatry* 1944; 101:141.
101. Litman T: The family as a basic unit in health and medical care: A social-behavioral overview. *Soc Sci Med* 1974; 8:495–519.
102. Long RT, Cope O: Emotional problems of burned children. *N Eng J Med* 1961; 264:1121–1127.
103. Lung RJ, et al: Recognizing burn injuries as child abuse. *Am Fam Physician* 1977; 15:134–135.
104. MacArthur JD, Francis M: Epidemiology of burns: The burn-prone patient. *JAMA* 1975; 231:259–263.
105. McCaffery M: Pain relief for the child: Problem areas and selected non-pharmacological methods. *Pediatr Nurs* 1977; 3:11–16.
106. MacGregor FC: *Transformation and Identity:*

The Face and Plastic Surgery. New York, Quadrangle Books Inc, 1974.
107. MacGregor FC: The facially disfigured child. *Pediatr Soc* 1980; 1:1–4.
108. McHugh ML, Dimitroff K, Dinsmor DN: Family support group in a burn unit. *Am J Nurs* 1979; 79:2148–2150.
109. McLoughlin E, Healer C, Crawford JD: Burn education intervention: A controlled study. *Burns* 1979; 6:26–29.
110. McNeese M, Hebler J: The abused child: A clinical approach to the identification and management. *Clin Symp* 1977; 2:1–34.
111. Margolis CG: Hypnosis in the treatment of burns. Presented at the American Burn Association Meetings, April 1977, Anaheim.
112. Marks RM, Sachar EJ: Undertreatment of medical inpatients with narcotic analgesics. *Ann Intern Med* 1973; 78:173–181.
113. Martin HL: Parent's and children's reactions to burns and scalds in children. *Br J Med Psychol* 1970; 43:183.
114. Mason EA: The hospitalized child: His emotional needs. *N Engl J Med* 2965; 8:406–414.
115. Mechanic D: Illness behavior, social adaptation and the management of illness. *J Ment Nerv Dis* 1977; 165:362–371.
116. Melzack R: Pain: Past, present and future, in Weisenberg M, Turskey B (eds): *Pain: New Perspectives in Therapy and Research*. New York, Plenum Press, 1976.
117. Melzack R, Torgerson WS: On the language of pain. *Anesthesiology* 1971; 34:50–55.
118. Montague FMA: *Touching: The Human Significance of Skin*. New York, Columbia University Press, 1971.
119. Noble E: *Play and the Sick Child*. London, Farber & Farber, 1967.
120. Nova J: Large dose morphine for pain control. Presented at the American Burn Association Meetings, April 1980, San Antonio.
121. Noyes R: Attitude changes following near-death experiences. *Psychiatry* 1980; 43:234–242.
122. Ofodile F, Norris J, Garnes A: Burns and child abuse. *East Afr Med J* 1979; 56:26–29.
123. Olness K, Gardner GG: Some guidelines for uses of hypnotherapy in pediatrics. *Pediatrics* 1978; 62:228–133.
124. Parkes CM: Psycho-social transitions: Comparison between reactions to loss of a limb and loss of a spouse. *Br J Psychiatry* 1975; 127:204–210.
125. Parks DH, Evans EB, Larson DL: Prevention and correction of deformity after severe burns. *Surg Clin North Am* 1978; 58(6).
126. Pavlovsky P: Occurrence and development of psychopathologic phenomena in burned persons and their relation to severity of burns, age and premorbid personality. *Acta Chir Plast* 1972; 14:2–8.
127. Perry S, Heidrich G: Management of pain during debridement: A survey of U.S. burn units. *Pain* 1982; 13:267–280.
128. Perry S, Heidrich G, Ramos E: Assessment of pain by burn patients. *J Burn Care Rehabil* 1981; 2:322–326.
129. Petrovich DV: The pain apperception test: Psychological correlates of pain perception. *J Clin Psychol* 1958; 14:367–374.
130. Pilisuk M, Froland C. Kinship, social networks, social support and health. *Soc Sci Med* 1978; 12B:173–280.
131. Pollock GH: Mourning and adaptation. *Int J Psychoanal* 1961; 42:341–361.
132. Quay NB, Alexander LL: Preparation of burned children and their families for discharge. *J Burn Care Rehabil* 1982; 4:288–290.
133. Quinby S, Bernstein NR: Identity problems and the adaptation of nurses to severely burned children. *Am J Psychiatr* 1971; 128:58–63.
134. Robinson SS: The causes of burns in children in Scotland. *Br J Plas Surg* 1968; 21:140–146.
135. Ronnebeck RW: A naturalistic investigation of community adjustment of facially disfigured burned teenagers, doctoral dissertation. University of Houston, December 1972.
136. Rosenberg M: *Conceiving the Self*. New York, Basic Books, 1979.
137. Roskies E, et al: Emergency hospitalization of young children: Some neglected psychological considerations. *Med Care* 1975; 13:570–581.
138. Sadler JE: The long-term hospitalization of asthmatic children. *Pediatr Clin North Am* 1975; 22.
139. Savedra M: Coping with pain: Strategies of severely burned children. *Matern Child Nurs J* 1976; 5:197–203.
140. Schaefer C, Coyne JC, Lazarus RS: The health-related functions of social support. *J Behav Med* 1981; 4:381–409.
141. Schafer DW: Hypnosis on a burn unit. *Int J Clin Exp Hypn* 1975; 23:1–14.
142. Schilder P: *The Image and Appearance of the Human Body*. New York, International University Press, 1950.
143. Schmitt RC: Some ecological variables of community adjustment in a group of facially disfigured burned children, doctoral dissertation. University of Houston, 1971.
144. Seligman R, MacMillan B, Carroll S: The

burned child: A neglected area of psychiatry. *Am J Psychiatry* 1971; 128:52–57.
145. Shontz FC: *Perceptual and Cognitive Aspects of Body Experience*. New York, Academic Press, 1969.
146. Shore MF (ed): Red is the color of hurting: Planning for children in the hospital, publication 1583. Public Health Service, 1965.
147. Shorkey CT, Taylor JE: Management of maladaptive behavior of a severely burned child. *Child Welfare* 1973; 52:543–547.
148. Silverstein AB: Age differences in pain apperception. *Percept Mot Skills* 1963; 16:169–170.
149. Simons RD, et al: Behavioral contracting in a burn care facility: A strategy for patient participation. *J Trauma* 1978; 18:257–260.
150. Slogoff S, et al: Clinical experience with subanesthetic Ketamine. *Anesth Analg* 1974; 53:354–358.
151. Sternbach RA: Pain: Psychophysiological analysis, in Weisenberg M, Tursky B (eds): *Pain: New Perspectives in Therapy and Research*. New York, Academic Press, 1968.
152. Sternbach RA, Tursky B: Ethnic differences among housewives in psychophysical skin potential responses to electric shock. *Psychophysiology* 1965; 1:241–246.
153. Suchman EA: Sociomedical variations among ethnic groups. *Am J Sociol* 1964; 70:319–331.
154. Tenbrince MS, Brewer PW: The stages of grief experienced by parents of handicapped children. *Ariz Med* 1976; 33:712–714.
155. Thiemer V: Individual approaches. *J Burn Care Rehabil* 1982; 3:101–105.
156. Vanderpool JP: Understanding death and the dying patient. *Contin Educ,* no. 77, 1976.
157. Visitainer MA, Wolfer JA: Psychological preparation for surgical pediatric patients: The effect on children's and parent's stress response and adjustment. *Pediatrics* 1975; 56:114–122.
158. Volicer BJ: Hospital stress and patient reports of pain physical status. *Am J Nurs* 1978; 4:28–37.
159. Wagner M: Pain and nursing care associated with burns, in Jacox A (ed): *Pain: A Source Book for Nurses and Health Professionals*. Boston, Little Brown & Co, 1977, pp 391–403.
160. Wakeman JR, Kaplan JZ: An experimental study of hypnosis in painful burns. *Am J Clin Hypn* 1978; 21:3–12.
161. Weinstein DJ: Imagery and relaxation in a burn patient. *Behav Res Ther* 1976; 14:481.
162. Weisenberg M, Tursky B: *Pain: New Perspectives in Therapy and Research*. New York, Plenum Press, 1975.
163. Wernick RL, Jaremko MW, Taylor PW: Pain management in severely burned adults: A test of stress innoculation. *J Behav Med* 1981; 4:103–110.
164. Woodward JM: Parental visiting of children with burns. *Br Med J* 1962; Dec 22.
165. Woodward JM, Jackson D: Emotional reactions in burned children and their mothers. *Br J Plast Surg* 1961; 13:316–324.
166. Wright L, Fulwiler R: Long-range emotional sequelae of burns: Effects on children and their mothers. *Br J Plast Surg* 1974; 8:931–934.
167. Zborowski M: *People in Pain*. San Francisco, Josey Bass, 1969.
168. Zide B, Pardoe R: The use of behavior modification. *Plast Reconstr Surg* 1976; 57:378–382.

27 / Discharge Planning for the Pediatric Burn Patient

LORY L. ALEXANDER, R.N., M.S.
NANCY B. QUAY, R.N., M.S.

Discharge planning is a crucial component in the effective care of children with burns. The most difficult part of being burned often begins at discharge.[7] Adjustment for reentry into the world outside the hospital requires advanced preparation as well as close follow-up (under supervision) of the burned child and family after discharge. Just as the injury creates a state of disequilibrium for the child and family, moving from one level of care (hospital) to another (home) creates disruption.[1]

The initial insult to the child and the subsequent shock and disbelief of the parents is often replaced by fear and anxiety, particularly when they realize the child is going to survive the injury and will soon be ready for discharge. The child and family may fear leaving the protective environment of the hospital, they may have doubts about the child's needs being met, or they may be apprehensive about the responsibility of home care.[4, 12] These feelings may interfere with comprehension and retention of discharge instructions.

DEFINITION OF DISCHARGE PLANNING

Discharge planning is a process and service in which patient and family needs are identified and assistance is provided in preparation for movement from one level of care to another.[2] The process should be centered on the patient and family and their needs and concerns. Effective discharge planning for the child with burns closely coordinates medical and nursing procedures with other essential activities such as physical therapy, occupational therapy, play therapy, and schoolwork.

The discharge planning program can be coordinated by any designated professional as long as everyone associated with the program contributes to the effort through sharing, negotiating, and compromising.[3] However, the nurse is often situated in the same environment as the patient and may be in the best position to coordinate team members' activities on a consistent basis. Members of all disciplines need to become involved early in the discharge planning process so that the child and family will perceive them as their allies and advocates.[9] The relationship that usually develops between the child, his family, and the burn team sets the stage for successful discharge planning.

GOALS OF DISCHARGE PLANNING

The following are the major goals of discharge planning.

1. Coordination of care between injury and recovery.
2. Teaching of self-care as early as possible.
3. Development of an individualized plan for continuing care.
4. Assisting the child in achieving a normal and productive role in society.

Accomplishment of these goals depends on three factors: (1) identification of patient and family needs, (2) education of the child and family, and (3) matching of appropriate resources to the identified needs.[5]

Identification of patient and family needs includes medical as well as psychological, sociological, and cultural characteristics of the child and family. The process begins with an initial assessment and continues with an ongoing assessment throughout hospitalization. Because the burn injury affects the entire family, identification of the child's needs requires assessment of the family as well as the child. Knowledge of the child's physical and emotional environment before and during hospitalization will help to determine unique and special needs after discharge.[7]

The child and family should know the purpose of discharge planning so that they will understand the activities that occur during hospitalization. Early discharge planning serves two purposes. First, problems regarding living arrangements can be solved prior to anticipated discharge. Second, since the future is emphasized, the patient and family can begin to acknowledge that the patient will be getting well and will be going home.[8] Early identification of existing and potential problems reduces the chances of unexpected posthospital problems for the child and his family.

There must be mutual awareness by the burn team, child, and family of the expected outcomes of discharge preparation. It is important to determine the child and family's feelings, concerns, strengths, and weaknesses regarding the planned discharge. The child and family should be assisted in identifying and finding ways to deal with potential problems. They can be helped to explore and assess their life situation in relation to new problems that are created by their child's recovery process. Questions should be asked regarding what they need to know or need to acquire before discharge, what their feelings and concerns are about body image and function, and how these needs will be met.[3]

EDUCATION IN DISCHARGE PLANNING

Educating the child and family is essential in meeting the goals of discharge planning. Discharge education involves more than teaching the skills necessary for home care; it also includes education and counseling throughout the hospitalization regarding the type and degree of injury, the treatments required during and after hospitalization, and accompanying psychosocial problems and resolutions. Discharge education enables the child and family to make informed decisions about the care and facilitates progress toward self-care.

Burned children's education must be planned in consideration of family, cultural, and environmental influences. Children want to know what is going on around them and what is happening to them. How well a child and family can be predicted to cope with the everyday routines at home depends on their understanding and acceptance of the burn and the reason for expected outcomes of treatment, as well as their adjustment in life-style to meet the child's special needs.[10]

Shortly after a child is admitted to the hospital and his condition is stable, the process of burn education must begin. Throughout the acute and intermediate phases of adaptation to hospitalization, the child and family will focus on survival and short-term psychological needs. The recuperative phase, extending through resocialization after discharge, involves largely discharge planning. At this point the focus must be on pressure garments, splints, and braces, which must be worn to prevent disfigurement and contractures.[7]

As discharge approaches, the family's knowledge of and ability to anticipate their child's physical and emotional needs after hospitalization are assessed. Specific teaching by the burn team should include information about wound care; splints, braces, and pressure bandages; medications; diet; exercise; potential problems; and psychosocial adjustment. Counseling in regard to posthospital adjustment may be facilitated through family support groups, adolescent "rap" sessions, and play for the younger child.

DEVELOPMENTAL STAGES AND DISCHARGE EDUCATION

Anticipatory guidance regarding expected behavioral changes that follow a lengthy hospitalization and factors that facilitate cooperation with home care must be provided. For example, the infant with a burn should have a limited number of caretakers. The parent should talk to the infant in a calm, quiet manner, and use a quick and gentle approach during care. With the toddler, deliberate and unhurried actions are effective. The parent can use distraction with conversation and toys.

Preparing the preschool child for discharge requires step-by-step explanations about what is to be done and where it is to be done, and emphasizes that the child will get better. The preschool child needs more than verbal explanations. Looking at pictures, handling equipment, imitation, and fantasy are useful techniques. A coloring book that depicts children with burns engaged in various activities and with necessary pressure garments is helpful (Figs 27–1 and 27–2).*

School-aged children can better understand what going home from the hospital will mean for them. Because of possible disfigurement and disability, there may be considerable anxiety as the child begins to think about going back to the world outside the hospital. These fears and anxiety must be anticipated and brought out for discussion.

School-aged children must be encouraged to actively participate and ensure responsibility and control for some aspects of their daily care. Adolescents are particularly concerned about returning to school and the reactions of peers. Parents should be aware of their need for privacy and achievement of self-care to encourage their self-identity and sense of control.[7, 10, 13]

Routine care for the burned child provides many opportunities for teaching. Activities

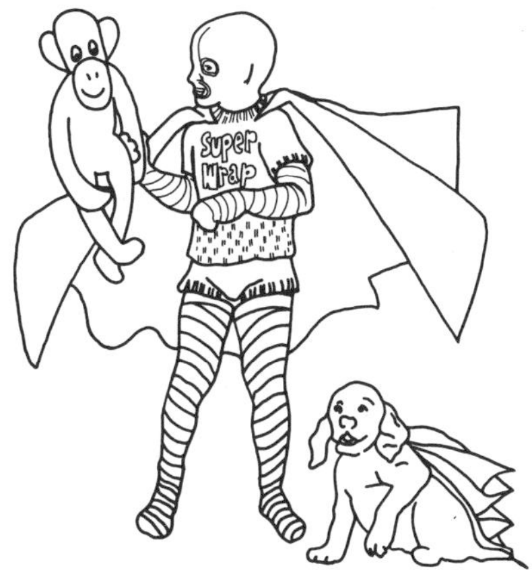

FIG 27–1.
"To prevent your burn from forming scars, you will have to wear 'wraps' on all the places that you were burned. Sometimes, you'll almost look and feel like a 'masked superhero.' The wraps press on the burned skin and help keep it from forming big, red, hard scars. They don't stop the scarring, but they help a lot! You must wear the wraps all the time, even to bed!"

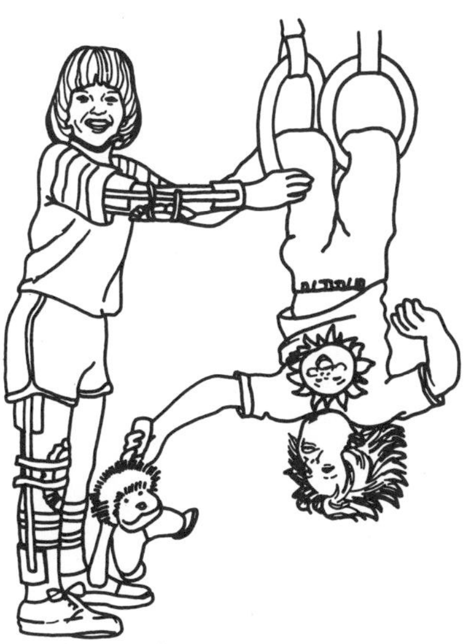

FIG 27–2.
"Splints and braces have to be worn at home, too! They will help make sure your arms, legs, neck, and hands will always work the way they should, so that you'll be able to do the things you did before you were burned."

*SBI Home Coloring Book was developed by Nancy Quay, R.N., M.S., and Edmond Stephenson for the Shriner's Burns Institute, Galveston, Texas.

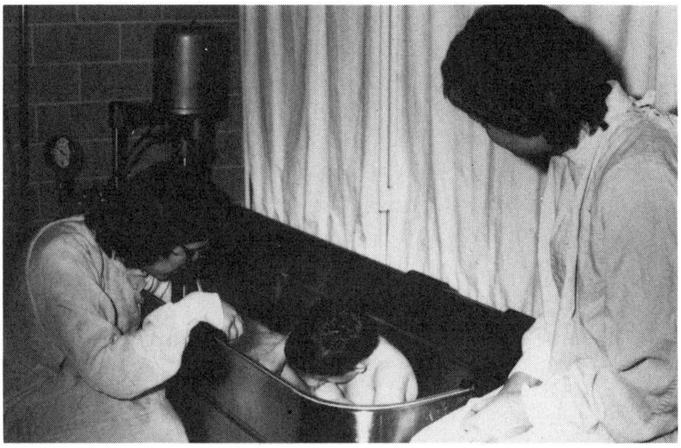

FIG 27–3.
An activity such as tubbing provides an excellent setting for teaching the child and family routine care skills.

such as medicating, tubbing, and changing dressings are excellent settings for explanations to children and their families (Fig 27–3). Involvement of the child and family in the care by handling supplies during the dressing change or application of splints allows them to observe, participate with assistance, and eventually perform the skill independently (Fig 27–4).

Studies have indicated that children who are allowed to be a part of burn care show increased cooperation and less depression, anxiety, and pain. It is important to inform the child when burn care is scheduled and emphasize the importance of the care. Discharge teaching may be facilitated if this is started at the first dressing change and continued throughout hospitalization.[6] In addition, discharge preparation started on admission has been effective in decreasing state anxiety at the time of the child's discharge and first clinic visit for parents of children with burns greater than 30% of total body surface area.[11]

For discharge teaching to be effective, consideration must be given to the child and family's readiness and ability to learn. Fostering the child and family's self-esteem is important for successful discharge preparation. By observing how the burn team members interact with their child, the parents usually learn the behavior that will be needed for caring for their child at home. A discharge checklist should be completed to ensure comprehensive planning and education (Fig 27–5).

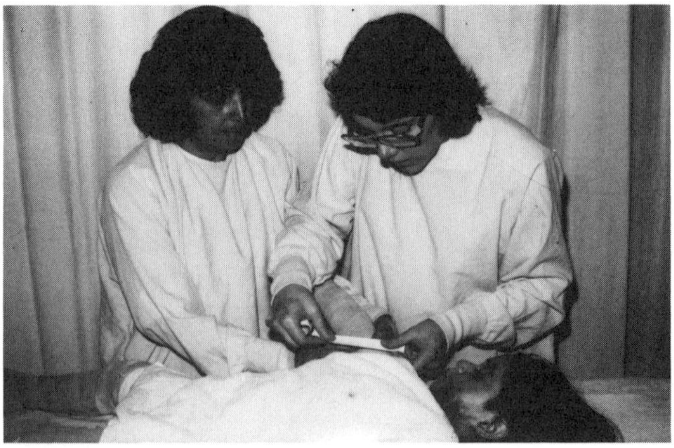

FIG 27–4.
Splinting also provides a good opportunity to apprise the burn patient and family of routine care continuing after discharge.

Name ____________________

The family is able to:

	Nurse	Parent
1. Discuss purpose of required treatments post discharge.		
2. Demonstrate performance of necessary treatments, procedures, and dressing changes.		
3. Obtain necessary items to provide the required treatments.		
4. Demonstrate proper administration of discharge medications and discuss possible side effects of those medications.		
5. Discuss dietary requirements after discharge.		
6. State who to contact for questions/concerns and how that person can be contacted.		
7. Discuss what community resources have been contacted to assist with adjustment and facilitate continuity of care.		

____________________ ____________________

Nurse/Discharge Coordinator Parent

FIG 27–5.
Example of discharge checklist for acute burn patient.

RESOURCES FOR DISCHARGE PLANNING

As the child and family's needs are identified or reassessed by the burn team, the appropriate resources must be matched with these needs. Many resources are found within the hospital setting, such as the social worker, psychologist, occupational therapist, physical therapist, and child life therapist. Other resource persons must be identified within the community and contacted as soon as the need is anticipated or identified to ensure continuity of care after discharge.

A local physician can be contacted to assess the child's ongoing physical needs and the family's compliance with the therapeutic regimen. He can also help with orders for visiting nurses, occupational therapy, physical therapy, and infant stimulation. A visiting nurse can assist directly with treatments, monitor the child's condition, and provide further education and reinforcement. Other community resource personnel who can be contacted are social workers for support and financial and transportation assistance, and mental health professionals for emotional problems—either the child's or family's—that interfere with functioning.

A final part of discharge planning is the provision for continuing rehabilitation after discharge. The child should be followed up by health care members experienced in burn care so that adjustments in pressure garments, splints, and braces, as well as plans for necessary corrective surgery, can be made as the child grows older. Careful planning will allow the child to resume and continue his home, school, and social activities with as little interruption as possible.

IMPORTANCE OF SCHOOL IN DISCHARGE PLANNING

Discharge planning for any child over the age of 3 years should include the school. Personnel in the child's school can assist in monitoring his progress and can have a major influence in helping the child with burns to adapt psychologically. This preparation involves the burned child himself and the staff and students who will be in direct contact with him. The disfigurement and disability that result from the burn injury and treatments required (such as scars, pressure bandages, and splints) can be frightening to both adults and to children not accustomed to interacting with people who have been burned. Preparing staff and students for interaction with a burned child can facilitate more positive relationships.

A member of the burn team should visit the school prior to the child's discharge from the hospital.* During that visit the "likes" or similarities, rather than the differences, between the schoolchildren and the burned child are stressed. Coloring or comic books, dolls with pressure bandages, and pictures or slides of the burned child engaged in normal activities in the community can be used to provide explanations to schoolchildren in terms they can understand (Figs 27–6 and 27–7). The children and teacher should be given a chance to apply pressure bandages and have their picture taken and developed immediately, so that they can become comfortable with the equipment and supplies they will see. Older children may be encouraged to form "buddy" systems with the burned child to encourage socialization (Fig 27–8).

*Preparing the Community Program was developed by Linda Crawford, R.N., B.S.N., C.R.R.N., for the Moody State School for Cerebral Palsy Children, Galveston, Texas.

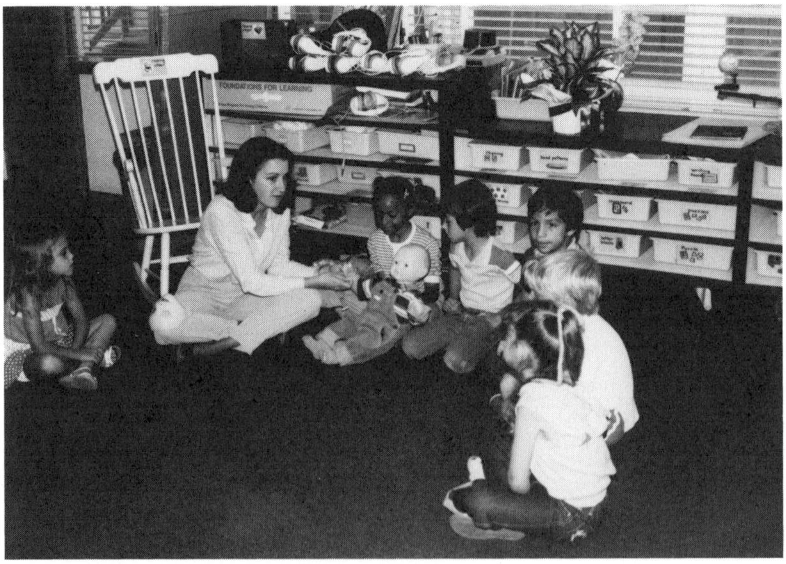

FIG 27–6.
A member of the burn team should visit the child's school prior to the child's discharge from the hospital.

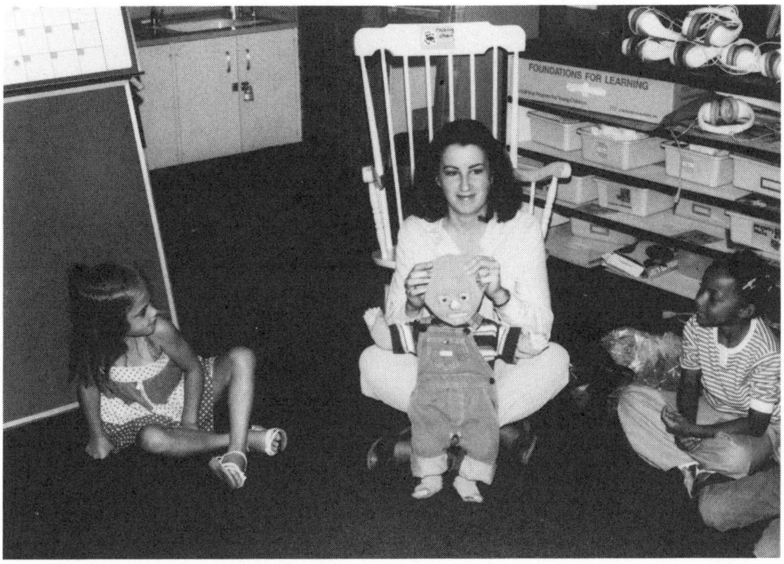

FIG 27–7.
Dolls with pressure bandages can be used to provide explanations to schoolchildren in terms that they can understand, which will help them acclimate to the burned child who is returning to their classroom.

SUMMARY

The key to successful discharge planning for the child with burns and his family is a multidisciplinary network, with the child and family at the center. This approach fosters communication among team members, child, and family, and prevents gaps in meeting the goals of discharge preparation. Each member of the burn care team is responsible for assisting with initial and ongoing assessment and planning for short- and long-term discharge needs. Systematically planning for a burned child's discharge encourages the child to

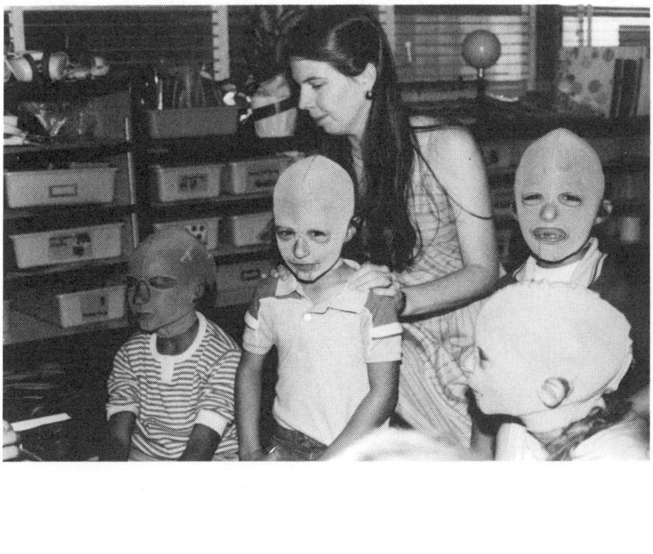

FIG 27–8.
The children and teacher should be given a chance to apply pressure bandages and to have their picture taken and developed immediately, so that they can become comfortable with the equipment they will see.

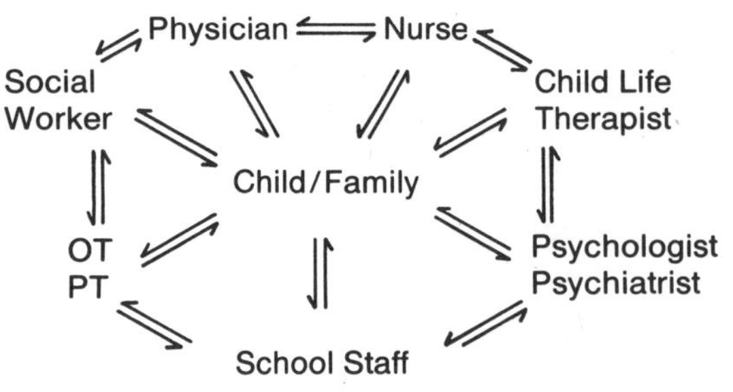

FIG 27–9.
Schematic representation of interrelationships of burned child and his family and support staff.

strive to meet his fullest potential with the least amount of discomfort and emotional stress (Fig 27–9).

REFERENCES

1. Bowden M, Feller I: Family reaction to a severe burn. *Am J Nurs* 1973; 73:317–319.
2. Bristow O, Stickney C, Thompson S: *Discharge Planning for Continuity of Care.* New York, National League of Nursing, 1976.
3. Crittenden FJ: *Discharge Planning for Health Care Facilities.* Bowie, Md, Robert J Bradley Co, 1983.
4. Hollingsworth C: Family conferences before discharge. *AORN Journal* 1978; 27:1224.
5. Hushower G, Gamberg D, Smith N: The nursing process in discharge planning. *Supervisor Nurse* 1978; 9:55–58.
6. Kavanagh C, Freeman R: Should children participate in burn care: *Am J Nurs* 1984; 84:601.
7. Knudson-Cooper MS: Emotional care of the hospitalized burned child. *J Burn Care Rehabil* 1982; 3:109–116.
8. Marvin J: Planning home care for burn patients. *Nursing '83* 1983; 13:65–67.
9. McKeehan KM: *Continuing Care: A Multidisciplinary Approach to Discharge Planning.* St Louis, CV Mosby Co, 1981.
10. Parker SS: *Pediatric Care: A Guide for Patient Education.* Norwalk, Conn, Appleton-Century-Crofts, 1983.
11. Quay NB, Alexander LL: Preparation of burned children and their families for discharge. *J Burn Care Rehabil* 1983; 4:288–290.
12. Savedra M: Moving from hospital to home. *Am J Maternal Child Nurs* 1977; 6:220–222.
13. Theimer V: Individual approaches. *J Burn Care Rehabil* 1982; 3:101–105.

Index

D

H